Experientia Supplementum

Volume 111

More information about this series at http://www.springer.com/series/4822

Peter Igaz • Attila Patócs
Editors

Genetics of Endocrine Diseases and Syndromes

Springer

Editors
Peter Igaz
2nd Department of Internal Medicine, Faculty of Medicine
Semmelweis University
Budapest, Hungary

MTA-SE Molecular Medicine Research Group
Hungarian Academy of Sciences and Semmelweis University
Budapest, Hungary

Attila Patócs
Department of Laboratory Medicine, Faculty of Medicine
Semmelweis University
Budapest, Hungary

"Lendület" Hereditary Endocrine Tumors Research Group
Hungarian Academy of Sciences and Semmelweis University
Budapest, Hungary

Department of Molecular Genetics
National Institute of Oncology
Budapest, Hungary

ISSN 1664-431X ISSN 2504-3692 (electronic)
Experientia Supplementum
ISBN 978-3-030-25904-4 ISBN 978-3-030-25905-1 (eBook)
https://doi.org/10.1007/978-3-030-25905-1

This Springer imprint is published by the registered company Springer Nature Switzerland AG.
The registered company address is: Gewerbestrasse 11, 6330 Cham, Switzerland

Preface

This book is intended for both clinicians and researchers to help in understanding the complexity and relevance of genetics in endocrinology.

Genetic factors are implicated in the disturbances of hormone homeostasis and diseases of hormone-producing endocrine organs. Some of them are primarily genetic diseases, such as monogenic diseases. Several but rare monogenic diseases are known which affect the function of the hormones and their receptors, e.g., hormone resistance syndromes. An important group of monogenic endocrine diseases increase the susceptibility to tumors. Several hereditary tumor syndromes are known, in which an individual suffers from multiple tumors in different organs. Genetic alterations in several endocrine tumors are known to contribute to disease manifestations. Apart from monogenic diseases, the most common diseases with endocrine relevance are polygenic, e.g., obesity, and there are chromosome alterations with endocrinological relevance, as well.

In this book, we present a synopsis of the most important diseases with endocrine relevance. The book comprises 20 chapters divided into five parts. In the first part, basic concepts of genetics, inheritance patterns, issues of family screening and genetic counseling, and the molecular methodology in genetics are discussed. The following three parts discuss monogenic diseases: in Part II, hormone resistance syndromes; in the most extensive Part III, monogenic diseases predisposing to tumor formation; and in Part IV, monogenic diseases predisposing to hormone deficiency and infertility are presented. In the fifth part, a prototype of polygenic inheritance, the genetics of obesity is discussed along with chromosomal aberrations. The list of authors includes leading international experts on these topics.

The book includes 70 figures and 34 tables to facilitate understanding.

The chapters discuss both molecular genetics and clinical issues, highlighting genetic counseling, and thereby aim to present a complex picture of these disease entities.

The editors are indebted to the late Professor Károly Rácz, the former director of the 2nd Department of Internal Medicine of Semmelweis University, who had the original idea to compile this book, but he unfortunately passed away in 2017.

We hope that the reader will find this book interesting, and the book will help to gain insights into this fascinating field of research and clinical medicine.

Budapest, Hungary

Peter Igaz
Attila Patócs

Contents

Part I Basics of Genetics

1 **Basic Concepts of Genetics** 3
Pál Perge and Peter Igaz

2 **Brief Description of Inheritance Patterns** 21
Annamária Kövesdi and Attila Patócs

3 **Family Screening and Genetic Counseling** 29
Pál Perge and Peter Igaz

4 **Brief Summary of the Most Important Molecular Genetic Methods (PCR, qPCR, Microarray, Next-Generation Sequencing, etc.)** 33
Henriett Butz and Attila Patócs

Part II Endocrine Diseases Inherited as Monogenic Traits: Hormone Resistance Syndromes

5 **Syndromes of Resistance to Thyroid Hormone Action** 55
Luca Persani and Irene Campi

6 **Glucocorticoid Resistance** 85
Nicolas C. Nicolaides and Evangelia Charmandari

Part III Endocrine Diseases Inherited as Monogenic Traits: Hereditary Diseases Predisposing to Endocrine Tumors

7 **Overview of Genetically Determined Diseases/Multiple Endocrine Neoplasia Syndromes Predisposing to Endocrine Tumors** 105
Abel Decmann, Attila Patócs, and Peter Igaz

8 **Hereditary Diseases Predisposing to Pheochromocytoma (VHL, NF-1, Paraganglioma Syndromes, and Novel Genes)** 129
Balázs Sarkadi and Attila Patócs

9 **Diseases Predisposing to Adrenocortical Malignancy (Li–Fraumeni Syndrome, Beckwith–Wiedemann Syndrome, and Carney Complex)** 149
Anne Jouinot and Jérôme Bertherat

10 **Genetics of Pituitary Tumours** 171
Paul Benjamin Loughrey and Márta Korbonits

11 **Timeline of Advances in Genetics of Primary Aldosteronism** 213
Lucie S. Meyer, Martin Reincke, and Tracy Ann Williams

12 **Congenital Adrenal Hyperplasia** 245
Dóra Török

Part IV Endocrine Diseases Inherited as Monogenic Traits: Monogenic Diseases Predisposing to Hormone Deficiency, Infertility and Diabetes Mellitus

13 **Pituitary Transcription Factor Mutations Leading to Hypopituitarism** 263
Peter Gergics

14 **Hereditary Neurohypophyseal Diabetes Insipidus** 299
Jonas Rutishauser, Nicole Beuret, Cristina Prescianotto-Baschong, and Martin Spiess

15 **Nephrogenic Diabetes Insipidus** 317
András Balla and László Hunyady

16 **Monogenic Forms of Male Infertility** 341
Csilla Krausz and Antoni Riera-Escamilla

17 **Genetic Causes of Female Infertility** 367
Artur Beke

18 **Monogenic Forms of Diabetes Mellitus** 385
Zsolt Gaál and István Balogh

Part V Example of a Multifactorial Disease and Chromosomal Alterations in Endocrine Diseases

19 **Genetics of Obesity** 419
Lotte Kleinendorst, Mieke M. van Haelst, and Erica L. T. van den Akker

20 **Chromosomal Aberrations with Endocrine Relevance (Turner Syndrome, Klinefelter Syndrome, Prader-Willi Syndrome)** 443
Irén Haltrich

Editors and Contributors

About the Editors

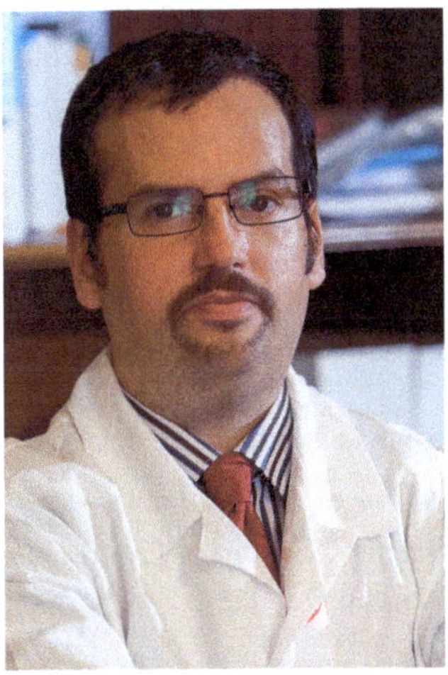

Peter Igaz, MD, MSc, PhD, DSc, is full professor of medicine and head of the 2nd Department of Internal Medicine at Semmelweis University and also the head of the MTA-SE Molecular Medicine Research Group of the Hungarian Academy of Sciences and Semmelweis University, Budapest. He has boarding exams in internal medicine, endocrinology, and clinical genetics. His research interests include adrenal tumors, multiple endocrine neoplasia syndromes, and neuroendocrine tumors focusing on classical genetics, microRNAs, and other noncoding RNA molecules. He has published over 140 scientific papers.

2nd Department of Internal Medicine, Faculty of Medicine, Semmelweis University, Budapest, Hungary
MTA-SE Molecular Medicine Research Group, Hungarian Academy of Sciences and Semmelweis University, Budapest, Hungary

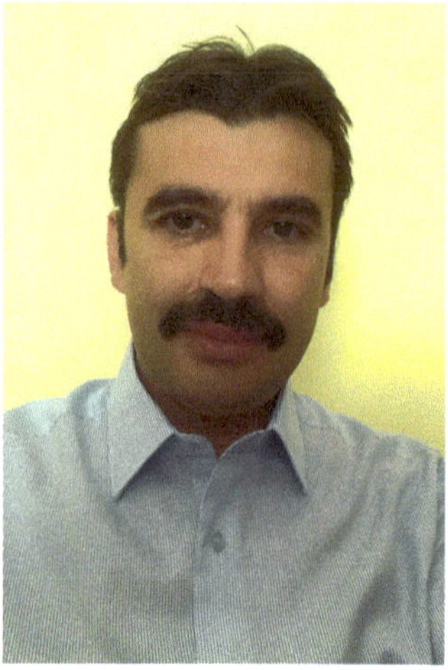

Attila Patócs, MD, MSc, PhD, DSc, is professor of molecular genetics and laboratory medicine at the Department of Laboratory Medicine of Semmelweis University and also the head of molecular genetics laboratory at the National Institute of Oncology in Budapest. He has boarding exams in laboratory medicine and molecular genetic diagnostics. His research is focused on hereditary cancer syndromes, endocrine tumors, and biomarkers. He has published over 180 scientific papers.

Department of Laboratory Medicine, Faculty of Medicine, Semmelweis University, Budapest, Hungary
"Lendulet" Hereditary Endocrine Tumors Research Group, Hungarian Academy of Sciences and Semmelweis University, Budapest, Hungary
Department of Molecular Genetics, National Institute of Oncology, Budapest, Hungary

Contributors

András Balla Department of Physiology, Semmelweis University, Budapest, Hungary
MTA-SE Laboratory of Molecular Physiology, Hungarian Academy of Sciences and Semmelweis University, Budapest, Hungary

István Balogh Division of Clinical Genetics, Department of Laboratory Medicine, Faculty of Medicine, University of Debrecen, Debrecen, Hungary

Artúr Beke Department of Gynecology and Obstretrics, Semmelweis University, Budapest, Hungary

Jérôme Bertherat Endocrinology Department, Cochin Hospital, APHP, Paris, France
Institut Cochin, INSERM U1016, Paris University, Paris, France

Nicole Beuret Biozentrum, University of Basel, Basel, Switzerland

Henriett Butz Department of Laboratory Medicine, Faculty of Medicine, Semmelweis University, Budapest, Hungary
"Lendület" Hereditary Endocrine Tumors Research Group, Hungarian Academy of Sciences and Semmelweis University, Budapest, Hungary
Department of Molecular Genetics, National Institute of Oncology, Budapest, Hungary

Irene Campi Department of Endocrine and Metabolic Diseases & Lab of Endocrine and Metabolic Research, San Luca Hospital, IRCCS Istituto Auxologico Italiano, Milan, Italy
Department of Pathophysiology and Transplantation, University of Milan, Milan, Italy

Evangelia Charmandari Division of Endocrinology, Metabolism and Diabetes, First Department of Pediatrics, National and Kapodistrian University of Athens Medical School, "Aghia Sophia" Children's Hospital, Athens, Greece
Division of Endocrinology and Metabolism, Center of Clinical, Experimental Surgery and Translational Research, Biomedical Research Foundation of the Academy of Athens, Athens, Greece

Ábel Decmann 2nd Department of Internal Medicine, Faculty of Medicine, Semmelweis University, Budapest, Hungary

Zsolt Gaál 4th Department of Medicine, Jósa András Teaching Hospital, Nyíregyháza, Hungary

Peter Gergics Department of Human Genetics, University of Michigan, Ann Arbor, Michigan, USA

Irén Haltrich 2nd Department of Pediatrics, Semmelweis University, Budapest, Hungary

László Hunyady Department of Physiology, Semmelweis University, Budapest, Hungary
MTA-SE Laboratory of Molecular Physiology, Hungarian Academy of Sciences and Semmelweis University, Budapest, Hungary

Peter Igaz 2nd Department of Internal Medicine, Faculty of Medicine, Semmelweis University, Budapest, Hungary
MTA-SE Molecular Medicine Research Group, Hungarian Academy of Sciences and Semmelweis University, Budapest, Hungary

Anne Jouinot Endocrinology Department, Cochin Hospital, APHP, Paris, France
Institut Cochin, INSERM U1016, Paris University, Paris, France

Lotte Kleinendorst Obesity Center CGG, Erasmus MC, University Medical Center, Rotterdam, The Netherlands
Department of Clinical Genetics, Amsterdam UMC, Amsterdam, The Netherlands

Annamária Kövesdi Department of Laboratory Medicine, Semmelweis University, Budapest, Hungary
"Lendület" Hereditary Endocrine Tumors Research Group, Hungarian Academy of Sciences and Semmelweis University, Budapest, Hungary

Márta Korbonits Centre for Endocrinology, William Harvey Research Institute, Barts and The London School of Medicine and Dentistry, Queen Mary University of London, London, UK

Csilla Krausz Department of Experimental and Clinical Biomedical Sciences "Mario Serio", University of Florence, Florence, Italy

Paul Benjamin Loughrey Regional Centre for Endocrinology and Diabetes, Royal Victoria Hospital, Belfast, Northern Ireland, UK

Lucie S. Meyer Medizinische Klinik und Poliklinik IV, Klinikum der Universität München, Ludwig-Maximilians-Universität München, Munich, Germany

Nicolas C. Nicolaides Division of Endocrinology, Metabolism and Diabetes, First Department of Pediatrics, National and Kapodistrian University of Athens Medical School, "Aghia Sophia" Children's Hospital, Athens, Greece
Division of Endocrinology and Metabolism, Center of Clinical, Experimental Surgery and Translational Research, Biomedical Research Foundation of the Academy of Athens, Athens, Greece

Attila Patócs Department of Laboratory Medicine, Faculty of Medicine, Semmelweis University, Budapest, Hungary
"Lendület" Hereditary Endocrine Tumors Research Group, Hungarian Academy of Sciences and Semmelweis University, Budapest, Hungary
Department of Molecular Genetics, National Institute of Oncology, Budapest, Hungary

Pál Perge 2nd Department of Internal Medicine, Faculty of Medicine, Semmelweis University, Budapest, Hungary

Luca Persani Department of Clinical Sciences and Community Health, University of Milan, Milan, Italy
Department of Endocrine and Metabolic Diseases & Lab of Endocrine and Metabolic Research, San Luca Hospital, IRCCS Istituto Auxologico Italiano, Milan, Italy

Cristina Prescianotto-Baschong Biozentrum, University of Basel, Basel, Switzerland

Martin Reincke Medizinische Klinik und Poliklinik IV, Klinikum der Universität München, Ludwig-Maximilians-Universität München, Munich, Germany

Antoni Riera-Escamilla Andrology Department, Fundació Puigvert, Instituto de Investigaciones Biomédicas Sant Pau (IIB-Sant Pau), Universitat Autònoma de Barcelona, Barcelona, Catalonia, Spain

Jonas Rutishauser Biozentrum, University of Basel, Basel, Switzerland

Balázs Sarkadi 2nd Department of Internal Medicine, Semmelweis University, Budapest, Hungary
MTA-SE Lendület Hereditary Endocrine Tumors Research Group, Budapest, Hungary

Martin Spiess Biozentrum, University of Basel, Basel, Switzerland

Dóra Török 2nd Department of Pediatrics, Semmelweis University, Budapest, Hungary

Erica L. T. van den Akker Obesity Center CGG, Erasmus MC, University Medical Center, Rotterdam, The Netherlands
Division of Endocrinology, Department of Pediatrics, Erasmus MC-Sophia Children's Hospital, University Medical Center, Rotterdam, The Netherlands

Mieke M. van Haelst Department of Clinical Genetics, Amsterdam UMC, Amsterdam, The Netherlands

Tracy Ann Williams Medizinische Klinik und Poliklinik IV, Klinikum der Universität München, Ludwig-Maximilians-Universität München, Munich, Germany
Division of Internal Medicine and Hypertension, Department of Medical Sciences, University of Turin, Turin, Italy

List of the Most Commonly Used Abbreviations

11-OHD	11β-Hydroxylase deficiency
17-OHD	17α-Hydroxylase deficiency
17-OHP	17-Hydroxyprogesterone
21-OHD	21-Hydroxylase deficiency
ACC	Adrenocortical carcinoma
aCGH	Array comparative genomic hybridization
ACTH	Adrenocorticotropic hormone
ADH	Antidiuretic hormone
AHR	Aryl hydrocarbon receptor
AIP	Aryl hydrocarbon receptor-interacting protein
AIS	Androgen insensitivity syndrome
AL	Anterior lobes of pituitary
AMH	Anti-Müllerian hormone
ANP	Atrial natriuretic peptide
APA	Aldosterone-producing adenoma
APC	Adenomatous polyposis coli
AQP	Aquaporin water channels
ARR	Aldosterone-to-renin ratio
AS	Angelman syndrome
AVP	Arginine vasopressin
BAH	Bilateral adrenal hyperplasia
BBB	Blood–brain barrier
BMI	Body mass index
BWS	Beckwith–Wiedemann syndrome
cAMP	Cyclic adenosine monophosphate
CAH	Congenital adrenal hyperplasia
CaSR	Calcium sensor
CAVD	Congenital absence of vas deferens
CDKN1C	Cyclin-dependent kinase inhibitor 1C
cDNA	Complementary DNA
CEL	Carboxyl ester lipase

CNC	Carney complex
cNDI	Congenital nephrogenic diabetes
CGH	Comparative genomic hybridization
circRNAs	Circular RNAs
CNS	Central nervous system
CNV	Copy number variations
CpG	Cytosine-guanine dinucleotides
CPHD	Combined pituitary hormone deficiency
CRH	Corticotropin-releasing hormone
CRP	C-reactive protein
CS	Cowden syndrome
cT	Cycle threshold
CT	Computed tomography
DHEA	Dehydroepiandrosterone
DHEAS	Dehydroepiandrosterone sulfate
DI	Diabetes insipidus
DIO	Deiodinase
DM	Diabetes mellitus
DNA	Deoxyribonucleic acid
dPCR	Digital polymerase chain reaction
DSD	Disorders of sexual development
dsDNA	Double-stranded DNA
ENaC	Amiloride-sensitive epithelial sodium channel
ER	Endoplasmic reticulum
FH	Familial hyperaldosteronism
FHH	Familial hypocalciuric hypercalcemia
FIPA	Familial isolated pituitary adenomas
FISH	Fluorescence In Situ Hybridization
FMR1	Fragile X Mental Retardation 1
FMTC	Familial medullary thyroid cancer
FSH	Follicle-stimulating hormone
FuH	Fumarate hydratase
GCK	Glucokinase
GDM	Gestational diabetes mellitus
GEP-NET	Gastroenteropancreatic neuroendocrine tumor
GH	Growth hormone
GHD	Growth hormone deficiency
GHRH	Growth hormone releasing hormone
GNAS1	Guanine nucleotide-binding protein, alpha-stimulating activity polypeptide 1
GPCR	G protein-coupled receptor
GR	Glucocorticoid receptor
GREs	Glucocorticoid response elements
GRTH	Generalized resistance to thyroid hormone

GWAS	Genome-wide association studies
HCG	Human chorionic gonadotropin
hGR	Human glucocorticoid receptor
HH	Hypogonadotropic hypogonadism
HIF1α	Hypoxia-inducible factor 1-α
HNF1A	Hepatic nuclear factor 1A
HNF1B	Hepatic nuclear factor 1B
HNF4A	Hepatic nuclear factor 4A
HNPGL	Head and neck paraganglioma
HPA axis	Hypothalamic–pituitary–adrenal axis
HPT-JT	Hyperparathyroidism-jaw tumor syndrome
IAD	Isolated ACTH deficiency
IC	Imprinting center
ICR	Imprinting control region
ID	Imprinting defects
IGF-1	Insulin-like growth factor-1
IGHD	Isolated growth hormone deficiency
i(X)	IsoXq chromosome
KS	Klinefelter syndrome
KSy	Kallmann syndrome
LFS	Li–Fraumeni syndrome
LH	Luteinizing hormone
lncRNA	Long noncoding RNA
LOH	Loss of heterozigosity
MAS	McCune–Albright syndrome
MC4R	Melanocortin 4 receptor
MEN	Multiplex endocrine neoplasia
MHC	Major histocompatibility complex
miRNA	microRNA
MLPA	Multiplex ligation-dependent probe amplification
MMR	Mismatch repair
MODY	Maturity-onset diabetes of the young
MRI	Magnetic resonance imaging
mRNA	Messenger ribonucleic acid
MTC	Medullary thyroid cancer
NCCAH	Non-classic CAH
NDI	Nephrogenic diabetes insipidus
NDM	Neonatal diabetes mellitus
NET	Neuroendocrine tumor
NF1	Neurofibromatosis type 1
NGS	Next-generation sequencing
NKCC	K^+-$2Cl^-$ cotransporter
NMD	Nonsense-mediated mRNA decay
NSHPT	Neonatal severe hyperparathyroidism

NSIAD	Nephrogenic syndrome of inappropriate diuresis
OMIM	Online Mendelian inheritance in man
PCOS	Polycystic ovary syndrome
PDE	Phosphodiesterase
PGGR	Primary generalized glucocorticoid resistance
PGL	Paraganglioma
Pheo	Pheochromocytoma
PHPT	Primary hyperparathyroidism
PJS	Peutz–Jeghers syndrome
PKA	Protein kinase A
PNDM	Permanent neonatal diabetes
pNET	Pancreatic neuroendocrine tumor
POF/POI	Premature ovarian failure/insufficiency
POMC	Proopiomelanocortin
PPNAD	Primary pigmented nodular adrenal disease
PRL	Prolactin
PRTH	Pituitary resistance to thyroid hormone
PTEN	Phosphatase and tensin homolog
PWS	Prader–Willi syndrome
REE	Resting energy expenditure
RNA	Ribonucleic acid
RTHα	Resistance to thyroid hormone alpha
RTHβ	Resistance to thyroid hormone beta
RT-qPCR	Reverse transcription quantitative polymerase chain reaction
SDH	Succinate dehydrogenase
SHOX	Short stature homeobox
SIADH	Syndrome of inappropriate ADH secretion
siRNA	Small interfering RNA
SNP	Single nucleotide polymorphism
SNV	Single nucleotide variants
SRY	Sex-determining region Y
SV, SV-CAH	Classic simple virilizing CAH
SW, SW-CAH	Classic salt-wasting CAH
TF	Transcription factor
THRA	Gene coding for thyroid hormone receptor alpha
THRB	Gene coding for thyroid hormone receptor beta
TNDM	Transient neonatal diabetes mellitus
TP53	Tumor protein 53
TR	Thyroid hormone receptor
TS	Turner syndrome
TSC	Tuberous sclerosis complex
TSH	Thyroid-stimulating hormone
UFC	Urinary free cortisol
UPD	Uniparental disomy

UTR	Untranslated region
VHL	von Hippel–Lindau disease
VUS	Variant of uncertain significance
V1R, V2R	Type 1 and type 2 arginine-vasopressin receptor
WES	Whole exome sequencing
WGS	Whole genome sequencing
Wnt	Wingless-type MMTV integration site family/beta-catenin
X-LAG	X-linked acrogigantism syndrome

Part I
Basics of Genetics

Chapter 1
Basic Concepts of Genetics

Pál Perge and Peter Igaz

Abstract Genetics is the study of heredity. In this introductory chapter of the book *Genetics of Endocrine Diseases and Syndromes*, we present the basic terms of genetics and basic physiological and pathogenic molecular processes that are implicated in the wide array of genetically determined diseases. Mutations, chromosomes, polymorphisms, and epigenetic terms are also briefly discussed.

Keywords Genetics · DNA · RNA · Gene · Genome · Genotype · Phenotype · Mutation · Chromosome · Polymorphism · Epigenetics

List of Abbreviations

DNA	Deoxyribonucleic acid
ICR	Imprinting control region
lncRNA	Long noncoding RNA
LOH	Loss of heterozygosity
MEN1	Multiplex endocrine neoplasia type 1
miRNA	microRNA
mRNA	Messenger ribonucleic acid
piRNA	Piwi-interacting RNA
RNA	Ribonucleic acid
rRNA	Ribosomal RNA

P. Perge
2nd Department of Internal Medicine, Faculty of Medicine, Semmelweis University, Budapest, Hungary

P. Igaz (✉)
2nd Department of Internal Medicine, Faculty of Medicine, Semmelweis University, Budapest, Hungary

MTA-SE Molecular Medicine Research Group, Hungarian Academy of Sciences and Semmelweis University, Budapest, Hungary
e-mail: igaz.peter@med.semmelweis-univ.hu

P. Igaz, A. Patócs (eds.), *Genetics of Endocrine Diseases and Syndromes*, Experientia Supplementum 111, https://doi.org/10.1007/978-3-030-25905-1_1

siRNA	Small interfering RNA
SNP	Single-nucleotide polymorphism
tRNA	Transfer RNA
UPD	Uniparental disomy
UTR	Untranslated region

1.1 Introduction

Genetics is the study of heredity. Heritable factors play major roles in the development and regulation of cells, tissues, organs, and the entire human organism. Besides their physiological and normal action, the disruption of genetic factors contributes to pathological conditions, including both heritable and sporadic diseases. In heritable diseases, the genetic disorders are the primary cause of disease, but genetic factors are involved in almost every disease. They affect not just the susceptibility of the person to different diseases but even the result of the treatment by influencing the individual reaction to the medical therapy, including any potential side effects, as well.

1.2 Basic Terms of Genetics

Deoxyribonucleic acid (DNA) is a molecule composed of two chains that coil around each other to form a double helix carrying the genetic information (Travers and Muskhelishvili 2015). To the core of the DNA (standing from a sugar called deoxyribose), four nitrogen-containing nucleobases can join together (adenine/A, thymine/T, cytosine/C, guanine/G). The monomeric unit of the DNA is called nucleotide (Lane and Fan 2015). Each monomer is composed of deoxyribose, nucleobase, and phosphate group. The order or in another term the sequence of the nitrogenous bases carries the genetic code. There are approximately 3.2 billion (3.2 Mb) nucleotide pairs in the human cell nucleus (Venter et al. 2001). The deoxyribose molecules are connected via phosphodiester bonds, which is the linkage between the fifth (5′) carbon atom of one sugar molecule and the third (3′) carbon atom of another. This linkage (5′–3′) is the direction of the information flow in the transcription. The DNA content of the cell (the nucleus) is called genome.

The genetic information from the DNA translates into proteins (polypeptides). The 20 standard amino acids (the monomers of the peptides) are encoded by the four bases, nucleotides in a three-letter combination (triplets, codons) (Shu 2017). The vast majority of the genome (more than 97%) does not encode protein sequences. However, the non-protein-coding regions have significant regulatory functions and contain structural elements too. Messenger RNA (ribonucleic acid) conveys the genetic information of the DNA that directs the synthesis of specific amino acids.

Table 1.1 The genetic code (mRNA level)

Name of the amino acid	Abbreviation of the amino acid (one letter)	Coding triplets
Alanine	Ala (A)	GCU, GCC, GCA, GCG
Arginine	Arg (R)	CGU, CGC, CGA, CGG, AGA, AGG
Asparagine	Asn (N)	AAU, AAC
Aspartic acid	Asp (D)	GAU, GAC
Cysteine	Cys (C)	UGU, UGC
Glutamine	Gln (Q)	CAA, CAG
Glutamic acid	Glu (E)	GAA, GAG
Glycine	Gly (G)	GGU, GGC, GGA, GGG
Histidine	His (H)	CAU, CAC
Isoleucine	Ile (I)	AUU, AUC, AUA
Leucine	Leu (L)	UUA, UUG, CUU, CUC, CUA, CUG
Lysine	Lys (K)	AAA, AAG
Methionine	Met (M)	AUG
Phenylalanine	Phe (F)	UUU, UUC
Proline	Pro (P)	CCU, CCC, CCA, CCG
Serine	Ser (S)	UCU, UCC, UCA, UCG, AGU, AGC
Threonine	Thr (T)	ACU, ACC, ACA, ACG
Tryptophan	Trp (W)	UGG
Tyrosine	Tyr (Y)	UGU, UGC
Valine	Val (V)	GUU, GUC, GUA, GUG
STOP codon		UAA, UAG, UGA

In contrast to DNA, the RNA contains ribose sugar molecules and uracil nucleobase instead of deoxyribose and thymine (Nachtergaele and He 2017). In contrast to DNA that is a very stable molecule, messenger RNA is highly instable and very susceptible to degradation. Table 1.1 shows the genetic code, the triplets that encode the amino acids. As it can be seen in this table, the majority of the amino acids is encoded by several triplets; thus the genetic code is degenerated. Besides messenger RNA, many other RNA molecules are also known. They play active roles in protein synthesis (transfer RNA, tRNA), build the ribosome (ribosomal RNA, rRNA), and have regulatory function of the gene expression (e.g., long noncoding RNA, lncRNA). The regulatory function of the small RNAs (e.g., microRNAs) was described recently (Romano et al. 2017). The three main classes of small RNAs are microRNAs (microRNAs), small interfering RNA (siRNAs), and Piwi-interacting RNAs (piRNAs). Small RNAs play pivotal roles in cellular processes such as cell differentiation, proliferation, apoptosis, metabolism, and immune function. Their altered expression has been described in several pathological conditions including cancer and cardiovascular, liver, and endocrinological diseases. Small

RNAs can be exploited as minimally invasive novel biomarkers and therapeutic targets for wide range of diseases (Storz 2002; Zhang 2009).

According to our current knowledge, the gene is the unit of the inheritance. The gene is the part of the DNA which is required to create a functional product (Pearson 2006). The classical products of genes are polypeptides, but more and more data underline the relevance of transcribed noncoding RNA molecules in genomic regulation. Every human gene has two copies, one from the mother and the other from the father. In a genetic locus, there can be alternative sequences of the given gene, which are different from each other just to a small extent. It has to be emphasized that one locus includes just one alternative variant; these are the so-called alleles (Benitez et al. 2017). The alleles that occur in the given locus constitute the genotype (Johannsen 2014). The phenotype results from the biochemical, physiological, and morphological effects of the genotype. In a wider concept, phenotype derives from all of the occurring human alleles (genotype) (Johannsen 2014).

According to our current concept, the human genome contains 20,000–30,000 genes that represent only about 3% of the whole genome. The rest of the genome was previously considered to be the "dark matter", even called junk DNA in the past. An ever-increasing amount of findings support that this huge part of the genome cannot be regarded as an inert, non-functional part; on the contrary, numerous non-protein-coding RNAs that contribute to genome maintenance and regulation are coded in this part (Lagos-Quintana et al. 2001).

In eukaryotic organisms, the DNA sequence of the genes does not code the amino acids continuously, but discontinuously. The DNA sections that code proteins are called exons (Schwartz et al. 2009). The introns do not code proteins, because their coded RNA sections are removed by the splicing process during the maturation of the final messenger RNA product (mRNA) (van den Hoogenhof et al. 2016). Several alternative methods of RNA splicing occur in nature; therefore the number of the mRNAs is far more bigger than the sum of the genes. All of these processes increase the biological complexity (Fig. 1.1).

The process of the transcription from the genes to RNA molecules is influenced by several factors. One of the most important factors is the promoter region of the gene, which is located in front of the protein-coding region of the gene on the 5′ end. The promoter includes different sequences which are able to bind transcriptional factors (Elkon et al. 2003). The transcriptional factors play a crucial role in the regulation of the transcription. Besides the promoters, other regulatory regions have also been described. They could have positive (enhancer) or negative (repressor) effect. Introns are not inactive parts; they can harbor non-protein-coding genes, e.g., microRNAs. The 5′ and 3′ ends of the gene [the so-called untranslated regions (UTR)] are also important in genetic regulation. A polyadenine tail binds to the 3′ end of the mature mRNA (Fig. 1.1).

The start codon is responsible for the initiation, while the stop codon induces the termination of the protein synthesis. In contrast with the transcription which takes place in the nucleus, this process happens in the cytoplasm. The ribosomes play fundamental roles in the regulation of the protein synthesis.

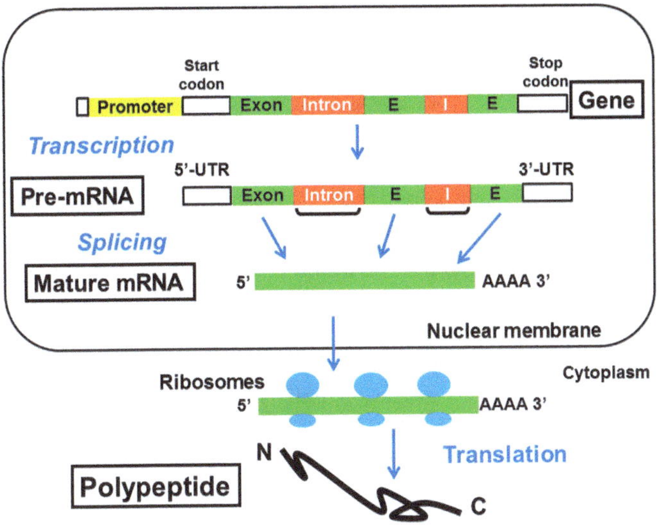

Fig. 1.1 The schematic representation of the gene, the transcription, and the splicing. The exons (E) are indicated by green whereas the introns (I) with red

The vast majority of the human DNA can be found in the nucleus. However, the mitochondria contain its own DNA proportion (Mounolou and Lacroute 2005). The magnitude of the mitochondrial DNA is far less than the size of the nuclear DNA. It contains only 16.5 kb and 37 genes. Among these genes, most of them play a crucial role in the protein synthesis. Besides these, a minor proportion codes for proteins which are responsible for the mitochondrial oxidative phosphorylation process. However, it has to be emphasized that the vast majority of the proteins which are crucial for the aforementioned process are encoded in the nucleus. The mitochondrial genome is circular and does not contain an exon-intron structure. Based on these observations, it can be assumed that the mitochondrion—the cellular energy creator—has evolved during the phylogenesis from bacteria which was internalized by a eukaryotic cell (Mounolou and Lacroute 2005).

1.3 Mutations

The alterations of the DNA are crucial in almost every genetic disease. Mutation is the permanent and irreversible alteration of the nucleotide sequence of the genome that occurs in less than 1% of the population and has pathogenic significance (Alexandrov et al. 2013). The mutation can affect genes—these are called gene mutations—or bigger structural units too such as chromosomes.

Point mutation is a type of mutation when only one nucleotide is altered. The silent or synonymous mutation means that the mutation does not induce amino acid modification. If a mutation leads to a change in the amino acid sequence, it is called missense mutation.

The nonsense mutation of the DNA sequence results in a stop codon. This leads to the early termination of the protein synthesis, and the resulting short, incomplete amino acid chains are quickly degraded via the process of nonsense-mediated decay. Short deletions and insertions—affecting just a couple of nucleotides—also occur. According to the triplet nature of gene expression by codons, a deletion or an insertion of a number of nucleotides in a DNA sequence that is not divisible by three can change the reading frame, resulting in a meaningless, completely different translational product in contrast to the original protein. This mutation is called frameshift mutation or in another term framing error. Nonsense and frameshift mutations lead to severely compromised or absent functional activity of the protein. On the other hand, activating mutations enhancing the activity of the protein are mostly missense mutations. Besides mutations which alter the amino acid-chain sequence, other point mutations are also known. These can affect the regulatory regions, the splicing process, and even the sequence of the small RNAs (mostly noncoding RNA molecules) too. All of these mutations can lead to severe pathogenetical conditions.

The point mutations in certain genes accumulate in particular regions. These regions are called mutational hotspots. The presence of the hotspots makes the genetical diagnosis easier, because it is recommended to investigate these hotspots at first for mutation screening. The evaluation of the other regions has to be performed just if the hotpots regions do contain mutation.

The mutation of an individual gene does not alter the phenotype of every patient, because the phenotype is affected by several factors. There are gene mutations which cause disease with high probability, even in every carrier, while other mutations' "effectivity" are far less in this term. The concept of penetrance shows the likelihood by which a certain mutation is manifested in the phenotype. The penetrance of multiplex endocrine neoplasia type 1 and type 2 is almost 100% (Bassett et al. 1998). In contrast, hemochromatosis—disturbance in iron homeostasis—has a very low penetrance (<1%); the vast majority of the carriers do not suffer from the disease. Expressivity is a similar but different concept. This concept quantifies variation in phenotype on a spectrum from mild to severe in the affected individual (e.g., how many fingers are affected in polydactyly).

The distinct mutations of an individual gene can lead to different phenotypes. Therefore in certain diseases, a genotype-phenotype correlation could be set up. These correlations have high clinical significance because different protocols can be required for the follow-up of the patients, and the prognosis of different mutations can also be established.

In connection with these concepts, we have to mention the phenomenon of phenocopy (Baum et al. 2010). Phenocopy describes that the person's phenotype matches a phenotype which is characteristic for a genetic disease. However in these cases, a genetic background cannot be identified, or the phenotype is caused by another genetic disease caused by mutations of other genes. In tumor syndromes, for example, the association of frequently observed sporadic tumors can mimic a hereditary tumor syndrome (e.g., combination of hyperparathyroidism and pituitary adenoma resembling MEN1 syndrome). Molecular genetic analysis has to be performed in order to exclude phenocopy.

The frequency of particular mutations is significantly higher in certain populations compared to the average population. The founder effect is often in the background of this phenomenon (Provine 2004). The founder effect can be interpretable at the populational genetic level. It means that a variation which is rare in the entire population but detectable in the ancestor becomes more and more frequent in the descendants of an originally small population.

1.4 Chromosomes

There are mutational forms besides gene mutations. They include genome mutations, which affect the number of the chromosomes and structural variations of the chromosomes (chromosome mutation). These alterations are investigated by cytogenetics. This was the first field of the genetics that reached historical discoveries in the diagnostic setting. The chromosomes are the transport forms of the genetic substance. They provide the proper cell division from the parent cell to the daughter cells. The centromere is the region of the chromosome where the arms of the chromosomes join (Pluta et al. 1995). The end region of the chromosome is named telomere. The centromeres have pivotal role in the cell division and in the fission of the chromosome. Four different types of the chromosomes are known according to the location of the centromere region (Hammond et al. 2017). These are the metacentric type (median location of the centromere with approximately equal long chromosomal arms), the submetacentric (a centromere located submedian resulting in slightly unequal length of chromosomal arms), and the acrocentric type (a centromere is severely offset from the center, leading to one very long and one very short section) (Fig. 1.2). The fourth type (telocentric chromosome) physiologically does not occur in human beings. The shorter chromosome arm is indicated with p (petit) while the longer with q. During meiosis the chromosome number is reduced by half and the homologous regions of the paternal and maternal chromosomes are switched (crossing over). This leads to the exchange of the genetic information and has a pivotal role in providing the genetic variability (Creighton and McClintock 1931).

There are different methods for the visualization of the chromosomes. These banding techniques are very important for the identification of the chromosome alteration. The most commonly used technique is the G-banding. By G-banding the light bands correspond to euchromatin, while the dark regions are named heterochromatin. The functionally active regions of the genome are located mainly in the euchromatin (Zheng and Hayes 2003).

The human genome contains 46 chromosomes, half of them derived from the mother and half of them from the father. The somatic cells are diploids, so they include 23 pairs of the chromosomes, while the germ cells are haploids, so they have

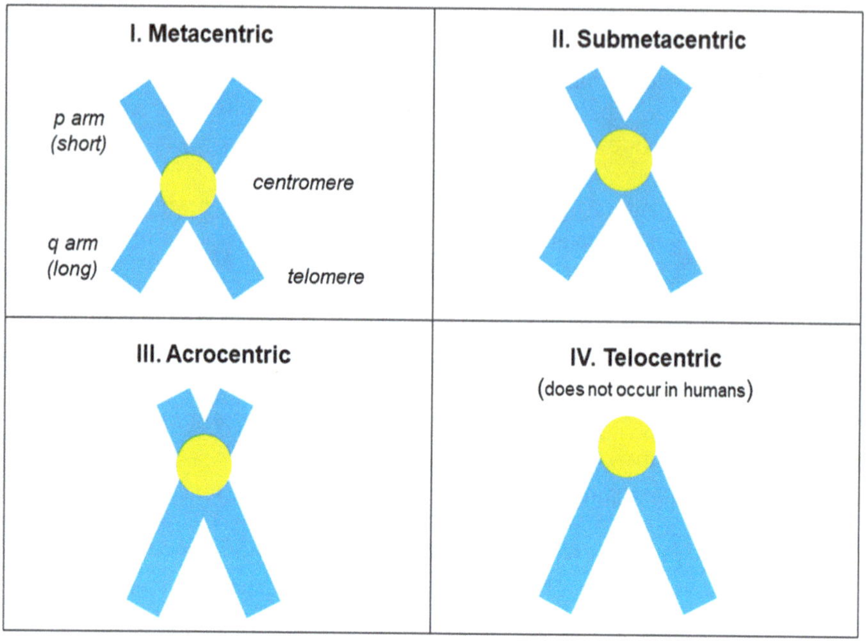

Fig. 1.2 The different types of the chromosomes

1 individual copy of a particular chromosome. The germ cells evolve during the meiosis. The fusion of the haploid germ cells is one of the most important factors of the genetic variability.

The two sex chromosomes play a dominant role in the determination of sex. 46XX (Fig. 1.3) is characteristic for females, while 46XY (Fig. 1.4) is for males (Ahmad et al. 2012). The karyotype is the distribution of the chromosomes of a particular person. The visualized depiction of the chromosomes is named karyogram. Among the structural alterations of the chromosome, several different forms, e.g., deletion, inversion, duplication, ring chromosome etc., occur. These variations could lead to severe conditions via the disturbed regulation or by the loss or gain of the genetic substance. Reciprocal (balanced) translocations are the exchange of material between nonhomologous chromosomes. In the vast majority of cases, the affected person is asymptomatic; however there are cases which lead to disease via the altered regulation (e.g., the presence of Philadelphia chromosome in chronic myeloid leukemia). In cases of balanced translocation, the parent's germ cell contains different forms of the chromosome; therefore the descendant can inherit a normal karyotype, balanced translocation just as the ancestor has, or deletion/insertion leading to severe morbidity. These translocations stand often in the background of habitual abortion.

Microdeletions which affect just some genes can also lead to serious consequences. The loss of more adjacent genes (contiguous gene syndrome) causes typical

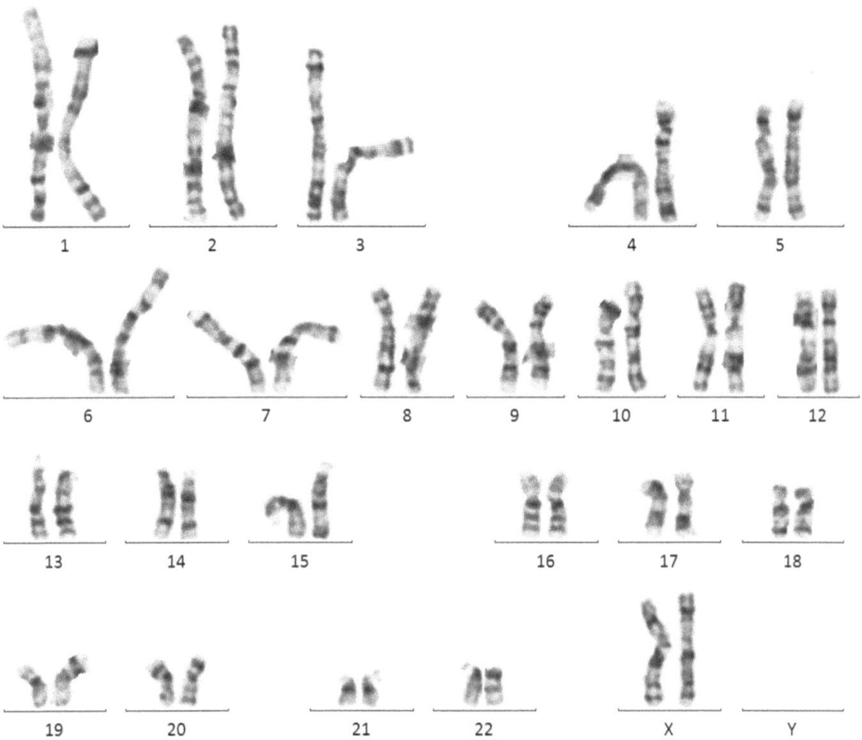

Fig. 1.3 The normal female karyotype (46XX). G-banding. Courtesy of Irén Haltrich PhD, Cytogenetic Laboratorium, 2nd Department of Pediatrics, Faculty of Medicine, Semmelweis University

syndromes. These syndromes have high significance in the recognition of the function of particular genes.

The abnormal number of chromosomes in a cell causes aneuploidy (Santaguida and Amon 2015). It means that a cell includes a difference of one or more incomplete sets of chromosomes. The integer multiple of the whole genome such as triploidy and tetraploidy is not compatible with life. In case of monosomy, the cell contains just one copy of the chromosome instead of two. Trisomy means three copies of the chromosomes. The number alteration of the somatic chromosomes leads to severe consequences and except for some chromosomes [e.g., chromosome 21—triploidy (Down syndrome)] is usually incompatible with life. In contrast, the numeric abnormalities of sex chromosomes are associated with milder phenotypes.

In certain cases, not every cell has the same karyotype (or genotype), but two or more types of karyotype (genotype) occur in the cell of the individual. This alteration is named mosaicism that can be the result of an early mutation (Taylor et al. 2014). Mosaicism appears not just at the level of chromosome alteration but in cases of point mutations, too.

Each gene has (at least) two copies in the genome. If both alleles are mutated of a diploid organism, the organism is homozygous at that locus. If the mutation affects

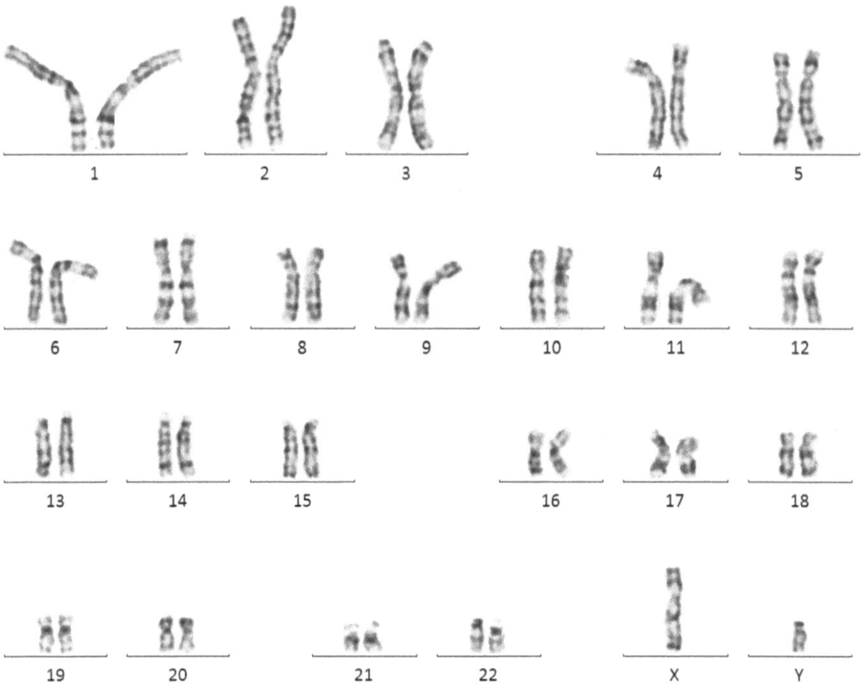

Fig. 1.4 The normal male karyotype (46XY). G-banding. Courtesy of Irén Haltrich PhD, Cytogenetic Laboratorium, 2nd Department of Pediatrics, Faculty of Medicine, Semmelweis University

just one allele, the organism is heterozygous at that locus. The X-chromosome has just one copy in males; therefore almost all X-linked genes are hemizygous in males. This topic is negotiated in more detail in the following chapter.

Two X-chromosomes are characteristic for females. One of them is inactivated and it could be visualized by cytological investigation as a form of Barr body (Barr and Bertram 1949). The inactivation of the chromosome is a random process. This could be the explanation to the fact that X-associated diseases can occur in females too.

The other classification of the mutations is based on the type of the affected cell. The mutation of the germ cell (germ-line mutation) is inherited to the descendants and can be detected in all of their somatic cells (Cinalli et al. 2008). Other mutations evolve in somatic cells during their lifetime; therefore these mutations are not detectable in every cell of the organism, just in the affected cell line. These mutations are named somatic mutations and play key role in the biology of tumorigenesis.

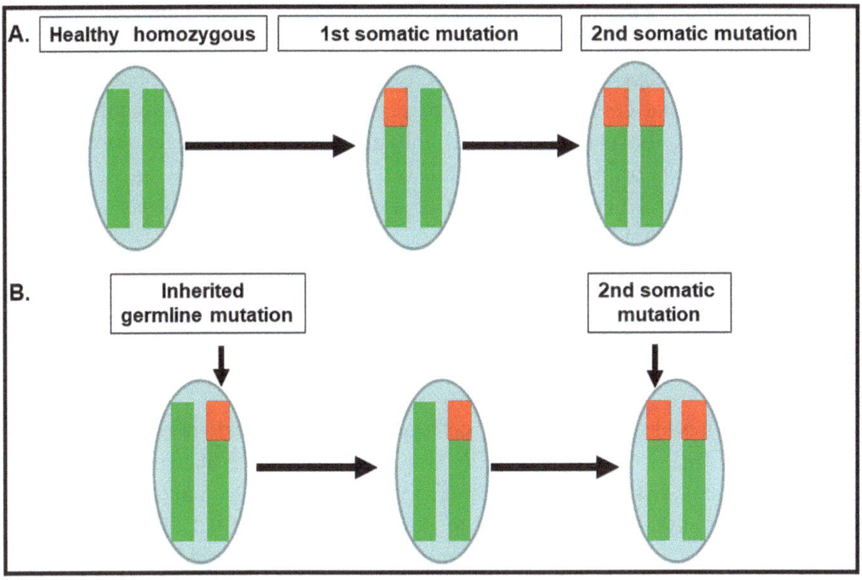

Fig. 1.5 The Knudson two-hit hypothesis of tumorigenesis. (**a**) The roles of tumor suppressor gene mutations in the formation of sporadic tumors. The loss of both alleles is caused by somatic mutations. (**b**) Germ-line mutation of one allele of the tumor suppressor gene is inherited in hereditary tumor syndromes. Therefore the affected person has an increased risk for malignancy. The other allele is inactivated in the given organ by a somatic mutation

1.5 Proto-oncogenes and Tumor Suppressors

There are two main groups of genes according to their function in the tumorigenesis. These are the proto-oncogenes and the tumor suppressor genes (Nordling 1953). The mutation of the proto-oncogenes leads to increased activity, while the inactivating mutations of tumor suppressor genes compromise their functions in controlling cell proliferation, apoptosis, etc. In the case of proto-oncogenes, the activation of one allele out of two is enough to cause cancer. On the other hand, both alleles of the tumor suppressor genes have to be mutated and inactivated to be tumorigenic in the cell. Somatic inactivating mutations of both alleles of the tumor suppressor genes are common in sporadic tumors. In hereditary tumor syndromes, one germ-line mutation is inherited. The Knudson hypothesis means that one allele of the tumor suppressor genes is affected by a germ-line mutation, while the other allele is inactivated in the tumor by a somatic mutation. (The germ-line mutation of both alleles of the tumor suppressor genes is usually incompatible with life.) The phenomenon of loss of heterozygosity (LOH) means the loss of the intact allele in the tumor (Lo et al. 2008) (Fig. 1.5).

The germ-line mutations are inheritable if the parent is a carrier. However, there are de novo mutations too; in these cases the mutations are not detectable in the parents and they are formed in the germ cell or in the zygote. Nevertheless, the de novo germ-line mutations are transmissible to the next generation as inherited mutations.

The germ-line mosaicism is a hardly certifiable but an important phenomenon. It means an individual carries two or more germ cell lines and a part of them are mutated, whereas the somatic cells of the individual are entirely normal. This phenomenon affects primarily the chromosomes. This could be the background for some clinical cases where the children of apparently healthy (normal karyotype) parents carry alterations in their genome.

1.6 DNA Variations

Besides mutations leading to severe consequences, more and more significance is attributed to DNA variability. The DNA sequence is not permanent; its change is important in the process of the evolution. The variation of the DNA nucleotides is rather common; every 1000th or according to novel data every 300th nucleotide can be different from the sequence of the majority (SNP: single-nucleotide polymorphism). Altogether, this results in an enormous variability of the DNA sequence.

The alterations of the DNA sequence are classified by their frequency. The most common form occurs in more than 1% in the population; these are called polymorphisms (Huxley et al. 1964). Most of them do not have clinical significance; however numerous polymorphisms are associated with diseases. Mutations are rare genetical variations, with an occurrence below 1% in the population (see above).

The vast majority of genetic diseases is caused by a mutation affecting a single gene; therefore these illnesses are called monogenic. Approximately 4000 monogenic diseases are described to date. Most of them are extremely rare and associated with slight clinical significance. The different types of the inheritance of the monogenic diseases are discussed in detail in the following chapter. Numerous basic pathogenic mechanisms were described by evaluating monogenic diseases; therefore these are not only important from a clinical but also from a research perspective.

Most of the clinically significant diseases (e.g., hypertension, diabetes mellitus) are associated with several genetic alterations. These diseases have complex, polygenic heredity. Polymorphisms and rare variations are common in the background of genetic alterations which lead to polygenic diseases. In contrast to monogenic diseases, the severity of the polygenic forms move on a wide scale and more parameters are measurable quantitatively.

1.7 Epigenetics

Besides the change of the nucleotide sequence, more and more significance is attributed to the secondary variations of DNA strand and the chromatin structure. We use the epigenetics term to all of the alterations that do not induce changes in the

DNA sequence but lead to heritable phenotypes (Dupont et al. 2009). The DNA methylation is one of the most important epigenetic processes (Rana and Ankri 2016), but regulation via microRNAs also belongs to this field.

We have to mention here a very interesting genetic phenomenon that plays crucial role in the pathogenesis of several diseases. This phenomenon is the genomic imprinting (Wilkins and Haig 2003). It is based on the different functional activities of the maternal and paternal chromosomes. In the case of maternal imprinting, only the paternal genes are active, and the maternal genes are not transcribed. On the other hand, in paternal imprinting, only the maternal genes are transcribed. The growth-stimulating genes (e.g., insulin-like growth factor 2) are usually regulated by maternal imprinting, whereas growth-inhibitory genes (e.g., cyclin-dependent kinase inhibitor 1C) are rather under the influence of paternal imprinting. To use a plastic however significantly simplified analogy, it can be said as if the father would like to have a big baby while the mother's interest is to decrease the size of the child in order to increase the chance of an easier child birth.

The imprinting control region (ICR) plays pivotal role in the formation of the methylation patterns governing the process of genomic imprinting. To date approximately 100 human genes are described to be regulated by genomic imprinting. Interestingly, a remarkable proportion of the gene loci affected by genomic imprinting is associated with the endocrine system. Therefore, it is not surprising that the disturbance of genomic imprinting is related to several endocrine diseases. The expression change of the genes—compared to the physiological condition—affected by the altered imprinting could lead to pathological conditions (Fig. 1.6). The expression of particular genes could vary from lack of expression to twofold higher expression. One pathologic mechanism leading to disturbed genomic imprinting is uniparental disomy (UPD) where both copies of the given chromosome are derived from one parent. The developmental biological background of this phenomenon could be that the zygote has to lose the chromosome from the other gamete to avoid the lethal trisomy caused by a supernumerary chromosome. As a consequence, both chromosomes originate from one parent (Fig. 1.7). The disturbance of the genomic imprinting is implicated in the background of Beckwith-Wiedemann and Prader-Willi syndrome (Knoll et al. 1989).

Following and based on the determination of the entire sequence of the human genome (Human Genome Project), more and more information about the structure and the variability of the genes have been gained (Green et al. 2015). In recent years novel bioinformatical methods have been developed which make it possible to investigate the expression of all known genes. Compared to classical genetics which evaluate just one or some genes and their changes, these methods lead to a new scientific field that studies the function of the whole genome. This field is called genomics and has two major branches: structural and functional genomics (Kadakkuzha and Puthanveettil 2013). The functional genomics evaluate the function of the genes or in wider meaning the entire genome. The expression of mRNAs alters in many pathological conditions including cancer. It makes possible to identify novel biomarkers to differentiate between benign and malignant tumors or even to predict prognosis. The evaluation of the short noncoding RNAs especially the

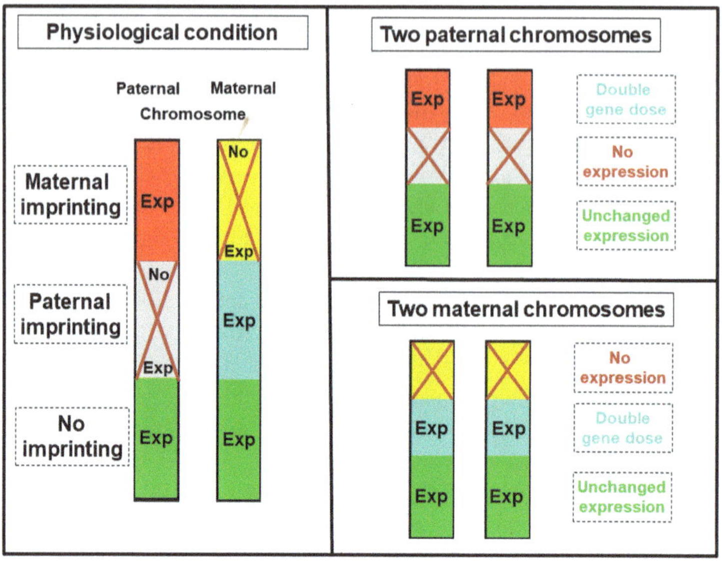

Fig. 1.6 The schematic representation of the disruption of the genomic imprinting. In case of maternal imprinting, only the paternal genes are active; the maternal genes are not transcribed. On the other hand, in paternal imprinting, only the maternal genes are transcribed. If both copies of the given locus affected by imprinting are derived from one parent, then in the case of maternal chromosomes, the genes influenced by paternal imprinting will be expressed twofold, while the genes affected by maternal imprinting will not be expressed. The expression of genes that is not influenced by the regulation of genomic imprinting—hence showing biallelic expression—is not affected

microRNA is one of the most highlighted field of contemporary medicine. The expression pattern of microRNAs is also altered in several diseases. However, it has to be emphasized that in some respects, they could be even more effective as biomarkers (Cortez et al. 2011). In applying novel bioinformatical approaches, it is not just the nucleic acids that are detectable but the proteins and the small-molecular-weight metabolites too (proteomics and metabolomics). These molecules may represent the determinative directions of the future diagnostics. However, the negotiation of these topics would be far beyond the frame of this book.

The extensive investigation of the aforementioned SNPs has become available; moreover it is possible to evaluate more thousands SNPs concurrently, which can open enormous perspectives in research. The investigation of SNP pattern could have particularly large relevance in the determination of susceptibility to diseases, prediction of side effects, and individualized therapy which is one of the most important perspectives of medicine.

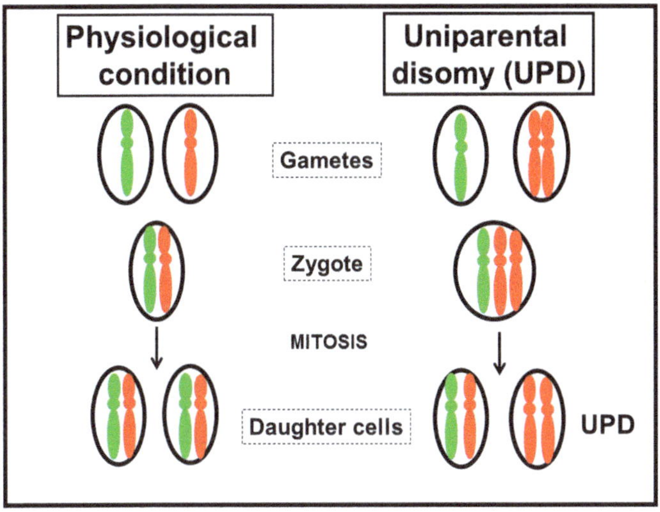

Fig. 1.7 The developmental mechanism of uniparental disomy (UPD). Just one chromosome is indicated for the sake of simplicity. (**a**) Physiological condition: one chromosome carrier zygote is formed by the fusion of haploid gametes. The daughter cells that are evolved during the process of mitosis carry both paternal and maternal chromosomes. (**b**) If a gamete carries one while the other carries two chromosomes, the zygote has to lose a chromosome to avoid the often lethal trisomy caused by a supernumerary chromosome. Therefore, one third of the diploid daughter cells carry chromosomes deriving from just one parent

Acknowledgments Supported by the Higher Education Institutional Excellence Programme of the Ministry of Human Capacities in Hungary, within the framework of the molecular biology thematic program of the Semmelweis University.

References

Ahmad A, Siddiqui MA, Goyal A, Wangnoo SK (2012) Is 46XX karyotype always a female? BMJCase Rep 2012:bcr2012006223-bcr2012006223. https://doi.org/10.1136/bcr-2012-006223

Alexandrov LB, Nik-Zainal S, Wedge DC et al (2013) Signatures of mutational processes in human cancer. Nature 500:415–421. https://doi.org/10.1038/nature12477

Barr ML, Bertram EG (1949) A morphological distinction between neurones of the male and female, and the behaviour of the nucleolar satellite during accelerated nucleoprotein synthesis. Nature 163:676

Bassett JH, Forbes SA, Pannett AA et al (1998) Characterization of mutations in patients with multiple endocrine neoplasia type 1. Am J Hum Genet 62:232–244. https://doi.org/10.1086/301729

Baum P, Schmid R, Ittrich C et al (2010) Phenocopy—a strategy to qualify chemical compounds during hit-to-lead and/or lead optimization. PLoS One 5:e14272. https://doi.org/10.1371/journal.pone.0014272

Benitez JA, Cheng S, Deng Q (2017) Revealing allele-specific gene expression by single-cell transcriptomics. Int J Biochem Cell Biol 90:155–160. https://doi.org/10.1016/j.biocel.2017.05.029

Cinalli RM, Rangan P, Lehmann R (2008) Germ cells are forever. Cell 132:559–562. https://doi.org/10.1016/j.cell.2008.02.003
Cortez MA, Bueso-Ramos C, Ferdin J et al (2011) MicroRNAs in body fluids—the mix of hormones and biomarkers. Nat Rev Clin Oncol 8:467–477. https://doi.org/10.1038/nrclinonc.2011.76
Creighton HB, McClintock B (1931) A correlation of cytological and genetical crossing-over in Zea mays. Proc Natl Acad Sci USA 17:492–497
Dupont C, Armant DR, Brenner CA (2009) Epigenetics: definition, mechanisms and clinical perspective. Semin Reprod Med 27:351–357. https://doi.org/10.1055/s-0029-1237423
Elkon R, Linhart C, Sharan R et al (2003) Genome-wide in silico identification of transcriptional regulators controlling the cell cycle in human cells. Genome Res 13:773–780. https://doi.org/10.1101/gr.947203
Green ED, Watson JD, Collins FS (2015) Human Genome Project: twenty-five years of big biology. Nature 526:29–31. https://doi.org/10.1038/526029a
Hammond CM, Strømme CB, Huang H et al (2017) Histone chaperone networks shaping chromatin function. Nat Rev Mol Cell Biol 18:141–158. https://doi.org/10.1038/nrm.2016.159
Huxley J, Mayr E, Osmond H, Hoffer A (1964) Schizophrenia as a genetic morphism. Nature 204:220–221
Johannsen W (2014) The genotype conception of heredity. Int J Epidemiol 43:989–1000. https://doi.org/10.1093/ije/dyu063
Kadakkuzha BM, Puthanveettil SV (2013) Genomics and proteomics in solving brain complexity. Mol BioSyst 9:1807. https://doi.org/10.1039/c3mb25391k
Knoll JHM, Nicholls RD, Magenis RE et al (1989) Angelman and Prader-Willi syndromes share a common chromosome 15 deletion but differ in parental origin of the deletion. Am J Med Genet 32:285–290. https://doi.org/10.1002/ajmg.1320320235
Lagos-Quintana M, Rauhut R, Lendeckel W, Tuschl T (2001) Identification of novel genes coding for small expressed RNAs. Science 294:853–858. https://doi.org/10.1126/science.1064921
Lane AN, Fan TW-M (2015) Regulation of mammalian nucleotide metabolism and biosynthesis. Nucleic Acids Res 43:2466–2485. https://doi.org/10.1093/nar/gkv047
Lo KC, Bailey D, Burkhardt T et al (2008) Comprehensive analysis of loss of heterozygosity events in glioblastoma using the 100K SNP mapping arrays and comparison with copy number abnormalities defined by BAC array comparative genomic hybridization. Genes Chromosomes Cancer 47:221–237. https://doi.org/10.1002/gcc.20524
Mounolou J-C, Lacroute F (2005) Mitochondrial DNA: an advance in eukaryotic cell biology in the 1960s. Biol Cell 97:743–748. https://doi.org/10.1042/BC20040128
Nachtergaele S, He C (2017) The emerging biology of RNA post-transcriptional modifications. RNA Biol 14:156–163. https://doi.org/10.1080/15476286.2016.1267096
Nordling CO (1953) A new theory on cancer-inducing mechanism. Br J Cancer 7:68–72
Pearson H (2006) What is a gene. Nature 441:398–401. https://doi.org/10.1038/441398a
Pluta AF, Mackay AM, Ainsztein AM et al (1995) The centromere: hub of chromosomal activities. Science 270:1591–1594
Provine WB (2004) Ernst Mayr: genetics and speciation. Genetics 167:1041–1046
Rana AK, Ankri S (2016) Reviving the RNA world: an insight into the appearance of RNA methyltransferases. Front Genet 7:99. https://doi.org/10.3389/fgene.2016.00099
Romano G, Veneziano D, Acunzo M, Croce CM (2017) Small non-coding RNA and cancer. Carcinogenesis 38:485–491. https://doi.org/10.1093/carcin/bgx026
Santaguida S, Amon A (2015) Short- and long-term effects of chromosome mis-segregation and aneuploidy. Nat Rev Mol Cell Biol 16:473–485. https://doi.org/10.1038/nrm4025
Schwartz S, Meshorer E, Ast G (2009) Chromatin organization marks exon-intron structure. Nat Struct Mol Biol 16:990–995. https://doi.org/10.1038/nsmb.1659
Shu J-J (2017) A new integrated symmetrical table for genetic codes. Biosystems 151:21–26. https://doi.org/10.1016/j.biosystems.2016.11.004

Storz G (2002) An expanding universe of noncoding RNAs. Science 296:1260–1263. https://doi.org/10.1126/science.1072249
Taylor TH, Gitlin SA, Patrick JL et al (2014) The origin, mechanisms, incidence and clinical consequences of chromosomal mosaicism in humans. Hum Reprod Update 20:571–581. https://doi.org/10.1093/humupd/dmu016
Travers A, Muskhelishvili G (2015) DNA structure and function. FEBS J 282:2279–2295. https://doi.org/10.1111/febs.13307
van den Hoogenhof MMG, Pinto YM, Creemers EE (2016) RNA splicing. Circ Res 118:454–468. https://doi.org/10.1161/CIRCRESAHA.115.307872
Venter JC, Adams MD, Myers EW et al (2001) The sequence of the human genome. Science 291:1304–1351. https://doi.org/10.1126/science.1058040
Wilkins JF, Haig D (2003) What good is genomic imprinting: the function of parent-specific gene expression. Nat Rev Genet 4:359–368. https://doi.org/10.1038/nrg1062
Zhang C (2009) Novel functions for small RNA molecules. Curr Opin Mol Ther 11:641–651
Zheng C, Hayes JJ (2003) Structures and interactions of the core histone tail domains. Biopolymers 68:539–546. https://doi.org/10.1002/bip.10303

Chapter 2
Brief Description of Inheritance Patterns

Annamária Kövesdi and Attila Patócs

Abstract Increasing data about the human genome and associations between certain genetic regions with various conditions and diseases positioned human genetics at the top of the most emerging fields in medicine. Many diagnostics algorithms and therapeutical approaches used in everyday practice are based on genetic data. Molecular genetic diagnostics covered by this book uses genetic data obtained using germline DNA. In this book, the role of somatic mutation testing will be not covered; however, in many chapters, i.e., on hereditary tumor syndromes, the role of somatic mutations as the second hit for tumorigenesis will be mentioned. Genetic variants (genotypes) identified in germline DNA are responsible for transmission of diseases (phenotypes). This chapter will briefly summarize classical inheritance patterns. Most of the heritable human diseases are transmitted in an autosomal recessive way, but others, i.e., inherited tumor syndromes, follow the autosomal dominant pattern. Nomenclature used for pedigree analysis as well as the main features of inheritance patterns are also briefly reviewed.

Keywords Inheritance · Dominant · Recessive · Allele · Mutation · Homozygous · Heterozygous

A. Kövesdi
Department of Laboratory Medicine, Semmelweis University, Budapest, Hungary

"Lendület" Hereditary Endocrine Tumors Research Group, Hungarian Academy of Sciences and Semmelweis University, Budapest, Hungary

A. Patócs (✉)
Department of Laboratory Medicine, Faculty of Medicine, Semmelweis University, Budapest, Hungary

"Lendület" Hereditary Endocrine Tumors Research Group, Hungarian Academy of Sciences and Semmelweis University, Budapest, Hungary

Department of Molecular Genetics, National Institute of Oncology, Budapest, Hungary
e-mail: patocs.attila@med.semmelweis-univ.hu

P. Igaz, A. Patócs (eds.), *Genetics of Endocrine Diseases and Syndromes*, Experientia Supplementum 111, https://doi.org/10.1007/978-3-030-25905-1_2

List of Abbreviations

CAH	Congenital adrenal hyperplasia
CYP21A2	Cytochrome P450 family 21 subfamily A member 2
DNA	Deoxyribonucleic acid
LOH	Loss of heterozygosity
MEN1	Multiple endocrine neoplasia type 1
MEN2	Multiple endocrine neoplasia type 2
NGS	Next-generation sequencing

2.1 Introduction

An increasing number of pathologic conditions have been associated with genetic alterations. Developing molecular genetic methods and mapping of the human genome allowed us to identify more and more gene loci in association with different disorders. In most cases, not a single gene (monogenic disease) but multiple—genomic and environmental—factors are responsible for the development of a disease (multifactorial disease). Genetic defects occurring in germ cells are transmitted to every single cell of the individual's offspring, while mutations in somatic cells lead to alterations in the tissue involved (Williams 1997; Oláh 2015).

One gene may have different forms, i.e., alleles. An allele that encodes the normal, most common phenotype in a population is called the wild-type allele. A gene defect that might cause disease results in a mutant allele. When two identical alleles are present at the same gene locus, the individual is homozygous for that gene; in the case of two different alleles of the gene, the individual is heterozygous. In monogenic diseases, a dominant allele can express its effect in one copy, i.e., in the presence of the other—recessive—allele at the same locus. The dominant allele is written with an upper case (e.g., *A*) and the recessive with lower case (e.g., *a*). The disorder is autosomal if the affected allele is on a non-sex chromosome and X- or Y-linked if it's on a sex chromosome (Aiello and Chiatti 2017).

The inheritance pattern of monogenic diseases can be assessed using a family tree. When an inherited condition is suspected, a detailed family history including a minimum of three generations is needed to construct a pedigree. Studying a pedigree helps us to identify the inheritance of the mutant allele and the disease. Figure 2.1 shows the commonly used nomenclature (Aiello and Chiatti 2017; Bennett et al. 2008). De novo mutations may also occur in germ cells. In this case, both parents of the proband have homozygous wild-type alleles, but the proband can transmit the de novo germline mutation to the offspring.

However, most disorders do not show the inheritance patterns discussed below. These disorders show multifactorial or complex inheritance: several genes that cause predisposition to disease in combination with environmental factors contribute to

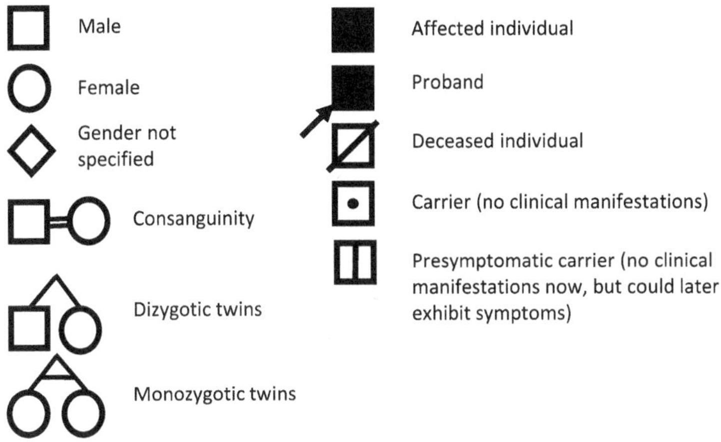

Fig. 2.1 The most commonly used pedigree symbols (Bennett et al. 2008)

their development. Some rare disorders are transmitted by mitochondrial genes, and these diseases are inherited only maternally (Oláh 2015).

Here we discuss the basic concepts of monogenic inheritance patterns first described by Mendel.

2.2 Autosomal Dominant Inheritance

The allele responsible for the trait or disease is located on an autosome. One copy of a dominant allele is enough to cause a phenotype or disorder in autosomal dominant inheritance. An individual will present the dominant feature both in heterozygous and homozygous states. Males and females have equal risk. There is 50% chance that the dominant allele will be passed from the affected parent to an offspring. One parent of the affected offspring also manifests the disease. The children of healthy parents are also unaffected; those that do not carry the dominant allele will not develop disease. The pedigree will show that the trait or disorder is present in each generation (Fig. 2.2). Clinical manifestations of the disease in members of the same family may vary, as seen in, e.g., multiple endocrine neoplasia type 1 (MEN1) syndrome. The difference can be attributable to the different expressions of the dominant allele as a result of several influencing factors. Autosomal dominant mutations tend to affect structural proteins or proteins regulating complex metabolic processes. Their reduced expression by 50% causes disease symptoms. In some autosomal dominantly inherited diseases, carrying the mutation in homozygous form may be minimally viable or lethal; thus in the clinical practice, the affected individuals are mostly heterozygous. Autosomal dominant diseases are common among the Mendelian diseases: their prevalence is approximately 1%. Some examples include achondroplasia, neurofibromatosis type 1, or polycystic kidney disease (Aiello and Chiatti 2017; Oláh 2015).

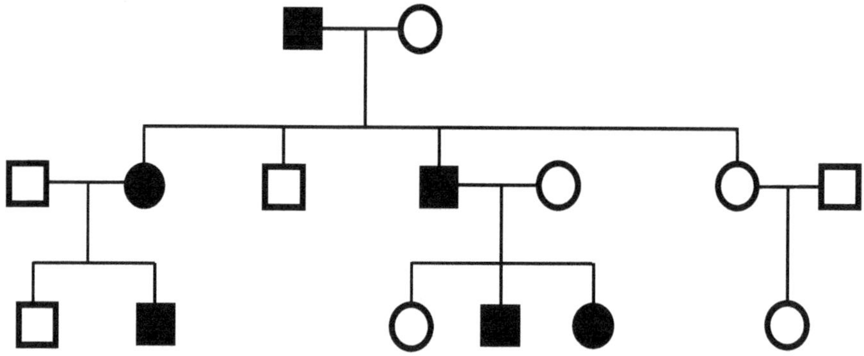

Fig. 2.2 Autosomal dominant inheritance

In the majority of cancer syndromes [e.g., Von Hippel-Lindau disease, multiple endocrine neoplasia type 2 (MEN2)], inherited genetic defects cause a predisposition to neoplastic transformation. Mutations of proto-oncogenes or tumor suppressor genes are inherited in an autosomal dominant manner, causing dysregulation of cell growth and cell proliferation or leading to activation of signaling pathways for cell survival. Tumor suppressor genes are recessive at cellular level: a second, somatic mutation causing loss of the other allele [loss of heterozygosity (LOH)] is needed for cancer development. However, variable expression and tissue specificity strongly contribute to carcinogenesis (Ponder 2001; Williams 1997).

2.3 Autosomal Recessive Inheritance

Contrary to the dominant diseases, the autosomal recessive alleles express their disease-causing effect only in homozygous form, when both copies are present. Individuals with only one copy are carriers of the disease, and they are clinically asymptomatic. The affected child inherits one copy of the recessive allele from each—usually heterozygous—parent. Unaffected parents may have affected children. Offsprings of two heterozygous parents have a 25% chance to inherit both recessive alleles, i.e., to be homozygous for the disease, 50% to be a heterozygous carrier, and 25% to be healthy. Both sexes are at equal risk. Pedigree analysis shows that not all generations are affected, but there may be more affected individuals in one generation (Fig. 2.3). The heterozygous carrier state of recessive diseases might be quite common; for instance, it reaches 4% of the population in case of cystic fibrosis. Recessive alleles usually affect enzyme proteins, which can still function in a reduced amount in heterozygous individuals, causing no or mild symptoms. Cystic fibrosis and phenylketonuria are inherited in autosomal recessive manner (Aiello and Chiatti 2017; Oláh 2015). The most important endocrinological condition showing recessive inheritance is congenital adrenal hyperplasia (CAH), which is caused by

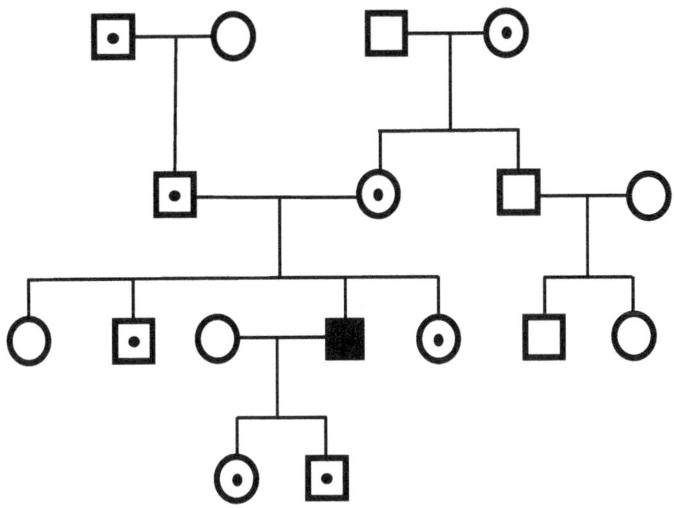

Fig. 2.3 Autosomal recessive inheritance

various mutations of the 21-hydroxilase (*CYP21A2*) gene (Chap. 12). Heterozygous carriers of mutations may present mild symptoms. Clinical and genetic heterogeneity is characteristic for CAH. Consanguinity increases the risk of giving birth to an offspring that carries an autosomal recessively inherited allele in a homozygous form, since both parents might carry the same recessive allele. In case of cystic fibrosis, the risk to inherit the disease is three times higher than in normal population (Stratakis 2017).

2.4 X-Linked Dominant Inheritance

The gene responsible for the disease is located on the X chromosome. Since males have only one X chromosome, they are hemizygous for X-linked diseases. In case of a dominant allele on X chromosome, both males and heterozygous females develop the disease. Based on clinical evidence, hemizygous males carrying one X chromosome with a mutated allele are more seriously affected than heterozygous females. Sons of an affected father are always healthy, because they inherit the Y chromosome from the father; in distinction, his daughters are always affected. Half of the offsprings of a heterozygous affected mother will also present the disease, independently of gender. Although this inheritance form is quite rare, diseases transmitted this way are usually severe or lethal. Most of the children in these families are females; males usually die in utero. According to the family tree, the disease is present in every generation (Fig. 2.4). Rare diseases including Fragile X syndrome and hereditary hypophosphatemic rickets show X-linked dominant inheritance (Aiello and Chiatti 2017; Oláh 2015).

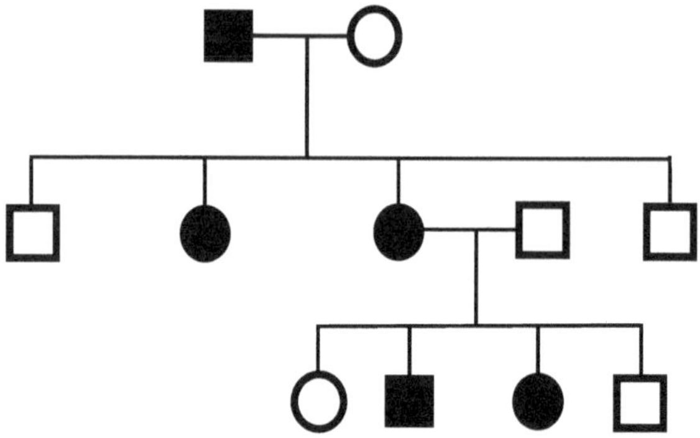

Fig. 2.4 X-linked dominant inheritance

2.5 X-Linked Recessive Inheritance

Most X-linked disorders are recessive. Disorders develop almost exclusively in hemizygotic males. Females are usually only heterozygous carriers of the mutation. Diseases develop extremely rarely in females, as they would need both affected alleles to manifest the disease. However, in some cases heterozygous females may present mild symptoms. Moreover, as a result of the physiological somatic inactivation of the chromosome X, some groups of cells of the body may present disease manifestations (mosaicism). Sons of the affected father will always be healthy, and all his daughters will carry the affected allele. Sons of a heterozygous mother have 50% chance for the disease and her daughters 50% chance to carry the disease. An affected male always inherits the disease from the mother. Some X-linked recessively inherited diseases may be severe; the affected males may not survive until the reproductive age. The pedigree is discontinuous; some generations are unaffected (Fig. 2.5). Hemophilia A and B and Duchenne muscular dystrophy are inherited as X-linked recessive traits (Aiello and Chiatti 2017; Oláh 2015).

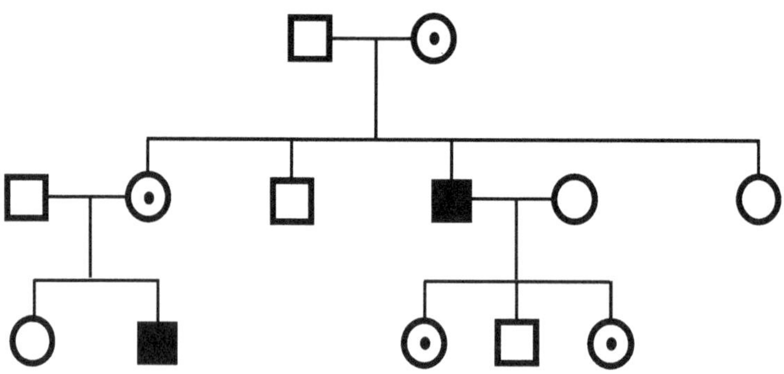

Fig. 2.5 X-linked recessive inheritance

Clinical significance of Y-linked inheritance and its role in the pathogenesis of diseases are not fully understood (Oláh 2015).

2.6 Conclusions

DNA transmitted through germline cells of the offspring may contain gene variants that already caused an altered phenotype or disease in the parents. When such a situation is likely, visualizing a pedigree helps us recognize the inheritance pattern. Nowadays, different software and algorithms are available not just to draw the family tree but also to identify the unknown gene responsible for the disease. Linkage analysis is based on the fact that genes located close to each other on the chromosome are most likely passed together to the descendant. It uses a map of known genetic markers and the inheritance pattern of the disease or phenotype from the pedigree and determines those markers nearest to the disease locus. The widespread use of next-generation sequencing (NGS) methods gives us even more opportunity to work with a huge amount of sequence data, thus improving our knowledge of hereditary conditions. However, during data analysis and finding the potential disease-causing algorithms, the knowledge on and computing the inheritance patterns are still in use.

Acknowledgments The authors acknowledge the financial support of the Higher Education Institutional Excellence Program of the Ministry of Human Capacities in Hungary, within the framework of the Molecular Biology thematic program of the Semmelweis University.

References

Aiello LB, Chiatti BD (2017) Primer in genetics and genomics, Article 4—Inheritance patterns. Biol Res Nurs 19(4):465–472. https://doi.org/10.1177/1099800417708616
Bennett RL, French KS, Resta RG, Doyle DL (2008) Standardized human pedigree nomenclature: update and assessment of the recommendations of the National Society of Genetic Counselors. J Genet Couns 17(5):424–433. https://doi.org/10.1007/s10897-008-9169-9
Oláh É (ed) (2015) Klinikai genetika [Clinical genetics]. Medicina, Budapest
Ponder BA (2001) Cancer genetics. Nature 411(6835):336–341. https://doi.org/10.1038/35077207
Stratakis C (ed) (2017) Genetics of endocrine disorders, an issue of endocrinology and metabolism clinics of North America. Elsevier, Philadelphia, PA
Williams JK (1997) Principles of genetics and cancer. Semin Oncol Nurs 13(2):68–73

Chapter 3
Family Screening and Genetic Counseling

Pál Perge and Peter Igaz

Abstract In this brief chapter, clinically very important topics of family screening and genetic counseling are discussed that are also pivotal in endocrine genetics. Genetic screening makes possible to diagnose a genetic disease at an early stage or to exclude its presence. Family members have to be screened if a heritable disease is diagnosed. Personal consultation with the patient and the relatives is inevitable in every genetically determined disease. The main function of genetic counseling is the transfer of important pieces of information to the patient about the congenital or later-manifesting diseases. This process via the informed consent should give enough information to the patient and the relatives to make decisions about the disease. Genetic data should be considered as special data; therefore the protection of the personal data and the confidentiality obligation should be prevailed intensively. The chief goal of the genetic counseling is the prevention of the conception or the birth of a person who would suffer from a severe genetic disease and/or to present information of the chance for having an affected descendant. If the prevention is not feasible, the alternative aim is to prevent the development of the consequences or to moderate its severity. Genetic counseling has important ethical aspects such as prenatal genetic investigations; hereditary, but treatable, nonlethal diseases; and genetic diseases that manifest late, predominantly in the adulthood.

Keywords Genetic screening · Heritable disease · Genetic counseling · Prevention · Ethical aspects

---

P. Perge
2nd Department of Internal Medicine, Faculty of Medicine, Semmelweis University, Budapest, Hungary

P. Igaz (✉)
2nd Department of Internal Medicine, Faculty of Medicine, Semmelweis University, Budapest, Hungary

MTA-SE Molecular Medicine Research Group, Hungarian Academy of Sciences and Semmelweis University, Budapest, Hungary
e-mail: igaz.peter@med.semmelweis-univ.hu

P. Igaz, A. Patócs (eds.), *Genetics of Endocrine Diseases and Syndromes*,
Experientia Supplementum 111, https://doi.org/10.1007/978-3-030-25905-1_3

Genetic screening makes possible to diagnose a genetic disease at an early stage or to exclude its presence, to predict the susceptibility or the resistance to the disease, and to identify the heritable genetic variant (Resta et al. 2006). The carriers of a genetic alteration, the individuals who have an increased risk to a disease, and the person who has extended chance to have an affected, sick child are identifiable by genetic screening (McCabe and McCabe 2004). The genetic screening can be performed at the populational level, such as the screening of the newborn or other age groups, or to screen the heterozygous people to determine the allele frequency (Jackson-Cook and Pandya 1995). Family screening has the biggest relevance regarding this book. If a heritable disease is diagnosed, the family members have to be screened in order to search for any affected person. The diseases caused by de novo mutations are also heritable; therefore the screening of descendants is indispensable. The investigation of the ancestors and the siblings is justifiable in order to explore the inheritance or to identify the affected individuals. The clinical significance of the family screening is outstanding. In case of a known mutation, if it is not detectable and therefore the disease can be excluded, then the expensive and time-consuming clinical screening procedures are unnecessary (Pletcher et al. 2007). In contrast, when the mutation is present, disease manifestation is probable; therefore the affected individuals have to be screened regularly in order to moderate or prevent the consequences of the disease. The procedures for clinical screening are different for every disease and in cases where genotype-phenotype correlations are established even for different mutations.

Personal consultation with the patient and the relatives is inevitable in every genetically determined disease. The communication with the patient and the family is especially important in the case of heritable/genetically determined diseases. Genetic counseling is a relatively new scientific field, dealing with heritable diseases and their potential effects in the descendants and relatives (Ormond et al. 2018).

During genetic counseling, the entitled person gives information to the affected patients and the family about the nature, the consequences, the causes, the inheritance, the risk of the manifestation, the prognosis, the diagnostic and therapeutical aspects, and the possibilities of prevention of the disease. Legally, the genetic counseling is a specialized process, accomplished during consultation and resulting in a detailed written summary. The participants are the legally entitled expert and the people who receive the guidance. The genetic counseling is enlisted mainly by families where genetic or developmental abnormalities have already occurred or have an increased risk to it.

The main function of genetic counseling is the transfer of important pieces of information to the patient about the congenital or later-manifesting diseases. This process via the informed consent should give enough information to the patient and the relatives to make decisions about the disease.

The cause and the inheritance of the disease are discussed during the guidance. It is extremely important that the council should be understandable for a nonprofessional person, and every question of the patients has to be answered clearly. The estimation or in some cases the determination of the genetic risk of the affected person or his/her relatives by a disease is one of the most momentous part of the counseling. A genetic counseling should precede any genetic test which would help to set up the diagnosis (Raymond et al. 2016). The advisor should inform the patient about the consequences of the expected results. Naturally, after the diagnosis, another counseling has to be performed in order to negotiate about the further possibilities.

The chief goal of the genetic counseling is the prevention of the conception or the birth of a person who would suffer from a severe genetic disease and/or to present information of the chance for having an affected descendant (Hodgson et al. 2010). If the prevention is not feasible, the alternative aim is to prevent the development of the consequences or to moderate its severity. The prevention has three levels. Primary prevention restrains the conception itself (contraception, sterilization, adoption, oocyte donation). Secondary prevention intervenes after the conception. It implies the termination of the pregnancy or chooses the healthy embryo in case of in vitro fertilization (prenatal, preimplantational diagnostics) (Benn et al. 2015). The aim of the tertiary prevention is to alleviate the symptoms of the manifested disease by diet or operation.

Genetic counseling is needed predominantly in the cases below (Ormond et al. 2018):

1. Genetic disease, developmental abnormality have occurred in the family
2. Agnation
3. The age of the mother is above 35
4. Teratogenic factors affect a pregnant female
5. In cases of habitual miscarriage and infertility that cannot be explained with any other cause

The genetic counseling is a nondirective process. It means that the consultant gives every information, but the decision has to be made by the patient only. The counselor should avoid to influence the patient with his/her personal opinion.

The genetic data should be considered as special data; therefore the protection of the personal data and the confidentiality obligation should be prevailed intensively. Sharing information from the genetic counseling to a third party is strictly prohibited.

Compared to other medical consultations, the genetic counseling is a time-consuming process, as it requires thorough preparation and multiple consultations. Only entitled experts have legal rights to give council.

The genetic counseling begins with the collection of the information. Firstly, a detailed family tree has to be recorded from the patient and the relatives. All known diseases and symptoms of the family members have to be listed. After all information are collected, the investigation of the patient follows. Thereafter begins the actual counseling about the nature, the consequences, and the chance of the recurrence of the disease, and the indications of the following examinations are also discussed. As the counseling is a nondirective process, it is expedient that the patient makes the decision after days-to-weeks lasting thinking time. The counseling happens in more sessions; therefore the affected person always has possibility to ask about the newly emerged questions also.

Compared to nonhereditary diseases, the recognition of a heritable sickness associates with higher psychological burden. Therefore, psychological consultational possibility should be provided besides genetic counseling (Grover 2003). The helper groups of the affected patients and their relatives play useful role to the newly diagnosed patients to cope with their disease.

The genetic counseling, the genetic examinations, and the clinical genetics have several important ethical aspects. The number of these questions is increasing steadily as the field evolves. Numerous problems with the prenatal genetic investigations and with the associated secondary prevention have emerged. The hereditary, but treatable, nonlethal diseases are perfect examples for this. Serious questions have to be answered for genetic diseases that manifest late, predominantly in the adulthood (Gilchrist 2002). These include endocrinological diseases that have genetical background: such as multiple endocrine neoplasia syndromes or particular forms of adrenoleukodystrophy. Several polymorphisms have been identified that play a role in the susceptibility to complex, polygenic, heritable diseases. Among them significant interindividual and populational differences are known in terms of the pathogenic role. Therefore, an unequivocal determination of the risk and far-reaching deduction for their consequences are cumbersome but necessary.

Acknowledgments Supported by the Higher Education Institutional Excellence Programme of the Ministry of Human Capacities in Hungary, within the framework of the molecular biology thematic program of the Semmelweis University.

References

Benn P, Borrell A, Chiu RWK et al (2015) Position statement from the Chromosome Abnormality Screening Committee on behalf of the Board of the International Society for Prenatal Diagnosis. Prenat Diagn 35:725–734. https://doi.org/10.1002/pd.4608

Gilchrist DM (2002) Medical genetics: 3. An approach to the adult with a genetic disorder. CMAJ 167:1021–1029

Grover S (2003) The psychological dimension of informed consent: dissonance processes in genetic testing. J Genet Couns 12:389–403

Hodgson JM, Gillam LH, Sahhar MA, Metcalfe SA (2010) "Testing times, challenging choices": an Australian study of prenatal genetic counseling. J Genet Couns 19:22–37. https://doi.org/10.1007/s10897-009-9248-6

Jackson-Cook C, Pandya A (1995) Strategies and logistical requirements for efficient testing in genetic disease. Clin Lab Med 15:839–857

McCabe LL, McCabe ERB (2004) Genetic screening: carriers and affected individuals. Annu Rev Genomics Hum Genet 5:57–69. https://doi.org/10.1146/annurev.genom.5.061903.175941

Ormond KE, Laurino MY, Barlow-Stewart K et al (2018) Genetic counseling globally: where are we now? Am J Med Genet C Semin Med Genet 178:98–107. https://doi.org/10.1002/ajmg.c.31607

Pletcher BA, Toriello HV, Noblin SJ et al (2007) Indications for genetic referral: a guide for healthcare providers. Genet Med 9:385–389. https://doi.org/10.1097GIM.0b013e318064e70c

Raymond VM, Gray SW, Roychowdhury S et al (2016) Germline findings in tumor-only sequencing: points to consider for clinicians and laboratories: Table 1. J Natl Cancer Inst 108:djv351. https://doi.org/10.1093/jnci/djv351

Resta R, Biesecker BB, Bennett RL et al (2006) A new definition of genetic counseling: National Society of Genetic Counselors' Task Force report. J Genet Couns 15:77–83. https://doi.org/10.1007/s10897-005-9014-3

Chapter 4
Brief Summary of the Most Important Molecular Genetic Methods (PCR, qPCR, Microarray, Next-Generation Sequencing, etc.)

Henriett Butz and Attila Patócs

Abstract Molecular genetic methods have become an organic part of everyday clinical practice. In the past, molecular diagnostic tests were carried out for genetic diagnosis of a particular monogenic disease. In these situations the tests itself were used for identification of one particular genetic alteration (e.g., point mutation or deletion) of the gene of interest. Later, parallel with the development of the technology, the focus has shifted by allowing investigating at once targeted gene panels and even the whole exome/genome behind a suspected genetic disorder. Historically for these purposes, array-based methods (oligonucleotide arrays) and then next-generation sequencing-based methods have been used. High-throughput methods have been fundamentally transforming the everyday, routine genetic diagnostics, but older molecular techniques still have a role in clinical genetics. Here, we summarize the most important molecular genetic methods and shed light to the advantages and disadvantages of their application in routine diagnostics. We mainly focus on methods used for detection of germline alterations.

Keywords Mutation · Genetic testing · Sequencing · Next-generation sequencing · Polymerase chain reaction

List of Abbreviations

aCGH	Array comparative genomic hybridization
ARMS	Amplification refractory mutation system

H. Butz · A. Patócs (✉)
Department of Laboratory Medicine, Faculty of Medicine, Semmelweis University, Budapest, Hungary

"Lendület" Hereditary Endocrine Tumors Research Group, Hungarian Academy of Sciences and Semmelweis University, Budapest, Hungary

Department of Molecular Genetics, National Institute of Oncology, Budapest, Hungary
e-mail: patocs.attila@med.semmelweis-univ.hu

P. Igaz, A. Patócs (eds.), *Genetics of Endocrine Diseases and Syndromes*, Experientia Supplementum 111, https://doi.org/10.1007/978-3-030-25905-1_4

AS-PCR	Allele-specific PCR
cDNA	Complementary DNA
CGH	Comparative genomic hybridization
CNV	Copy number variations
cT	Cycle threshold
DDGE	denaturing gradient gel electrophoresis
ddNTP	Dideoxyribonucleotide triphosphate
DNA	Deoxyribonucleic acid
dNTP	Deoxyribonucleotide triphosphate (adenine, cytosine, guanine, and thymine triphosphate: dATP, dCTP, dGTP, and dTTP, respectively)
dPCR	Digital polymerase chain reaction
dsDNA	Double-stranded DNA
EDTA	Ethylenediaminetetraacetic acid
FRET	Fluorescence resonance energy transfer
HA	Heteroduplex analysis
HRM	High-resolution melting analysis
IVD	In vitro diagnosis
MLPA	Multiplex ligation-dependent probe amplification
NGS	Next-generation sequencing
OD	Optical density
PASA	PCR amplification of specific alleles
PCR	Polymerase chain reaction
qPCR	Quantitative polymerase chain reaction
RFLP	Restriction fragment length polymorphism
RT-qPCR	Reverse transcription quantitative polymerase chain reaction
SNP	Single-nucleotide polymorphism
SNV	Single-nucleotide variants
SSCP	Single-strand conformation polymorphism (SSCP)
STR	Small tandem repeat
UPD	Uniparental disomy
VAF	Variant allele frequency
VUS	Variant of uncertain significance
WES	Whole-exome sequencing
WGS	Whole-genome sequencing

4.1 Introduction

Formerly, genetic testing was confined to rare genetic disorders due to their complexity, labor intensity, and cost. With the appearance of the idea of personalized and later precision medicine and technological development, molecular genetic tests are now widely available regarding different fields of medicine. There are utilized for newborn screening (mostly targeted tests for recessively inherited diseases), diagnostic and carrier testing, predictive and pre-symptomatic testing, or pharmacogenetics (Katsanis and Katsanis 2013).

Genetic methods are often categorized as indirect and direct tests (Katsanis and Katsanis 2013). While direct genetic tests investigate the presence or the absence of known genetic variants that can contribute to the pathogenic condition, indirect tests compare DNA characteristics between patients and healthy controls. For instance, linkage analysis based on single-nucleotide array or short tandem repeat data can identify potential candidate region of interest of a particular condition. Single-strand conformation polymorphism (SSCP), denaturing gradient gel electrophoresis (DDGE), and heteroduplex analysis (HA) are also classical indirect mutation screening methods. When classical sequencing was labor-intensive and costly, these methods were used as screening tools and their role was to decrease the mutation screening cost. Due to the fact that their sensitivity fails 100%, nowadays their application cannot be permitted in diagnostic settings. In addition, as these techniques required validation using another method (almost exclusively Sanger sequencing), these techniques practically disappeared from today's genetic diagnostics. Current molecular diagnostics prefers direct genetic tests including PCR and qPCR-based methods, array CGH, genome-wide SNP arrays, and sequencing (classical Sanger and next-generation sequencing) (Table 4.1).

4.2 DNA Isolation and Quality Control

Before any genetic tests, genomic deoxyribonucleic acid (DNA) has to be extracted from blood (white blood cells containing nucleus) or tissue sample. As the first step of DNA extraction, cells have to be broken to obtain purified DNA molecules, e.g., by homogenizing or lysing (mechanically or enzymatically). The lysis buffer contains detergents which dissolve lipid membranes and denature proteins while it protects the DNA during isolation. DNA is a very long, negatively charged molecule. Therefore cations in the lysis buffer (e.g., $Na+$) stabilize the negatively charged DNA and separate it from proteins such as histones. Other chemicals like ethylenediamine-tetraacetic acid (EDTA) are also included in the lysis buffer in order to sequester $Mg2+$ ions (necessary cofactor for nucleases) hence to protect DNA integrity. As a result of the homogenization process, double-stranded DNA molecules are released from the chromatin into the lysis buffer. Then the free DNA molecules have to be separated and purified. Proteins can be removed either by proteinase enzymes (e.g., Proteinase K is used to digest protein components) or by precipitation (through adjusting the salt concentration). The supernatant (containing DNA and other small molecules) is then mixed with ethanol in order to precipitate DNA which can be pelleted by centrifugation. After further ethanol washing steps, the DNA pellet can be dissolved in water or EDTA buffer. These steps can be made manually; however DNA extraction in molecular diagnostics is fully automated using commercially available kits. Taking advantage of negative charge, the unique characteristic of DNA, it is bound to columns containing silica membranes or magnetic beads which help DNA separation from other components of the cell during the extraction process.

DNA quantity and quality have to be controlled in order to get reliable result of a genetic test. As the result depends on the quality of the input material, DNA integrity should be revealed by electrophoresis (traditional agarose gel electrophoresis or on microfluidic chips provided by several suppliers), and DNA degradation has to be excluded. Also, DNA yield can be assessed using the absorbance (optical density) measurement method or by the use of fluorescent DNA-binding dyes.

The most common and simple technique used to determine DNA yield and purity is measurement of absorbance (optical density, OD) using spectrophotometry. As at 260 nm nucleic acids absorb light most strongly, the result allows one to estimate the DNA concentration of the solution (adjusting the A260 measurement for turbidity measured by absorbance at 320 nm). As a nucleic acid, RNA and isothiocyanate (used for RNA isolations) also absorb at 260 nm, and proteins (aromatic amino acids) have absorbance at 280 nm and they contribute to the measurement at 260 nm as contaminants if present in the solution (after correcting for absorbance at 320 nm). Therefore, DNA quantity can be overestimated if contaminants are present.

To evaluate DNA purity, measurement of absorbance of 230–320 nm is also used to detect contaminants such as organic compounds or chaotropic salts (e.g., guanidine HCL used for DNA extraction, EDTA, carbohydrates). Phenol that was used for DNA extraction in former times and even today for RNA isolation have absorbance

Table 4.1 Molecular genetic methods and their application in clinical genetics

Method	Small nucleotide variants (SNV)	Small deletion/ insertion	Copy number variants (CNV)	Repeat expansion	Uniparental disomy
PCR-RFLP	X	X			
AS-PCR	X				
HRM	X	X			
Probe-based RT-PCR	X	X			
Fluorescent PCR			X	X	
Multiplex ligation-dependent probe amplification			X		
Sanger sequencing	X	X			
SNP array	X		X		
aCGH			X		X
WGS	X	X	X		
WES	X	X	X		
Targeted panel NGS	X	X			

PCR-RFLP PCR product restriction fragment length polymorphism, *AS-PCR* allele-specific PCR, *HRM* high-resolution melting, *RT-PCR* real-time PCR, *MLPA* multiplex ligation-dependent probe amplification, *SNP* small nucleotide polymorphism, *aCGH* array comparative genomic hybridization, *WGS* whole-genome sequencing, *WES* whole-exome sequencing, *NGS* next-generation sequencing

both at 230 nm and around 270 nm. Therefore, DNA purity factor is investigated by A260/280 and A230/280 ratios.

$$A260/A280 = (A260 - A320)/(A280 - A320) \text{ and } A230/A280 \\ = (A230 - A320)/(A230 - A320)$$

Good-quality DNA would have an A260/A280 ratio between 1.7 and 2.0, and the expected A260/A230 ratios are commonly in the range of 2.0–2.2.

Fluorescence methods are also becoming popular as they are more sensitive compared to the absorbance measurement; hence these techniques are particularly important for samples where low concentration is expected. The use of DNA-binding dyes (binding selectively double-stranded DNA) allows more specific measurement of DNA compared to spectrophotometric methods. Fluorescence measurements are done at excitation and emission values that depend on the dye. The DNA concentration is calculated using a standard curve generated from samples with known concentration. (Logically, genomic, fragment, and plasmid DNA require their own standard curves.) This method is predominantly recommended for next-generation sequencing where low amount of DNA is used.

DNA quality and integrity have to be considered with respect to the downstream application. Salts can inhibit restriction enzymes, and methods using modifying enzymes (e.g., ligation, cloning) can be interfered by the presence of not only salts but organic solvents and EDTA. Similarly, cycle sequencing is also inhibited by salts, organic solvents, EDTA, and nuclease enzymes. As polymerase enzymes are inhibited by heparin, EDTA, detergents, organic solvents, or hemoglobin, only good-quality DNA guarantees the best results in PCR amplification. In quantitative PCR methods, RNA contamination can be an interfering factor especially in case of absolute quantification. Acceptable DNA integrity is important in sequencing and particularly in long-PCR-based methods.

4.3 Polymerase Chain Reaction (PCR)

The invention of polymerase chain reaction technique brought a Nobel Prize in Chemistry for Kary Mullis in 1993. Indeed, PCR revolutionized biochemistry, starting a new era of molecular genetic tests. Since then, it has been the essential technique giving a solid base for further molecular genetic methods. PCR is a simple in vitro chemical reaction allowing the synthesis of extensive quantities of a targeted nucleic acid sequence. The reaction mixture consists of target DNA, oligonucleotide primers, a thermostable DNA polymerase, a mixture of deoxyribonucleotide triphosphates (dATP, dCTP, dGTP, and dTTP), $MgCl_2$, KCl, and a Tris-HCl buffer. The target DNA sequence is flanked by the two primers that are usually 18–30 nucleotide bases long and are complementary to opposite strands of the target DNA. The PCR reaction consists of three steps: denaturation, annealing, and extension that

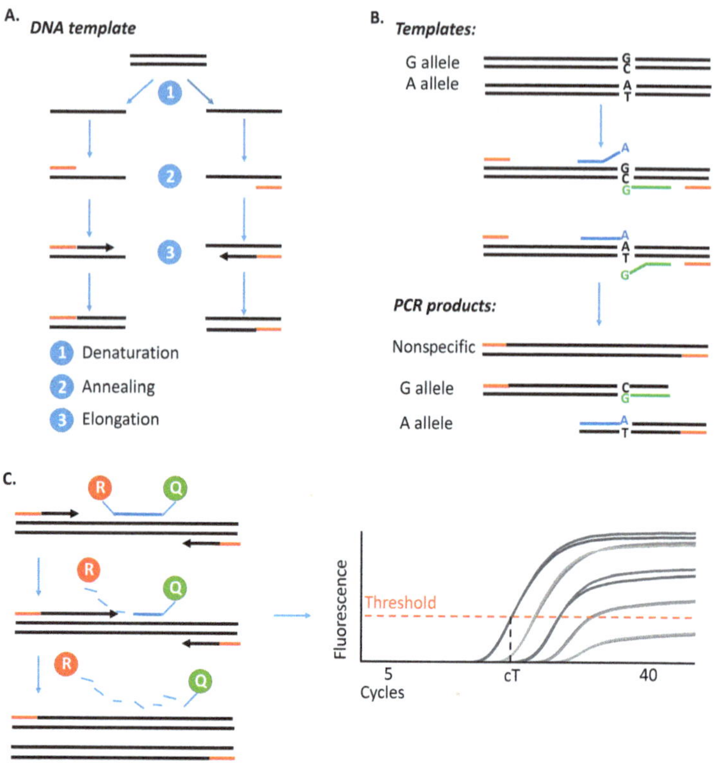

Fig. 4.1 (**a**) Steps of polymerase chain reaction (PCR). (**b**) Allele-specific PCR. (**c**) Hydrolysis probe and quantitative PCR (*R* reporter dye, *Q* quencher, *cT* cycle threshold). See details in the text

are repeated in cycles. As the first step, target DNA has to be denatured by heating (usually at 95 °C) to separate the two strands. Then by cooling, the mixture primers are allowed to anneal to the target DNA in a sequence-specific manner at the annealing temperature determined by the primer sequences. In the third step, the DNA polymerase initiates the chain extension of each primer at its 3′ end (Fig. 4.1a). Finally, the extension products are dissociated from the target DNA by heating that is already the first step (denaturation) of the next cycle. Each new PCR product and the original target as well can serve as a template for subsequent cycles. This cycle is usually repeated 30–35 times. Optimally, at the end of each cycle, the PCR products are doubled; therefore after 20 cycles of PCR a millionfold and after 30 cycles a billionfold amplification is achieved.

In conventional PCR, amplified products are analyzed at the end of the reaction using, e.g. gel electrophoresis (end-point measurement). For instance, if the product is specific, it can be further used, for example, for sequencing by Sanger dideoxynucleotide chain termination method (see below) or digested by restriction enzymes. *PCR-RFLP* (restriction fragment length polymorphism) was used to detect single-nucleotide (or small deletion/insertion) variation affecting a digestion site of a restriction enzyme. When the variant destroys or creates a new digestion site for a restriction enzyme, then it can be used as indirect detection. However, this method was cheap and simple, and it has been replaced the easier and faster (and today cheaper) qPCR methods (see below).

Correspondingly, *allele-specific PCR* (AS-PCR) is a method used for detection of known single-nucleotide (or small deletion/insertion) variation. This method is also known as amplification refractory mutation system (ARMS) or PCR amplification of specific alleles (PASA). In AS-PCR specific primers are designed to permit amplification only if the nucleotide at the 3′ end of the primer is perfectly complementary to the wild type or the variant sequences. After electrophoresis of the PCR product, the patterns of specific PCR products permit the differentiation of the SNPs. The product of the nonspecific primers serves as an internal control for the quality of the reaction (Fig. 4.1b). The reaction of primers specific to each allele can be run in different or even in the same tube if the primers are designed to yield products with different lengths. Although this method is smart and easy, today it is replaced by the fast, less labor-intensive, high-throughput, automatable, and cheap qPCR (genotyping) method (see below).

Another type of PCR is *nested PCR*. It was developed to increase both the sensitivity and specificity of the reaction. In nested PCR, two pairs of primers are applied in two rounds of PCR. The first primer pair is used in the first PCR for usually 15–30 cycles. Then the product of the first round of amplification is subjected to a second round of PCR with the second set of primers. Typically, the second set of primers anneal to a sequence internal to the sequence amplified. Again, in routine diagnostic testing (especially in testing for conditions of clinical genetics), the enhanced sensitivity offered by nested PCR is not required, and it is replaced by the automatable qPCR methods.

It is possible to detect multiple targets at the same time in a single tube using *multiplex PCR*. It is more complicated to develop primers for multiplex PCR, and it is often less sensitive than single-primer-set PCR. However, it is widely used in microbial molecular testing in a fully automated way where usually different fluorescent probes are used for detection. It is also an essential tool used in library preparation for next-generation sequencing (see below).

When the template is not DNA but RNA, *reverse-transcription PCR* (RT-PCR) can be applied. This application is mainly used for determination of gene expression level (in research) or in microbial (viral) detection in routine diagnostics many times in an absolute quantification manner. Here, RNA has to be transcribed to complementary DNA (cDNA) in a first step followed by a second often quantitative PCR reaction. As it is not applied in the molecular genetic methods for clinical genetic conditions, the detailed description of RT-PCR is beyond the aims of this chapter.

During *real-time PCR*, the target amplification and detection steps occur simultaneously. The detection is performed by fluorescence measurement in every cycle. It results in the amplification plot representing the exponential increase in PCR products. At the initial cycles, the change of fluorescence is below the detection limit, and it defines the so-called baseline. After the fluorescence level reaches the lower detection limit exponential increase of the signal can be detectable. The PCR cycle at which the fluorescence signal passes the detection limit is defined as the cycle threshold (cT) (Fig. 4.1c). Reasonably, there is an inverse relationship between the initial input DNA (cDNA) concentration and the cT values. This gives the basis of the quantitative characteristic of the real-time PCR (RT-qPCR). In clinical genetics, RT-qPCR is not applied in contrast to research and microbial testing.

The detection is based on emission of fluorescent dyes. One example is the use of intercalating dyes (e.g., SYBR Green) that preferentially bind to any double-stranded DNA (dsDNA). In the unbound state of the intercalating dyes, the fluorescence is relatively low, but when bound to dsDNA, the fluorescence is greatly enhanced. As they are able to bind any dsDNA molecule, both specific and unspecific PCR products and primer dimers can be detected at the same time. Therefore, the specificity is usually enhanced by performing melting curve analysis. In melting curve analysis when temperature is increased, the two strands of PCR product separated and the fluorescence decreases. Each PCR product has its own melting point determined by the nucleotide composition and length; therefore potential unspecific products can be identified.

High-resolution melting analysis (HRM) is another option to detect small variants. It requires improved instrumentation and the application of new DNA-binding dyes. Simple intercalating dyes do not saturate entirely the whole dsDNA fragment. This leads to dye redistribution during melting that decreases specificity in discrimination. The use of highly saturating dyes that have been developed to achieve highly homogeneous staining of the available PCR products and do not inhibit PCR resulted in the success of HRM analysis (Erali et al. 2008).

Still, the major drawback of DNA-binding dyes is their lack of specificity as mentioned before; they bind to any dsDNA (specific, nonspecific product and primer dimers). Due to the same fact, DNA-binding dyes are not suited for multiplex reactions either, as fluorescence signals from different products cannot be distinguished. Also, HRM is an indirect detection method, and in clinical diagnostics, the application of direct detection is preferred.

Direct detection of small nucleotide variations (mutation, deletion/insertion regarding one or a couple of nucleotides) can be achieved by using *specific probes*. In real-time PCR, fluorescent probes and primers represent two advantages over DNA-binding dyes. On the one hand, probes specifically detect the target sequence; therefore nonspecific products are not detected which would affect the accuracy of quantification. On the other hand, the use of fluorescent probes and DNA primers enables single-tube multiplexing of qPCR reactions for multiple target sequences due to the application of different fluorescent dyes. Probably, the mostly used probe type is the *hydrolysis probe* applied in TaqMan assays. This assay includes a sequence-specific, fluorescently labeled oligonucleotide probe in addition to a sequence-specific PCR primer. Certain polymerase enzymes have a $5' \rightarrow 3'$ exonuclease activity that ensures the hydrolysis of the probe in the assay. The TaqMan or hydrolysis probe is labeled with a fluorescent reporter (usually FAM but not necessarily) at the $5'$ end and a quencher at the $3'$ end. When the probe is intact, the fluorescent signal of the reporter is blocked by the close proximity of the quencher molecule. During the amplification, the DNA polymerase cleaves the reporter that is now able to provide the fluorescent signal (Fig. 4.1c). Although the assay design is not always easy, it represents a highly specific method with a high signal-to-noise ratio. The use of different fluorescent dyes allows to perform multiplex reactions. In addition to TaqMan assays, in molecular genetic testing *dual hybridization probes* are also preferred. In this assay, besides the sequence-specific PCR primer pair, two sequence-specific oligonucleotide probes are used which are labeled with two dyes that exhibit the phenomenon of fluorescence resonance energy transfer (FRET). The two probes are designed to bind (hybridize) to adjacent sequences in the target during the annealing step of the PCR allowing FRET to occur as the two probes are located in close proximity. During detection, excitation is performed at a wavelength of the donor dye, and the emission is monitored at the emission wavelength of the acceptor dye. The two hybridization probes assure the specificity, while the amount of fluorescence is proportional to the PCR product synthetized. This approach is a highly reliable method and its only disadvantage is the cost. Many other types of probes are also available (e.g., molecular beacons, Eclipse probes, Amplifluor, LUX, snake assay, Plexor primers, etc.), but these are beyond of the frame of this chapter, and detailed description of them can be found elsewhere (Navarro et al. 2015). In routine diagnostics, hydrolysis and hybridization probes are the most widely applied methods due to their high specificity, cost, and the possibility for multiplexing. In diagnostics for clinical genetic conditions, these are mainly used for genotyping where different alleles (wild type, mutant) can be differentiated using probes labeled with different fluorescent dyes.

PCR has other applications in clinical genetics using fluorescently labeled primers (*fluorescent PCR*). In a multiplex PCR reaction using different fluorescent primers specific for highly polymorphic small tandem repeat (STR) regions, it is possible to detect possible aneuploidy from, e.g., DNA obtained by amniocentesis or chorionic villus biopsy following fragment analysis in prenatal diagnostics. STRs are small repeat polymorphisms that show high polymorphism among individuals in copy numbers. Among STR markers, only heterozygote markers are appropriate for the analysis. Fluorescent primers are used to amplify STR markers. In the case of a heterozygote marker, two PCR products will be amplified with different lengths that can be separated on capillary electrophoresis, and it can be detected by the fluorescent label of the product. Therefore, for example, in the case of a chromosomal trisomy genotype, STR marker will either show three peaks of equal intensity or two fragments at a 2:1 dosage ratio. With the use of several STR markers from different chromosomes, STR patterns obtained from fetus with trisomy or monosomy of any chromosomes can be distinguished from controls. Even in Turner syndrome (45, X0) DNA can be differentiated from normal male DNA (46, XY) because it does not amplify the Y-chromosome-specific STR marker and still contains only a single dose of X-specific STR markers (Mansfield 1993). With the use of high-enough STR marker, this approach is used for DNA fingerprinting in forensics to investigate paternity or personal identification. The gold standard method in prenatal testing for chromosomal abnormality is still karyotyping, and the application of STR markers (fluorescent PCR fragment analysis) is supplementary. Next-generation sequencing revolutionized prenatal testing mainly due to the opportunity of investigation of fetal

DNA from maternal blood. Besides prenatal testing, fluorescent PCR followed by fragment length analysis is also used for detection of microdeletion and microduplication syndromes in the pediatric field (Stofanko et al. 2013). Additionally, fluorescent PCR has another important application regarding clinical genetics: the detection of repeats. In *repeat-primed PCR*, the repeat region is amplified by PCR using a fluorescently labeled forward primer and a chimeric reverse primer located partially within the repeat. The forward primer is located upstream of the repeat region. During PCR the chimeric reverse primer can hybridize to multiple locations within the repeat region, resulting in PCR products of varying sizes. PCR products then are separated by capillary electrophoresis. Because the chimeric reverse primer is located partially within the repeat and partially in 3′ direction of the repeat, the true allele is identified as the highest peak, and so-called stutter peaks are detected according to the repeat region (Bean and Bayrak-Toydemir 2014).

Digital polymerase chain reaction (dPCR) is a novel method for the absolute quantification of target DNA sequence. In dPCR, the sample is first partitioned (diluted) into many independent PCR microreactors (cells) until that each partition contains either one (few) or no target sequences. After amplification the fraction of amplification-positive cells is used to quantify the concentration of the target sequence with a statistically defined accuracy using Poisson's statistics (Quan et al. 2018). Different platforms are available for partitioning based on direct mechanical shearing, viscous shearing or droplet generators, etc. [see detailed review in Quan et al. (2018)], generating 10^3–10^6 partitions per sample in nanoliters or picoliters depending on platform. Similarly to qPCR, dPCR can use intercalating DNA dyes and hydrolysis-based probes for detection. Assay multiplexing is possible, but dPCR platforms currently lack the possibility of sample multiplexing as one sample is distributed (partitioned) to the whole chip. The main difference between qPCR and dPCR is that dPCR collects fluorescence signals at the end of PCR reaction (end-point measurement) while qPCR detects signal real time.

The advantage of dPCR is that due to the sample dilution (low template input), template competition is reduced, and it allows the detection of rare mutations in a background of wild-type sequences (especially important in detection of somatic mutations in tumor specimens regarding tumor heterogeneity). Additionally, the low sample dilution results in higher tolerance to inhibitors potentially present in the particular sample. It provides reliable detection even with specimens containing very low concentration of the nucleic acids of interest (e.g., liquid biopsies or microbe detection). It is also extensively used to detect genetic imbalances or copy number variants (CNVs) (Quan et al. 2018). However, dPCR has lower sensitivity for absolute quantification, which is attributed to its smaller reaction volume, the detection range is narrower compared to conventional qPCR, and sample multiplexing is still not available in one run.

4.4 Multiplex Ligation-Dependent Probe Amplification (MLPA)

Multiplex ligation-dependent probe amplification (MLPA) is a semi-high-throughput method developed to detect copy number alteration of up to 50 genomic DNA sequences in a single multiplex PCR-based reaction. The MLPA reaction consists of five steps. After DNA denaturation (1) MLPA probes are hybridized (2) to the target regions of the DNA. Each MLPA probe consists of two separate oligonucleotides, each containing one of the PCR primer sequences. Following hybridization, the two separate oligonucleotide parts of the probes are ligated (3). One MLPA probe usually covers 50–100 bp of the target sequence (depending on the probe). Then, MLPA probes are amplified using their primer binding sites by an universal primer set labeled with fluorescent dye (4). Only hybridized and ligated probes can be amplified during the subsequent PCR reaction. The PCR products are then subjected to fragment analysis (separated using capillary electrophoresis). Because each probe has an unique length, the fragment length determines the probe localization. Both internal control probes and positive-negative control samples have to be used during the analysis. First normalizing to internal controls (probes that are hardly suffers copy number alteration) in each sample and then normalizing to control samples yield the relatively quantitative result of the dosage of the regions in the localization of each probe. MLPA is an essential method for detection of large deletion even in hemizygote state. Of endocrine disorders, MLPA extends Sanger sequencing for mutation identification of hereditary endocrine tumor syndromes (von Hippel-Lindau disease, hereditary pheochromocytoma/paraganglioma syndrome, multiple endocrine neoplasia type 1, etc.) and other endocrine diseases including congenital adrenal hyperplasia.

4.5 Sanger Sequencing

Sanger sequencing is a targeted sequencing method, and it is still the gold standard method in determining the nucleotide sequence of DNA. It was developed by two-time Nobel Laureate Frederick Sanger and his colleagues in 1977. It is also called "chain termination method" as it is based on irreversible chain termination in the sequencing PCR using dideoxynucleotides (ddNTP). After amplification of a certain region of interest by conventional PCR, the purified PCR product is used as a template in the sequencing PCR reaction. In the sequencing PCR reaction, sequencing primers are added to designate the region to be sequenced. After denaturation, the sequencing primers are annealed to single-stranded DNA template and it is elongated using a mixture of deoxynucleotide triphosphates (dNTPs) to build the new double-stranded structure. In addition, a small quantity of dideoxynucleotide triphosphates (ddNTPs) for each nucleotide is included. Where ddNTP is incorporated into the chain, the reaction terminates as the polymerase enzyme could not continue chain elongation due to the lack of hydroxyl group at 3′ carbons of the sugar moiety. A much smaller amount of dideoxynucleotides is used than the amount of regular nucleotides, and at the end of reaction, each sequence will terminate at varying lengths. Additionally, a fluorescent marker dye is attached to each ddNTP (ddATP, ddGTP, ddCTP, ddTTP); therefore each PCR product is labeled with a fluorescent dye as well at the end position. Each ddNTP has its own emission spectra (detected as different colors), and conventionally, adenine is indicated by green fluorescence, T by red, G by black, and C by blue. Following the sequencing PCR reaction, PCR products are then separated by capillary gel electrophoresis. The shorter fragments move faster than the longer fragments. Then a laser within the automated instrument excites the label on the nucleotide at the end of each sequence, and the light emitted by each excited nucleotide can be tied to the correct base. The fluorescent intensity then is translated into a peak on the chromatogram. When a heterozygous variant occurs within a sequence, two fluorescent signals appear at the same position with equal intensity. When a homozygous variant is present, the expected fluorescent color is replaced completely by the new base pair's color.

Sanger sequencing is the gold standard testing method able to determine point mutations and small deletions/duplications. It has been widely used for several decades in diagnostic testing. Primers can be easily created to cover several regions of 100–1000 bp region of interest.

However, when long regions or multiple genes have to be tested, this approach can be costly compared with other multiplex testing systems. Therefore, most of the time, Sanger sequencing tests are gene-specific and/or analyze a small subset of genes. Sanger sequencing is able to identify mosaic mutations too present as low as in 20% of the cells. However, this method is hardly quantifiable; therefore it is not used in somatic testing (e.g., tumor heterogeneity), and for these purposes, next-generation sequencing and digital PCR emerge in clinical practice.

4.6 Array-Based Methods

Microarrays belong to high-throughput methods, and they are used to analyze the expression, genotype, or copy number of multiple genes simultaneously. In clinical genetics gene expression microarrays are not the main interest, but array-based genotyping is routinely used. The three main applications are the following (Katsanis and Katsanis 2013): phenotype-specific SNP panels, genome-wide SNP panels, and array comparative genomic hybridization (array CGH, aCGH).

SNP microarrays are small glass slides containing tens of thousands of probes specific to single nucleotide variant alleles. For each there is a specific probe to accurately identify the exact genotype. During the test after DNA extraction, the DNA is digested, denatured, and labeled with fluorescent dye marker. Then the test DNA is hybridized with the probes of the array slide, and a laser scans the amount of fluorescence at each position. As there is a probe for each possible genotype for each

SNP location, heterozygous and homozygous wild-type or mutant state of each variant can be identified. Additionally, further analysis for copy number variation can also be performed by normalizing the fluorescence signal of the test DNA to a reference sample. Therefore, using SNP arrays not only small nucleotide variants (SNV) but copy number variations (CNV), uniparental disomy (UPD), and large regions of homozygosity can be also investigated.

Phenotype-specific SNP panels contain alleles that are known to drive specific phenotypes, e.g., epilepsy, or retinal degeneration. It is a promising approach by investigating well-known variants of multiple genes in high quality. However, it focuses only on individual variants and not on whole sequence, and the continuous discovery of novel variants and novel genes and the clinical utility of phenotype-specific SNP array panels are restrained, especially in the light of variable penetrance and expressivity of certain mutations. Genome-wide SNP panels offer a larger-scale option usually used to assess risk of multiple disorders, such as cancers; ophthalmologic, cardiac, renal, and neurological disorders or pharmacogenetic variants. Similarly to phenotype-specific panels, genome-wide SNP panels confines analysis to preselected variants of the genome and not whole sequence. Also, as SNP-based diagnostics are probabilistic (assessing risk) not deterministic, the clinical validity is variable, and the result should be interpreted with caution.

Array CGH method also uses a small glass slide (chip) that contains a grid consisting of thousands of probes specific for certain regions of the genome. The DNA sample is digested into fragments that are labeled with a fluorescent dye. The sample is then combined with a reference DNA sample fragmented the same way and labeled with another fluorescent dye. The mixed samples are denaturated and hybridized with the DNA probes of the array slide. By detecting the two fluorescent signals, the results are given as the ratio of test DNA to reference DNA at each available probe.

Depending on platform (design and probe density), the resolution of aCGH can vary from whole chromosomes to a few kilobases in size. It is designed to detect genomic rearrangements (except of balanced inversions and translocations) and uniparental disomy (UPD), which are not detectable through chromosomal CGH. Parallel with increase of resolution, detection of submicroscopic genomic rearrangements with unclear importance are also increases. Result interpretation is supported by resources such as Database of Chromosomal Imbalance and Phenotype in Humans using Ensembl Resources (DECIPHER) and International Standards for Cytogenomic Arrays Consortium (ISCA Consortium).

Array-based technologies are useful for patients presenting with a phenotype that overlaps with several possible genetic etiologies or giving a starting point for diagnosis to the clinician when the clinical picture and syndromatology are complicated. Apart from clinical genetics investigating somatic alterations, it can be helpful in classifying and guiding treatment and the prognosis of neoplastic diseases. However, array-based platforms can be expensive and its options for identifying mutational spectrum are limited. SNP arrays are also unable to identify CNVs smaller than ~80 kb and balanced translocations. In somatic testing (tumor heterogeneity), the detection of mosaicism is also restrained (only mutation present in more than 20–30% of the cells can be identified).

4.7 Next-Generation Sequencing

Next-generation sequencing (NGS) is a high-throughput technology allowing simultaneous sequencing of multiple DNA samples. While in Sanger method the nucleotide sequence is determined after sequencing PCR on fluorescently labeled PCR products, during NGS, nucleotide sequence is detected "real time" during synthesis. Due to its time and cost-effectiveness, it has been rapidly integrated into laboratory diagnostics. Both in identification of germline mutations in inherited diseases and somatic alterations in sporadic tumors, NGS gives more opportunity to improve personalized patient care through more precise diagnosis, prognosis, and initation of dedicated therapy.

Although whole-genome (WGS, sequencing of the entire genome) and whole-exome sequencing (WES, sequencing all of the protein-coding genes) are available, the most prevalent applications of NGS in clinical practice are testing of certain genes using targeted panels specific for a multigenic disease (i.e., hypogonadotrop hyopogonadism, pheochromocytoma/paraganglioma syndrome etc.).

NGS is comprised of three steps (Fig. 4.2): library preparation, sequencing, and data analysis. As a first step, following DNA extraction, some approaches (targeted panels and exome sequencing) include enrichment steps to focus on the selected regions of interest. During *library preparation*, DNA fragments of a certain size range are prepared and amplified. Also, adapters that are complementary of platform-specific PCR and sequencing primers are included by ligation to the DNA fragments. Barcodes are unique, 3–5-base-length sequences that are used to label different samples, therefore enabling pooling patients' samples into one reaction and decreasing per-sample cost. Barcodes can be part of the adapters or can be added during the PCR enrichment step of the library preparation. Unless whole-genome sequencing is performed, selected regions of interest have to be enriched. The target enrichment can be either multiplex PCR-based or oligonucleotide hybridization based. For the second *sequencing step*, several platforms are available. The common characteristic is that they perform massively parallel reactions yielding millions of sequence reads. Sequencing chemistry is depending on the platform; there is sequencing by synthesis, by pyrophosphate detection, or by ion sensing (Table 4.2). Each platform can be characterized by general parameters (read length, output read number, cost and run time) which are needed to be taken into consideration when an NGS platform initiated. During NGS, a huge amount of sequence data is produced that requires special *bioinformatics handling and analysis* (Biesecker and Green 2014). Appropriate hardware, software and expert personnel are required for data analysis and for obtaining valid results (Oliver et al. 2015). Data analysis can be divided into four dedicated steps: base calling, read alignment, variant calling and variant annotation. Base calling is a process that allows

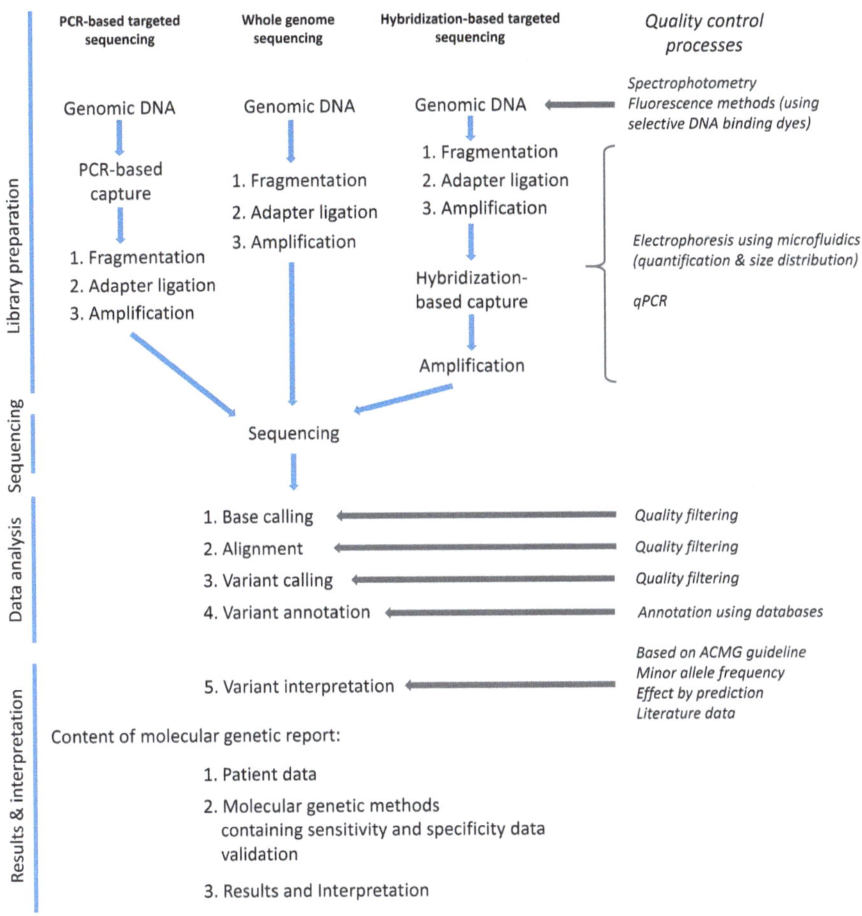

Fig. 4.2 Steps of next-generation sequencing. See details in the text

identification of nucleotides at each position based on certain quality filters. Usually base calling is integrated into the instrument's software and is platform-specific. After quality filtering, raw reads are aligned to the reference human genome. Variant calling is performed to identify alterations compared to the reference sequence, followed by variant analysis and interpretation. The entire process needs verification and validation. As in vitro diagnosis (IVD) proved NGS-based assays are not widely available, each laboratory has to develop and validate their own protocols including from sample and library preparation, bioinformatics analysis, and quality assurance (Rehm et al. 2013).

Quality filtering of read alignment defines sensitivity and specificity of the test. Using very strong filtering could lead to loss of variants present at low level which can be problematic for identification of mutations present at low level, i.e., somatic mutations due to the tumor heterogeneity. Alternatively, inclusive filters can

Table 4.2 Current next-generation sequencing platforms

Platform	Library amplification	Sequencing principle	Read length (bp)	Accuracy (%)
Illumina	Cluster amplification by bridge PCR on the flow cell	Sequencing by cyclic reversible termination. Fluorescent detection	25–250	>99
Thermofisher ion torrent	On-bead emulsion PCR	Ion semiconductor sequencing. Detection of hydrogen ions that are released during the polymerization of DNA	35–400	>99
454/Roche[a]	On-bead emulsion PCR	Pyrosequencing. Optical detection of pyrophosphate when it is released as a result of nucleotide incorporated by polymerase	700	>99
Pacific bioscience SMRT[a]	Library is composed of double-stranded DNA templates capped by hairpin loops at both ends	Single-molecule real-time sequencing. Detection of fluorescent tags that are cleaved off when a single nucleotide is being incorporated by DNA polymerase	3000	84–85
Oxford nanopore	Library is prepared without amplification	Detection of changes in ionic current as nucleotides pass through the nanopore	Hundreds of kb	96

[a]Recently not available

minimize false-negative results, but it will increase the burden of confirmatory analysis. The accuracy depends on the depth of sequence coverage; increased coverage improves variant calling. In molecular pathology 300–500 reads/target has been suggested to be enough for diagnostics, and variants present with <5 reads are usually considered likely false calls. During variant calling and analysis, it is important to identify false sequence variants and to determine variant allele frequency (VAF) (Lee et al. 2014; Deans et al. 2017). VAF is the percentage of sequence reads divided by the overall coverage of the particular locus. In germline testing, VAF represents diploid zygosity (near 0 and 100% for homozygosity and near 50% for heterozygosity) (Fig. 4.3). In somatic testing due to the abovementioned factors (contamination with normal tissue, neoplastic cell ratio, and tumor heterogeneity), VAF can be unpredictable. Also, in case of indels, it is recommended to confirm the variants by visualization of sequencing to reduce the risk of false positive or incorrect calls.

After bioinformatics, in order to maintain technical validity, confirmatory tests are recommended and needed. In germline testing, Sanger sequencing is generally accepted, but due to its 10–20% VAF sensitivity in case of somatic tumor mutations,

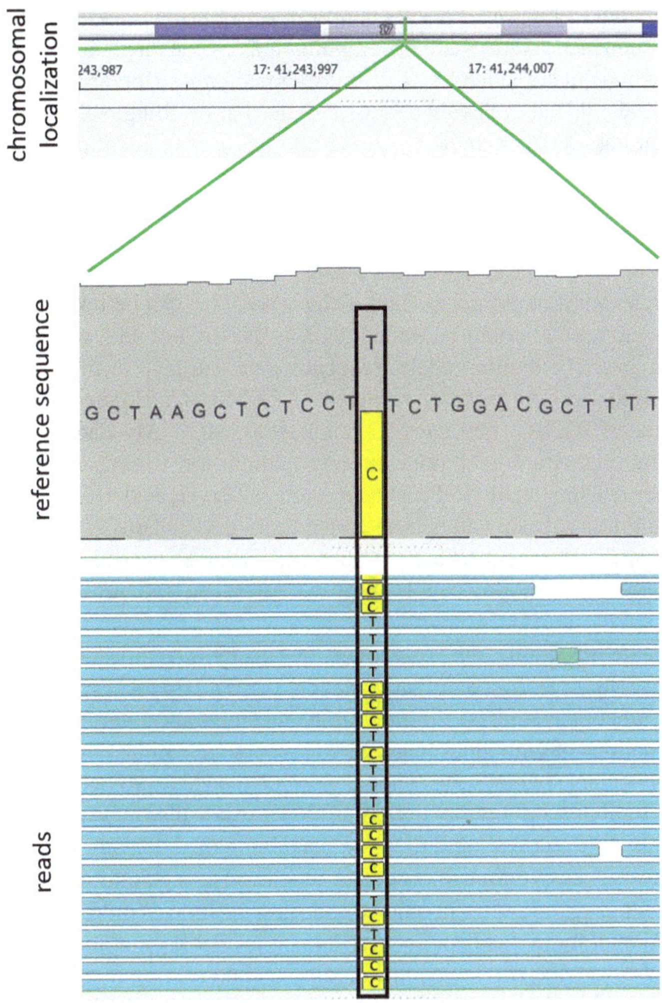

Fig. 4.3 Visualization of read alignment. Light blue bars represent reads generated by NGS instrument that are aligned to reference sequence. In germline setting, a heterozygous variant is called when approximately 50% of reads show nucleotide of Allele 1 (e.g., "T" on the figure) and another 50% of aligned reads show nucleotide of Allele 2 (e.g., "C") highlighted by yellow. (*Mapped reads are visualized by GoldenHelix GenomeBrowse 3.0*)

it is not the ideal method for confirmation of all variants revealed. Some recommend duplicate sequencing of the entire panels using other methodologies or perform single-locus test for every targeted gene that obviously increase the cost of analysis. It is also needed to be kept in mind that some alterations are not well detectable by NGS methods due to its methodology. Repetitive sequences, copy-number variations, long insertion-deletions, structural variants, aneuploidy, or epigenetic alterations are usually missed by NGS. In summary, handling large data sets generated by high-throughput technologies results in false-positive results and incidental findings. As a consequence, some authors highlighted overtesting, overdiagnosis and overtreatment as major side effects of translational omics (Ibrahim et al. 2016).

To achieve clinically relevant results of molecular profiling, validation with large independent data sets is mandatory. It is important to pay attention to other factors such as tumor type (different mutations can have different impacts in different tumors) and clinical questions (diagnosis, prognosis, and recommendation for targeted therapy). Both somatic and germline tissues can be assessed at the same time, and the tumor tissue-specific variant subtraction can be helpful to find the clinically relevant mutation or variant. Otherwise VAF can be taken into consideration. Generally, any variant presented >1% is usually not relevant for cancer, and various databases containing allele frequency data can help in filtering of relevant variants. Tumor-specific mutation resources (COSMIC, Catalogue of Somatic Mutations in Cancer; TCGA, The Cancer Genome Atlas; MCG, My Cancer Genome) and literature mining could add relevant information for variant interpretation. At germline level ClinVar, dbSNP, Exome Variant Server, and HGMD (the Human Gene Mutation Database) can help the interpretation (Richards et al. 2015). Hence, the continual development of high-quality and as far as possible freely accessible databases will have a profoundly positive effect on the progress of genomic medicine.

To estimate the significance of variants of uncertain significance (VUS) is more challenging. Multiple source of information (variant frequency, predictions, and subsidiary functional studies) is needed to be taken into account in order to achieve recommendations of guidelines (e.g. ACMG recommendations) in categorization of a particular variant. Laboratories should also have a clear protocol about reporting secondary findings. Laboratory report of NGS result also has special obligatory requirements. The report should focus on containing the clinically relevant information, but a brief description of technical characteristics, bioinformatics pipelines, validation reports, variant annotations and classification should also be included while additional, more detailed, data have to be available on request.

As *WGS* covers the whole genome (coding and noncoding regions), it may seem the most preferable choice to perform. Indeed, one advantage of WGS is that library preparation is straightforward as it does not require PCR or hybridization-based target enrichment. Moreover, WGS data can easily be used for detection of CNVs or structural alterations that are outside of coding regions. However, among NGS approaches, it gives the least average depth of coverage, and it is the most costly technology. Also, from the clinical point of view, the interpretation of noncoding variants and VUSs make its utility limited. *WES* aims to cover all coding regions in the genome. Exome contains all of the protein-coding region of genes, and it comprises ~1–2% of the genome, yet contains ~85% of known disease-causing mutations. Therefore, it is a more feasible option comparing to WGS. During library preparation, targeted enrichment of coding regions is required. Usually, the average exome coverage of a WES test is 90–95% due to sequence complexity. WES is sometimes used by clinical laboratories by interpreting only genes that are already known to be associated with any disease (clinical exome). When no mutation is identified, data analysis can be extended to the remaining regions. It has been shown that when there is no clinical direction for searching genetic background of certain diseases, WES provides diagnosis for approximately 20% of the tested cases. Furthermore, because the depth of coverage for WES is not uniform, the sensitivity is usually lower compared to targeted disease panels. *Targeted panels* are therefore the most widely used NGS approach currently in clinical practice. By focusing on a limited set of genes selected for certain clinical condition, it provides high coverage that increases analytical sensitivity even in detection of mosaicism, low-level heteroplasmy in mitochondrial diseases, or in somatic mutation detection in oncology. Also, because the role of genes included in these panels is known to be associated with the particular condition, the detection rate (positive finding) is also higher compared to WES. In certain cases, due to sequence complexity, 1–2% of the targeted region may not be covered, but laboratories used to fill in these gaps by Sanger sequencing to ensure proper result.

4.8 Conclusion

As technology rapidly improves and brings newer and easier methods to detect genetic alterations on a high-throughput manner, the need to increase efficiency of genetic tests emerges. First of all, indications of a genetic test should be considered. Without proper clinical indications, genetic tests turn out as useless cost in health care as the results most probably will be negative. NGS approaches for standard screening are also not recommended as identification variants of unknown significance would not improve patient quality of life, only makes it more complicated. One approach that is recently suggested to increase cost-effectiveness is the application of targeted disease panels with proper indication. Establishing genotype-phenotype correlations will also improve the value of genetic tests. In certain cases, establishment of genetic diagnosis when the clinical diagnosis is already clear can be also just an additional information without any clinical value for the patient if the genetic diagnosis lacks any consequences regarding prognosis or therapy. Only investigation of genetic alterations with clinical significance should be included in clinical practice.

Acknowledgments This work has been supported by the National Excellence Program to Attila Patócs and ÚNKP-18-4-SE-8 New National Excellence Program of The Ministry of Human Capacities to Henriett Butz. Henriett Butz is a recipient of Bolyai Research Fellowship of Hungarian Academy of Sciences.

References

Bean L, Bayrak-Toydemir P (2014) American College of Medical Genetics and Genomics standards and guidelines for clinical genetics laboratories, 2014 edition: technical standards and guidelines for Huntington disease. Genet Med 16:e2. https://doi.org/10.1038/gim.2014.146

Biesecker LG, Green RC (2014) Diagnostic clinical genome and exome sequencing. N Engl J Med 370:2418–2425. https://doi.org/10.1056/NEJMra1312543
Deans ZC, Costa JL, Cree I et al (2017) Integration of next-generation sequencing in clinical diagnostic molecular pathology laboratories for analysis of solid tumours; an expert opinion on behalf of IQN Path ASBL. Virchows Arch 470:5–20. https://doi.org/10.1007/s00428-016-2025-7
Erali M, Voelkerding KV, Wittwer CT (2008) High resolution melting applications for clinical laboratory medicine. Exp Mol Pathol 85:50–58. https://doi.org/10.1016/j.yexmp.2008.03.012
Ibrahim R, Pasic M, Yousef GM (2016) Omics for personalized medicine: defining the current we swim in. Expert Rev Mol Diagn 16:719–722. https://doi.org/10.1586/14737159.2016.1164601
Katsanis SH, Katsanis N (2013) Molecular genetic testing and the future of clinical genomics. Nat Rev Genet 14:415–426. https://doi.org/10.1038/nrg3493
Lee H, Deignan JL, Dorrani N et al (2014) Clinical exome sequencing for genetic identification of rare Mendelian disorders. JAMA 312:1880–1887. https://doi.org/10.1001/jama.2014.14604
Mansfield ES (1993) Diagnosis of Down syndrome and other aneuploidies using quantitative polymerase chain reaction and small tandem repeat polymorphisms. Hum Mol Genet 2:43–50
Navarro E, Serrano-Heras G, Castaño MJ, Solera J (2015) Real-time PCR detection chemistry. Clin Chim Acta 439:231–250. https://doi.org/10.1016/j.cca.2014.10.017
Oliver GR, Hart SN, Klee EW (2015) Bioinformatics for clinical next generation sequencing. Clin Chem 61:124–135. https://doi.org/10.1373/clinchem.2014.224360
Quan P-L, Sauzade M, Brouzes E (2018) dPCR: a technology review. Sensors 18:1271. https://doi.org/10.3390/s18041271
Rehm HL, Bale SJ, Bayrak-Toydemir P et al (2013) ACMG clinical laboratory standards for next-generation sequencing. Genet Med 15:733–747. https://doi.org/10.1038/gim.2013.92
Richards S, Aziz N, Bale S et al (2015) Standards and guidelines for the interpretation of sequence variants: a joint consensus recommendation of the American College of Medical Genetics and Genomics and the Association for Molecular Pathology. Genet Med 17:405–424. https://doi.org/10.1038/gim.2015.30
Stofanko M, Gonçalves-Dornelas H, Cunha PS et al (2013) Simple, rapid and inexpensive quantitative fluorescent PCR method for detection of microdeletion and microduplication syndromes. PLoS One 8:e61328. https://doi.org/10.1371/journal.pone.0061328

Part II
Endocrine Diseases Inherited as Monogenic Traits: Hormone Resistance Syndromes

Chapter 5
Syndromes of Resistance to Thyroid Hormone Action

Luca Persani and Irene Campi

Abstract Thyroid hormone (TH) action is crucial for the development of several tissues.

A number of syndromes are associated with reduced responsiveness to thyroid hormones, expanding the original definition of thyroid hormone resistance, firstly described by Refetoff and collaborators in 1967, which is characterized by elevated circulating levels of T4 and T3 with measurable serum TSH concentrations, as a consequence of mutations of thyroid hormone receptor beta (TRβ), recently named as RTHβ. More recently, another form of insensitivity to TH has been identified due to mutations in the thyroid hormone receptor alpha (TRα), named RTHα. In this chapter we will focus the discussion on the phenotype of RTHβ and RTHα. These diseases share the same pathogenic mechanism caused by dominant negative mutations in TH receptor genes that reduce T3 binding or affect the recruitment of cofactors. As a consequence, thyroid hormone actions are impaired at the tissue level. The phenotypic manifestations of RTHβ and RTHα are to some extent correlated with the degree of disruption and the tissue distribution of the TRs being characterized by variable coexistence of hypothyroid or thyrotoxic manifestations in RTHβ or by a congenital hypothyroid features in RTHα despite normal TSH and borderline low free T4.

Keywords THRA · THRB · Thyroid hormone receptor · RTHβ · RTHα · Resistance to thyroid hormone · Thyroid hormone action · Mental retardation · Metabolic disorder

---

L. Persani (✉)
Department of Clinical Sciences and Community Health, University of Milan, Milan, Italy

Department of Endocrine and Metabolic Diseases, Lab of Endocrine and Metabolic Research, San Luca Hospital, IRCCS Istituto Auxologico Italiano, Milan, Italy
e-mail: luca.persani@unimi.it

I. Campi
Department of Endocrine and Metabolic Diseases, Lab of Endocrine and Metabolic Research, San Luca Hospital, IRCCS Istituto Auxologico Italiano, Milan, Italy

Department of Pathophysiology and Transplantation, University of Milan, Milan, Italy

P. Igaz, A. Patócs (eds.), *Genetics of Endocrine Diseases and Syndromes*, Experientia Supplementum 111, https://doi.org/10.1007/978-3-030-25905-1_5

List of Abbreviations

ADHD	Attention deficit hyperactivity disorders
BBB	Blood–brain barrier
BMR	Basal metabolic rate
CNS	Central nervous system
DIO1	Type 1 deiodinase
DIO2	Type 2 deiodinase
DIO3	Type 3 deiodinase
GRTH	Generalized resistance to thyroid hormone
α-GSU	Alpha subunit of glycoprotein hormones
ICTP	Serum carboxy-terminal telopeptide of type 1 collagen
LAT1	L-Type amino acid transporter 1
LAT2	L-Type amino acid transporter 2
LT4	Levothyroxine
MCT8	Monocarboxylate transporter 8
MCT10	Monocarboxylate transporter 10
MRI	Magnetic resonance imaging
OATP1C1	Organic anion-transporting polypeptide 1c1
PRTH	Pituitary resistance to thyroid hormone
REE	Resting energy expenditure
RTHα	Resistance to thyroid hormone alpha
RTHβ	Resistance to thyroid hormone beta
RXR	Retinoid X receptor
SECISBP	Selenocysteine insertion sequence (SECIS)-binding protein 2
SHBG	Sex hormone-binding globulin
TH	Thyroid hormone
THRA	Gene coding for thyroid hormone receptor alpha
THRB	Gene coding for thyroid hormone receptor beta
TRE	Thyroid hormone-responsive elements
TRIAC	Triiodothyroacetic acid
TSHomas	TSH-secreting pituitary adenomas
TR	Thyroid hormone receptor

5.1 Background

Different molecular mechanisms regulate the biological actions of TH on their target tissues. These mechanisms include the cell surface transporters, the deiodinases system controlling the metabolism of TH, and the nuclear TH receptors that in concert with specific cofactors mediate the TH actions in the nucleus (Van Gucht et al. 2017; Dumitrescu and Refetoff 2012; Cheng et al. 2010; Visser et al. 2011).

Here, we briefly summarize these processes and their significance in the pathogenesis of human syndromes of reduced thyroid hormone sensitivity (Refetoff et al. 2014).

5.1.1 Cell Surface Transporters

The actions of TH are mainly intracellular; thus an efficient mechanism of transport of iodothyronines across the plasma membrane is required in order to increase the cytoplasmic availability of TH.

The majority of the transporters identified up to now, such as the Na+/taurocholate cotransporting polypeptide (SLC10A1), multidrug resistance-associated proteins, the heterodimeric L-type amino acid transporters (LAT1 and LAT2), the organic anion-transporting polypeptide (OATP) family, and the MCTs family bind to several different ligands, while MCT8 (*SLC16A2*), MCT10 (*SLC16A10*), and OATP1C1 (*SLCO1C1*) are specific for T3 (Visser et al. 2011; Refetoff and Dumitrescu 2007).

MCT8 is expressed in the heart, liver, kidney, adrenal glands, and thyroid, but its function appears to be critical especially in the brain: in fact, genetic defects of this transporter are involved in the pathogenesis of the Allan–Herndon–Dudley syndrome and of the Pelizaeus–Merzbacher-like disease, which are associated with severe neurological phenotypes. THs enter in neurons by two mechanisms, mediated by OATP1C1 and MTC8, respectively. In the first case, TH uptake occurs from the endothelial cells into the astrocytes, with a greater efficiency for T4 than T3. Thereafter, DIO2 converts T4 locally to T3, which enters in the neurons by binding to MCT8. Alternatively, TH may also enter directly in the neurons through gaps in the astrocytes processes via MTC8, which exhibits a higher affinity for T3 compared to T4 (Refetoff and Dumitrescu 2007).

Data about the role of MCT10 and OATP1C1 in human physiology are limited (Visser et al. 2011). However, T3 concentrations in the CNS are roughly the 20% of serum levels (Schroeder and Privalsky 2014). In order to reach the brain, the TH need to cross the blood–brain barrier (BBB).

5.1.2 Deiodination System

The intracellular concentrations of T3 are regulated by three deiodinases, selenocysteine-containing enzymes, which activate or inactivate the iodothyronines through the removal of iodide from thyroxine and its metabolites.

Type 1 deiodinase (DIO1) deiodinates T4 (3,5,3′,5′-tetraiodothyronine) into T3 (3,5,3′-triiodothyronine) and of T3 into T2 (3,3′-diiodothyronine); *DIO1* is highly expressed in the liver and kidney and contributes to the production of plasma T3 by deiodination of T4. The type 2 deiodinase (DIO2) converts T4 to T3 intracellularly;

it is highly expressed in the thyroid, being responsible for the increased intrathyroidal production of T3 in Graves' disease and toxic thyroid nodules.

Finally, type 3 deiodinase (DIO3) degrades T4 to rT3 and T3 to 3,3′-diiodothyronine (T2), thus downregulating the local T3 production and protecting tissues from TH excess.

In the CNS, *DIO2* is mainly expressed in glial-derived cells, such as the astrocytes and the tanycytes, while DIO3 is primarily found in neurons. In order to maintain adequate levels of T3 in neural tissues, the deiodinases function is finely regulated. In particular, recent data suggest that astrocytes produce active T3, which enters in neurons via MCT-8. In these cells, DIO3 controls the local bioavailability of T3 by the production of rT3 and T2 from T4 and T3, respectively (Schroeder and Privalsky 2014).

DIO3 has a critical role during development, as suggested by high expression of this enzyme in the pregnant uterus, placenta, and fetal and neonatal tissues, and regulates the maturation of the pituitary–thyroid axis. Consistently, the DIO3-KO mouse model displays neonatal thyrotoxicosis followed by central hypothyroidism that persists throughout life (Hernandez et al. 2006). In humans, an increased methylation profile of the imprinted DLK1-DIO3 domain in the placenta is associated in neonates with a reduced weight and length in the first postnatal year (Prats-Puig et al. 2017).

At present, no pathogenic variants in the DIOs genes have been identified in patients with reduced sensitivity to TH. However, an abnormal thyroid hormone function is associated with genetic mutations in proteins belonging to the multiprotein complex of incorporation of selenium such as the selenocysteine insertion sequence-binding protein 2 (*SECISBP2*). Mutations in this gene cause a deficient production of all the selenoproteins, including DIOs. The biochemical consequence is an abnormal thyroid metabolism characterized by high serum levels of FT4, low-normal FT3, and a slightly increased TSH (Schoenmakers et al. 2010).

5.1.3 Nuclear Receptors

Thyroid hormone receptors (TRs) belong to the nuclear receptor superfamily. In humans, TRs are encoded by two different genes: *THRA* and *THRB* located on chromosomes 17 and 3, respectively.

Two different isoforms are generated from both the *THRB* and *THRA* loci: TRβ1 and TRβ2, which diverge in their amino-terminal regions and TRα1 and TRα2 which differ in the C-terminal domain. TRβ1 is the major isoform in the brain, liver, kidney, and thyroid (Fig. 5.1). The TRβ2 is mainly expressed in the pituitary, the inner ear, and the retina where it mediates overlapping functions with TRβ1 (Ng et al. 2015). On the contrary, TRα1 is ubiquitously expressed in the central nervous system (CNS), bone, heart, skeletal muscle, and gastrointestinal tract.TRα2 is a non-T3-binding isoform preserving the DNA-binding properties and is considered a modulator of TH action. It is expressed in various tissues, but its functions

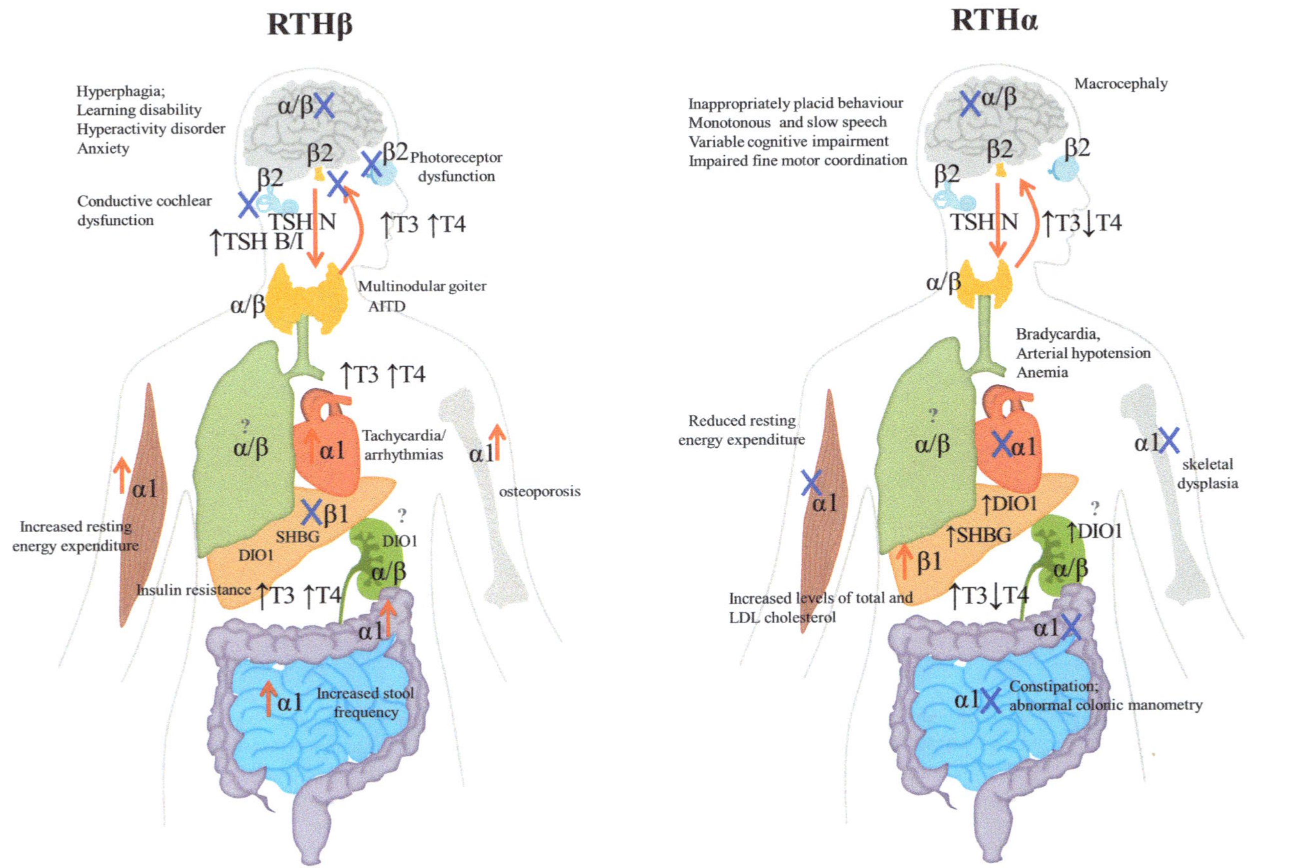

Fig. 5.1 Pathogenesis of resistance to thyroid hormone syndromes. The different tissue expression of TH receptors isoforms causes the divergent phenotype of RTHβ (on the left) and RTHα (on the right). In RTHβ, the inappropriate secretion of TSH is due to the reduced sensitivity of the pituitary gland to T3 leading to

Fig. 5.1 (continued) increased thyroid stimulation and production of T4/T3 by the thyroid to overcome the affected TRβ2 pathway. Such modification partially compensates for the tissue resistance of RTHβ and is obtained by the secretion of TSH with increased bioactivity (high TSH bioactivity/immunoreactivity ratio, TSH B/I). In RTHα, the pituitary-thyroid axis is not affected and the imbalanced T4/T3 ratio is likely due to the increased DIO1 activity in the liver where the TRβ1 isoform is predominantly expressed. The blue crosses indicate the impaired function of the mutated receptors, the red arrows represent the hyperstimulation of the unaffected receptors, and the question marks represent unclear pathogenetic mechanisms. *α1* Thyroid hormone receptor alpha isoform 1, *β1/2* Thyroid hormone receptor beta isoform 1/2, *DIO1* Type 1 deiodinase, *SHBG* Sex hormone-binding globulin

have not been clearly deciphered (Bradley et al. 1992; Hodin et al. 1989; Lechan et al. 1994).

TRs functions are crucial in the development of CNS. Compared to TRα, the TRβ is expressed at a later stage of brain development. TRβ1 and TRβ2 isoforms are expressed in a neurogenic subpopulation and located in the hippocampus are apparently involved in the proliferation of neuronal progenitors (Desouza et al. 2005). In particular, it has been suggested that unliganded TRβ isoforms may exert an inhibitory effect on hippocampal cellular growth (Kapoor et al. 2011). A similar role has been hypothesized for unliganded TRα1 in the cerebellum (Fauquieret al. 2014; Heuer and Mason 2003) and hippocampus (Kapoor et al. 2010).

TRs bind as heterodimers to retinoid X receptor (RXR), or less frequently as homodimers to regulatory DNA sequences, known as thyroid response elements (TRE) located in the promoter of target genes. A number of cofactors (proteins acting as coactivators and corepressors) are involved in TH receptor signaling.

On positively regulated genes, in the absence of T3, the heterodimers/homodimers are associated to corepressors and bind to TREs repressing transcription. The arrival of T3 and its binding to TRs results in dissociation of corepressors, recruitment of coactivators, and transcriptional activation. Conversely, negatively regulated TH target genes show transcriptional activation in the absence of TH and repression in the presence of the ligand T3.

The two major corepressors, the nuclear receptor corepressor (NCoR) and the silencing mediator of retinoic acid and thyroid hormone receptors (SMRT), are crucial regulators of nuclear receptor signaling (Astapova et al. 2008). They form a complex with other repressors, such as Sin 3, and histone deacetylases (Hu and Lazar 2000), thus leading to shut down basal transcription. Several coactivators interact with TRs, such as the steroid receptor coactivator complex (SRC) and the vitamin D receptor interacting protein–TR-associated protein complex (DRIP–TRAP), which enhance the T3-dependent transcription. SRC complex interacts with CREB-binding protein (CBP), responsible for cAMP-stimulated transcription, interacting with the phosphorylated form of CREB (cAMP-regulated enhancer binding protein) and with the related protein p300. CBP/P300 interact with P/CAF (p300/CBP-associated factor) which has an intrinsic histone acetyltransferase (HAT) activity and with the RNA pol II (Torchia et al. 1998). Several interacting components associate with RNA Pol II, thus connecting nuclear receptors to the basal transcriptional machinery (Ito and Roeder 2001).

5.2 Molecular Mechanisms Causing Resistance to Thyroid Hormone

Both RTHα and RTHβ share a similar underlying pathogenic mechanism caused by heterozygous mutations in the *TR*s (Fig. 5.1). These syndromes are inherited in an autosomal dominant manner.

This inheritance depends on the so-called dominant negative effect, due to the inhibition of the activity of the wild-type receptors, by the mutant TRs. The most frequent genetic variants associated with RTHα and β are single-nucleotide changes or small in/dels causing three different receptor defects: missense mutations, with a single nucleotide substitution; frameshift/premature stop mutations, in which a deletion or insertion of one or several nucleotides results in a truncated receptor; and nonsense mutations, in which a nucleotide substitution results in a premature stop codon (see Chap. 1).

The TRβ mutations are distributed in the carboxyl terminus of the TRβ. Typically, three CpG-rich "hot spots" regions, located in the ligand-binding domain and in the contiguous hinge domain of the protein, have been identified. At present, only 21 mutations in *THRA* have been described in RTHα patients, but it is possible that a similar pattern of distribution in LBD domain might be recognized in the future. This hypothesis is supported by the observation of a high homology (95%) of their thyroid hormone-binding domains, so that corresponding mutations in human TRα can be predicted. Indeed, some already-reported mutations correspond to a mutation of the homologous residue in TRβ1 (Tylki-Szymanska et al. 2015).

Mutant receptors display either a reduced affinity for T_3 or an impaired interaction with the cofactors (coactivators and corepressors), thus losing its ability to modulate target gene expression in different tissues. Different mechanisms have been evoked to explain this dominant negative effect (Dumitrescu and Refetoff 2012; Van Gucht et al. 2017):

1. Formation of inactive dimers between mutant TRs and wild-type TRs
2. Competition between mutant and wild-type (wt) receptors for essential cofactors
3. Competition between mutant TR and wild-type TR for DNA-binding sites

In vitro, some mutant receptors exhibit a transcriptional activity similar to wild-type when treated with high T3 concentrations with reversal of their dominant-negative inhibitory activity. Interestingly, for RTHβ no clear genotype-phenotype correlation was described; thus patients harboring the same mutation may display different degrees of disease severity. On the contrary, RTHα patients harboring missense mutations, rescued in vitro by T3, seem to have a milder phenotype and benefit from TH treatment (Van Gucht et al. 2017).

In contrast to what is observed for other nuclear receptors (such as vitamin D, androgen receptor or PPARγ), no mutations have been identified in the DNA-binding domain or in other regions of the receptor.

In the original RTHβ family, in which a deletion of exons 4–10 resulted in the abolition of the dimerization and DNA-binding properties of TRβ, the disease segregated as an autosomal recessive trait. The homozygous patients had goiter and deaf-mutism together with high TH levels; conversely, the heterozygous subjects were phenotypically normal, supporting the hypothesis that reduced amount of TRβ does not produce haploinsufficiency (Dumitrescu and Refetoff 2012; Takeda et al. 1992) and that the mutant receptor must conserve its DNA-binding and dimerization properties, in order to cause the biochemical phenotype of RTHβ, i.e., high free TH in the presence of unsuppressed TSH levels.

None of the RTHα patients described about up to now harbor large gene deletions.

The majority of the RTHβ cases (nearly 85%) are associated with heterozygous mutations in the *THRB* gene, while in 10–15% of the cases with the biochemical phenotype of RTHβ, no mutation could be found in the TRβ gene, and this situation is defined as "non-TR-RTH." It is speculated that these patients may have an abnormality in one of the cofactors or TH transporters into the cells. However, screening of several families with non-TR-RTH excluded the involvement of coactivators (SRC-1/NcoA-1 and NcoA-3/SRC-3/AIB1/RAC-3), two corepressors (NCoR and SMRT), and two coregulators (RXRγ and TRIP1) as well as the cell transporter LST-1 (OATP1B1) (Reutrakul et al. 2000).

It is unclear if a similar condition might be found also in RTHα. Interestingly, in the Polish cohort described by Tylki-Szymanska, one case sharing the same clinical phenotype as the affected probands, no mutations in *THRA* were found. Additional genetic studies (exome sequencing, high-resolution microarray copy number variation analysis) were not able to identify any potential pathogenic variants in any candidate genes.

5.3 Resistance to Thyroid Hormones Syndrome Due to Mutations in the THRB Gene (RTHβ)

5.3.1 General Clinical Features

Resistance to thyroid hormones syndrome (RTHβ) is a rare condition (OMIM ID # 188570). More than 3000 cases have been published worldwide from about 1200 different families with a wide geographic and ethnic distribution (Van Gucht et al. 2017; Dumitrescu and Refetoff 2012; Refetoff et al. 2014). The prevalence of the disease is indefinite, since most of the screening programs for congenital hypothyroidism are based on the sole TSH determination which is typically normal in this condition. A limited survey in a cohort of 80,000 newborns found one case among 40,000 live births, but a more recent work in Basque Country reported an incidence of RTHβ in 1:18,750 newborns (Vela et al. 2019).

The majority of the cases (nearly 85%) are associated with heterozygous mutations in the TRβ gene and the condition is inherited in an autosomal dominant fashion (Dumitrescu and Refetoff 2012).

As other rare heritable conditions, RTHβ presents with the biochemical picture of raised TH associated with inappropriately unsuppressed TSH concentrations (Table 5.1). The clinical picture of RTHβ ranges from thyrotoxic manifestations to the absence of any signs of TH excess. Differences in the degree of hormonal resistance are probably due to the different TRβ and TRα expression in different tissues (Table 5.2).

TRβ mainly is expressed in the hypothalamus, kidney, liver, anterior pituitary gland, hypothalamus, retina, and cochlea, whereas TRα predominates in the skeletal

Table 5.1 Genetic disorders characterized by increased serum thyroid hormones levels and detectable TSH concentrations

	Gene	Free T4	Free T3	TSH	Total reverse T3	SHBG[a]
Familial dysalbuminemic Hyperthyroxinemia (FDH)	*ALB*	N[b]	N[b]	N	↑	N
Resistance to thyroid Hormone (RTHβ)	*THRB*	↑	↑	Nor slightly ↑	↑	N
Defect of THRA gene (RTH α)	*THRA*	Borderline or slightly↓	↑	N	↓	↑
Defect of thyroid hormones transport (Allan–Herndon–Dudley syndrome)	*MCT8*	Slightly ↓	↑	Nor slightly ↑	↓	↑
Defect of thyroid hormones metabolism (SBP2 deficiency)	*SBP2*	↑	Nor slightly ↓	Nor slightly ↑	↑	N

[a]*SHBG* Sex hormone-binding globulin
[b]As measured by equilibrium dialysis or direct "two-step" measurement methods. Interferences leading to spuriously high levels of FT4 and/or FT3 may be present by using other methods

and cardiac muscle, brain, brown fat, intestine, spleen, and vascular endothelial cells. Consequently, symptoms of TH deficiency and excess could coexist in the different tissues of one subject. As an example, hypercholesterolemia, delayed bone maturation, growth retardation, and learning disabilities (suggestive of hypothyroidism) may coexist with weight loss, osteoporosis, heat intolerance, hyperactivity, and tachycardia (typical of thyrotoxicosis).

Classically, RTHβ subjects have been classified into two subgroups according to the absence or presence of symptoms of thyrotoxicosis, selective pituitary resistance (PRTH), and generalized thyroid hormone resistance (GRTH), respectively. Patients with PRTH display variable symptoms of hyperthyroidism (Beck-Peccoz and Chatterjee 1994). Conversely, subjects with GRTH exhibit a sort of "compensated hypothyroidism," being the genetic defect of TH responsiveness balanced by the high circulating TH concentrations; the efficiency of this compensatory mechanism is variable in each individual, in different tissues, as well as in different periods of life.

In addition, TRβ mutations found in both GRTH and PRTH may be the same and patients of the same family may present with either form. Indeed, PRTH patients have normal levels of sex hormone-binding globulin, a marker of peripheral thyroid hormone action, elevated in the case of hyperthyroidism, thus suggesting that insensitivity to TH action is present not only in the hypothalamic-pituitary region but also in the liver. Therefore, this clinical distinction may be loose and more theoretical than actual.

The main clinical features of patients with RTHβ are summarized in Table 5.2 and in the following paragraphs.

Table 5.2 The main clinical characteristics of the patients with RTHα or RTHß

	RTHβ	RTHα
Thyroid morphology	Thyroid volume: increased (50–75%) Nodules: frequent Prevalence thyroid autoimmunity: 15–22% Serum thyroglobulin: increased 99Tc uptake: increased	Thyroid volume: normal Nodules: not reported Prevalence thyroid autoimmunity: unknown Serum thyroglobulin: increased/normal 99Tc uptake: unknown
Pituitary	TSH response to TRH: normal/brilliant TSH is suppressed by high doses (100–200 μg) of T3	TSH response to TRH: not specific (reported as normal/delayed/reduced) TSH is suppressed by levothyroxine
Cardiovascular system	*Heterozygous patients*: Subjective tachycardia. Increased heart rate, stroke Volume and cardiac output (less evident than conventional hyperthyroidism) Increased systemic vascular resistance and arterial stiffness *Homozygous patients*: tachycardia, congenital heart malformations *Patients with THRB deletions*: tachycardia	Bradycardia (some patients) Arterial hypotension (some patients) Hypertrophic obstructive cardiomyopathy (only in the patient with the C380fs387X mutation)
Dysmorphic face	*Heterozygous patients*: have no specific features except for a patient with the T426I variant who had a triangular face appearance (Menzaghi et al. 1998) *Homozygous patients*: birdlike facies with prominent nasal bridge *Patients with THRB deletions*: birdlike facies with prominent nasal bridge	Large coarse face, macrocephaly, large, short and upturned nose with a flat nasal bridge wide forehead, hypertelorism, eyelid ptosis, multiple skin tags, short neck
Skeletal abnormalities	*Heterozygous patients*: accelerated bone in childhood (rare) Osteoporosis/osteopenia in adults *Homozygous patients*: Growth delay, delayed bone maturation *Patients with THRB deletions*: Stippled epiphyses. Growth delay. Delayed bone maturation, pigeon breast, winged scapulae	Retarded bone age Delayed dentition and ossification Disproportionate short stature (unclear if partially reversible with L-T4 Skull abnormalities: macrocephaly, multiple Wormian bones; thickening of the calvarium Lower limbs abnormalities: short limbs, club feet, valgus foot, coxa valga, femoral epiphyseal dysgenesis Spine: lumbar kyphosis
Metabolism	Low body mass index Hyperphagia and enhanced energy intake. Basal metabolic rate normal or increased. Enhanced resting energy expenditure (REE) Reduced insulin sensitivity and dyslipidemia (some patients)	Obesity (two patients) Low basal metabolic rate Increased levels of total and LDL cholesterol (some patients)

(continued)

Table 5.2 (continued)

	RTHβ	RTHα
Immune system	Increased frequency of respiratory infections (pulmonitis and infections of the upper respiratory tract) Unclear if related to reduced immunoglobulin concentrations or abnormal regulation of granulocytes and lymphocytes	Normal macrophage functions (phagocytosis and cytokine induction), elevated IL-8 levels
Neurological system	*Heterozygous patients*: Severe mental retardation (IQ < 60) is uncommon (3% and reported in truncated form of TRβ) 30% of affected subjects display a mild learning disability (IQ < 85) in the verbal and performance components and impairment on an attention auditory discrimination task Attention deficit hyperactivity disorder (ADHD)/hyperactive behavior (some pediatric patients, responsive to TRIAC) Delayed developmental milestones and language disorders (some pediatric patients) Brain anatomical reported in a single study (in male patients extra or missing gyri in the parietal bank of the Sylvian fissure or multiple Heschl's transverse gyri in the primary auditory cortex) *Homozygous patients*: mild to severe intellectual impairment, hearing loss neuropsychomotor retardation *Patients with THRB deletions* deaf-mutism without mental retardation	Inappropriately placid behavior Monotonous and low speech Variable cognitive impairment (normal intelligence in few patients, selective cognitive difficulties in most, severe cognitive impairment in some patients) Motor dyspraxia Difficulties in fine motor coordination Ataxic gait Muscular hypotonia Seizures Delayed developmental milestones also in patients without mental retardation autism spectrum disorder (one case) Structural abnormalities such as reduced cerebellar and hippocampal volume, diminished white matter
Visual system	*Heterozygous patients*: decrease of the L/M photoreceptor (red/green) waves associated with an impaired rod response in electrophysiological studies *Homozygous patients*: color blindness, at electrophysiology normal scotopic response and a reduced photopic response resembling the enhanced S cone syndrome *Patients with THRB deletions* color blindness	Not impaired

(continued)

Table 5.2 (continued)

	RTHβ	RTHα
Hearing system	*Heterozygous patients*: conductive (susceptibility to infections); cochlear dysfunction (defective TRβ expression) *Homozygous patients*: hearing loss *Patients with THRB deletions* deaf-mutism	Not impaired
Other features	Non-diarrheal increased frequency of bowel movements (uncommon) Higher rate of miscarriage and intrauterine growth retardation of unaffected fetuses	Constipation due to delayed intestinal transit (common) Abnormal colonic manometry and reduced peristalsis Low or low-normal IGF-1 Normocytic normochromic anemia

Noteworthy, the frequency of the different signs and symptoms RTHβ are assumed from studies performed on a limited number of patients. Moreover, it is possible that the spectrum of the certain manifestations of the disease may change over time.

As an example, the prevalence of nodular goiter may be influenced by the iodine status of a certain country or by the inappropriate administration of thionamides in these patients that was more common in the past due to misdiagnosis. Data from our cohort suggest a reduction of the prevalence of goiter during the decades (Campi, personal communication AIT 2016). These observations are supported by data from Amor et al. on a cohort of Mediterranean RTHβ patients diagnosed after 1997, in which the prevalence of goiter was 50%, thus much lower than previously reported (Amor et al. 2014). In the same study, tachycardia was reported in less than 30% of the patients. This result can be influenced by the mean age of patients included in this survey (Hauser et al. 1993). However, in this cohort, there was a low prevalence of mutations-positive patients (50/166) so it was possible that patients with assays interferences or even TSHomas might be included in these series. In our experience, the heart manifestations are more frequent and tend to worsen with increasing age. The early administration of beta-blockers seems to reduce the risk of development of arrhythmias, such as atrial fibrillation.

Unfortunately, there are several limitations of these studies including the lack of a disease registry, the extreme fragmentations of the cohorts, and, most importantly, the lack of prospective data. Future studies are warranted to define if RTHβ has an impact on patients' quality of life, reproductive function, and life expectancy.

5.3.2 *Detailed Clinical Picture of RTHβ*

5.3.2.1 Thyroid Morphology

Diffuse or multinodular goiter is a common finding in RTHβ, independently from the presence of clinical symptoms. An increased biological activity of circulating

TSH molecules may favor the formation of goiter in RTHβ subjects with normal TSH levels (Persani et al. 1994). In RTHβ patients treated with surgical ablation, the goiter commonly relapses with nodular alterations and gross asymmetries, requiring additional surgery or radioiodine treatment.

5.3.2.2 Cardiovascular Symptoms

Approximately 75% of RTHβ patients exhibit palpitations and tachycardia at rest. Predominance of TRα may explain the presence of partially hyperthyroid response in the heart, as the dominant negative effect exerted by mutant TRβs on the normal receptors should be weaker than in other tissues. The finding that some indices of cardiac systolic and diastolic function (e.g., heart rate, stroke volume, cardiac output, diastolic filling, maximal aortic flow velocity) showed values that are intermediate between normal and hyperthyroid subjects supports this hypothesis. However, the normal values of other parameters (e.g., ejection and shortening fractions of the left ventricle, systolic diameter, and left ventricle wall thickness) suggest an incomplete response of the heart to the high TH concentrations. In addition, systemic vascular resistance and arterial stiffness are increased in RTHβ, as seen in subclinical hypothyroidism, thus indicating a more complex derangement of cardiovascular function. A reduced insulin sensitivity and dyslipidemia have been documented in a number of patients, suggesting an increased cardiovascular risk in RTHβ (Kahaly et al. 2002; Pulcrano et al. 2009; Owen et al. 2009; Mitchell et al. 2010).

5.3.2.3 Skeletal Abnormalities

Similarly to the cardiovascular system, also the bone is affected by a mixed of hypothyroid and thyrotoxic manifestations in RTHβ. Studies performed in animal models suggest that skeletal thyrotoxicosis, due to elevated circulating thyroid hormone levels which overstimulate the intact TRα1 signaling pathway, may be responsible for bone abnormalities in RTHβ (O'Shea et al. 2006).

In humans, dysmorphic skeletal features, such as "stippled epiphyses," dysmorphic facies, and winged scapulae, have been documented only in the cases harboring complete TRβ resistance due to homozygous deletion of TRβ gene. Delayed bone maturation and growth are present in about one third of children with RTHβ; however the final adult height seems unaffected.

A decreased bone mineral density has been reported in adult RTHβ. Conversely, the normal levels of the markers of bone turnover may imply a reduced bone formation rate resulting in a low peak bone mass similar to that observed in childhood hypothyroidism. At present, it is unclear if these abnormalities may increase the overall risk of hip or vertebral fractures compared to controls.

In a small group of 14 patients with RTHβ, biochemical abnormalities in calcium homeostasis were seen in RTHβ subjects of all ages. In particular, RTHβ was associated with hypophosphatemia with urinary phosphate loss and "inappropriately" increased serum FGF-23 levels in childhood; this suggests a sort of renal resistance to the action of TH. Higher serum calcium levels not associated with increased urinary excretion were present at any age but associated with PTH levels comparable to those of controls. In adult life, a low BMD was seen (Cardoso et al. 2014).

5.3.2.4 Metabolism

Low body mass index (BMI) is reported in about 30% of RTHβ children, in spite of the hyperphagia and the enhanced energy intake.

Basal metabolic rate (BMR) has been found normal or even increased. Indirect calorimetry assessment showed enhanced resting energy expenditure (REE), either in adults or children with TRβ mutations. This increase was intermediate between euthyroid and thyrotoxic subjects. The skeletal muscle and myocardium, in which the TRα isoform expression is prevalent, seem responsible of increased energy expenditure, as suggested by the correlation between mean heart rate and REE in both RTH and thyrotoxicosis. In both these conditions, TH excess was associated with uncoupling between tricarboxylic acid cycle activity and ATP synthesis in vivo, as measured by magnetic resonance spectroscopy (Mitchell et al. 2010).

5.3.2.5 Immune System

An increased frequency of respiratory infections (pulmonitis and infections of the upper respiratory tract) has been reported in RTHβ patients, compared to their unaffected relatives. This susceptibility has been related to reduced immunoglobulin concentrations but may also derive from an abnormal regulation of granulocytes and lymphocytes that express TH receptors.

5.3.2.6 Neurological System

It has been hypothesized that in RTHβ an uncompensated hypothyroidism at an early stage may be responsible for defects of neuroanatomical development.

Few data are available about the brain anatomical abnormalities associated with RTHβ. A single MRI study in 43 RTHβ patients found, in male patients, an increased frequency of cerebral anomalies of the left hemisphere, particularly extra or missing gyri in the parietal bank of the Sylvian fissure or multiple Heschl's transverse gyri in the primary auditory cortex when compared to unaffected relatives. No abnormalities were found in female patients (Leonard et al. 1995).

Although severe mental retardation ($IQ < 60$) is uncommon (only 3%), about 30% of affected subjects display a mild learning disability ($IQ < 85$). In particular, either the verbal or the performance component was impaired compared with controls (Brucker-Davis et al. 1995). Some authors have reported in their RTHβ cohort a high frequency of attention deficit hyperactivity disorder (ADHD). This finding has not been confirmed by other groups, but it is possible that the low IQ may be responsible for ADHD manifestations, more than RTHβ per se. In addition, an increased frequency of delayed developmental milestones and language disorders have been found in RTHβ patients, compared to their unaffected relatives (Brucker-Davis et al. 1995; Stein et al. 1995; Hauser et al. 1993; Weiss et al. 1997).

The neuroanatomical regions involved in attention and vigilance are located in the right lateral prefrontal cortex, in the parietal lobe and in the anterior cingulate. Consistently, Matochik et al. found a severe impairment on an attention auditory discrimination task, in adults with RTHβ compared to controls. The PET scan performed during this task demonstrated the presence of an increased metabolic activation of the anterior cingulate in RTHβ. The reduction of the functional activity in this brain area and the subsequent activation of other structures, such as the frontal cortex, is required for an efficient performance on complex attention tasks. However, it is not clear whether these functional anomalies are related to a defect in brain development or may be a consequence of the elevated levels of thyroid hormones via overstimulation of the TR-α (Matochik et al. 1996).

Patients with homozygous deletion of *THRB* display a phenotype characterized by deaf-mutism due to sensorineural hearing loss, delayed bone maturation, stippled epiphyses, goiter, and high levels of circulating thyroid hormone in the presence of a normal TSH (Dumitrescu and Refetoff 2012; Takeda et al. 1992).

Interestingly, these patients with deletions do not display growth delay, mental retardation, or cognitive impairment, while the five cases homozygous for missense mutations of *THRB* are invariably associated with a mild to severe intellectual impairment, neuropsychomotor retardation, goiter, hyperactivity, tachycardia, and hearing loss, as the extreme manifestations of resistance (Ono et al. 1991; Frank-Raue et al. 2004; Ferrara et al. 2012).

"Conventional" heterozygous mutations, resulting in a premature stop codon with the consequent production of a TR-β lacking a number of residues in the C- terminal, also display a strong dominant-negative effect in vitro and are often associated with a severe clinical phenotype, including mental retardation (Behr et al. 1997; Phillips et al. 2001; Gurgel et al. 2008).

5.3.2.7 Visual System

In animal models, the deletion of the TRβ2 isoform produces a selective loss of M-cone photoreceptors resulting in abnormal color vision. In particular, during embryogenesis, TR-β seems responsible for the photoreceptor distribution in the retina, inhibiting the S-opsin and committing the differentiation of M-opsin photoreceptor. Patients with homozygous deletion of *THRB* gene (Dumitrescu and Refetoff 2012; Takeda et al. 1992) are color blind, while in one patient with compound heterozygous mutation (R338W in exon 9 and R429W in exon 10 of *THRB* gene), an abnormal electroretinographic pattern was found, characterized by a normal scotopic response and a reduced photopic response. In particular, this patient showed a small amplitude b-wave to a red flash and a larger amplitude b-wave to the blue flash, similar to what is commonly described in the enhanced S cone syndrome (Weiss et al. 2012). Although no abnormalities of color sensitiveness have been identified in "conventional" RTHβ patients with heterozygous TRβ mutations, electrophysiological studies have shown a decrease of the L/M photoreceptor (red/green) waves associated with an impaired rod response (Campi et al. 2017).

5.3.2.8 Hearing System

An increased incidence of conductive or sensorineural hearing impairment, which may contribute to the defective speech development, has been reported in some RTHβ children. The pathophysiology of these abnormalities is composite, being the conductive defect due to the higher susceptibility to upper airways infection of RTHβ children, whereas the defective TRβ expression may be responsible for the cochlear dysfunction (Brucker-Davis et al. 1996).

Noteworthy, mice with targeted disruption of the TRβ locus develop profound sensorineural hearing loss, thus suggesting an important role of TH in the development of the hearing system.

5.3.2.9 Other Features

In mothers affected with RTHβ, there is a higher rate of miscarriage and intrauterine growth retardation of unaffected offspring, thus suggesting that intrauterine exposure to high TH levels does have adverse effects on the unaffected fetus (Weiss et al. 2010).

Prenatal diagnosis of RTHβ is not usually suggested; however, there are reports suggesting that a short course of propylthiouracil later in pregnancy may be beneficial in RTHβ mothers carrying fetuses with a normal *THRB* genotype (Anselmo et al. 2004). In particular, in the second and third trimesters, it seems to be a prudent approach keeping the maternal fT_4 levels not above 50% of the upper limit of normal. Obviously, no treatment is required in RTHβ-carrying affected fetuses (Pappa et al. 2017).

In case of prenatal diagnosis, it should be kept in mind that amniocentesis and chorionic villus sampling might be associated with an additional overall risk of miscarriage from 1 to 2%. Thus, pros and cons of these procedures should be clearly discussed with the patients.

There is only one patient, homozygous for TRβ mutations, in whom RTHβ may have contributed to death: this patient had resting pulse of 190 beats/min and died from cardiogenic shock complicated by septicemia.

Coexistence of TSH-secreting pituitary adenomas (TSHomas) and RTHβ has been suggested in only two cases. The impaired TH feedback in the pituitary may lead to a continuous stimulus to thyrotropes to synthesize and secrete TSH molecules, which may play a role in the development of pituitary tumors. However, the pituitary lesions associated to RTHβ appear to be pituitary "incidentalomas" (Beck-

Peccoz and Persani 2010). Interestingly, somatic mutations of TR-beta have been found in two TSH-secreting pituitary adenomas (Ando et al. 2001a, b) but never on the germinal DNA of patients with TSHomas.

Occasionally, RTHβ occurs in association with autoimmune thyroid disorders, such as Graves' disease or Hashimoto's thyroiditis. The occurrence of anti-TPO or anti-TSH receptor autoantibodies in RTH subjects has been described. Recent data suggest that the individuals with RTHβ due to TRβ gene mutations have an increased likelihood of AITD compared to unaffected relatives (Barkoff et al. 2010). The reason of this association seems to be related with the hyperstimulation, via TR-alpha, of the cells of the immune system.

The RTH patients, who develop Graves' disease, undergo a progressive increase in goiter size along with frank symptoms of thyrotoxicosis. The further elevation of TH levels causes TSH secretion to be totally inhibited. Conversely, hypothyroidism may occur in the presence of normal serum TH concentrations, as consequence of Hashimoto's thyroiditis. Treatment with L-T4 should be carefully monitored in order not to determine thyrotoxicosis.

5.3.3 *Differential Diagnosis of RTHβ*

RTHβ share the same biochemical features of several heritable conditions (Table 5.1), as well as of patients with TSH-secreting pituitary adenomas (TSHomas). Since these two diseases have completely different therapeutic and management approaches, their differential diagnosis is mandatory (Beck-Peccoz and Persani 2010).

The first step of the differential diagnosis is the exclusion of assay interferences that may be a common source of misdiagnosis, if not recognized. The identification of the same abnormal biochemical pattern of thyroid function in other first-degree relatives supports the diagnosis of RTHβ, since familiar cases of TSHoma have never been reported (except for four families in a setting of multiple endocrine neoplasia 1). In these cases, molecular analysis of the THRB gene makes a definitive diagnosis in 85–90% of cases of RTHβ.

Although different clinical parameters have been proposed (basal metabolic rate, systolic time intervals, Achilles reflex time) in order to discriminate among these two conditions, the clinical presentation of patients with RTHβ may be similar to those with TSHoma (Beck-Peccoz and Persani 2010), though the onset of central hyperthyroidism generally occurs beyond 30 years of age in the latter condition.

In patients with TSHomas, serum levels of glycoprotein hormone α-subunit (α-GSU) and α-GSU/TSH molar ratio are elevated, whereas in RTHβ patients, both indices are in the normal range.

To assess the degree of resistance in specific target tissues, different in vitro parameters have been proposed. Particularly, Sex Hormone Binding Globulin (SHBG) and serum carboxy-terminal telopeptide of type 1 collagen (ICTP) are in the hyperthyroid range in patients with TSHoma and within the normal range in RTHβ. The sensitivity and specificity of these tests are improved, when assessed after T3 suppression test, performed with oral administration of supraphysiological doses of T3 (50 μg/day for 3 days, followed by 100 μg/day for another 3 days and then 200 μg/day for another 3 days) (Refetoff and Dumitrescu 2007). In RTHβ patients, the increase of peripheral markers of TH actions and heart rate is blunted in comparison to normal subjects, thus definitively confirming the presence of resistance to TH action.

The TRH test (IV injection of TRH 200 μg) has been also widely used: in the majority of patients affected with TSHoma, TSH and α-GSU levels do not increase after TRH injection, whereas RTHβ subjects show normal response of TSH.

T3 inhibitory test, performed as reported above or administering T3 for 8–10 days at the dose of 80–100 μg/day, may show a full inhibition of TSH levels in RTHβ patients but persistent TSH response to TRH, carried out at the end of T3 administration. Since none of these tests have a clear diagnostic cut-off value, the combination of them, if possible, increases the specificity and sensitivity of the diagnostic process.

The administration of long-acting somatostatin analogs (e.g., long-acting octreotide-LAR 30 mg intramuscularly every 28 days) for at least 2 months can be useful in the differential diagnosis in problematic cases of central hyperthyroidism. Chronic administration of long-acting somatostatin analog in patients with central hyperthyroidism caused a marked decrease of FT3 and FT4 levels in patients with TSHoma (>30% of pretreatment values), while patients with PRTH did not respond at all.

Pituitary MRI is required in case of not univocal results with other tests; however the detection of pituitary lesion does not definitely rule out the diagnosis of RTHβ. In fact, pituitary lesions are quite common findings (20–25% of MRI performed for other reasons) in the general population. These lesions are usually considered as "pituitary incidentalomas," especially when a hypothalamic-pituitary dysfunction has been excluded. The presence of a microadenoma, in combination with lack of TSH response to dynamic tests and high levels of α-GSU or α-GSU/TSH molar ratio strongly sustains the diagnosis of a TSHoma.

5.3.4 Therapy

There is currently no definite therapy to correct the molecular defect causing RTHβ, and in most patients, a specific treatment is even not necessary, as goiter may be the only sign of the disease. The high levels of circulating free TH may be able to compensate for the resistance in several of the peripheral tissues but may create a thyrotoxic state in several others.

Patients with tachycardia and palpitations at rest may benefit by the use of a cardioselective β-blockers (atenolol or others). In the event of severe thyrotoxic symptoms, not responding to β-blockers, a reduction of thyroid hormone levels may be beneficial. This can't be achieved using antithyroid drugs, because the consequent increase of TSH levels may determine goiter enlargement. The treatment of choice in such cases is the administration of thyromimetic compounds, such as 3,5,3-′-triiodothyroacetic acid (TRIAC), which through the feedback mechanism reduces TSH secretion and causes a slight decrease of circulating T4 levels (values of T3 are unreliable as TRIAC cross-react in T3 measurement methods). As a consequence of its weaker effects on peripheral tissues, TRIAC reduces the thyrotoxic signs and symptoms, particularly at the heart level. TRIAC has been shown to be beneficial in both children and adult patients with RTHβ at the dose of 1.4–2.8 mg/day, fractionated in two or three administrations (Beck-Peccoz et al. 1983).

The use of dopaminergic drugs and somatostatin analogs has limited success because TSH secretion rapidly escapes the inhibitory effects of both drugs, as the T4 reduction triggers the much more potent stimulatory effect of TH negative feedback mechanism.

Although controversial, in children with signs of growth or mental retardation, the administration of supraphysiological doses of L-T4 to overcome the high degree of resistance present in some tissues can be beneficial. Supraphysiological doses of thyroid hormones are also necessary in patients treated with total thyroidectomy for a missed diagnosis of RTHβ. The use of high doses of L-T4 requires a careful monitoring of patients, assessing not only the TSH as in conventional autoimmune hypothyroidism but also the indices of peripheral thyroid hormones action. Very often in patients needing to suppress their TSH (as an example for a differentiated thyroid cancer), L-T4 treatment might be associated with TRIAC.

Recently, TRβ selective agonists (GC1 or sobetirome, eprotirome) have been developed and they could be beneficial for some abnormalities (dyslipidemia) found in RTHβ. Unfortunately, the development program on these drugs has been discontinued after the evidence of cartilage damage after 12 months' administration in dogs. In addition, there is evidence that eprotirome may induce liver injury in humans (Sjoukeet al. 2014). More recently, sobetirome has been proposed as a potential therapeutic for X-linked adrenoleukodystrophy (Hartley et al. 2017).

5.4 T3 Resistance to Thyroid Hormones Due to THRA Mutations

5.4.1 General Features of RTHα

RTHα patients retain normal hormone responsiveness in the hypothalamic–pituitary axis and liver, but they display manifestations (e.g., neurological, skeletal, gastrointestinal, and myocardial) due to resistance in TRα-specific tissues (Table 5.2).

The biochemical hallmark of this syndrome is the presence of an abnormally high T3/T4 ratio, associated with a higher serum T3/reverse T3 (rT3) ratio due to the reduction of the latter, and a normal TSH (Table 5.1). The thyroid biochemical abnormality is variable between patients with different mutations and may also change over time in the same patient. A rise in FT4 levels into the normal range might be observed during follow-up, and the FT3 levels might be high or high-normal or even normal (Moranet al. 2017; Demir et al. 2016).

The increased T3 and decreased rT3 levels could be due to upregulation of liver DIO1 or reduced DIO3 activity. This is supported by the observation that TRα-PV mutant mice have markedly increased activity of DIO1 in the kidney and liver and a reduced T3-induced DIO3 expression in the cortex, resulting in a decreased clearance of T3 (Zavacki et al. 2005; Barca-Mayo et al. 2011; Kaneshige et al. 2001). These alterations in deiodinase activities are characteristics also in the zebra fish model of RTHα (Marelli et al. 2017). Interestingly and similarly to what was reported in humans, the abnormalities in thyroid function are variable among the different mouse models. Indeed, the TRα-PV and TRα1-P398H mice have an overt thyroid dysfunction, while normal T3 and t4 levels are found in the TRα1-R384C and TRα1-L400R animals (Van Gucht et al. 2017).

Common features of this syndrome are growth retardation, which might transiently improve after L-T4 administration, disproportionate short stature characterized by femoral epiphyseal dysgenesis, and macrocephaly due to delayed closure of skull sutures, together with delayed tooth eruption, hypotension, subnormal heart, and basal metabolic rate. Similar to what is described in animal models (O'Shea et al. 2006), these subjects present variable features of hypothyroidism associated with normal TSH levels. Several of these manifestations had been also reported in mice with TRα1-PV mutation (O'Shea et al. 2006; Bochukova et al. 2012).

The clinical presentation of RTHα is characterized by abnormalities in tissues in which the TRα is the major isoform expressed. Free T4 levels were described at the lower limit of the normal range or slightly below, while free T3 levels were above the upper level of normal, resulting in a reduced FT4/FT3 ratio. Interestingly, the four affected individuals of the three first families described showed a truncated form of the receptor (E403X, F397fs406X, and Ala382ProfsX7) with a premature stop codon located in exon 9, thus affecting the only TRα1 isoform and not the other transcript (TRα2, Rev-erbα) generated from the *THRA* locus. All these mutations showed in vitro a reduced transcriptional activity and a strong dominant negative effect on the wild-type receptor. More recently, other missense mutations involving a domain common to TRα1 and TRα2 have also been described. The biochemical and clinical features did not differ from those described in the other cases (Moranet al. 2014).

The clinical phenotype is highly variable being severe in patients with truncated form of the receptor as the first identified patients and milder other cases such as p. A263S or the p.A263V.

5.4.2 *Detailed Clinical Picture of RTHα*

5.4.2.1 Thyroid Morphology

No abnormalities in the thyroid gland morphology have been documented in all the patients reported up to now. The patient harboring the p.E395X mutation had a normal thyroid US scan although a slightly elevated thyroglobulin was present (Sun et al. 2019).The response to TRH stimulation test is variable being normal in one patient harboring the mutations p.C380fs387X, (Moran et al. 2017), delayed in one case harboring the p.R384H mutation (Moran et al. 2017), and reduced in two patients with the F397fs406X mutation (van Mullem et al. 2012). The reduced response to TRH has been justified with high FT3 levels. Of note, the administration of levothyroxine caused in all patients a TSH suppression, suggesting an integrity of the pituitary-thyroid axis.

5.4.2.2 Cardiovascular Symptoms

Except for two patients described by Bochukova et al. and Sun et al. (p.E403X and p. E395X) who displayed bradycardia and arterial hypotension, most of the RTHα patients have a normal heart rate and blood pressure, although inappropriate for the Ft3 levels (van Mullem et al. 2012; Moran et al. 2017). In one patient with the C380fs387X variant (Moran et al. 2017), a hypertrophic obstructive cardiomyopathy associated with pericardial effusion was found. These signs were not rescued by T4 administration.

5.4.2.3 Skeletal Abnormalities

Macrocephaly due to late closure of skull fissures and retarded skeletal growth seem the most common signs associated with RTHα. Disproportionate short stature is another common finding, although patients with milder mutations such as A263V have a normal and proportionate stature (Moran et al. 2014). Noteworthy, these patients were all treated with L-T4 since childhood although the syndrome was correctly diagnosed later in life, because of symptoms of hypothyroidism. Conversely, an untreated 8-year-old patient harboring the P398R mutation (Tylki-Szymanska et al. 2015) had a disproportionate normal stature, suggesting that L-T4 treatment might improve the linear growth of long bones. Other skeletal abnormalities have been documented, including club feet (C392X), valgus foot (E403X, E403K, and P398R), lumbar kyphosis (C392X and E403X), coxa valga (L274P), multiple Wormian bones (E403X, L274P, R384H, C380fs387X), and femoral epiphyseal dysgenesis (E403X, L274P) and thickening of the calvarium (E403X, L274P, A263V, Ala382ProfsX7, C380fs387X, and R384H). Delayed dentition and ossification with retarded bone age are frequently observed (Tylki-Szymanska et al. 2015; Moran et al. 2017).

Skull abnormalities cause a dysmorphic face: all patients are characterized by resembling untreated patients with congenital hypothyroidism with a large coarse face; macrocephaly; a large, short, and upturned nose with a flat nasal bridge; wide forehead; hypertelorism; multiple skin tags; eyelid ptosis; and short neck.

5.4.2.4 Metabolism

In several patients, including the first pediatric case reported, a low basal metabolic rate measured by indirect calorimetry was found consistent to hypothyroidism. Increased levels of total and LDL cholesterol may be present (Bochukovaet al. 2012; Moran et al. 2013, 2014), and this may increase the overall cardiovascular risk. However, long-term data are needed to establish if a long-term treatment with L-T4 may improve dyslipidemia. Two adult patients were obese.

5.4.2.5 Immune System

Although one patient with the A263S mutation had frequent infections, further studies on this and other seven patients (with the C380fs387X, R384H, and D211G mutations) (Demir et al. 2016; Van Gucht et al. 2016) have shown a macrophage function similar to that of controls, as measured by phagocytosis and cytokine induction after LPS treatment (Demir et al. 2016; van der Spek et al. 2017). Elevated Il-8 levels were also found in these patients as seen in subjects with hyperthyroidism.

5.4.2.6 Neurological System

In the first pediatric case described, the cognitive deficits were consistent with a congenital hypothyroidism (Bochukova et al. 2012). She was inappropriately placid and her speech was slow and monotonous. A neuropsychological assessment showed selective cognitive difficulties in the adaptive behavior, short-term memory, and visuoperceptual function, and conversely the verbal comprehension was normal. In addition, motor dyspraxia and difficulties in fine motor coordination resulted in the inability to write or draw. In addition, she had a broad-based ataxic gait. Finally, muscular hypotonia but no weakness was present. A similar phenotype, thus associated with a more severe cognitive impairment, has been described in another female patient harboring the Ala382ProfsX7 mutation (Demir et al. 2016). The patient was unable to read and her IQ was around 52. In addition, this patient was affected with epilepsy, confirmed by the electroencephalographic demonstration of bilateral theta waves during hyperventilation; seizures decreased in frequency with sodium valproate administration (Moran et al. 2013). More recently, childhood seizures have been also described in a patient harboring the D211G missense variant (Van Gucht et al. 2016). The proband of the second family (TRα1-F397fs406X) and her affected father had a mild cognitive deficit with an IQ of 90 and 85, respectively (van Mullem et al. 2012). Also, in the two cohorts of patients reported by Tylki-Szymańska and Demir, the cognitive impairment was variable spanning from patients with severe mental retardation (pC392X and C380fs387X) to patients with a normal cognitive function and a normal IQ (p.P398R and p.A263S). However, also in patients without mental retardation, a delay in reaching developmental milestones (including delayed speech development, dysarthric speech, slow initiation of motor movement, impaired fine and gross motor coordination, hypotonia dyspraxia, and ataxic gait) is invariably present. Interestingly, in a cohort of 170 individuals (parents and two ASD-affected siblings) with autism spectrum disorder, a de novo variant in the THRA gene was found in a (pR384C) (Yuen et al. 2015). The observed neurocognitive deficits seem associated with structural abnormalities such as reduced cerebellar and hippocampal volume, diminished white matter density and accord with the known developmental actions of TH, and substantiate the critical role of TRα1 in CNS (Moran et al. 2014; BES meeting, personal communication).

5.4.2.7 Other Features

The *visual and the hearing systems* do not seem to be affected by the THRA mutation. In one family, the affected father of the proband had an acquired hearing loss, due to otosclerosis and thus not related with the presence of the F397fs406X mutation in the TRα1.

Constipation due to delayed intestinal transit is a common feature of the syndrome, and in the family with the TRα1-F397fs406X, the administration of L-T4 improved the intestinal manifestations in both father and affected daughter (Schoenmakers et al. 2013). Abdominal radiography and colonic manometry may show a delayed intestinal transit with bowel dilatation and a reduced peristalsis, respectively (Bochukova et al. 2012; Moran et al. 2013). An adult patient with the E403X had no constipation that was however present in his affected daughter.

Interestingly, in most affected patients low or low-normal levels of IGF-1 were found. One patient was treated with rh-GH, without a significant improvement of the growth retardation (Schoenmakers et al. 2013). Also, the L-T4 administration was only transiently beneficial on the growth delay.

Normocytic normochromic anemia is a constant finding in the RTHα patients described up to now. Iron, vitamin B12, folate, reticulocyte count, circulating haptoglobin, and lactate dehydrogenase are usually in the normal range. The pathogenic mechanisms underlying anemia in RTHα patients is unclear; however, several studies have shown an association between hypothyroidism and anemia. In addition, animal models have suggested a direct role of TRα in erythropoiesis. It has been suggested that mutations in human TRα may alter the balance between proliferation and differentiation of progenitor cells during erythropoiesis (Van Gucht et al. 2017).

5.4.3 Differential Diagnosis of RTHα

The normal TSH and borderline low FT4 typical of RTHα patients are similar to those found in several forms of central hypothyroidism (Persani et al. 2018).

However, the abnormal FT4/FT3 ratio associated with the typical manifestations of congenital hypothyroidism should raise the suspect of RTHα.

In patients with milder biochemical abnormalities, RTHα diagnosis may become more difficult as several pathological conditions may be associated with similar dysmorphic presentations. As an example, patients with *PTEN* mutations have macrocephaly, short stature, and a short and depressed nasal bridge along with autism, developmental delay, and mental retardation. *SHOX* mutations are associated with disproportionate short stature; *CUL4B* mutations associate with hyperactivity, mental retardation, ataxic gait, and dysmorphic face (coarse face, macrocephaly, short stature, mental retardation), speech delay, and decreased fine-motor coordination.

It is noteworthy that one case was "incidentally" found by exome sequence while studying a specific cohort of patients with autism in which *THRA* was not the primary researched gene (Yuenet al. 2015), suggesting that the clinical phenotype is not so obvious to recognize.

5.4.4 Therapy

The administration of L-T4 results in a normalization of FT4, with a further increase of FT3 and a suppression of the TSH levels, suggesting a conserved negative feedback of TH on TSH secretion. The peripheral markers of TH action also change during LT4 therapy, in particular SHBG and IGF1 levels increase, while serum creatine kinase and LDL cholesterol levels decrease.

In general, LT4 therapy has no beneficial effects on anemia. Also the cardiac function did not change significantly in patients with bradycardia at clinical presentation (Van Gucht et al. 2017).

The response to treatment is variable, depending on the type of mutation and on the age on which L-T4 was started. Although positive effects of L-T4 have been described also in adults, RTHα identified by familiar screening, it seems that an early treatment in infancy results in a better response with an improved final height and amelioration of the disproportionate body proportion, especially in the case of a milder mutation (A263V) (Moran et al. 2017).

In the patient with E403X mutant TRα, the levels of IGF-1 normalized, with a minimal improvement in growth velocity, growth rate, and intestinal transit. In the family with the F397fs406X mutation, L-T4 treatment caused an improvement of constipation with a persistence of growth retardation in both subjects. In other cases, LT4 therapy had a positive effect on constipation. In the child harboring the D211G mutation, LT4 treatment improved muscle hypotonia and motor development (Van Gucht et al. 2016). In contrast, LT4 treatment did not rescue the growth retardation and cardiac and renal problems in a girl with the C380fs387X (the most short form of mutant TRa described), suggesting persistent tissue hypothyroidism (Demir et al. 2016).

Higher-dose thyroxine therapy could possibly overcome TH resistance in organs expressing the TRα1 isoform (bone, skeletal muscle, gastrointestinal tract, myocardium, brain). Unfortunately, this may result in unwanted toxicities in TRβ-expressing tissues (hypothalamus, pituitary, liver) as suggested by the raised levels of SHBG and the TSH suppression.

The design of novel TH analogs targeting the TRα mutations may open novel therapeutic perspectives in these subjects. In fact, the use of TRα-selective thyromimetic agents may be helpful to avoid hyperthyroidism in TRβ-expressing tissues (Schoenmakers et al. 2013).

5.5 Conclusions

RTHβ and RTHα are rare disorders to be considered in patients with inappropriate TSH secretion. These diseases are caused by heterozygous mutations in TRs that reduce T3 binding or affect the recruitment of cofactors. These mutant TRs exert dominant negative effects on the activities of the coexisting wild-type receptors. Despite compensatory mechanisms (such as increased thyroid stimulation in RTHβ or modifications in TH metabolism in RTHα), the thyroid hormone actions are pathological at several tissue levels. The phenotypic manifestations of these syndromes are correlated with the degree of disruption and the tissue distribution of the TRs being characterized by variable coexistence of hypothyroid or thyrotoxic manifestations in RTHβ or by a congenital hypothyroid features in RTHα despite normal TSH and borderline low free T4.

Although the pathogenesis of these syndromes is well established, only symptomatic or partially effective treatments are currently available thus frequently leading to severe complications. Further research is warranted to find a suitable therapeutic strategy of the affected patients.

Acknowledgments This work was partially supported by the Italian Ministry of Health, Rome (Fund RF-2010-2309484).

References

Amor AJ, Halperin I, Alfayate R et al (2014) Identification of four novel mutations in the thyroid hormone receptor-β gene in 164 Spanish and 2 Greek patients with resistance to thyroid hormone. Hormones 13:74–78

Ando S, Sarlis NJ, Krishnan J et al (2001a) Aberrant alternative splicing of thyroid hormone receptor in a TSH-secreting pituitary tumor is a mechanism for hormone resistance. Mol Endocrinol 15:1529–1538

Ando S, Sarlis NJ, Oldfield EH, Yen PM (2001b) Somatic mutation of TRbeta can cause a defect in negative regulation of TSH in a TSH-secreting pituitary tumor. J Clin Endocrinol Metab 86:5572–5576

Anselmo J, Cao D, Karrison T, Weiss RE, Refetoff S (2004) Fetal loss associated with excess thyroid hormone exposure. JAMA 292:691–695

Astapova I, Lee LJ, Morales C, Tauber S, Bilban M, Hollenberg AN (2008) The nuclear corepressor, NCoR, regulates thyroid hormone action in vivo. Proc Natl Acad Sci USA 105:19544–19549

Barca-Mayo O, Liao XH, Alonso M et al (2011) Thyroid hormone receptor alpha and regulation of type 3 deiodinase. Mol Endocrinol 25:575–583

Barkoff MS, Kocherginsky M, Anselmo J, Weiss RE, Refetoff S (2010) Autoimmunity in patients with resistance to thyroid hormone. J Clin Endocrinol Metab 95:3189–3193

Beck-Peccoz P, Chatterjee VKK (1994) The variable clinical phenotype in thyroid hormone resistance syndrome. Thyroid 4:225–231

Beck-Peccoz P, Persani L (2010) TSH-producing adenomas. In: Jameson LJ, DeGroot LJ (eds) Endocrinology, adult and pediatric, 6th edn. Sauderns Elsevier, Philadelphia, PA, pp 324–332

Beck-Peccoz P, Piscitelli G, Cattaneo MG, Faglia G (1983) Successful treatment of hyperthyroidism due to nonneoplastic pituitary TSH hypersecretion with 3,5,3′-triiodothyroacetic acid (TRIAC). J Endocrinol Investig 6:217–223

Behr M, Ramsden DB, Loos U (1997) Deoxyribonucleic acid binding and transcriptional silencing by a truncated c-erbA beta 1 thyroid hormone receptor identified in a severely retarded patient with resistance to thyroid hormone. J Clin Endocrinol Metab 82:1081–1087

Bochukova E, Schoenmakers N, Agostini M et al (2012) A mutation in the thyroid hormone receptor alpha gene. N Engl J Med 19:243–249

Bradley DJ, Towle HC, Young WS 3rd (1992) Spatial and temporal expression of α- and β-thyroid hormone receptor mRNAs, including the β2-subtype, in the developing mammalian nervous system. J Neurosci 12:2288–2302

Brucker-Davis F, Skarulis MC et al (1995) Genetic and clinical features of 42 kindreds with resistance to thyroid hormone. The National Institutes of Health Prospective Study. Ann Intern Med 15:572–583

Brucker-Davis F, Skarulis MC, Pikus A et al (1996) Prevalence and mechanisms of hearing loss in patients with resistance to thyroid hormone. J Clin Endocrinol Metab 81:2768–2772

Campi I, Cammarata G, Bianchi Marzoli S et al (2017) Retinal photoreceptor functions are compromised in patients with resistance to thyroid hormone syndrome (RTHβ). J Clin Endocrinol Metab 102:2620–2627

Cardoso LF, de Paula FJ, Maciel LM (2014) Resistance to thyroid hormone due to mutations in the THRB gene impairs bone mass and affects calcium and phosphorus homeostasis. Bone 67:222–227

Cheng SY, Leonard JL, Davis PJ (2010) Molecular aspects of thyroid hormone actions. Endocr Rev 31:139–170

Demir K, van Gucht AL, Büyükinan M et al (2016) Diverse genotypes and phenotypes of three novel thyroid hormone receptor alpha mutations. J Clin Endocrinol Metab 101:2945–2954

Desouza LA, Ladiwala U, Daniel SM, Agashe S, Vaidya RA, Vaidya VA (2005) Thyroid hormone regulates hippocampal neurogenesis in the adult rat brain. Mol Cell Neurosci 29:414–426

Dumitrescu AM, Refetoff S (2012) The syndromes of reduced sensitivity to thyroid hormone. Biochim Biophys Acta 1830:3987–4003

Fauquier T, Chatonnet F, Picou F et al (2014) Purkinje cells and Bergmann glia are primary targets of the TRα1 thyroid hormone receptor during mouse cerebellum postnatal development. Development 141:166–175

Ferrara AM, Onigata K, Ercan O, Woodhead H, Weiss RE, Refetoff S (2012) Homozygous thyroid hormone receptor β-gene mutations in resistance to thyroid hormone: three new cases and review of the literature. J Clin Endocrinol Metab 97:1328–1336

Frank-Raue K, Lorenz A, Haag C et al (2004) Severe form of thyroid hormone resistance in a patient with homozygous/hemizygous mutation of T3 receptor gene. Eur J Endocrinol 150:819–823

Gurgel MH, Montenegro Junior RM, Magalhaes RA et al (2008) E449X mutation in the thyroid hormone receptor beta associated with autoimmune thyroid disease and severe neuropsychomotor involvement. Arq Bras Endocrinol Metabol 52:1205–1210

Hartley MD, Kirkemo LL, Banerji T, Scanlan TS (2017) A thyroid hormone-based strategy for correcting the biochemical abnormality in X-linked adrenoleukodystrophy. Endocrinology 158:1328–1338

Hauser P, Zametkin AJ, Martinez P et al (1993) Attention deficit-hyperactivity disorder in people with generalized resistance to thyroid hormone. N Engl J Med 8:997–1001

Hernandez A, Martinez ME, Fiering S et al (2006) Type 3 deiodinase is critical for the maturation and function of the thyroid axis. J Clin Invest 116:476–484

Heuer H, Mason CA (2003) Thyroid hormone induces cerebellar Purkinje cell dendritic development via the thyroid hormone receptor alpha1. J Neurosci 19:10604–10612

Hodin RA, Lazar MA, Wintman BI et al (1989) Identification of a thyroid hormone receptor that is pituitary-specific. Science 7:76–79

Hu X, Lazar MA (2000) Transcriptional repression by nuclear hormone receptors. Trends Endocrinol Metab 11:6–10

Ito M, Roeder RG (2001) The TRAP/SMCC/mediator complex and thyroid hormone receptor function. Trends Endocrinol Metab 12:127–134

Kahaly GJ, Matthews CH, Mohr-Kahaly S, Richards CA, Chatterjee VK (2002) Cardiac involvement in thyroid hormone resistance. J Clin Endocrinol Metab 87:204–212

Kaneshige M, Suzuki H, Kaneshige K et al (2001) A targeted dominant negative mutation of the thyroid hormone alpha 1 receptor causes increased mortality, infertility, and dwarfism in mice. Proc Natl Acad Sci USA 98:15095–15100

Kapoor R, van Hogerlinden M, Wallis K et al (2010) Unliganded thyroid hormone receptor alpha1 impairs adult hippocampal neurogenesis. FASEB J 24:4793–4805

Kapoor R, Ghosh H, Nordstrom K, Vennstrom B, Vaidya VA (2011) Loss of thyroid hormone receptor β is associated with increased progenitor proliferation and NeuroD positive cell number in the adult hippocampus. Neurosci Lett 7:199–203

Lechan RM, Qi Y, Jackson IM, Mahdavi V (1994) Identification of thyroid hormone receptor isoforms in thyrotropin-releasing hormone neurons of the hypothalamic paraventricular nucleus. Endocrinology 135:92–100

Leonard CM, Martinez P, Weintraub BD, Hauser P (1995) Magnetic resonance imaging of cerebral anomalies in subjects with resistance to thyroid hormone. Am J Med Genet 19:238–243

Marelli F, Carra S, Rurale G, Cotelli F, Persani L (2017) In vivo functional consequences of human THRA variants expressed in the zebrafish. Thyroid 27:279–291

Matochik JA, Zametkin AJ, Cohen RM, Hauser P, Weintraub BD (1996) Abnormalities in sustained attention and anterior cingulate metabolism in subjects with resistance to thyroid hormone. Brain Res 3:23–28

Menzaghi C, Di Paola R, Corrias A et al (1998) T426I a new mutation in the thyroid hormone receptor beta gene in a sporadic patient with resistance to thyroid hormone and dysmorphism. Mutations in brief no. 192. Hum Mutat 12:289

Mitchell CS, Savage DB, Dufour S et al (2010) Resistance to thyroid hormone is associated with raised energy expenditure, muscle mitochondrial uncoupling, and hyperphagia. J Clin Invest 120:1345–1354

Moran C, Schoenmakers N, Agostini M et al (2013) An adult female with resistance to thyroid hormone mediated by defective thyroid hormone receptor α. J Clin Endocrinol Metab 98:4254–4261

Moran C, Agostini M, Visser WE et al (2014) Resistance to thyroid hormone caused by a mutation in thyroid hormone receptor TRα1 and TRα2: clinical, biochemical, and genetic analyses of three related patients. Lancet Diabetes Endocrinol 2:619–626

Moran C, Agostini M, McGowan A et al (2017) Contrasting phenotypes in resistance to thyroid hormone alpha correlate with divergent properties of thyroid hormone receptor α1 mutant proteins. Thyroid 27:973–982

Ng L, Cordas E, Wu X, Vella KR, Hollenberg AN, Forrest D (2015) Age-related hearing loss and degeneration of cochlear hair cells in mice lacking thyroid hormone receptor β1. Endocrinology 156:3853–3865

Ono S, Schwartz ID, Mueller OT, Root AW, Usala SJ, Bercu BB (1991) Homozygosity for a dominant negative thyroid hormone receptor gene responsible for generalized resistance to thyroid hormone. J Clin Endocrinol Metab 73(5):990–994.
O'Shea PJ, Bassett JH, Cheng SY, Williams GR (2006) Characterization of skeletal phenotypes of TRalpha1 and TRbeta mutant mice: implications for tissue thyroid status and T3 target gene expression. Nucl Recept Signal 4:1–5
Owen PJ, Chatterjee VK, John R, Halsall D, Lazarus JH (2009) Augmentation index in resistance to thyroid hormone (RTH). Clin Endocrinol 70:650–654
Pappa T, Anselmo J, Mamanasiri S, Dumitrescu AM, Weiss RE, Refetoff S (2017) Prenatal diagnosis of resistance to thyroid hormone and its clinical implications. J Clin Endocrinol Metab 102:3775–3782
Persani L, Asteria C, Tonacchera M et al (1994) Evidence for the secretion of thyrotropin with enhanced bioactivity in syndromes of thyroid hormone resistance. J Clin Endocrinol Metab 78:1034–1039
Persani L, Brabant G, Dattani M et al (2018) 2018 European Thyroid Association (ETA) guidelines on the diagnosis and management of central hypothyroidism. Eur Thyroid J 7(5):225–237
Phillips SA, Rotman-Pikielny P, Lazar J et al (2001) Extreme thyroid hormone resistance in a patient with a novel truncated TR mutant. J Clin Endocrinol Metab 86:5142–5147
Prats-Puig A, Carreras-Badosa G, Bassols J et al (2017) The placental imprinted DLK1-DIO3 domain: a new link to prenatal and postnatal growth in humans. Am J Obstet Gynecol 217:350.e1–350.e13
Pulcrano M, Palmieri EA, Mannavola D et al (2009) Impact of resistance to thyroid hormone on the cardiovascular system in adults. J Clin Endocrinol Metab 94:2812–2816
Refetoff S, Dumitrescu AM (2007) Syndromes of reduced sensitivity to thyroid hormone: genetic defects in hormone receptors, cell transporters and deiodination. Best Pract Res Clin Endocrinol Metab 21:277–305
Refetoff S, Bassett JH, Beck-Peccoz P et al (2014) Classification and proposed nomenclature for inherited defects of thyroid hormone action, cell transport, and metabolism. Eur Thyroid J 3:7–9
Reutrakul S, Sadow PM, Pannain S et al (2000) Search for abnormalities of nuclear corepressors, coactivators, and a coregulator in families with resistance to thyroid hormone without mutations in thyroid hormone receptor beta or alpha genes. J Clin Endocrinol Metab 85:3609–3617
Schoenmakers E, Agostini M, Mitchell C et al (2010) Mutations in the selenocysteine insertion sequence-binding protein 2 gene lead to a multisystem selenoprotein deficiency disorder in humans. J Clin Invest 120:4220–4235
Schoenmakers N, Moran C, Peeters RP, Visser T, Gurnell M, Chatterjee K (2013) Resistance to thyroid hormone mediated by defective thyroid hormone receptor alpha. Biochim Biophys Acta 1830:4004–4008
Schroeder AC, Privalsky ML (2014) Thyroid hormones, T3 and T4, in the brain. Front Endocrinol 31:5–40
Sjouke B, Langslet G, Ceska R et al (2014) Eprotirome in patients with familial hypercholesterolaemia (the AKKA trial): a randomised, double-blind, placebo-controlled phase 3 study. Lancet Diabetes Endocrinol 2:455–463
Stein MA, Weiss RE, Refetoff S (1995) Neurocognitive characteristics of individuals with resistance to thyroid hormone: comparisons with individuals with attention-deficit hyperactivity disorder. J Dev Behav Pediatr 16:406–411
Sun H, Wu H, Xie R et al (2019) New case of thyroid hormone resistance α caused by a mutation of THRA/TRα1. J Endocr Soc 3:665–669
Takeda K, Sakurai A, DeGroot LJ, Refetoff S (1992) Recessive inheritance of thyroid hormone resistance caused by complete deletion of the protein-coding region of the thyroid hormone receptor-beta gene. J Clin Endocrinol Metab 74:49–55
Torchia J, Glass C, Rosenfeld MG (1998) Co-activators and co-repressors in the integration of transcriptional responses. Curr Opin Cell Biol 10:373–383

Tylki-Szymanska A, Acuna-Hidalgo R, Krajewska-Walasek M et al (2015) Thyroid hormone resistance syndrome due to mutations in the thyroid hormone receptor alpha gene (THRA). J Med Genet 52:312–316
van der Spek AH, Surovtseva OV, Aan S et al (2017) Increased circulating interleukin-8 in patients with resistance to thyroid hormone receptor α. Endocr Connect 6:731–740
van Gucht A, Meima M, Zwaveling-Soonawala N et al (2016) Resistance to thyroid hormone alpha in an 18 months old girl; clinical, therapeutic and molecular characteristics. Thyroid 26:338–346
Van Gucht ALM, Moran C, Meima ME et al (2017) Resistance to thyroid hormone due to heterozygous mutations in thyroid hormone receptor alpha. Curr Top Dev Biol 125:337–355
van Mullem A, van Heerebeek R, Chrysis D et al (2012) Clinical phenotype and mutant TRα1. N Engl J Med 12:1451–1453
Vela A, Pérez-Nanclares G, Ríos I, Rica I, Portillo N, Castaño L, Spanish Group for the Study of RTH (2019) Thyroid hormone resistance from newborns to adults: a Spanish experience. J Endocrinol Investig. https://doi.org/10.1007/s40618-019-1007-4
Visser WE, Friesema EC, Visser TJ (2011) Minireview: thyroid hormone transporters: the knowns and the unknowns. Mol Endocrinol 25:1–14
Weiss RE, Stein MA, Refetoff S (1997) Behavioral effects of liothyronine (L-T3) in children with attention deficit hyperactivity disorder in the presence and absence of resistance to thyroid hormone. Thyroid 7:389–393
Weiss RE, Dumitrescu A, Refetoff S (2010) Approach to the patient with resistance to thyroid hormone and pregnancy. J Clin Endocrinol Metab 95:3094–3102
Weiss AH, Kelly JP, Bisset D, Deeb SS (2012) Reduced L- and M- and increased S-cone functions in an infant with thyroid hormone resistance due to mutations in the THRβ2 gene. Ophthalmic Genet 33:187–195
Yuen RK, Thiruvahindrapuram B, Merico D et al (2015) Whole-genome sequencing of quartet families with autism spectrum disorder. Nat Med 21:185–191
Zavacki AM, Ying H, Christoffolete MA, Aerts G, So E, Harney J (2005) Type 1 iodothyronine deiodinase is a sensitive marker of peripheral thyroid status in the mouse. Endocrinology 146:1568–1575

Chapter 6
Glucocorticoid Resistance

Nicolas C. Nicolaides and Evangelia Charmandari

Abstract Primary generalized glucocorticoid resistance or Chrousos syndrome is a rare disorder, which affects all tissues expressing the human glucocorticoid receptor. It is characterized by generalized, partial tissue insensitivity to glucocorticoids caused by genetic defects in the *NR3C1* gene. We and others have applied standard methods of molecular and structural biology to investigate the molecular mechanisms and conformational alterations through which the mutant glucocorticoid receptors lead to the broad spectrum of clinical manifestations of Chrousos syndrome. The ever-increasing application of novel technologies, including the next-generation sequencing, will enhance our knowledge in factors that influence the glucocorticoid signal transduction in a positive or negative fashion.

Keywords Chrousos syndrome · Glucocorticoid receptor · Glucocorticoid signaling · Glucocorticoids · *NR3C1* mutations · Primary generalized glucocorticoid resistance

List of Abbreviations

ACTH	Adrenocorticotropic hormone
AP-1	Activator protein-1
AVP	Arginine vasopressin
CpG	Cytosine-guanine dinucleotides
CRH	Corticotropin-releasing hormone

N. C. Nicolaides (✉) · E. Charmandari
Division of Endocrinology, Metabolism and Diabetes, First Department of Pediatrics, National and Kapodistrian University of Athens Medical School, "Aghia Sophia" Children's Hospital, Athens, Greece

Division of Endocrinology and Metabolism, Center of Clinical, Experimental Surgery and Translational Research, Biomedical Research Foundation of the Academy of Athens, Athens, Greece
e-mail: nnicolaides@bioacademy.gr

P. Igaz, A. Patócs (eds.), *Genetics of Endocrine Diseases and Syndromes*, Experientia Supplementum 111, https://doi.org/10.1007/978-3-030-25905-1_6

DHEA	Dehydroepiandrosterone
DHEAS	Dehydroepiandrosterone-sulfate
GR	Glucocorticoid receptor
GREs	Glucocorticoid response elements
GRIP1	Glucocorticoid receptor-interacting protein 1
GST	Glutathione-S-transferase
hGR	Human glucocorticoid receptor
hGRα	Human glucocorticoid receptor alpha
hGRβ	Human glucocorticoid receptor beta
HPA axis	Hypothalamic-pituitary-adrenal axis
HSP	Heat-shock proteins
LBD	Ligand-binding domain
MAPK	Mitogen-activated protein kinase
NF-κB	Nuclear factor-κB
PGGR	Primary generalized glucocorticoid resistance
PI3K	Phosphatidylinositol 3-kinase
STATs	Signal transducers and activators of transcription
UFC	Urinary free cortisol

6.1 Introduction

Glucocorticoids are steroid hormones secreted by the *zona fasciculata* of the adrenal cortex (Nicolaides et al. 2015a). These lipophilic molecules are the end products of the hypothalamic-pituitary-adrenal (HPA) axis and play a fundamental role in the maintenance of resting and stress-related homeostasis by influencing almost every physiologic function in living organisms (Charmandari et al. 2005a, b, c). In addition to proliferation, differentiation, and programmed cell death (apoptosis), a growing body of evidence suggests that glucocorticoids can cause epigenetic modifications in a large number of cytosine-guanine dinucleotides (CpG) located in the regulatory regions of several genes (Zannas and Chrousos 2017). All these myriad effects of glucocorticoids are mediated by the glucocorticoid receptor (GR), a ubiquitously expressed protein that belongs to the steroid receptor subfamily of the nuclear receptor family of transcription factors (Nicolaides et al. 2010). Interestingly, GR influences the expression of 1 in 5 genes expressed in human leukocytes, indicating a pivotal role of the receptor in the transcription process (Galon et al. 2002). Since glucocorticoids have potent immunomodulating effects, an ever-increasing number of synthetic analogues have been developed for the treatment of autoimmune, inflammatory, and malignant disorders (Rhen and Cidlowski 2005).

6.2 The Human Glucocorticoid Receptor (hGR)

The hGR is encoded by the *NR3C1* gene, which is located on chromosome 5. The *NR3C1* gene consists of 10 exons; exon 1 contains several regulatory regions, whereas exons 2–9α/9β are responsible for protein expression (Ramamoorthy and Cidlowski 2016). Through several molecular mechanisms, including alternative splicing, insertions, deletions, and alternative translation initiation, the *NR3C1* gene encodes a large number of protein isoforms that differ in terms of subcellular localization and transcriptional activity (Oakley and Cidlowski 2011). Indeed, the alternative usage of exon 9α or 9β generates the two main protein isoforms, the hGRα and the hGRβ. The hGRα represents the classical hGR isoform, which is expressed in all tissues apart from the suprachiasmatic nucleus. In addition, the hGRα is primarily localized in the cytoplasm, binds natural and synthetic glucocorticoids, and mediates most of the glucocorticoid effects. On the other hand, the hGRβ is expressed in specific cell types, is localized in the nucleus, and exerts inhibitory (dominant negative) effects on the transcriptional activity of hGRα (Bamberger et al. 1995; Charmandari et al. 2005a, b, c; Yudt et al. 2003). A growing body of evidence suggests that the hGRβ has an important role in insulin signaling, in glioma formation, as well as in the migration of bladder cancer cells (Stechschulte et al. 2014; Yin et al. 2013; Wang et al. 2015; McBeth et al. 2016).

In addition to hGRα and hGRβ, there are three splice hGR isoforms, which are expressed both in cancer cells and normal tissues, the hGR-γ, hGR-A, and hGR-P (Ramamoorthy and Cidlowski 2016). In hGR-γ, an arginine residue is inserted at amino acid position 452 in the ligand-binding domain (LBD) of the receptor (Ray et al. 1996). This isoform has been implicated in glucocorticoid resistance in acute lymphoblastic leukemia, small-cell lung carcinoma, and pituitary corticotroph adenomas (Beger et al. 2003). In hGR-A, a large fragment between amino acid positions 490 and 674 has been deleted, thereby forming a defective LBD (Ramamoorthy and Cidlowski 2016). Finally, exons 7 and 8 have been deleted in hGR-P, which is overexpressed in non-Hodgkin lymphoma, acute lymphoblastic leukemia, and multiple myeloma (Krett et al. 1995). An additional cohort of hGR isoforms have been suggested by Lu and Cidlowski, more than 10 years ago (Lu and Cidlowski 2005). Through alternative initiation of hGRα mRNA translation, the eight start codons in exon 2 of the hGR transcript could give rise to eight receptor isoforms with progressively shorter aminoterminal domain. These hGRα isoforms, termed hGRα-A, hGRα-B, hGRα-C1, hGRα-C2, hGRα-C3, hGRα-D1, hGRα-D2, and hGRα-D3, are currently under intense investigation in terms of localization and function (Lu et al. 2007; Wu et al. 2013).

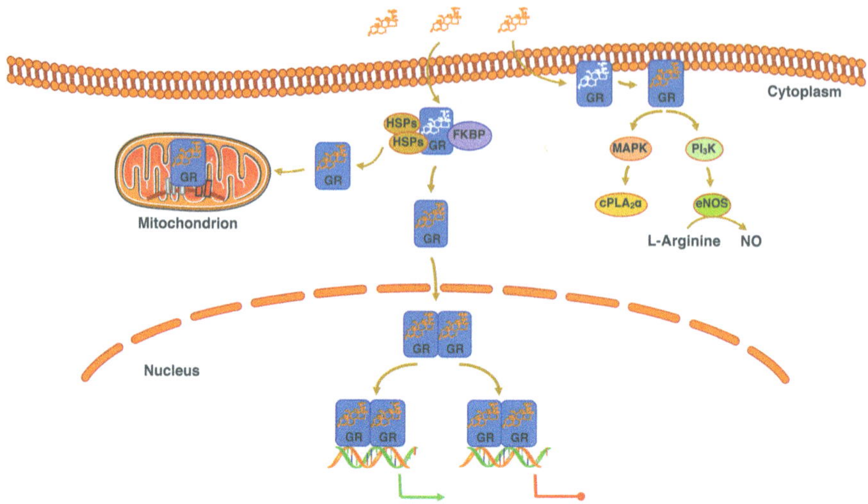

Fig. 6.1 Glucocorticoid signal transduction. *cPLA2α* cytosolic phospholipase A2 alpha, *eNOS* endothelial nitric oxide synthetase, *FKBP* immunophilins, *GR* glucocorticoid receptor, *HSP* heat-shock proteins, *MAPK* mitogen-activated protein kinases, *NO* nitric oxide, *PI3K* phosphatidylinositol 3-kinase

6.3 The Glucocorticoid Signaling Pathway

At the cellular and molecular level, the hGRα resides primarily in the cytoplasm and interacts with heat-shock proteins (HSP90, HSP70) and immunophilins (FKBP51 and FKBP52) (Grad and Picard 2007). In the presence of glucocorticoids, the receptor undergoes conformational changes, dissociates from the multiprotein complex, and translocates to the nucleus forming homo- or heterodimers (Fig. 6.1). These dimers bind to specific DNA sequences, termed "glucocorticoid response elements" (GREs), located in the regulatory regions of glucocorticoid-responsive genes. Upon hGRα binding to GREs, the dimers recruit coactivators and chromatin-remodeling complexes, which induce the activity of RNA polymerase II, therefore enabling gene transcription (Ramamoorthy and Cidlowski 2016). Moreover, the hGRα may regulate gene expression by physically interacting, possibly as monomer, with other important transcription factors, such as the activator protein-1 (AP-1), the nuclear factor-κB (NF-κB), and signal transducers and activators of transcription (STATs), influencing the transcriptional activity of the latter in a positive or negative fashion (Fig. 6.1) (Chrousos and Kino 2005; Nicolaides et al. 2015a; Ramamoorthy and Cidlowski 2016).

In addition to genomic actions, accumulating evidence suggests that glucocorticoids can induce some effects in a short time frame, independently of transcription/translation processes (Groeneweg et al. 2012). These effects are referred to as "nongenomic" and are mediated by ligand-activated membrane-bound GRs that trigger the activation of kinase signaling cascades, including the mitogen-activated protein kinase (MAPK) or the phosphatidylinositol 3-kinase (PI3K) pathways (Fig. 6.1) (Samarasinghe et al. 2012). However, the nature of this membrane-anchoring GR has not been clarified, yet (Deng et al. 2015; Nicolaides et al. 2017). Furthermore, GREs have been identified within the regulatory sites (D-loop) of the mitochondrial genome, suggesting a genomic interrelation between mitochondria and the nucleus (Fig. 6.1) (Demonacos et al. 1995). In addition to mitochondrial GR-GRE interaction, the mitochondrial gene expression is regulated indirectly by nuclear GR-GRE interactions, which lead to the transcription of genes encoding nuclear respiratory factors, mitochondrial RNA-processing enzymes, or mitochondrial transcription factors (Lee et al.2013).

6.4 Primary Generalized Glucocorticoid Resistance (PGGR) or "Chrousos Syndrome"

Primary generalized glucocorticoid resistance (PGGR) or "Chrousos syndrome" is a rare endocrinologic condition, which affects almost all tissues, and is characterized by generalized, partial tissue insensitivity to glucocorticoids (Charmandari et al. 2008, 2013; Charmandari and Kino 2010; Charmandari 2011, 2012; Chrousos 2011; Nicolaides et al. 2014a; Nicolaides and Charmandari 2017). Chrousos syndrome may be sporadic or can be inherited in an autosomal recessive or dominant fashion (OMIM ID: 615962, ORPHA: 786) (Charmandari et al. 2008) (Fig. 6.2). Patients with Chrousos syndrome have defective glucocorticoid negative feedback loops, which lead to compensatory hyperactivation of the HPA axis. The elevated plasma adrenocorticotropic hormone (ACTH) concentrations result in adrenal hyperplasia and increased production of steroid precursors with mineralocorticoid activity (deoxycorticosterone and corticosterone) and adrenal androgens (androstenedione, dehydroepiandrosterone (DHEA), and DHEA-sulfate (DHEAS)) (Charmandari et al. 2008, 2013; Charmandari and Kino 2010; Charmandari 2011, 2012; Chrousos 2011; Nicolaides et al. 2014a; Nicolaides and Charmandari 2017). According to the underlying pathophysiology, patients with this syndrome may be asymptomatic with only biochemical alterations or present with clinical manifestations and laboratory findings suggestive of mineralocorticoid excess (hypertension and/or hypokalemic alkalosis) and/or androgen excess (ambiguous genitalia at birth in karyotypic females, acne, hirsutism, precocious puberty, male-pattern hair loss, and hypofertility in both sexes, oligo-amenorrhea and menstrual irregularities in women, and oligospermia in men). Moreover, the increased production of corticotropin-releasing hormone (CRH) and arginine vasopressin (AVP) may result in profound anxiety and depression in some patients (Nicolaides and Charmandari 2015a, b).

The molecular basis of Chrousos syndrome has been ascribed to genetic defects in the *NR3C1* gene, such as inactivating point mutations, insertions, or deletions (Table 6.1; Fig. 6.3). Most of these defects, which have been identified in patients with this condition, were heterozygous. The tremendous progress of molecular and

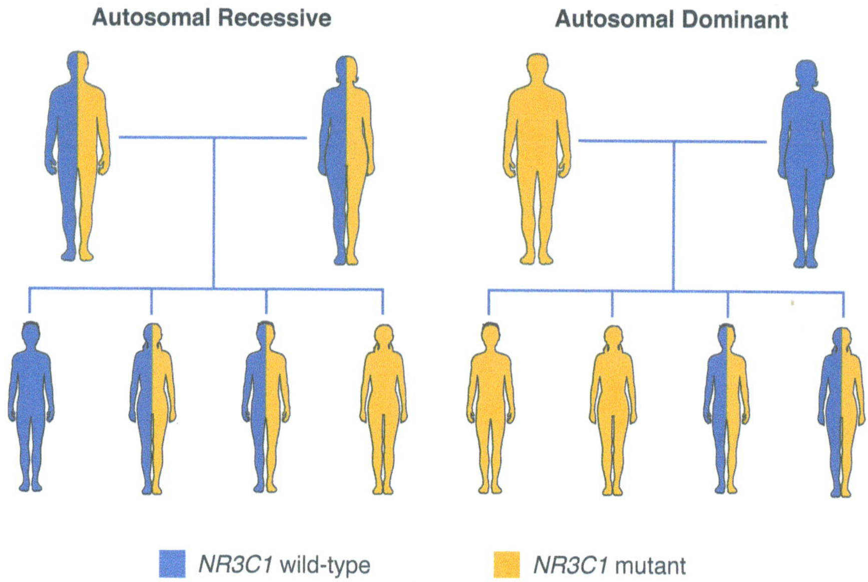

Fig. 6.2 Typical family trees demonstrating the inheritance pattern of Chrousos syndrome. The *NR3C1* wild-type allele is depicted with blue color, whereas the *NR3C1* mutant allele is shown with orange color

structural biology has enabled us and others to systematically investigate the molecular mechanisms through which the mutant hGRs cause Chrousos syndrome (listed in Table 6.1). Our research team investigated (1) the transcriptional activity of the mutant receptors, (2) the protein expression, (3) the ability of the mutant receptors to exert a dominant negative effect upon the hGRαWT-mediated transcriptional activity, (4) the affinity of the mutant receptors for the ligand, (5) the subcellular localization of the mutant receptors and the time required to complete cytoplasmic-to-nuclear translocation following exposure to the ligand, (6) the ability of the mutant receptors to bind to GREs, and (7) the interaction of the mutant receptors with the glucocorticoid receptor-interacting protein 1 (GRIP1) coactivator using glutathione-S-transferase (GST)-pull-down assays. Finally, we performed structural biology assays to investigate the mechanism through which the conformational changes of mutant receptors cause glucocorticoid resistance (Roberts et al. 2013; Nicolaides et al. 2014b, 2015b, 2016a, b).

Al Argan and collaborators recently described a new case of Chrousos syndrome (Al Argan et al. 2018). This was a 55-year-old woman who underwent a surgical removal of a paraovarian benign serous adenofibroma and a benign adrenal multinodular mass, with background changes suggestive of adrenocortical hyperplasia. Two months after the surgical procedure, the patient complained of anorexia and severe fatigue while she was unable to regain weight. Her past medical history revealed a long-standing anxiety disorder treated with benzodiazepines, chronic fatigue, acne, hirsutism, and hypomenorrhea (Al Argan et al. 2018). Her serum

Table 6.1 Mutations of the *NR3C1* gene causing Chrousos syndrome: molecular mechanisms and clinical manifestations

References	cDNA	Amino acid	Molecular mechanisms	Genotype	Phenotype
Chrousos et al. (1982), Hurley et al. (1991), and Charmandari et al. (2004)	1922 (A → T)	641 (D → V)	Transactivation ↓ Affinity for ligand ↓ (× 3) Nuclear translocation: 22 min Abnormal interaction with GRIP1	Homozygous	Hypertension Hypokalemic alkalosis
Karl et al. (1993)	4 bp deletion in exon-intron 6		hGRα number: 50% of control Inactivation of the affected allele	Heterozygous	Hirsutism Male-pattern hair-loss Menstrual irregularities
Malchoff et al. (1993), Charmandari et al. (2004)	2185 (G → A)	729 (V → I)	Transactivation ↓ Affinity for ligand ↓ (× 2) Nuclear translocation: 120 min Abnormal interaction with GRIP1	Homozygous	Precocious puberty Hyperandrogenism
Karl et al. (1996), Kino et al. (2001), and Charmandari et al. (2004)	1676 (T → A)	559 (I → N)	Transactivation ↓ Decrease in hGR binding sites Transdominance (+) Nuclear translocation: 180 min Abnormal interaction with GRIP1	Heterozygous	Hypertension Oligospermia Infertility

(continued)

Table 6.1 (continued)

References	cDNA	Amino acid	Molecular mechanisms	Genotype	Phenotype
Ruiz et al. (2001), Charmandari et al. (2006)	1430 (G → A)	477 (R → H)	Transactivation ↓ No DNA binding Nuclear translocation: 20 min	Heterozygous	Hirsutism Fatigue Hypertension
Ruiz et al. (2001), Charmandari et al. (2006)	2035 (G → A)	679 (G → S)	Transactivation ↓ Affinity for ligand ↓ (× 2) Nuclear translocation: 30 min Abnormal interaction with GRIP1	Heterozygous	Hirsutism Fatigue Hypertension
Mendonca et al. (2002), Charmandari et al. (2004)	1712 (T → C)	571 (V → A)	Transactivation ↓ Affinity for ligand ↓ (× 6) Nuclear translocation: 25 min Abnormal interaction with GRIP1	Homozygous	Ambiguous genitalia Hypertension Hypokalemia Hyperandrogenism
Vottero et al. (2002), Charmandari et al. (2004)	2241 (T → G)	747 (I → M)	Transactivation ↓ Transdominance (+) Affinity for ligand ↓ (× 2) Nuclear translocation ↓ Abnormal interaction with GRIP1	Heterozygous	Cystic acne Hirsutism Oligo-amenorrhea
Charmandari et al. (2005a, b, c)	2318 (T → C)	773 (L → P)	Transactivation ↓ Transdominance (+) Affinity for ligand ↓	Heterozygous	Fatigue Anxiety Acne

			(× 2.6) Nuclear translocation: 30 min Abnormal interaction with GRIP1		Hirsutism Hypertension
Charmandari et al. (2007)	2209 (T → C)	737 (F → L)	Transactivation ↓ Transdominance (+) Affinity for ligand ↓ (× 1.5) Nuclear translocation: 180 min	Heterozygous	Hypertension Hypokalemia
McMahon et al. (2010)	2 bp deletion at nt 2318-9	773	Transactivation ↓ Affinity for ligand: absent No suppression of IL-6	Homozygous	Hypoglycemia Fatigability with feeding Hypertension
Nader et al. (2010)	2141 (G → A)	714 (R → Q)	Transactivation ↓ Transdominance (+) Affinity for ligand ↓ (× 2) Nuclear translocation ↓ Abnormal interaction with GRIP1	Heterozygous	Hypoglycemia Hypokalemia Hypertension Mild clitoromegaly Advanced bone age Precocious pubarche
Bouligand et al. (2010)	1405 (C → T)	469 (R → X)	Transactivation ↓ Ligand-binding sites ↓ No DNA binding No nuclear translocation	Heterozygous	Adrenal hyperplasia Hypertension Hypokalemia
Zhu Hui-juan et al. (2011), Nicolaides et al. (2016a, b)	1667 (G → T)	556 (T → I)	Transactivation ↓ Transrepression ↑	Heterozygous	Adrenal incidentaloma

(continued)

Table 6.1 (continued)

References	cDNA	Amino acid	Molecular mechanisms	Genotype	Phenotype
			Affinity for ligand ↓ Nuclear translocation ↓ Abnormal interaction with GRIP1		
Roberts et al. (2013)	1268 (T → C)	423 (V → A)	Transactivation ↓ Affinity for ligand: Normal No DNA binding Nuclear translocation: 35 min Interaction with GRIP1: Normal	Heterozygous	Fatigue Anxiety Hypertension
Nicolaides et al. (2014b)	1724 (T → G)	575 (V → G)	Transactivation ↓ Transrepression ↑ Affinity for ligand ↓ (× 2) Nuclear translocation ↓ Abnormal interaction with GRIP1	Heterozygous	Melanoma Asymptomatic daughters
Nicolaides et al. (2015b)	2177 (A → G)	726 (H → R)	Transactivation ↓ Transrepression ↓ Affinity for ligand ↓ (× 2) Nuclear translocation ↓ Abnormal interaction with GRIP1	Heterozygous	Hirsutism Acne Alopecia Anxiety Fatigue Irregular menstrual cycles
Velayos et al. (2016)	1429 (C → T)	477 (R → C)	Not studied yet	Heterozygous	Mild hirsutism Asymptomatic mother

Velayos et al. (2016)	1762_1763insTTAC	588 (H → L*5)	Not studied yet	Heterozygous	Hirsutism Anxiety Chronic fatigue
Vitellius et al. (2016)	1429 (C → A)	477 (R → S)	No transactivation Affinity for ligand: Normal No DNA binding Nuclear translocation ↓	Heterozygous	Adrenal incidentaloma
Vitellius et al. (2016)	1433 (A → G)	478 (Y → C)	Transactivation ↓ Affinity for ligand: Normal DNA binding ↓ Nuclear translocation ↓	Heterozygous	Adrenal incidentaloma
Vitellius et al. (2016)	2015 (T → C)	672 (L → P)	No transactivation No affinity for ligand No DNA binding No nuclear translocation	Heterozygous	Adrenal incidentaloma
Al Argan et al. (2018)	1392del	465 (I → S)	Not studied yet	Heterozygous	Chronic fatigue Acne Hirsutism Hypomenorrhea
Molnár et al. (2018)	2141G → A	714 (R → Q)	Studied in Nader et al. (2010)	Heterozygous	Infertility Asymptomatic sister

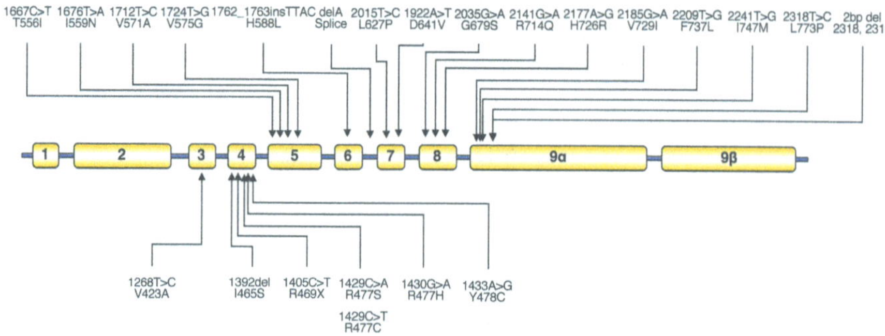

Fig. 6.3 Schematic representation of the mutations of the *NR3C1* gene causing Chrousos syndrome. Mutations in the upper panel are located in the LBD (ligand-binding domain) of the receptor, while mutations in the lower panel are located in the DBD (DNA-binding domain) of the receptor

cortisol and plasma ACTH concentrations as well as the urinary free cortisol (UFC) excretion were elevated at subsequent postoperative follow-up visits, and the patient failed to suppress the HPA axis following a 1 mg-dexamethasone suppression test. MRI of the sella turcica showed a normal pituitary. All the abovementioned findings were suggestive of Chrousos syndrome. Sequencing analysis of the *NR3C1* gene revealed a novel heterozygous frameshift defect, which resulted in a substitution of isoleucine to serine at amino acid position 465 and the formation of a stop codon (p. Ile465Serfs∗ 22). This mutation, located in exon 4, led to a truncated protein and was predicted to be pathogenic (Al Argan et al. 2018).

To the best of our knowledge, 24 genetic defects have been identified so far in the *NR3C1* gene in patients with a broad spectrum of clinical manifestations. Indeed, the hGRαV575G was found in a 70-year-old man who presented with bilateral adrenal hyperplasia during follow-up for melanoma. He was otherwise asymptomatic without any clinical manifestations of Cushing syndrome. Interestingly, his two daughters had mild hirsutism and carried the same genetic defect (Nicolaides et al. 2014b). In addition, we have described a 30-year-old woman with severe clinical manifestations of Chrousos syndrome, including hirsutism, acne, alopecia, anxiety, fatigue, and irregular menstrual cycles, who carried a heterozygous mutation at nucleotide position 2177, leading to arginine (R) to histidine (H) substitution at amino acid position 726 (hGRαH726R) (Nicolaides et al. 2015b). These cases indicate that a specific genetic defect in the *NR3C1* gene may lead to a very broad spectrum of clinical manifestations of the syndrome. Given this, as well as the fact that the number of cases that have been described thus far is small, genotype-phenotype correlations cannot be accurate.

Patients with Chrousos syndrome, who present with clinical manifestations of mineralocorticoid and/or androgen excess, have to be treated with daily high doses of mineralocorticoid-sparing synthetic glucocorticoids, such as dexamethasone (1–3 mg) (Charmandari et al. 2008, 2013; Charmandari 2011, 2012; Chrousos 2011; Nicolaides et al. 2016a, b). The goal of treatment is to decrease the excess secretion of ACTH, thereby decreasing the concentrations of adrenal steroids with mineralocorticoid and/or androgenic activity. The dose of dexamethasone should be carefully adjusted according to clinical manifestations and biochemical profile of each patient. It is important to note that the HPA axis should be adequately suppressed by dexamethasone to prevent the development of ACTH-dependent adenomas (Charmandari et al. 2008, 2013; Charmandari 2011, 2012; Chrousos 2011; Nicolaides et al. 2016a, b).

6.5 Beyond *NR3C1* Genetic Defects

Interestingly, many patients with Chrousos syndrome do not harbor a *NR3C1* genetic defect, suggesting that other genes encoding factors, which participate directly or indirectly in the glucocorticoid signal transduction, might be defective. Indeed, Gossain and coworkers presented a patient with Chrousos syndrome who did not have any mutations in the *NR3C1* gene (Gossain et al. 2018). This patient was a 41-year-old female with hirsutism. Endocrinologic evaluation revealed elevated plasma ACTH and serum cortisol concentrations and increased UFC excretion. In addition, the patient had resistance to dexamethasone suppression and normal findings in pituitary and adrenal imaging (Gossain et al. 2018). On the other hand, the same genetic defect can be found in patients with completely different clinical manifestations (Nader et al. 2010; Molnár et al. 2018). Nader et al. identified the pathologic Arg714Gln mutation in the *NR3C1* gene in a 2-year-old child with generalized seizure, hypertension, premature pubarche, hypoglycemia, and hypokalemia (Nader et al. 2010). The Arg714Gln mutation was also found in a 31-year-old woman, who was evaluated for infertility, as well as in her asymptomatic sister (Molnár et al. 2018). In such cases, the ever-increasing application of next-generation sequencing will undoubtedly reveal defects in genes that encode partners of hGR.

6.6 *NR3C1* Polymorphisms

In addition to the *NR3C1* mutations (Table 6.1), three *NR3C1* polymorphisms have been associated with alterations in glucocorticoid sensitivity (van Rossum et al. 2004; Marti et al. 2006; Quax et al. 2013; Kino 2018). Their frequency reaches up to 10% in various populations, and they do not have a preferential distribution in the functional domains of hGR (Kino 2018). Two of them, the N363S and B*clI* polymorphisms, have been associated with glucocorticoid hypersensitivity, whereas the ER22/23EK has been linked to glucocorticoid resistance (Kino 2018).

In the N363S polymorphism, aspartic acid has been replaced by serine at amino acid position 363, leading to an altered GR protein with slightly increased transcriptional activity (Huizenga et al. 1998). Carriers of the N363S polymorphism display higher sensitivity to glucocorticoids in vivo, increased insulin response to exogenous dexamethasone administration, higher BMI, higher waist-to-hip ratio, and a tendency toward lower bone mineral density in trabecular bone (Charmandari 2011). They also have elevated cholesterol and triglyceride concentrations and higher incidence of coronary artery disease independent of weight (Dobson et al. 2001; Lin et al. 2003a, b; van Rossum and Lamberts 2004; Charmandari 2011).

In addition to the N363S polymorphism, the *BclI* has also been associated with increased sensitivity to glucocorticoids (Kino 2018). This polymorphism is due to a cytosine-to-guanine nucleotide substitution located at 646 bp downstream of exon 2. Subjects with this polymorphism have central obesity, hyperinsulinism, and increased response to exogenous dexamethasone (van Rossum et al. 2003). They also have increased susceptibility to hypertension, bronchial asthma, and mood disorders (Manenschijn et al. 2009; Charmandari 2011; van Moorsel et al. 2015).

The ER22/23EK polymorphism has been associated with glucocorticoid resistance. This polymorphism consists of two linked, single-nucleotide mutations in codons 22 and 23 in exon 2 of the hGR gene. The first mutation in codon 22 is silent, not resulting in an amino acid change (GAG to GAA, both coding for glutamic acid (E)), but the second mutation in codon 23 (AGG to AAG) results in arginine (R) to lysine (K) substitution (Kino 2018). Carriers of the ER22/23EK polymorphism display relative glucocorticoid resistance, lower fasting insulin concentrations and improved insulin sensitivity, lower total and LDL cholesterol concentrations, and lower CRP concentrations (van Rossum et al. 2002). These effects lead to a healthier metabolic profile, decreased incidence of cardiovascular disease and dementia, and increased longevity (van Rossum et al. 2004; Charmandari 2011).

6.7 Concluding Remarks

Primary generalized glucocorticoid resistance or Chrousos syndrome is a rare endocrinologic condition caused by genetic defects in the *NR3C1* gene. Affected patients may be asymptomatic or present with clinical manifestations and laboratory findings suggestive of mineralocorticoid and/or androgen excess. The concurrent progress of molecular and structural biology has enabled us to have a deeper understanding of how a mutant receptor leads to partial tissue glucocorticoid resistance. The ever-increasing application of next-generation sequencing technologies will uncover novel defects in genes encoding proteins that influence directly or indirectly the glucocorticoid signaling cascade.

References

Al Argan R, Saskin A, Yang JW, D'Agostino MD, Rivera J (2018) Glucocorticoid resistance syndrome caused by a novel NR3C1 point mutation. Endocr J 65(11):1139–1146
Bamberger CM, Bamberger AM, de Castro M, Chrousos GP (1995) Glucocorticoid receptor β, a potential endogenous inhibitor of glucocorticoid action in humans. J Clin Invest 95:2435–2441
Beger C, Gerdes K, Lauten M et al (2003) Expression and structural analysis of glucocorticoid receptor isoform gamma in human leukaemia cells using an isoform-specific real-time polymerase chain reaction approach. Br J Haematol 122(2):245–252
Bouligand J, Delemer B, Hecart AC et al (2010) Familial glucocorticoid receptor haploinsufficiency by non-sense mediated mRNA decay, adrenal hyperplasia and apparent mineralocorticoid excess. PLoS One 5:e13563
Charmandari E (2011) Primary generalized glucocorticoid resistance and hypersensitivity. Horm Res Paediatr 76:145–155
Charmandari E (2012) Primary generalized glucocorticoid resistance and hypersensitivity: the end-organ involvement in the stress response. Sci Signal 5:pt5
Charmandari E, Kino T (2010) Chrousos syndrome: a seminal report, a phylogenetic enigma and the clinical implications of glucocorticoid signaling changes. Eur J Clin Investig 40:932–942
Charmandari E, Kino T, Vottero A, Souvatzoglou E, Bhattacharyya N, Chrousos GP (2004) Natural glucocorticoid receptor mutants causing generalized glucocorticoid resistance: molecular genotype, genetic transmission and clinical phenotype. J Clin Endocrinol Metab 89(4):1939–1949
Charmandari E, Chrousos GP, Ichijo T et al (2005a) The human glucocorticoid receptor (hGR) β isoform suppresses the transcriptional activity of hGRα by interfering with formation of active coactivator complexes. Mol Endocrinol 19:52–64
Charmandari E, Raji A, Kino T et al (2005b) A novel point mutation in the ligand-binding domain (LBD) of the human glucocorticoid receptor (hGR) causing generalized glucocorticoid resistance: the importance of the C terminus of hGR LBD in conferring transactivational activity. J Clin Endocrinol Metab 90:3696–3705
Charmandari E, Tsigos C, Chrousos GP (2005c) Endocrinology of the stress response. Annu Rev Physiol 67:259–284
Charmandari E, Kino T, Ichijo T, Zachman K, Alatsatianos A, Chrousos GP (2006) Functional characterization of the natural human glucocorticoid receptor (hGR) mutants hGRαR477H and hGRαG679S associated with generalized glucocorticoid resistance. J Clin Endocrinol Metab 91:1535–1543
Charmandari E, Kino T, Ichijo T et al (2007) A novel point mutation in helix 11 of the ligand-binding domain of the human glucocorticoid receptor gene causing generalized glucocorticoid resistance. J Clin Endocrinol Metab 92:3986–3990
Charmandari E, Kino T, Ichijo T, Chrousos GP (2008) Generalized glucocorticoid resistance: clinical aspects, molecular mechanisms, and implications of a rare genetic disorder. J Clin Endocrinol Metab 93:1563–1572
Charmandari E, Kino T, Chrousos GP (2013) Primary generalized familial and sporadic glucocorticoid resistance (Chrousos syndrome) and hypersensitivity. Endocr Dev 24:67–85
Chrousos G (2011) Q&A: primary generalized glucocorticoid resistance. BMC Med 9:27
Chrousos GP, Kino T (2005) Intracellular glucocorticoid signaling: a formerly simple system turns stochastic. Sci STKE 2005(304):pe48
Chrousos GP, Vingerhoeds A, Brandon D et al (1982) Primary cortisol resistance in man. A glucocorticoid receptor-mediated disease. J Clin Invest 69:1261–1269
Demonacos C, Djordjevic-Markovic R, Tsawdaroglou N, Sekeris CE (1995) The mitochondrion as a primary site of action of glucocorticoids: the interaction of the glucocorticoid receptor with mitochondrial DNA sequences showing partial similarity to the nuclear glucocorticoid responsive elements. J Steroid Biochem Mol Biol 55(1):43–55
Deng Q, Waxse B, Riquelme D, Zhang J, Aguilera G (2015) Helix 8 of the ligand binding domain of the glucocorticoid receptor (GR) is essential for ligand binding. Mol Cell Endocrinol 408:23–32

Dobson MG, Redfern CP, Unwin N, Weaver JU (2001) The N363S polymorphism of the glucocorticoid receptor: potential contribution to central obesity in men and lack of association with other risk factors for coronary heart disease and diabetes mellitus. J Clin Endocrinol Metab 86 (5):2270–2274
Galon J, Franchimont D, Hiroi N et al (2002) Gene profiling reveals unknown enhancing and suppressive actions of glucocorticoids on immune cells. FASEB J 16(1):61–71
Gossain VV, El-Rifai M, Krishnan P, Bhavsar B (2018) Cushing's syndrome with no clinical stigmata - a variant of glucocorticoid resistance syndrome. Clin Diabetes Endocrinol 4:23
Grad I, Picard D (2007) The glucocorticoid responses are shaped by molecular chaperones. Mol Cell Endocrinol 275(1–2):2–12
Groeneweg FL, Karst H, de Kloet ER, Joëls M (2012) Mineralocorticoid and glucocorticoid receptors at the neuronal membrane, regulators of nongenomic corticosteroid signalling. Mol Cell Endocrinol 350(2):299–309
Huizenga NA, Koper JW, De Lange P et al (1998) A polymorphism in the glucocorticoid receptor gene may be associated with and increased sensitivity to glucocorticoids in vivo. J Clin Endocrinol Metab 83(1):144–151
Hurley DM, Accili D, Stratakis CA et al (1991) Point mutation causing a single amino acid substitution in the hormone binding domain of the glucocorticoid receptor in familial glucocorticoid resistance. J Clin Invest 87:680–686
Karl M, Lamberts SW, Detera-Wadleigh SD et al (1993) Familial glucocorticoid resistance caused by a splice site deletion in the human glucocorticoid receptor gene. J Clin Endocrinol Metab 76:683–689
Karl M, Lamberts SW, Koper JW et al (1996) Cushing's disease preceded by generalized glucocorticoid resistance: clinical consequences of a novel, dominant-negative glucocorticoid receptor mutation. Proc Assoc Am Physicians 108:296–307
Kino T (2018) Single nucleotide variations of the human GR gene manifested as pathologic mutations or polymorphisms. Endocrinology 159(7):2506–2519
Kino T, Stauber RH, Resau JH, Pavlakis GN, Chrousos GP (2001) Pathologic human GR mutant has a transdominant negative effect on the wild-type GR by inhibiting its translocation into the nucleus: importance of the ligand-binding domain for intracellular GR trafficking. J Clin Endocrinol Metab 86:5600–5608
Krett NL, Pillay S, Moalli PA, Greipp PR, Rosen ST (1995) A variant glucocorticoid receptor messenger RNA is expressed in multiple myeloma patients. Cancer Res 55(13):2727–2729
Lee SR, Kim HK, Song IS et al (2013) Glucocorticoids and their receptors: insights into specific roles in mitochondria. Prog Biophys Mol Biol 112(1–2):44–54
Lin RC, Wang XL, Dalziel B et al (2003a) Association of obesity, but not diabetes or hypertension, with glucocorticoid receptor N363S variant. Obes Res 11(6):802–808
Lin RC, Wang XL, Morris BJ (2003b) Association of coronary artery disease with glucocorticoid receptor N363S variant. Hypertension 41(3):404–407
Lu NZ, Cidlowski JA (2005) Translational regulatory mechanisms generate N-terminal glucocorticoid receptor isoforms with unique transcriptional target genes. Mol Cell 18:331–342
Lu NZ, Collins JB, Grissom SF, Cidlowski JA (2007) Selective regulation of bone cell apoptosis by translational isoforms of the glucocorticoid receptor. Mol Cell Biol 27(20):7143–7160
Malchoff DM, Brufsky A, Reardon G et al (1993) A mutation of the glucocorticoid receptor in primary cortisol resistance. J Clin Invest 91:1918–1925
Manenschijn L, van den Akker EL, Lamberts SW, van Rossum EF (2009) Clinical features associated with glucocorticoid receptor polymorphisms an overview. Ann N Y Acad Sci 1179 (1):179–198
Marti A, Ochoa MC, Sánchez-Villegas A et al (2006) Meta-analysis on the effect of the N363S polymorphism of the glucocorticoid receptor gene (GRL) on human obesity. BMC Med Genet 7 (1):50
McBeth L, Nwaneri AC, Grabnar M, Demeter J, Nestor-Kalinoski A, Hinds TD Jr (2016) Glucocorticoid receptor beta increases migration of human bladder cancer cells. Oncotarget 7 (19):27313–27324

McMahon SK, Pretorius CJ, Ungerer JP et al (2010) Neonatal complete generalized glucocorticoid resistance and growth hormone deficiency caused by a novel homozygous mutation in Helix 12 of the ligand binding domain of the glucocorticoid receptor gene (NR3C1). J Clin Endocrinol Metab 95:297–302

Mendonca BB, Leite MV, de Castro M et al (2002) Female pseudohermaphroditism caused by a novel homozygous missense mutation of the GR gene. J Clin Endocrinol Metab 87:1805–1809

Molnár Á, Patócs A, Likó I, Nyírő G, Rácz K, Tóth M, Sármán B (2018) An unexpected, mild phenotype of glucocorticoid resistance associated with glucocorticoid receptor gene mutation case report and review of the literature. BMC Med Genet 19(1):37

Nader N, Bachrach BE, Hurt DE et al (2010) A novel point mutation in the helix 10 of the human glucocorticoid receptor causes generalized glucocorticoid resistance by disrupting the structure of the ligand-binding domain. J Clin Endocrinol Metab 95:2281–2285

Nicolaides NC, Charmandari E (2017) Novel insights into the molecular mechanisms underlying generalized glucocorticoid resistance and hypersensitivity syndromes. Hormones (Athens) 16 (2):124–138

Nicolaides NC, Galata Z, Kino T, Chrousos GP, Charmandari E (2010) The human glucocorticoid receptor: molecular basis of biologic function. Steroids 75:1–12

Nicolaides NC, Charmandari E, Chrousos GP, Kino T (2014a) Recent advances in the molecular mechanisms determining tissue sensitivity to glucocorticoids: novel mutations, circadian rhythm and ligand-induced repression of the human glucocorticoid receptor. BMC Endocr Disord 14:71

Nicolaides NC, Roberts ML, Kino T et al (2014b) A novel point mutation of the human glucocorticoid receptor gene causes primary generalized glucocorticoid resistance through impaired interaction with the LXXLL motif of the p160 coactivators: dissociation of the transactivating and transreppressive activities. J Clin Endocrinol Metab 99:E902–E907

Nicolaides NC, Kyratzi E, Lamprokostopoulou A, Chrousos GP, Charmandari E (2015a) Stress, the stress system and the role of glucocorticoids. Neuroimmunomodulation 22:6–19

Nicolaides NC, Geer EB, Vlachakis D et al (2015b) A novel mutation of the hGR gene causing Chrousos syndrome. Eur J Clin Investig 45:782–791

Nicolaides N, Lamprokostopoulou A, Sertedaki A, Charmandari E (2016a) Recent advances in the molecular mechanisms causing primary generalized glucocorticoid resistance. Hormones (Athens) 15(1):23–34

Nicolaides NC, Skyrla E, Vlachakis D et al (2016b) Functional characterization of the hGRαT556I causing Chrousos syndrome. Eur J Clin Investig 46(1):42–49

Nicolaides NC, Kino T, Roberts ML et al (2017) The role of S-Palmitoylation of the human glucocorticoid receptor (hGR) in mediating the nongenomic glucocorticoid actions. J Mol Biochem 6(1):3–12

Oakley RH, Cidlowski JA (2011) Cellular processing of the glucocorticoid receptor gene and protein: new mechanisms for generating tissue-specific actions of glucocorticoids. J Biol Chem 286:3177–3184

Quax RA, Manenschijn L, Koper JW et al (2013) Glucocorticoid sensitivity in health and disease. Nat Rev Endocrinol 9(11):670–686

Ramamoorthy S, Cidlowski JA (2016) Corticosteroids: mechanisms of action in health and disease. Rheum Dis Clin N Am 42(1):15–31

Ray DW, Davis JR, White A, Clark AJ (1996) Glucocorticoid receptor structure and function in glucocorticoid-resistant small cell lung carcinoma cells. Cancer Res 56(14):3276–3280

Rhen T, Cidlowski JA (2005) Anti-inflammatory action of glucocorticoids–new mechanisms for old drugs. N Engl J Med 353(16):1711–1723

Roberts ML, Kino T, Nicolaides NC et al (2013) A novel point mutation in the DNA-binding domain (DBD) of the human glucocorticoid receptor causes primary generalized glucocorticoid resistance by disrupting the hydrophobic structure of its DBD. J Clin Endocrinol Metab 98: E790–E795

Ruiz M, Lind U, Gafvels M et al (2001) Characterization of two novel mutations in the glucocorticoid receptor gene in patients with primary cortisol resistance. Clin Endocrinol 55:363–371
Samarasinghe RA, Witchell SF, DeFranco DB (2012) Cooperativity and complementarity: synergies in non-classical and classical glucocorticoid signaling. Cell Cycle 11(15):2819–2827
Stechschulte LA, Wuescher L, Marino JS, Hill JW, Eng C, Hinds TD Jr (2014) Glucocorticoid receptor β stimulates Akt1 growth pathway by attenuation of PTEN. J Biol Chem 289:17885–17894
van Moorsel D, van Greevenbroek MM, Schaper NC et al (2015) BclI glucocorticoid receptor polymorphism in relation to cardiovascular variables: the Hoorn and CODAM studies. Eur J Endocrinol 173(4):455–464
van Rossum EF, Lamberts SW (2004) Polymorphisms in the glucocorticoid receptor gene and their associations with metabolic parameters and body composition. Recent Prog Horm Res 59:333–357
van Rossum EF, Koper JW, Huizenga NA et al (2002) A polymorphism in the glucocorticoid receptor gene, which decreases sensitivity to glucocorticoids in vivo, is associated with low insulin and cholesterol levels. Diabetes 51(10):3128–3134
van Rossum EF, Koper JW, van den Beld AW et al (2003) Identification of the BclI polymorphism in the glucocorticoid receptor gene: association with sensitivity to glucocorticoids in vivo and body mass index. Clin Endocrinol 59(5):585–592
van Rossum EF, Voorhoeve PG, te Velde SJ et al (2004) The ER22/23EK polymorphism in the glucocorticoid receptor gene is associated with a beneficial body composition and muscle strength in young adults. J Clin Endocrinol Metab 89(8):4004–4009
Velayos T, Grau G, Rica I, Pérez-Nanclares G, Gaztambide S (2016) Glucocorticoid resistance syndrome caused by two novel mutations in the NR3C1 gene. Endocrinol Nutr 63(7):369–371
Vitellius G, Fagart J, Delemer B et al (2016) Three novel heterozygous point mutations of NR3C1 causing glucocorticoid resistance. Hum Mutat 37(8):794–803
Vottero A, Kino T, Combe H, Lecomte P, Chrousos GP (2002) A novel, C-terminal dominant negative mutation of the GR causes familial glucocorticoid resistance through abnormal interactions with p160 steroid receptor coactivators. J Clin Endocrinol Metab 87:2658–2667
Wang Q, Lu PH, Shi ZF et al (2015) Glucocorticoid receptor β acts as a co-activator of T-cell factor 4 and enhances glioma cell proliferation. Mol Neurobiol 52(3):1106–1118
Wu I, Shin SC, Cao Y et al (2013) Selective glucocorticoid receptor translational isoforms reveal glucocorticoid-induced apoptotic transcriptomes. Cell Death Dis 4:e453
Yin Y, Zhang X, Li Z et al (2013) Glucocorticoid receptor β regulates injury-mediated astrocyte activation and contributes to glioma pathogenesis via modulation of β-catenin/TCF transcriptional activity. Neurobiol Dis 59:165–176
Yudt MR, Jewell CM, Bienstock RJ, Cidlowski JA (2003) Molecular origins for the dominant negative function of human glucocorticoid receptor β. Mol Cell Biol 23:4319–4330
Zannas AS, Chrousos GP (2017) Epigenetic programming by stress and glucocorticoids along the human lifespan. Mol Psychiatry 22(5):640–646
Zhu HJ, Dai YF, Wang O et al (2011) Generalized glucocorticoid resistance accompanied with an adrenocortical adenoma and caused by a novel point mutation of human glucocorticoid receptor gene. Chin Med J 124:551–555

Part III
Endocrine Diseases Inherited as Monogenic Traits: Hereditary Diseases Predisposing to Endocrine Tumors

Chapter 7
Overview of Genetically Determined Diseases/Multiple Endocrine Neoplasia Syndromes Predisposing to Endocrine Tumors

Abel Decmann, Attila Patócs, and Peter Igaz

Abstract In this chapter, we present an overview of multiple endocrine neoplasia syndromes including their most important clinical and molecular features. Multiple endocrine neoplasia type 1 and 2 syndromes (MEN1 and MEN2) are discussed in detail. Syndromes that are presented in other chapters are only briefly mentioned. We discuss the relevance of germline gene alterations in apparently sporadic endocrine tumors, e.g., medullary thyroid cancer, primary hyperparathyroidism, and neuroendocrine tumors. McCune-Albright syndrome that only exists in non-hereditary, sporadic forms is also discussed in detail, as tumors of several endocrine organs can develop in the same individual.

Keywords Multiple endocrine neoplasia · MEN1 · MEN2 · Mutation · Sporadic tumors · McCune-Albright syndrome

A. Decmann
2nd Department of Internal Medicine, Faculty of Medicine, Semmelweis University, Budapest, Hungary

A. Patócs
Department of Laboratory Medicine, Faculty of Medicine, Semmelweis University, Budapest, Hungary

"Lendület" Hereditary Endocrine Tumors Research Group, Hungarian Academy of Sciences and Semmelweis University, Budapest, Hungary

Department of Molecular Genetics, National Institute of Oncology, Budapest, Hungary

P. Igaz (✉)
2nd Department of Internal Medicine, Faculty of Medicine, Semmelweis University, Budapest, Hungary

MTA-SE Molecular Medicine Research Group, Hungarian Academy of Sciences and Semmelweis University, Budapest, Hungary
e-mail: igaz.peter@med.semmelweis-univ.hu

P. Igaz, A. Patócs (eds.), *Genetics of Endocrine Diseases and Syndromes*, Experientia Supplementum 111, https://doi.org/10.1007/978-3-030-25905-1_7

List of Abbreviations

ACTH	Adrenocorticotropic hormone
CaSR	Calcium sensor
CNS	Central nervous system
CS	Cowden syndrome
FHH	Familial hypocalciuric hypercalcemia
FMTC	Familial medullary thyroid cancer
GEP-NET	Gastroenteropancreatic neuroendocrine tumor
GH	Growth hormone
GNAS1	Guanine nucleotide-binding protein, alpha-stimulating activity polypeptide 1
HD	Hirschsprung's disease
HPT-JT	Hyperparathyroidism-jaw tumor syndrome
MAS	McCune-Albright syndrome
MEN	Multiple endocrine neoplasia syndrome (1, 2A, 2B, 4)
MTC	Medullary thyroid cancer
NET	Neuroendocrine tumor
NF1	Neurofibromatosis type 1
NSHPT	Neonatal severe hyperparathyroidism
OMIM	Online Mendelian Inheritance in Man
PHPT	Primary hyperparathyroidism
PJS	Peutz-Jeghers syndrome
pNET	Pancreatic neuroendocrine tumor
RET	Rearranged during transfection
TSC	Tuberous sclerosis complex
VHL	von Hippel-Lindau syndrome
VIP	Vasoactive intestinal peptide

7.1 Introduction

Multiple endocrine neoplasia syndromes include mostly rare diseases where tumors of different endocrine organs occur in the same individual both as familial and sporadic cases. The prototypes of multiple endocrine neoplasia (MEN) syndromes are MEN1 and MEN2, but there are many more syndromes with endocrine manifestations that can be thus regarded as multiple endocrine neoplasia syndromes.

The vast majority of multiple endocrine neoplasia syndromes is linked to mutations of tumor suppressor genes, and thus their pathogenesis follows the classical Knudson's model with an inherited affected allele with a germline mutation and a second somatic mutation leading to the loss of heterozygosity and disease. Mutations of tumor suppressor genes are inactivating. On the other hand, multiple endocrine neoplasia type 2 (MEN2) syndrome is caused by activating mutations of a proto-oncogene. Whereas mutations of tumor suppressor genes have severe consequences on gene functioning (e.g., nonsense or frameshift point mutations, insertions, deletions), activating mutations are mostly missense mutations leading to amino acid replacements.

In this chapter, we present an overview of hereditary diseases/multiple endocrine neoplasia syndromes and highlight differences and similarities.

7.2 Multiple Endocrine Neoplasia Syndromes

The term "multiple endocrine neoplasia" syndrome cannot be defined easily. Hereditary or genetically determined syndromes predispose patients to endocrine neoplasia, often affecting several organs in the same individual or in different members of affected families. Some syndromes, e.g., MEN1, include several endocrine manifestations (e.g., hyperparathyroidism, pituitary tumors, duodenopancreatic tumors), whereas others have only one endocrine tumor manifestation (e.g., familial medullary thyroid cancer (FMTC, as part of MEN2) or hyperparathyroidism-jaw tumor syndrome) (Table 7.1). In this chapter, we briefly present these syndromes which are inherited, or in other words, familial syndromes with the exception of the also discussed McCune-Albright syndrome that exists only as a sporadic syndrome. Most of these syndromes have autosomal dominant inheritance with high penetrance.

MEN1 and MEN2 will be discussed in more details, whereas other tumor syndromes that are presented in detail in other chapters will only be briefly mentioned or not be covered here.

7.2.1 *Multiple Endocrine Neoplasia Type 1*

Multiple endocrine neoplasia type 1 (MEN1; OMIM: 131100) is caused by inactivating mutations of the *MEN1* tumor suppressor gene. To date, more than 1300 different mutations have been described (Lemos and Thakker 2008). MEN1 syndrome is inherited in an autosomal dominant trait, and there are no recognized genotype-phenotype correlations so far. It has a prevalence of 2–3 per 100,000 population (Giusti et al. 2013). *MEN1* encodes a protein, called menin, consisting of 610 amino acids. The exact function of menin is unknown, but it is a putative tumor suppressor. It is a nuclear protein that regulates multiple signaling pathways (transforming growth factor beta (TGFβ) (Kaji et al. 2001), bone morphogenetic protein (BMP) (Naito et al. 2005), Wnt/β-catenin (Cao et al. 2009), Ras (Gallo et al. 2002), etc. but is also regulated by proteins, signaling pathways, and posttranslational modifications (prolactin, TGFβ, somatostatin, etc.); thus it is considered as a scaffold protein. These mechanisms appear to be highly tissue-specific (Matkar et al. 2013). *MEN1* mutations can result in a truncated protein, which lacks nuclear localization signals or some missense mutations which can reduce the stability of

Table 7.1 Overview of hereditary diseases/multiple endocrine neoplasia syndromes predisposing to endocrine tumor formation

Manifestation	Disease	Syndromes
Thyroid glands	MTC	MEN2A, MEN2B, FMTC
	Thyroid nodules, adenoma or carcinoma	Carney complex, Peutz-Jeghers syndrome, Cowden syndrome, McCune-Albright syndrome
Parathyroid glands	PHPT	MEN1, MEN4, MEN2A, HP-JT
Neuroendocrine tumors	BP-NET	MEN1
	Thymic	MEN1
	pNET	MEN1 (40–80%), NF1 (<10%), VHL 10–17%), TSC1 (rare), TSC2 (rare)
Adrenal gland	Pheochromocytoma	MEN2A, MEN2B, NF1, VHL, familial PPGL syndromes
	Adrenocortical adenoma or cancer	MEN1, McCune-Albright syndrome
	Hyperplasia	Carney complex
Gonads	Ovarian	Peutz-Jeghers syndrome
	Testicular	Peutz-Jeghers syndrome, Carney complex, McCune-Albright syndrome
Pituitary	Adenomas	Carney complex, MEN1, McCune-Albright syndrome, FIPA

BP-NET bronchopulmonary neuroendocrine tumor, *FIPA* familial isolated pituitary adenoma syndrome, *FMTC* familial medullary thyroid carcinoma syndrome, *HP-JT* hyperparathyroidism-jaw tumor syndrome, *MEN1* multiple endocrine neoplasia syndrome type 1, *MEN2A* multiple endocrine neoplasia syndrome type 2A, *MEN2B* multiple endocrine neoplasia syndrome type 2B, *MEN4* multiple endocrine neoplasia syndrome type 4, *MTC* medullary thyroid carcinoma, *NF1* neurofibromatosis type 1, *PHPT* primary hyperparathyroidism, *pNET* pancreatic neuroendocrine tumor, *PPGL* pheochromocytoma/paraganglioma, *TSC1* tuberous sclerosis complex type 1, *TSC2* tuberous sclerosis complex type 2, *VHL* von Hippel-Lindau syndrome

menin and enhance its degradation. About 42% of mutations are frameshift mutations, 25.5% are missense mutations, 14% are nonsense mutations, 10.5% are splice-site mutations, 5.5% are in-frame indel mutations, and 2.5% are gross deletions (Concolino et al. 2016). The effects of missense mutations of *MEN1* are inactivation of menin, alteration of menin's capacity to regulate the target promoters, reduced stability of the menin protein, or enhanced proteolytic degradation (Lemos and Thakker 2008; Matkar et al. 2013; Concolino et al. 2016).

MEN1 has over 90% penetrance for primary hyperparathyroidism (mostly parathyroid hyperplasia) by the age of 40 years. Other common endocrine manifestations are gastroenteropancreatic neuroendocrine tumors (GEP-NETs) with up to 80–90% penetrance [gastrinoma (30–40%), insulinoma, glucagonoma, VIPoma], foregut carcinoids (bronchial, thymic), anterior pituitary tumors (prolactinoma, ACTH producing, etc.), or adrenocortical tumors (mostly benign) (Doherty 2003; Ito et al. 2013). Non-endocrine features are facial angiofibromas (85%), lipomas (30%), and collagenomas (70%) (Brandi et al. 2001; Saggini and Brandi 2011; Vashi et al. 2012). Usually, patients develop two or more tumors mainly in the parathyroid

Table 7.2 When and how to screen confirmed MEN1 patients? Based on Brandi et al. (2001)

Tumor	Subtype	When to start screening (years)	Biochemical tests yearly (plasma or serum)	Imaging (time interval)
Parathyroid adenoma		8	Calcium, PTH	
	Insulinoma	5	Fasting glucose and insulin	
	Gastrinoma	20	Gastrin (± gastric pH)	
	Other	<10	Chromogranin-A, pancreatic polypeptide, glucagon, VIP	MRI or CT or EUS (yearly) or ^{111}In-DTPA-octreotide scan
Anterior hypophysis		5	Prolactin, IGF-1	MRI (3 yearly)
Adrenal		<10	Only functional tumors and/or tumors smaller than 1 cm diagnosed by imaging	MRI or CT (yearly)
Foregut (thymic, bronchus) carcinoid		15		CT or MRI (1–2 yearly)

CT computed tomography, *IGF-1* insulin-like growth factor 1, *MRI* magnetic resonance imaging, *PTH* parathyroid hormone, *VIP* vasoactive intestinal polypeptide

glands, pancreas, and pituitary gland. Patients with malignant duodenopancreatic NETs and thymic or bronchial NETs have the most severe variants of this disease.

MEN1 syndrome should be considered, if there is a family history of endocrine tumors of the pancreas, as about 20–25% of all patients with sporadic gastrinoma (Zollinger-Ellison syndrome) have MEN1, family members with pituitary or parathyroid disease or renal colic with NETs, patient with a young age onset of pNET (pancreatic NET), and with multiple pNETs (Jensen et al. 2008; Thakker et al. 2012; Norton et al. 2015). Genetic screening is recommended for MEN1 if an individual has two or more MEN1-related tumors, multiple abnormal parathyroid glands before the age of 30 years, recurrent hyperparathyroidism at a young age, gastrinoma and hyperparathyroidism or multiple pNETs at any age or a family history of kidney stones, and first-degree relatives of a known MEN1 mutation carrier (either symptomatic or asymptomatic) (Marx et al. 1986; Vasen et al. 1989; Brandi et al. 2001). Eighty-three percent of patients develop clinical manifestations of MEN1 after age of 21 years (Goudet et al. 2015). Clinical screening in a MEN1 mutation carrier should be performed following the most recent guidelines (Table 7.2). Commencing tumor screening is important from the recommended age, because following regular screening, the tumors might be potentially well treatable.

The preferred parathyroid operation is subtotal parathyroidectomy with or without autograft implantation (usually under the forearm skin) along with simultaneous transcervical near-total thymectomy (Brandi et al. 2001). Thymectomy is aimed to prevent the development of the potentially malignant thymic neuroendocrine tumor, which represents the only prophylactic operation in MEN1.

In 5–25% of clinically diagnosed MEN1 patients, a pathogenic mutation could not be identified in the *MEN1* gene. Some of these cases are phenocopies that arise either as only a coincidence of two relatively common sporadic endocrine tumors (e.g., hyperparathyroidism and pituitary microadenoma) or caused by other gene mutations like the MEN4 syndrome or familial isolated pituitary adenomas (FIPA) (Lemos and Thakker 2008; Thakker et al. 2012; De Laat et al. 2018).

Children of patients with *MEN1* mutation have 50% chance to inherit the MEN1 syndrome. Genetic screening should be performed in members of affected families. Since mutations can affect the whole gene, all exons and exon-intron boundaries should be sequenced. MLPA (multiplex ligation-dependent probe amplification) might be needed in cases with strong clinical suspicion to detect the deletion of the *MEN1* gene. Affected children should be screened for clinical manifestations (Table 7.2). However, it is still a matter of debate whether young children with *MEN1* mutations should be screened from early childhood or not. An argument for postponed routine screening is that symptomatic or severe manifestations of MEN1 occur rarely below the age of 16 years. Considering psychological burden and cost-effectiveness, some authors propose the postponement of routine screening in asymptomatic children until the age of 16 years (Manoharan et al. 2017).

7.2.2 Multiple Endocrine Neoplasia Type 4

Multiple endocrine neoplasia type 4 (MEN4; OMIM: 610755) is similar to the MEN1 syndrome which is also following an autosomal dominant inheritance. The inactivating mutations of cyclin-dependent kinase inhibitor 1B (*CDKN1B*) are responsible for this syndrome that is very rare (less than 20 cases described in the literature) and was and only differentiated from MEN1 in 2008 (Alrezk et al. 2017). Almost all of the affected patients have primary hyperparathyroidism. Pituitary adenomas (growth hormone or adrenocorticotropin-secreting and nonfunctioning) are also common features of MEN4 syndrome (Pellegata 2012). Less than half of the reported patients had GEP-NETs (Alrezk et al. 2017). In contrast to MEN1, adrenal neoplasias have not been reported so far.

7.2.3 Multiple Endocrine Neoplasia Type 2

Multiple endocrine neoplasia type 2 syndrome (MEN2) has three subtypes based on phenotypic variants of activating mutations of *RET* proto-oncogene: MEN2A (~55%), MEN2B (~10%), and FMTC (~35%) (Eng et al. 1996; Frank-Raue et al. 2010). The *RET* gene encodes a tyrosine-kinase receptor consisting of three parts (extracellular, transmembrane, intracellular) that functions as a part of a receptor complex for the glial cell line-derived neurotrophic factors (GDNF, e.g., neurturin, artemin, persephin) and has physiological roles in the development, maturation, and maintenance of the nervous (central, peripheral) and excretory (mainly urinary) systems. The receptor complex is complete with the glial cell-derived neurotrophic factor receptor α-1 (GFRα-1). It is expressed in thyroid parafollicular C-cells along with other neural crest-derived cells, e.g., in adrenal medulla (Hofstra et al. 1994; Moline and Eng 2011; Castellone and Melillo 2018). Migration disorders of neurons expressing RET/GFRα-1 complex in the gastrointestinal system can explain the connection between *RET* mutations and Hirschsprung's disease or mucosal neuromas (MEN2B). However, the relevance of the RET/GFRα-1 complex in the endocrine neoplasms of MEN2 syndrome is not fully clarified.

The *RET* gene mutations responsible for MEN2 syndromes cause constitutive activation of the receptor. Mutations causing the MEN2A phenotype affect the extracellular part of the protein, while MEN2B phenotype causing mutations affect the intracellular (tyrosine kinase domain) part of the receptor (Eng et al. 1996). Ninety percent of oncogenic mutations of *RET* responsible for MEN2 syndromes are located mainly in codons encoding cysteine amino acid in exons 10 and 11 (codons 609, 611, 618, 620, 630, 634). Mutations of codon 634 are the most frequent, causing 80% of MEN2A syndromes. Rarely, mutations causing MEN2 syndromes are in exons 8, 13, 14, 15, and 16. Ninety percent of MEN2B patients carry mutation in codon 918 of exon 16 (Hofstra et al. 1994). Medullary thyroid cancer (MTC) is the most characteristic feature shared by all subtypes with variable aggressiveness.

MEN2A (OMIM: 171400) is autosomal dominantly inherited with an almost complete penetrance for MTC. Ninety-five percent of MEN2A patients are carriers of codon 634, 620, and 618 mutations (Cui et al. 2013). MEN2A syndrome accounts for 80% of hereditary MTCs (Wells et al. 2013). Pheochromocytoma (50%) and parathyroid adenoma (20–30%) are also characteristic for MEN2A (Table 7.3). Occasionally, cutaneous lichen amyloidosis and Hirschsprung's disease (HD) are present (Gagel et al. 1989). MEN2A is rare with an incidence of 10–28 per million

Table 7.3 Subcategories of MEN2

Subtype	Clinical manifestations
MEN2A	Medullary thyroid carcinoma Pheochromocytoma Hyperparathyroidism (parathyroid adenoma)
MEN2A/FMTC + Hirschprung's disease	MEN2A/FMTC + Hirschprung's disease
FMTC	Medullary thyroid carcinoma
FMTC + Cutaneous lichen amyloidosis	FMTC + itching dermatoses on the surface of the back
MEN2B	Medullary thyroid carcinoma Pheochromocytoma Mucosal neuromas Intestinal ganglioneuromatosis Marfanoid habitus

FMTC familial medullary thyroid carcinoma, *MEN* multiple endocrine neoplasia

population and prevalence of 24–25 per million (Steiner et al. 1968; Hoff et al. 2000; Traugott and Moley 2010; Machens et al. 2013; Opsahl et al. 2016; Mathiesen et al. 2018). The association of MEN2A with Hirschsprung's disease in patients with RET mutations represents a very interesting phenomenon. Whereas activated RET is involved in the pathogenesis of MEN2A-associated MTC, RET proteins bearing the same amino acid change behave as loss-of-function mutants in the intestinal peripheral nervous system, leading to Hirschsprung's disease (Fialkowski et al. 2008; Moore and Zaahl 2010; Tomuschat and Puri 2015). HD was found in about 50% of children with codon 620 mutation (Bütter et al. 2007). The same mutant protein thus behaves quite differently in different organs.

MEN2B (OMIM: 162300, formerly also called MEN3) is a very rare syndrome, with a prevalence of 0.9–1.65 per million population and an incidence of 2.6 per million population (Znaczko et al. 2014; Mathiesen et al. 2017). The syndrome is most commonly caused by a methionine-to-threonine substitution at codon 918 in the tyrosine-kinase domain of *RET* (Hofstra et al. 1994). This mutation (M918T RET) is the most frequent cause of MEN2B (Hansford 2000). MEN2B often comes with an early-onset and aggressive presentation of MTC. Depending on the genotype, patients have a 50% lifetime risk of pheochromocytoma. The syndrome is also associated with intestinal (megacolon, constipation) and ophthalmologic (e.g., alacrima in infants, hypertrophy of corneal nerves) manifestations (Cohen et al. 2002; Brauckhoff et al. 2008). Patients develop a marfanoid habitus including taller stature, long limbs, arachnodactyly, joint hypermobility, high-arched palate, pectus excavatum, kyphosis, scoliosis, etc. Mucosal neuromas, seen as multiple soft papules in or around the oral cavity (tip of tongue, lips), are often present in MEN2B. MTC is often the first manifestation of this syndrome and can develop in very early ages; therefore, prophylactic thyroidectomy by an expert surgeon in children with MEN2B is recommended before the age of 1 year (Wells et al. 2015). Variable forms of marfanoid habitus can be seen in these patients. Intestinal signs of MEN2B are recognizable in infant age as constipation or as Hirschsprung's disease (Castinetti et al. 2018).

FMTC (OMIM: 255240) is exclusively characterized by MTC that is mostly less aggressive than in the other forms of MEN2 syndrome. MTC is usually not fatal in FMTC. FMTC should be suspected when at least four family members have MTC without other tumor findings.

Genotype-phenotype correlations are well-known in MEN2, and these can be exploited to plan the time for prophylactic thyroidectomy (discussed in Sect. 7.3.1). Due to the presence of mutation hotspots, the genetic diagnosis of MEN2 is easier and has a higher sensitivity than that of MEN1.

7.2.4 Tuberous Sclerosis Complex

Two types of the rare tuberous sclerosis complex exist. Type 1 (OMIM: 191100) and type 2 (OMIM: 613254) have a 166:1,000,000 and 100:1,000,000 incidence, respectively (Northrup et al. 2013). TSC patients have neurologic (epilepsy, cortical brain malformations, mental retardation), dermatologic (hypomelanotic macules, facial angiofibromas, shagreen patches), renal (renal angiomyolipomas), cardiac (rhabdomyomas), ocular (retinal abnormalities), pulmonary (lymphangioleiomyomatosis), and endocrine (neuroendocrine tumor) manifestations (Randle 2017). Manifestations in patients harboring TSC2 mutations are more severe (Au et al. 2007). Common initial manifestations are cardiac rhabdomyomas and hypomelanotic macules. Endocrine tumors in TSC are rare and include ACTH- and GH-producing pituitary adenomas, benign and malignant parathyroid neoplasms, insulinomas, and gastrinomas based mostly on case reports (Osborne et al. 1991; Rosser et al. 2006; Dworakowska and Grossman 2009; Nelson and Wild 2018).

7.2.5 Hyperparathyroidism-Jaw Tumor Syndrome

Hyperparathyroidism-jaw tumor syndrome (OMIM: 145001) is a rare autosomal dominant familial cancer syndrome. Inactivating mutation of *CDC73(/HRPT2)* is the main causative factor. Patients mainly have adenomatous or malignant lesions of the parathyroids and fibro-ossifying tumors of the maxilla and mandibula, along with renal and uterine tumors (Bradley et al. 2005). Ninety-five percent of patients have primary hyperparathyroidism, whose onset is in the late adolescence or early adulthood (Hyde et al. 1993). Penetrance for these tumors is incomplete; therefore, patients can present with a spectrum of phenotypes: seemingly sporadic parathyroid cancer, familial isolated hyperparathyroidism (FIHP) with or without parathyroid cancer, or full expression of HPT-JT (Li and Simonds 2016). No clear genotype-phenotype correlations have been established so far. However, a study reports that missense mutations in *CDC73* gene are more likely associated with the FIHP phenotype (Cardoso et al. 2017). As parathyroid cancer is a very rare disease, suspicion for hyperparathyroidism-jaw tumor syndrome should be raised in young affected individuals (Sharretts and Simonds 2010; Mehta et al. 2014).

7.2.6 Peutz-Jeghers Syndrome

Peutz-Jeghers syndrome (PJS; OMIM: 175200) is a rare hamartomatosis with an incidence of 5–6:1,000,000 (Lindor and Greene 1998; Tchekmedyian et al. 2013). Although mostly related to gastroenterology, as being associated with gastrointestinal hamartomatous polyps and also a significantly increased risk for gastrointestinal cancers, it has also some endocrine tumor manifestations. PJS is characterized by pigmented spots on the lips or oral mucosa presenting in childhood. The gastrointestinal hamartomatous polyps can lead to severe complications, such as gastrointestinal bleeding, bowel obstruction, or intussusception (Duan et al. 2018). The responsible genetic event for this syndrome is an inactivating mutation in the *STK11* (Serine threonine kinase 11) tumor suppressor gene. Genotype-phenotype correlations are not fully explored yet. The endocrine manifestations occurring in this syndrome include thyroid nodules and differentiated carcinoma, ovarian sex cord tumors with annular tubules (SCTAT), endometrium and cervix adenocarcinoma, and Leydig and Sertoli cell cancer (Beggs et al. 2010; Van Lier et al. 2011; Lodish and Stratakis 2011; Gondak et al. 2012; Sammour et al. 2015).

7.2.7 Cowden Disease

Cowden disease or Cowden syndrome (CD/CS; OMIM: 158350) is an autosomal dominantly inherited disease caused by mutations of the *PTEN* (phosphatase and tensin homolog) tumor suppressor gene. The syndrome is associated with hamartomas and tumors of ecto-, meso-, and endodermal origin affecting multiple organs. Most of its features are listed in the diagnostic criteria: (a) pathognomonic criteria, mucocutaneous lesions (facial trichilemmomas, acral keratosis, papillomatous papules, mucosal lesions); (b) major criteria, breast cancer, non-medullary thyroid cancer, macrocephaly, endometrial cancer, and Lhermitte-Duclos disease (dysplastic cerebellar gangliocytoma); (c) minor criteria, benign thyroid lesions (goiter/nodules), mental retardation, hamartomatous intestinal polyps, lipomas, fibrocystic breast disease, fibromas, and genitourinary tumors or malformations (Pilarski 2009; Mester and Eng 2015; Stratakis 2016).

7.2.8 McCune-Albright Syndrome

McCune-Albright syndrome (MAS; OMIM: 174800) is a rare multiorgan disorder involving non-endocrine and endocrine manifestations that are non-inherited. We will discuss this syndrome here in more detail. Its prevalence varies between 1:100,000 and 1:1,000,000. MAS is a sporadic, non-hereditary disease; however, a single somatic mutation was identified in most patients. The mutation responsible for MAS is gain-of-function that perturbs the GNAS1 gene coding for the alpha subunit of G-proteins (Gsα). The mutation can be found in some organs and cells of the individual, but not all. This condition, i.e., the presence of the genetic alteration in some cells and its absence in others, is termed genetic mosaicism. MAS is hypothesized to be due to an early postzygotic mutation that may explain the disease of organs deriving from different germ layers (Weinstein et al. 1991).

7.2.8.1 Clinical Features

The original description of MAS involved polyostotic fibrous dysplasia of the bone, café-au-lait spots on the skin, and precocious puberty. Later, however, several other endocrine manifestations were observed in MAS patients including acromegaly, hyperthyroidism, renal phosphate wasting, etc. At present, a broader definition is favored: fibrous dysplasia + at least one of the typical hormonal hyperfunction syndromes and/or café-au-lait spots (Dumitrescu and Collins 2008).

The most frequent manifestations of MAS are café-au-lait spots, polyostotic fibrous dysplasia, and precocious puberty. Fibrous dysplasia most commonly affects the skull, the axial skeleton, and the proximal femoral bones (Hart et al. 2007; Ippolito et al. 2014). Bone pain, fractures, and deformities are the most common clinical features. Facial asymmetry can develop that can be more severe in patients with concomitant acromegaly (Subbiah et al. 2011; Salenave et al. 2014). Neurological complications including blindness due to the compression of nerves by dysplastic bones may rarely develop. Children may complain about being tired, but rarely pathologic fractures may be the first symptoms. Deformation of the femur or tibia may result in a "shepherd's crook" appearance. Bones may present a "ground-glass" appearance on X-ray due to endosteal scalloping and thinning of the cortex with the matrix of the intramedullary tissue (Ippolito et al. 2014). It should be mentioned that fibrous dysplasia is much more common than MAS itself. Malignant transformation of fibrous dysplasia is rare; however, external beam irradiation may predispose these patients to sarcoma formation (Ruggieri et al. 1994; Davies et al. 2014). Radiotherapy should be therefore carefully considered in patients with fibrous dysplasia (Qu et al. 2015). The concomitant presence of growth hormone excess might further worsen the danger of malignant transformation. Fibrous dysplasia alone is much more frequent than MAS; only about 5% of patients with fibrous dysplasia belong to the group of MAS (Chapurlat and Orcel 2008; Dumitrescu and Collins 2008).

Gonadotropin-independent (hypogonadotropic) precocious puberty is the most frequent endocrine manifestation. Girls are more frequently affected. Early development of secondary sexual characteristics in both genders (growth of pubic hair), precocious vaginal bleeding and breast growth (early thelarche) in girls and testicular and penile enlargement in boys, can develop (Collins et al. 2012; Boyce et al. 2012). Acromegaly due to growth hormone excess is rare, but characteristic in MAS (Bhansali et al. 2003). Prolactin hypersecretion may also occur, often together with growth hormone (Madsen et al. 2011).

Overt hyperthyroidism was observed in up to 40% of all patients, but subclinical forms are even more common, reaching almost 60% of patients tested. Thyroid nodules may turn malignant (Celi et al. 2008).

Adrenocortical hyperactivity resulting in Cushing's syndrome is a rare manifestation and is mostly observed in neonates. It may be transient, resolving spontaneously before the end of the first year (Brown et al. 2010).

Table 7.4 Clinical features of McCune-Albright syndrome

Skin	Bone	Endocrine	Non-endocrine tumor	Other
Café-au-lait spots	Fibrous dysplasia	Precocious puberty	Myxoma[a]	Cardiomyopathy
Alopecia		Testicular tumor	Cholestatic liver disease	Myelofibrosis
		Pituitary tumors (GH, PRL, non-secreting)	Thymic hyperplasia	
		Adrenal adenomas and hyperplasia	Gastrointestinal polyps	
		Thyroid nodule (hyperthyroidism)		

[a]The association of fibrous dysplasia with intramuscular myxomas is also called Mazabraud syndrome

Renal phosphate wasting can occur with or without hypophosphatemia and/or osteomalacia/rickets. Renal phosphate wasting is due to a proximal tubulopathy and is probably caused by the secretion of the phosphaturic fibroblast growth factor 23 (FGF23) by the dysplastic bone tissue (Leet et al. 2006; Boyce et al. 2013).

The clinical manifestations of MAS are presented in Table 7.4.

The prognosis of MAS is very variable. Possible therapeutical approaches of fibrous dysplasia include bisphosphonates, calcium, vitamin D, and phosphorus supplementation. Severe bone deformities may require surgical intervention. The therapy of the other endocrine and non-endocrine manifestations does not differ from that used to treat their non-syndromic counterparts (Robinson et al. 2016).

7.2.8.2 Genetics and Pathogenesis

The GNAS locus exhibits one of the most complex genetic regulations in humans. It is an imprinted locus with several promoters. Both activating and inactivating mutations are known. Whereas activating (gain-of-function) mutations are implicated in fibrous dysplasia and MAS, several inactivating mutations were associated with Albright's hereditary osteodystrophy and pseudohypoparathyroidism (Lania et al. 2001). The various diseases associated with GNAS mutations are summarized in Table 7.5.

Two codons were found to be affected by activating missense mutations in MAS patients. Codon 201 codes for an arginine that has pivotal functions in the activity of the enzyme's catalytic center. It is interesting to note that the Cholera vibrio exotoxin targets this amino acid by ADP-ribosylation and thus leads to excessive intestinal fluid loss. Two mutations of codon201 have been described, Arg201Cys and Arg201His. In less than 5% of cases, Gln227 is affected (Masters et al. 1989; Weinstein et al. 1991). The resulting molecular phenotype displays hormone-independent activation of adenyl-cyclase due to GTPase inhibition; therefore, the

Table 7.5 Endocrine diseases related to GNAS1 (Gsα) mutations

Type of mutation	Disease	Mechanism
Inactivating mutations	Pseudohypoparathyroidism 1a	Germline point mutations, deletions, insertions
	Pseudohypoparathyroidism 1b	Imprinting defects (germline)
Gain-of-function mutations	McCune-Albright syndrome	Postzygotic mutation
	Pituitary, thyroid and Leydig cell tumors	Somatic mutations

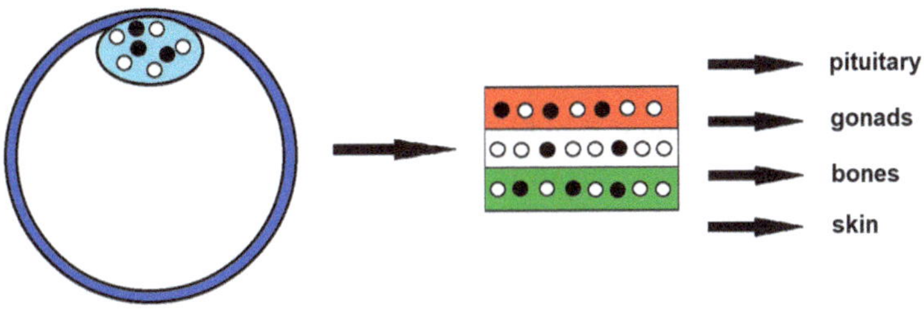

Fig. 7.1 Schematic representation of McCune-Albright syndrome pathogenesis. Mutations arising in the postzytogic stage result in mosaicism of the inner cell mass. Cells harboring GNAS1 mutations are depicted black, normal cells as white. Mutant cells are present in all three germ layers (ectoderm, mesoderm, endoderm) giving rise to diseases of several organs

production of cyclic AMP is increased in the cells harboring the mutant alleles. Activation of the Gsα/protein kinase A/CREB (cAMP response element binding protein) results in the overactivation of the transcription factor c-fos. Overexpression of c-fos results in the extensive proliferation of bone marrow stromal cells and disturbance of the differentiation of osteoblasts. Transgenic mice overexpressing c-fos exhibit a phenotype that is reminiscent of that found in patients with fibrous dysplasia (Rüther et al. 1987; Riminucci et al. 2006; Piersanti et al. 2010).

GNAS1 mutations leading to MAS are postzygotic and occur probably before gastrulation as organs deriving from all three germ layers may be affected (Fig. 7.1). According to this hypothesis, the earlier the mutation develops, the more severe the manifestations are. Germline-activating mutations of *GNAS1* are thought to be incompatible with life. Due to its postzygotic nature and the resulting genetic mosaicism, the clinical picture of MAS is highly variable: ranging from asymptomatic carriers to severely affected patients. It is of interest to note that activating, somatic *GNAS1* mutations were described in sporadic pituitary, thyroid, and Leydig cell tumors underlining the tumor-promoting activities of these mutations. Somatic mutations of Arg201 are frequent among these mutations (Happle 1986; Riminucci et al. 2002; Collins et al. 2003; Diaz et al. 2007).

The diagnosis of MAS should be clinical. Genetic diagnosis is possible with DNA isolated from peripheral mononuclear cells, melanocytes, bone, and endocrine cells. The likelihood of finding the mutation increases with the severity of the disease. Genetic diagnosis, however, is not proposed, since being a mosaic disease, it is difficult, laborious, and unreliable: a negative result may not exclude the disease (Boyce et al. 2015).

7.3 Suspicion for Multiple Endocrine Neoplasia in Case of Sporadic Tumors

In this section, we present characteristic endocrine tumors which are not covered in other chapters of the book, where multiple endocrine neoplasia syndromes might be suspected.

7.3.1 Medullary Thyroid Carcinoma

Medullary thyroid carcinoma develops from the neural crest-derived calcitonin-secreting parafollicular or C-cells of the thyroid gland. Approximately 70–80% of MTCs are sporadic, whereas in 20–30% of cases represent hereditary MTC caused by germline *RET* mutations responsible for MEN2A, MEN2B, and FMTC syndromes. About 6.5% of apparently sporadic MTC are in fact caused by germline *RET* mutations (Romei et al. 2011). Somatic mutations were also described in sporadic MTCs (Hofstra et al. 1994). Hereditary forms tend to present as bilateral, multifocal, and associated with C-cell hyperplasia (Pappa and Alevizaki 2016). MEN2A accounts for 80%, MEN2B for 5%, and FMTC for 15% of hereditary MTCs (Wells et al. 2013).

Genotype-phenotype analysis showed that genotype determines the time of presentation and aggressiveness of MTCs. MTC develops most probably in the second decade of life, in the third decade of life, or in middle age in MEN2B, MEN2A, and FMTC, respectively (Marquard and Eng 2015). Early manifestation and very high risk of aggressiveness are associated with MEN2B syndrome and/or mutations of codons 883, 918, or 922. High risk of aggressiveness is associated with mutations of codons 611, 618, 620, and 634. The least aggressive phenotypes are associated with mutations of codons 609, 768, 790, 791, 804, or 891 (Hofstra et al. 1994). Accordingly, the recent ATA guideline classifies *RET* mutation in high, moderate, and low risk for MTC (Wells et al. 2015).

Different mutations have different therapeutic consequences. According to the American Thyroid Association's (ATA) guideline, prophylactic thyroidectomy should be carried out in patients with *RET* mutations, as it can prevent MTC. Genotype-phenotype connections make codon-specific genetic counseling possible and are helpful to determine the most appropriate time for operation. Thyroidectomy in the first 6 month of life is recommended in patients with the most aggressive M918T (or other MEN2B specific) mutation. Patients with high-risk C634 mutation (or other mutations characteristic for MEN2A) should undergo prophylactic thyroidectomy around the fifth year of age or earlier if calcitonin level is elevated. If the risk is moderate—practically, all remaining mutations—the thyroidectomy should be planned upon elevated calcitonin levels, or around 5 years if parents do not wish to embark on a lengthy period of evaluation which might last for years or decades (Wells et al. 2015; Pappa and Alevizaki 2016).

7.3.2 *Primary Hyperparathyroidism (PHPT)*

Genetic background of primary hyperparathyroidism should be suspected in young patients (>30–35 years), patients with multiple gland involvement, recurrent disease, or associated tumors. In most patients, parathyroid gland hyperplasia or adenoma is present; parathyroid cancer is very rare. Hereditary cases comprise 2–5% of all primary hyperparathyroidism (Li and Simonds 2016).

Hyperparathyroidism is usually the earliest and most common endocrine manifestation of MEN1 syndrome. Almost all patients have hypercalcemia at the time of the diagnosis (Marx et al. 1986). Patients usually are diagnosed with parathyroid gland hyperplasia affecting all glands. MEN4 syndrome has a very similar phenotype, but parathyroid adenomas are mostly seen in the majority of patients (Pellegata 2012).

Among MEN2 syndromes, only MEN2A is associated with parathyroid disease (Steiner et al. 1968). It is usually a mild manifestation and is usually due to parathyroid adenoma (Simonds 2017).

Primary hyperparathyroidism is the most penetrant and usually the presenting manifestation in hyperparathyroidism-jaw tumor syndrome. Parathyroid carcinoma is present approximately in one fifth of the patients (Jackson et al. 1990; Chen et al. 2003; Bradley et al. 2005; Mehta et al. 2014). The vast majority of these malignant tumors are functioning, so signs related to severe primary hyperparathyroidism and hypercalcemia are often present (joint pain, fatigue, nephrolithiasis, muscle weakness, constipation, reduced bone mass, and psychiatric abnormalities). Parathyroid carcinomas can often cause compressive symptoms such as dysphagia, dyspnea, dysphonia, and dysarthria (Asare et al. 2015).

7.3.2.1 Disorders Associated with Mutations of the *CaSR* (Calcium Sensing Receptor) Gene

Unique forms of primary hyperparathyroidism can be caused by mutations of the *CaSR* (calcium sensing receptor) gene.

Neonatal severe hyperparathyroidism (NSHPT, OMIM: 239200) is caused by homozygous or compound heterozygous inactivating mutations of the *CaSR* gene. This syndrome, if it is undiagnosed, can be life-threatening. Severe hypercalcemia (>3.5 mmol/L), respiratory distress, hypotonia, and spontaneous bone fractures could develop in the affected neonates, and bone fractures can be observed even in utero. Based on the genetic background, it is important to clarify whether the disease-causing mutation is a homozygous or compound heterozygous inherited from both parents or if it occurs de novo or from the paternal side. This has major impact on disease course and therapy. In this latter case, secondary hyperparathyroidism will develop during the intrauterine life which later, after delivery, will be resolved by setting the CaSR set point and consequently the parathormone secretion will return to normal (Glaudo et al. 2016).

Inactivating mutations of *CaSR* cause familial hypocalciuric hypercalcemia (FHH, OMIM: 145980) too. This disease is characterized by mild, usually symptomless, hypercalcemia and relative hypocalciuria. Most mutations are missense mutations and cause amino acid changes in the N-terminal and extracellular domain of the receptor. The mutant receptor is responsible for the decreased capacity of calcium binding and receptor dimerization (Bai et al. 1996). Clinically, the syndrome is characterized by lifelong mild hypercalcemia without no clinical signs, detected usually incidentally. In clinical practice, FHH should be differentiated from mild forms of PHPT, and parathyroidectomy should not be performed in FHH. The clinical diagnosis bases on determining calcium to creatinine clearance ratio (Christensen et al. 2011), but there are numerous overlaps between these two clinical entities. Mutational analysis of the *CaSR* gene would be useful in diagnosis of all FHH cases to avoid unnecessary parathyroidectomy. In addition, genetic counseling and germline testing of the *CaSR* gene may be offered to adult patients diagnosed with asymptomatic mild hypercalcemia and hypocalciuria, in whom there is high suspicion of a genetic etiology (familial aggregation of asymptomatic hypercalcemia, young age at the diagnosis), and it is recommended for patients and their parents with NSHPT. In this latter case, prenatal genetic test or genetic test at birth is also proposed.

7.3.3 Neuroendocrine Tumors

Functional and nonfunctional duodenopancreatic NETs (pNETs) represent major manifestations of the MEN1 syndrome. 40–80% of MEN1 patients have pNET, and in 80–100% of affected patients, postmortem examination reports these kind of tumors (Goudet et al. 2010). Nonfunctioning pNET are more prevalent (50%) and have higher malignancy rate than functional pNETs (Yates et al. 2015). Functional pNETs such as insulinoma, gastrinoma, glucagonoma, or VIPoma are often present with the respective clinical syndromes. MEN1-associated pNETs are more aggressive than their sporadic counterparts. Young patients suffering from these tumors, especially gastrinoma, should be screened for MEN1. 15–30% of all gastrinomas arise in the context of MEN1 (Deveney et al. 1983; Mignon et al. 1986; Soga and Yakuwa 1998; Roy et al. 2000; Hopper et al. 2018).

Less than 10% of NF1 patients can also develop functional (duodenal somatostatinoma) or nonfunctional duodenpancreatic NET, which are also included in the diagnostic criteria of NF1 (Guilmette and Nosé 2018). 5–17% of individuals with von Hippel-Lindau syndrome develop pNETs, which are mainly nonfunctioning tumors, but 8% of them can become malignant and metastatic. Compared to the sporadic pNETs, VHL-associated tumors have better long-term outcome (Lonser et al. 2003; Maher et al. 2011; Varshney et al. 2017; Guilmette and Nosé 2018). Development of pNETs in TSC syndromes is known and is relatively common in affected children and young adults (Koc et al. 2017; Guilmette and Nosé 2018).

Bronchial NETs are also observed in MEN1 but are less common than duodenopancreatic NET (Brandi et al. 2001).

Thymic carcinoids are present in approximately 5% of MEN1 patients (Trump et al. 1997), and 25% of thymic carcinoids are observed in MEN1 patients (Sakurai et al. 2012). In MEN1 patients, thymic carcinoids are the most aggressive tumors with approx. fourfold increase in mortality. They are mainly due to the increased metastatic activity of these tumors (Giusti et al. 1993; Gibril et al. 2003; Goudet et al. 2010). Thymic carcinoid patients should be screened for MEN1. The potential development of thymic carcinoid in MEN1 represents the only form of prophylactic surgery in this syndrome, as patients undergoing parathyroidectomy should be considered to undergo thymectomy (Litvak and Pietanza 2016; Li and Simonds 2016).

References

Alrezk R, Hannah-Shmouni F, Stratakis CA (2017) MEN4 and CDKN1B mutations: the latest of the MEN syndromes. Endocr Relat Cancer 24:T195–T208

Asare EA, Sturgeon C, Winchester DJ et al (2015) Parathyroid carcinoma: an update on treatment outcomes and prognostic factors from the National Cancer Data Base (NCDB). Ann Surg Oncol 22:3990–3995. https://doi.org/10.1245/s10434-015-4672-3

Au KS, Williams AT, Roach ES et al (2007) Genotype/phenotype correlation in 325 individuals referred for a diagnosis of tuberous sclerosis complex in the United States. Genet Med 9:88–100. https://doi.org/10.1097/GIM.0b013e31803068c7

Bai M et al (1996) Expression and characterization of inactivating and activating mutations in the human Ca2+o-sensing receptor. J Biol Chem 271:19537–19545

Beggs AD, Latchford AR, Vasen HFA et al (2010) Peutz-Jeghers syndrome: a systematic review and recommendations for management. Gut 59:975–986

Bhansali A, Sharma BS, Sreenivasulu P et al (2003) Acromegaly with fibrous dysplasia: McCune-Albright syndrome – clinical studies in 3 cases and brief review of literature. Endocr J 50:793–799

Boyce AM, Chong WH, Shawker TH et al (2012) Characterization and management of testicular pathology in McCune-Albright syndrome. J Clin Endocrinol Metab 97:E1782–E1790. https://doi.org/10.1210/jc.2012-1791

Boyce AM, Bhattacharyya N, Collins MT (2013) Fibrous dysplasia and fibroblast growth factor-23 regulation. Curr Osteoporos Rep 11:65–71. https://doi.org/10.1007/s11914-013-0144-5

Boyce AM, Florenzano P, de Castro LF, Collins MT (2015) Fibrous dysplasia/McCune-Albright syndrome. In: Adam MP, Ardinger HH, Pagon RA, Wallace SE, LJH B, Stephens K, Amemiya A (eds) GeneReviews® [Internet]. University of Washington, Seattle (WA). 1993–2019 [updated 2018 Aug 16]

Bradley KJ, Hobbs MR, Buley ID, et al (2005) Uterine tumours are a phenotypic manifestation of the hyperparathyroidism-jaw tumour syndrome. J Intern Med. 257 (1) 18–26

Brandi ML, Gagel RF, Angeli A et al (2001) Consensus: guidelines for diagnosis and therapy of MEN type 1 and type 2. J Clin Endocrinol Metab 86(12):5658–5671

Brauckhoff M, Machens A, Hess S et al (2008) Premonitory symptoms preceding metastatic medullary thyroid cancer in MEN 2B: an exploratory analysis. Surgery 144:1044–1051. https://doi.org/10.1016/j.surg.2008.08.028

Brown RJ, Kelly MH, Collins MT (2010) Cushing syndrome in the McCune-Albright syndrome. J Clin Endocrinol Metab 95:1508–1515. https://doi.org/10.1210/jc.2009-2321

Bütter A, Gagné J, Al-Jazaeri A et al (2007) Prophylactic thyroidectomy in pediatric carriers of multiple endocrine neoplasia type 2A or familial medullary thyroid carcinoma: mutation in C620 is associated with Hirschsprung's disease. J Pediatr Surg 42:203–206. https://doi.org/10.1016/j.jpedsurg.2006.09.019

Cao Y, Liu R, Jiang X et al (2009) Nuclear-cytoplasmic shuttling of menin regulates nuclear translocation of -catenin. Mol Cell Biol 29:5477–5487. https://doi.org/10.1128/MCB.00335-09

Cardoso L, Stevenson M, Thakker RV (2017) Molecular genetics of syndromic and non-syndromic forms of parathyroid carcinoma. Hum Mutat 38:1621–1648

Castellone MD, Melillo RM (2018) RET-mediated modulation of tumor microenvironment and immune response in multiple endocrine neoplasia type 2 (MEN2). Endocr Relat Cancer 25: T105–T119

Castinetti F, Moley J, Mulligan L, Waguespack SG (2018) A comprehensive review on MEN2B. Endocr Relat Cancer 25:T29–T39

Celi FS, Coppotelli G, Chidakel A et al (2008) The role of type 1 and type 2 5′-deiodinase in the pathophysiology of the 3,5,3′-triiodothyronine toxicosis of McCune-Albright syndrome. J Clin Endocrinol Metab 93:2383–2389. https://doi.org/10.1210/jc.2007-2237

Chapurlat RD, Orcel P (2008) Fibrous dysplasia of bone and McCune-Albright syndrome. Best Pract Res Clin Rheumatol 22:55–69

Chen JD, Morrison C, Zhang C et al (2003) Hyperparathyroidism-jaw tumour syndrome. J Intern Med 253(6):634–642

Christensen SE, Nissen PH, Vestergaard P, Mosekilde L (2011) Familial hypocalciuric hypercalcaemia: a review. Curr Opin Endocrinol Diabetes Obes 18:359–370

Cohen MS, Phay JE, Albinson C et al (2002) Gastrointestinal manifestations of multiple endocrine neoplasia type 2. Ann Surg 235:648–655. https://doi.org/10.1097/00000658-200205000-00006

Collins MT, Sarlis NJ, Merino MJ et al (2003) Thyroid carcinoma in the McCune-Albright syndrome: contributory role of activating Gsα mutations. J Clin Endocrinol Metab 88:4413–4417. https://doi.org/10.1210/jc.2002-021642

Collins MT, Singer FR, Eugster E (2012) McCune-Albright syndrome and the extraskeletal manifestations of fibrous dysplasia. Orphanet J Rare Dis 7(Suppl 1):S4. https://doi.org/10.1186/1750-1172-7-S1-S4

Concolino P, Costella A, Capoluongo E (2016) Multiple endocrine neoplasia type 1 (MEN1): an update of 208 new germline variants reported in the last nine years. Cancer Genet 209:36–41. https://doi.org/10.1016/j.cancergen.2015.12.002

Cui Q, Wang W, Fu Z et al (2013) Integrated DNA-based/biochemical screening for early diagnosis of multiple endocrine neoplasia type 2A (MEN2A). J Biomed Res 27:145–150. https://doi.org/10.7555/JBR.27.20120121

Davies BW, Prescott CR, Said SA et al (2014) Radiation-induced dedifferentiated chondrosarcoma with orbital invasion. Ophthal Plast Reconstr Surg 30:205–208

De Laat JM, Van Leeuwaarde RS, Valk GD (2018) The importance of an early and accurate MEN1 diagnosis. Front Endocrinol (Lausanne) 9:533

Deveney CW, Deveney KE, Stark D et al (1983) Resection of gastrinomas. Ann Surg 198:546–553. https://doi.org/10.1097/00000658-198310000-00015

Diaz A, Danon M, Crawford J (2007) McCune-Albright syndrome and disorders due to activating mutations of GNAS1. J Pediatr Endocrinol Metab 20:853–880

Doherty GM (2003) Multiple endocrine neoplasia type 1: duodenopancreatic tumors. Surg Oncol 12:135–143

Duan F-X, Gu G-L, Yang H-R et al (2018) Must Peutz-Jeghers syndrome patients have the LKB1/ STK11 gene mutation? A case report and review of the literature. World J Clin Cases 6:224–232. https://doi.org/10.12998/wjcc.v6.i8.224

Dumitrescu CE, Collins MT (2008) McCune-Albright syndrome. Orphanet J Rare Dis 3:12. https://doi.org/10.1186/1750-1172-3-12

Dworakowska D, Grossman AB (2009) Are neuroendocrine tumours a feature of tuberous sclerosis? A systematic review. Endocr Relat Cancer 16:45–58

Eng C, Clayton D, Schuffenecker I et al (1996) The relationship between specific ret proto-oncogene mutations and disease phenotype in multiple endocrine neoplasia type 2: international RET mutation consortium analysis. J Am Med Assoc 276:1575–1579. https://doi.org/10.1001/jama.276.19.1575

Fialkowski EA, DeBenedetti MK, Moley JF, Bachrach B (2008) RET proto-oncogene testing in infants presenting with Hirschsprung disease identifies 2 new multiple endocrine neoplasia 2A kindreds. J Pediatr Surg 43:188–190. https://doi.org/10.1016/j.jpedsurg.2007.09.043

Frank-Raue K, Rondot S, Raue F (2010) Molecular genetics and phenomics of RET mutations: impact on prognosis of MTC. Mol Cell Endocrinol 322:2–7

Gagel RF, Levy ML, Donovan DT et al (1989) Multiple endocrine neoplasia type 2a associated with cutaneous lichen amyloidosis. Ann Intern Med 111:802–806. https://doi.org/10.7326/0003-4819-111-10-802

Gallo A, Cuozzo C, Esposito I et al (2002) Menin uncouples Elk-1, JunD and c-Jun phosphorylation from MAP kinase activation. Oncogene 21:6434–6445. https://doi.org/10.1038/sj.onc.1205822

Gibril F, Chen YJ, Schrump DS et al (2003) Prospective study of thymic carcinoids in patients with multiple endocrine neoplasia type 1. J Clin Endocrinol Metab 88:1066–1081. https://doi.org/10.1210/jc.2002-021314

Giusti F, Marini F, Brandi ML (1993) Multiple endocrine neoplasia Type 1. In: Adam MP, Ardinger HH, Pagon RA, Wallace SE, LJH B, Stephens K, Amemiya A (eds) GeneReviews® [Internet]. University of Washington, Seattle. 1993–2019. 2005 Aug 31 [updated 2017 Dec 14]

Giusti F, Cavalli L, Cavalli T, Brandi ML (2013) Hereditary hyperparathyroidism syndromes. J Clin Densitom 16:69–74. https://doi.org/10.1016/j.jocd.2012.11.003

Glaudo M et al (2016) Heterozygous inactivating CaSR mutations causing neonatal hyperparathyroidism: function, inheritance and phenotype. Eur J Endocrinol 175:421–431

Gondak RO, da Silva-Jorge R, Jorge J et al (2012) Oral pigmented lesions: clinicopathologic features and review of the literature. Med Oral Patol Oral Cir Bucal 17:e919–e924

Goudet P, Murat A, Binquet C et al (2010) Risk factors and causes of death in MEN1 disease. A GTE (Groupe d'etude des Tumeurs Endocrines) cohort study among 758 patients. World J Surg 34:249–255. https://doi.org/10.1007/s00268-009-0290-1

Goudet P, Dalac A, Le Bras M et al (2015) MEN1 disease occurring before 21 years old: a 160-patient cohort study from the Groupe d'étude des Tumeurs Endocrines. J Clin Endocrinol Metab 100:1568–1577. https://doi.org/10.1210/jc.2014-3659

Guilmette JM, Nosé V (2018) Neoplasms of the neuroendocrine pancreas: an update in the classification, definition, and molecular genetic advances. Adv Anat Pathol 26(1):13–30. https://doi.org/10.1097/PAP.0000000000000201

Hansford JR (2000) Multiple endocrine neoplasia type 2 and RET: from neoplasia to neurogenesis. J Med Genet 37:817–827. https://doi.org/10.1136/jmg.37.11.817

Happle R (1986) The McCune-Albright syndrome: a lethal gene surviving by mosaicism. Clin Genet 29:321–324. https://doi.org/10.1111/j.1399-0004.1986.tb01261.x

Hart ES, Kelly MH, Brillante B et al (2007) Onset, progression, and plateau of skeletal lesions in fibrous dysplasia and the relationship to functional outcome. J Bone Miner Res 22:1468–1474. https://doi.org/10.1359/jbmr.070511

Hoff AO, Cote GJ, Gagel RF (2000) Multiple endocrine neoplasias. Annu Rev Physiol 62:377–411. https://doi.org/10.1146/annurev.physiol.62.1.377

Hofstra RMW, Landsvater RM, Ceccherini I et al (1994) A mutation in the RET proto-oncogene associated with multiple endocrine neoplasia type 2B and sporadic medullary thyroid carcinoma. Nature 367:375–376. https://doi.org/10.1038/367375a0

Hopper AD, Jalal M, Munir A (2018) Recent advances in the diagnosis and management of pancreatic neuroendocrine tumours. Frontline Gastroenterol 10:269–274. https://doi.org/10.1136/flgastro-2018-101006

Hyde SM, Rich TA, Waguespack SG et al (1993) CDC73-related disorders. University of Washington, Seattle

Ippolito E, Farsetti P, Boyce AM et al (2014) Radiographic classification of coronal plane femoral deformities in polyostotic fibrous dysplasia. Clin Orthop Relat Res 472:1558–1567. https://doi.org/10.1007/s11999-013-3380-1

Ito T, Igarashi H, Uehara H et al (2013) Causes of death and prognostic factors in multiple endocrine neoplasia type 1: a prospective study:comparison of 106 men1/zollinger-ellison syndrome patients with 1613 literature MEN1 patients with or without pancreatic endocrine tumors. Med (United States) 92:135–181. https://doi.org/10.1097/MD.0b013e3182954af1

Jackson CE, Norum RA, Boyd SB et al (1990) Hereditary hyperparathyroidism and multiple ossifying jaw fibromas: a clinically and genetically distinct syndrome. Surgery 108:1003–1006

Jensen RT, Berna MJ, Bingham DB, Norton JA (2008) Inherited pancreatic endocrine tumor syndromes: advances in molecular pathogenesis, diagnosis, management, and controversies. Cancer 113:1807–1843

Kaji H, Canaff L, Lebrun JJ et al (2001) Inactivation of menin, a Smad3-interacting protein, blocks transforming growth factor type beta signaling. Proc Natl Acad Sci U S A 98:3837–3842. https://doi.org/10.1073/pnas.061358098

Koc G, Sugimoto S, Kuperman R et al (2017) Pancreatic tumors in children and young adults with tuberous sclerosis complex. Pediatr Radiol 47:39–45. https://doi.org/10.1007/s00247-016-3701-0

Lania A, Mantovani G, Spada A (2001) G protein mutations in endocrine diseases. Eur J Endocrinol 145:543–559

Leet AI, Wientroub S, Kushner H et al (2006) The correlation of specific orthopaedic features of polyostotic fibrous dysplasia with functional outcome scores in children. J Bone Joint Surg Ser A 88:818–823. https://doi.org/10.2106/JBJS.E.00259

Lemos MC, Thakker RV (2008) Multiple endocrine neoplasia type 1 (MEN1): analysis of 1336 mutations reported in the first decade following identification of the gene. Hum Mutat 29:22–32. https://doi.org/10.1002/humu.20605

Li Y, Simonds WF (2016) Endocrine neoplasms in familial syndromes of hyperparathyroidism. Endocr Relat Cancer 23:R229–R247. https://doi.org/10.1530/ERC-16-0059

Lindor NM, Greene MH (1998) The concise handbook of family cancer syndromes. J Natl Cancer Inst 90:1039–1071. https://doi.org/10.1093/jnci/90.14.1039

Litvak A, Pietanza MC (2016) Bronchial and thymic carcinoid tumors. Hematol Oncol Clin North Am 30:83–102

Lodish MB, Stratakis CA (2011) The differential diagnosis of familial lentiginosis syndromes. Fam Cancer 10(3):481–490

Lonser RR, Glenn GM, Walther M et al (2003) von Hippel-Lindau disease. Lancet 361:2059–2067. https://doi.org/10.1016/S0140-6736(03)13643-4

Machens A, Lorenz K, Sekulla C et al (2013) Molecular epidemiology of multiple endocrine neoplasia 2: implications for RET screening in the new millenium. Eur J Endocrinol 168:307–314. https://doi.org/10.1530/EJE-12-0919

Madsen H, Borges MT, Kerr JM et al (2011) McCune-Albright syndrome: surgical and therapeutic challenges in GH-secreting pituitary adenomas. J Neuro-Oncol 104:215–224. https://doi.org/10.1007/s11060-010-0461-9

Maher ER, Neumann HP, Richard S (2011) Von Hippel-Lindau disease: a clinical and scientific review. Eur J Hum Genet 19:617–623

Manoharan J, Raue F, Lopez CL et al (2017) Is routine screening of young asymptomatic MEN1 patients necessary? World J Surg 41:2026–2032. https://doi.org/10.1007/s00268-017-3992-9

Marquard J, Eng C (2015) Multiple endocrine Neoplasia type 2. In: Adam MP, Ardinger HH, Pagon RA, Wallace SE, Bean LJH, Stephens K, Amemiya A (eds) GeneReviews® [Internet]. University of Washington, Seattle. 1993–2019. 1999 Sep 27 [updated 2015 Jun 25], Seattle (WA), pp 315–325

Marx SJ, Vinik AI, Santen RJ et al (1986) Multiple endocrine neoplasia type I: assessment of laboratory tests to screen for the gene in a large kindred. Medicine (United States) 65:226–241. https://doi.org/10.1097/00005792-198607000-00003

Masters SB, Miller RT, Chi MH et al (1989) Mutations in the GTP-binding site of G(sα) alter stimulation of adenylyl cyclase. J Biol Chem 264:15467–15474

Mathiesen JS, Kroustrup JP, Vestergaard P et al (2017) Incidence and prevalence of multiple endocrine neoplasia 2B in Denmark: a nationwide study. Endocr Relat Cancer 24:L39–L42. https://doi.org/10.1530/ERC-17-0122

Mathiesen JS, Kroustrup JP, Vestergaard P et al (2018) Incidence and prevalence of multiple endocrine neoplasia 2A in Denmark 1901–2014: a nationwide study. Clin Epidemiol 10:1479–1487. https://doi.org/10.2147/CLEP.S174606

Matkar S, Thiel A, Hua X (2013) Menin: a scaffold protein that controls gene expression and cell signaling. Trends Biochem Sci 38:394–402. https://doi.org/10.1016/j.tibs.2013.05.005

Mehta A, Patel D, Rosenberg A et al (2014) Hyperparathyroidism-jaw tumor syndrome: results of operative management. Surgery 156:1315–1324. discussion 1324–5. https://doi.org/10.1016/j.surg.2014.08.004

Mester J, Eng C (2015) Cowden syndrome: recognizing and managing a not-so-rare hereditary cancer syndrome. J Surg Oncol 111:125–130

Mignon M, Ruszniewski P, Haffar S et al (1986) Current approach to the management of tumoral process in patients with gastrinoma. World J Surg 10:703–710. https://doi.org/10.1007/BF01655562

Moline J, Eng C (2011) Multiple endocrine neoplasia type 2: an overview. Genet Med 13:755–764

Moore SW, Zaahl M (2010) Familial associations in medullary thyroid carcinoma with Hirschsprung disease: the role of the RET-C620 "Janus" genetic variation. J Pediatr Surg 45:393–396. https://doi.org/10.1016/j.jpedsurg.2009.10.080

Naito J, Kaji H, Sowa H et al (2005) Menin suppresses osteoblast differentiation by antagonizing the AP-1 factor, JunD. J Biol Chem 280:4785–4791. https://doi.org/10.1074/jbc.M408143200

Nelson SL, Wild BM (2018) Tuberous sclerosis complex: early diagnosis in infants. Pediatr Neurol Briefs 32:12. https://doi.org/10.15844/pedneurbriefs-32-12

Northrup H, Krueger DA, Roberds S et al (2013) Tuberous sclerosis complex diagnostic criteria update: recommendations of the 2012 international tuberous sclerosis complex consensus conference. Pediatr Neurol 49:243–254. https://doi.org/10.1016/j.pediatrneurol.2013.08.001

Norton JA, Krampitz G, Jensen RT (2015) Multiple endocrine neoplasia: genetics and clinical management. Surg Oncol Clin N Am 24:795–832. https://doi.org/10.1016/j.soc.2015.06.008

Opsahl EM, Brauckhoff M, Schlichting E et al (2016) A nationwide study of multiple endocrine Neoplasia type 2A in Norway: predictive and prognostic factors for the clinical course of medullary thyroid carcinoma. Thyroid 26:1225–1238. https://doi.org/10.1089/thy.2015.0673

Osborne JP, Fryer A, Webb D (1991) Epidemiology of tuberous sclerosis. Ann N Y Acad Sci 615:125–127. https://doi.org/10.1111/j.1749-6632.1991.tb37754.x

Pappa T, Alevizaki M (2016) Management of hereditary medullary thyroid carcinoma. Endocrine 53:7–17. https://doi.org/10.1007/s12020-016-0873-1

Pellegata N (2012) MENX and MEN4. Clinics 67:13–18. https://doi.org/10.6061/clinics/2012(Sup01)04

Piersanti S, Remoli C, Saggio I et al (2010) Transfer, analysis, and reversion of the fibrous dysplasia cellular phenotype in human skeletal progenitors. J Bone Miner Res 25:1103–1116. https://doi.org/10.1359/jbmr.091036

Pilarski R (2009) Cowden syndrome: a critical review of the clinical literature. J Genet Couns 18:13–27

Qu N, Yao W, Cui X, Zhang H (2015) Malignant transformation in monostotic fibrous dysplasia: clinical features, imaging features, outcomes in 10 patients, and review. Medicine (United States) 94:e369. https://doi.org/10.1097/MD.0000000000000369

Randle SC (2017) Tuberous sclerosis complex: a review. Pediatr Ann 46:e166–e171. https://doi.org/10.3928/19382359-20170320-01

Riminucci M, Collins MT, Lala R et al (2002) An R201H activating mutation of the GNAS1 (Gsα) gene in a corticotroph pituitary adenoma. J Clin Pathol Mol Pathol 55:58–60. https://doi.org/10.1136/mp.55.1.58

Riminucci M, Saggio I, Gehron Robey P, Bianco P (2006) Fibrous dysplasia as a stem cell disease. J Bone Mineral Res 21(Suppl 2):P125–P131

Robinson C, Collins MT, Boyce AM (2016) Fibrous dysplasia/McCune-Albright syndrome: clinical and translational perspectives. Curr Osteoporos Rep 14:178–186

Romei C, Cosci B, Renzini G et al (2011) RET genetic screening of sporadic medullary thyroid cancer (MTC) allows the preclinical diagnosis of unsuspected gene carriers and the identification of a relevant percentage of hidden familial MTC (FMTC). Clin Endocrinol 74:241–247. https://doi.org/10.1111/j.1365-2265.2010.03900.x

Rosser T, Panigrahy A, McClintock W (2006) The diverse clinical manifestations of tuberous sclerosis complex: a review. Semin Pediatr Neurol 13:27–36. https://doi.org/10.1016/j.spen.2006.01.008

Roy PK, Venzon DJ, Shojamanesh H et al (2000) Zollinger-Ellison syndrome: clinical presentation in 261 patients. Medicine (Baltimore) 79:379–411. https://doi.org/10.1097/00005792-200011000-00004

Ruggieri P, Sim FH, Bond JR, Krishnan Unni K (1994) Malignancies in fibrous dysplasia. Cancer 73:1411–1424. https://doi.org/10.1002/1097-0142(19940301)73:5<1411::AID-CNCR2820730516>3.0.CO;2-T

Rüther U, Garber C, Komitowski D et al (1987) Deregulated c-fos expression interferes with normal bone development in transgenic mice. Nature 325:412–416. https://doi.org/10.1038/325412a0

Saggini A, Brandi M (2011) Skin lesions in hereditary endocrine tumor syndromes. Endocr Pract 17:47–57. https://doi.org/10.4158/EP11055.RA

Sakurai A, Suzuki S, Kosugi S et al (2012) Multiple endocrine neoplasia type 1 in Japan: establishment and analysis of a multicentre database. Clin Endocrinol 76:533–539. https://doi.org/10.1111/j.1365-2265.2011.04227.x

Salenave S, Boyce AM, Collins MT, Chanson P (2014) Acromegaly and Mccune-albright syndrome. J Clin Endocrinol Metab 99:1955–1969. https://doi.org/10.1210/jc.2013-3826

Sammour T, Hayes IP, Hill AG et al (2015) Familial colorectal cancer syndromes: an overview of clinical management. Expert Rev Gastroenterol Hepatol 9:757–764. https://doi.org/10.1586/17474124.2015.1026328

Sharretts JM, Simonds WF (2010) Clinical and molecular genetics of parathyroid neoplasms. Best Pract Res Clin Endocrinol Metab 24:491–502. https://doi.org/10.1016/j.beem.2010.01.003

Simonds WF (2017) Genetics of hyperparathyroidism, including parathyroid Cancer. Endocrinol Metab Clin N Am 46:405–418

Soga J, Yakuwa Y (1998) The gastrinoma/Zollinger-Ellison syndrome: statistical evaluation of a Japanese series of 359 cases. J Hepato-Biliary-Pancreat Surg 5:77–85. https://doi.org/10.1007/PL00009955

Steiner AL, Goodman AD, Powers SR (1968) Study of a kindred with pheochromocytoma, medullary thyroid carcinoma, hyperparathyroidism and Cushing's disease: multiple endocrine neoplasia, type 2. Medicine (United States) 47:371–409. https://doi.org/10.1097/00005792-196809000-00001

Stratakis CA (2016) Hereditary syndromes predisposing to endocrine tumors and their skin manifestations. Rev Endocr Metab Disord 17:381–388

Subbiah S, Palikhe G, Bhadada SK et al (2011) Acrogigantism and facial asymmetry: McCune-Albright syndrome. J Pediatr Endocrinol Metab 24:835–837. https://doi.org/10.1515/JPEM.2011.274

Tchekmedyian A, Amos CI, Bale SJ et al (2013) Findings from the Peutz-Jeghers syndrome registry of Uruguay. PLoS One 8:e79639. https://doi.org/10.1371/journal.pone.0079639

Thakker RV, Newey PJ, Walls GV et al (2012) Clinical practice guidelines for multiple endocrine neoplasia type 1 (MEN1). J Clin Endocrinol Metab 97:2990–3011

Tomuschat C, Puri P (2015) RET gene is a major risk factor for Hirschsprung's disease: a meta-analysis. Pediatr Surg Int 31:701–710. https://doi.org/10.1007/s00383-015-3731-y

Traugott AL, Moley JF (2010) Multiple endocrine neoplasia type 2: clinical manifestations and management. Cancer Treat Res 153:321–337. https://doi.org/10.1007/978-1-4419-0857-5_18

Trump D, Farren B, Wooding C et al (1997) Clinical studies of multiple endocrine neoplasia type 1 (MEN1). Q J Med 90:19–25. https://doi.org/10.2307/2327868

Van Lier MGF, Westerman AM, Wagner A et al (2011) High cancer risk and increased mortality in patients with Peutz-Jeghers syndrome. Gut 60:141–147

Varshney N, Kebede AA, Owusu-Dapaah H et al (2017) A review of Von Hippel-Lindau syndrome. J Kidney Cancer VHL 4:20–29. https://doi.org/10.15586/jkcvhl.2017.88

Vasen HFA, Lamers CBHW, Lips CJM (1989) Screening for the multiple endocrine neoplasia syndrome type I. A study of 11 kindreds in the Netherlands. Arch Intern Med 149:2717–2722. https://doi.org/10.1001/archinte.149.12.2717
Vashi N, Hunt R, Fischer M et al (2012) Angiofibromas in multiple endocrine neoplasia type 1. Dermatol Online J 18:20
Weinstein LS, Shenker A, Gejman PV et al (1991) Activating mutations of the stimulatory G protein in the McCune–Albright syndrome. N Engl J Med 325:1688–1695. https://doi.org/10.1056/NEJM199112123252403
Wells SA, Pacini F, Robinson BG, Santoro M (2013) Multiple endocrine neoplasia type 2 and familial medullary thyroid carcinoma: an update. J Clin Endocrinol Metab 98:3149–3164. https://doi.org/10.1210/jc.2013-1204
Wells SA, Asa SL, Dralle H et al (2015) Revised American Thyroid Association guidelines for the management of medullary thyroid carcinoma. Thyroid 25:567–610. https://doi.org/10.1089/thy.2014.0335
Yates CJ, Newey PJ, Thakker RV (2015) Challenges and controversies in management of pancreatic neuroendocrine tumours in patients with MEN1. Lancet Diabetes Endocrinol 3:895–905
Znaczko A, Donnelly DE, Morrison PJ (2014) Epidemiology, clinical features, and genetics of multiple endocrine neoplasia type 2B in a complete population. Oncologist 19:1284–1286. https://doi.org/10.1634/theoncologist.2014-0277

Chapter 8
Hereditary Diseases Predisposing to Pheochromocytoma (VHL, NF-1, Paraganglioma Syndromes, and Novel Genes)

Balázs Sarkadi and Attila Patócs

Abstract Pheochromocytomas (Pheo) and paragangliomas (PGL) are rare tumors originating from catecholamine-producing chromaffin cells. They occur approximately in 0.1% of patients affected with hypertonia. Pheo/PGL may manifest itself at any age; in 10% of the patients, the disease is bilateral, and also in 10% it occurs outside of the adrenal medulla. From a genetic aspect, a considerable proportion of these tumors represents a prototype for an autosomal dominantly inherited syndrome with incomplete penetrance. In addition, to date more than 15 genes have been identified representing genetic susceptibility for Pheo/PGL and accounting for 40% of all cases. In general, in familiar cases, the tumor manifests at younger age, and they are often occurring as multiplex tumors. Permanent recovery can be achieved with an early diagnosis and with a successful surgical removal of the tumor tissue. On the other hand, undiagnosed, hormonally active Pheos may lead to severe, or even lethal, consequences. This chapter will summarize our recent knowledge about the genetics of Pheo/PGL, focusing on tumor syndromes where Pheo/PGLs are among the main manifestations.

Keywords Pheochromocytoma · Paraganglioma · Hereditary tumor syndromes

B. Sarkadi
2nd Department of Medicine, Semmelweis University, Budapest, Hungary

MTA-SE Lendület Hereditary Endocrine Tumors Research Group, Budapest, Hungary

A. Patócs (✉)
Department of Laboratory Medicine, Faculty of Medicine, Semmelweis University, Budapest, Hungary

"Lendület" Hereditary Endocrine Tumors Research Group, Hungarian Academy of Sciences and Semmelweis University, Budapest, Hungary

Department of Molecular Genetics, National Institute of Oncology, Budapest, Hungary
e-mail: patocs.attila@med.semmelweis-univ.hu

P. Igaz, A. Patócs (eds.), *Genetics of Endocrine Diseases and Syndromes*, Experientia Supplementum 111, https://doi.org/10.1007/978-3-030-25905-1_8

List of Abbreviations

CT	Computed tomography
FuH	Fumarate hydratase
GAP	GTPase-activating protein
GLUT1	Glucose transporter 1
HIF-1	Hypoxia-inducible factor type 1
HNPGL	Head and neck paraganglioma
KIF1	Kinesin-like protein 1
LDH	Lactate dehydrogenase
MAX	MYC-associated factor X
MDH2	Malate dehydrogenase type 2
MIBG	Meta-iodobenzylguanidine
MLPA	Multiple ligation probe amplification
MRI	Magnetic resonance imaging
NF1	Neurofibromatosis type 1
PDGF	Platelet-derived growth factor
PGL	Paraganglioma
PHD1,2	Prolyl-hydroxylases 1 and 2
Pheo	Pheochromocytoma
RT-PCR	Reverse transcription polymerase chain reaction
SDH	Succinate dehydrogenase
SLC25A11	Solute carrier family 25 member 11
TCA	Tricarboxylic acid cycle
TMEM127	Transmembrane protein 127
VEGF	Vascular endothelial growth factor
VHL	von Hippel-Lindau

8.1 Introduction

Pheochromocytomas (Pheo) and paragangliomas (PGL) are tumors arising from neural crest cells. There are some discrepancies in terminology, but in this chapter we use the term "Pheo" for tumors located in the adrenal gland (adrenal medulla), while the term "PGL" is used for tumors located both at the head and neck (HNPGL) or intra-abdominal but extra-adrenal PGL. For PGLs, the most prominent location is the carotid body, but tumors in the vagal, jugular, and tympanic glomus are also observed. Usually, both Pheos and PGLs are benign, slowly growing tumors. Hormonal activity is related to their catecholamine synthesis and release, and major clinical manifestations and symptoms are also caused by catecholamines. Pheo are more hormonally active compared to head and neck PGL. For evaluation of hormone activity, collected urine for determination of catecholamine and catecholamine metabolites as well as serum chromogranin A assay are recommended (Lenders et al. 2014).

Hormonally inactive tumors are usually detected incidentally through imaging studies of the abdomen, thorax, or skull. On the other hand, in patients with suspicion for Pheo and PGL, imaging studies are important part of the diagnosis. Computed tomography (CT) and magnetic resonance imaging (MRI) as well as carotid ultrasound for head and neck PGLs, while for intra-abdominal tumors abdominal ultrasound, CT and MRI, and meta-iodobenzylguanidine (MIBG) scan are used. In many cases, most often in the case of extra-adrenal tumors, PET is the most effective diagnostic tool. In familial cases, tumors may be multifocal, and their localization is best identified by MIBG. The definitive diagnosis of PGL is achievable by histological examination. It must be noted that malignancy of Pheo/PGL cannot be established by histological diagnosis, and malignancy can only be based on clinical criteria, i.e., presence of metastases. Metastases can appear several years after tumor removal. Thus, although malignancy is rare, all Pheo/PGLs should be considered potentially malignant and should be followed up regularly (Plouin et al. 2016).

In general, these tumors are rare; an annual incidence is approximately 1 per 100,000. HNPGL represents less than 0.5% of all head and neck tumors. 20% of Pheo and PGLs are diagnosed in children, where usually symptomatic, bilateral, and extra-adrenal tumors are typical. Of note, many Pheos were unidentified during life and were diagnosed during autopsies. The prevalence of Pheo is about 1:2000 in autopsy series. Therefore, clinical diagnosis in many cases is missed. The main reason behind this phenomenon is the lack of specific clinical symptoms or lack of biochemical evidence. Genetics and developments of diagnostic procedures from the past decade might help in improving the diagnostics.

Genetic background is well established in Pheo/PGLs. Some of these tumors develop within a classical tumor syndrome including multiple endocrine neoplasia type 2 (MEN2), von Hippel-Lindau disease, neurofibromatosis type 1, and hereditary PGL syndromes (PGL1-5). Patients with hereditary Pheo have a lifelong risk of second primary tumors and relapse. The recent findings about their pathogenesis and phenotypic characteristics help to reduce their morbidity and mortality. In many cases gene- or even codon/mutation-specific preventive medical management has been described (Frank-Raue et al. 2011; Bausch et al. 2017).

Early onset of disease, bilateral, multifocal, extra-adrenal, and malignant tumors are clinical hallmarks of hereditary disease. Pheo/PGLs are the most genetically determined tumors. Except for *RET* proto-oncogene, other genes involved in genetic susceptibility for Pheo/PGLs are classical tumor suppressor genes. The tumorigenesis mechanism in these cases follows the Knudson described mechanism. The first mutation (first hit) appears germline, but for the development of the tumor, an additional somatic mutation or loss of wild type allele (second hit) is necessary. Tumor suppressor genes associated to date with development of Pheo/PGLs are the following: *SDHD*, *SDHC*, *SDHB*, *SDHAF2*, *SDHA*, *VHL*, *HIF2*, *FuH*, *EGLN1*, *EGLN2*, *KIF1ß*, *NF1*, *MAX*, *TMEM127*, *GOT2*, *MDH2*, and *SLC25A11* (Bausch et al. 2017; Buffet et al. 2018). *RET* mutations cause multiple endocrine neoplasia type 2. This syndrome was discussed in the previous chapter (Chap. 7), but all other genes will be presented in detail in this current chapter.

8.2 von Hippel-Lindau Syndrome (VHL) (OMIM NM_000551.3)

8.2.1 Prevalence, Phenotype

The VHL syndrome was first described by Eugen von Hippel and Arvid Lindau. Generally it manifests with central nervous system's vessel-related tumors (hemangioblastomas of the cerebellum, spinal cord, and retina), renal cell carcinoma, endolymphatic cancer and Pheo. Moreover, it is often accompanied by cystic lesions of the kidney, the pancreas, and the epididymis. Pancreatic neuroendocrine tumor also occurs, and it represents significant morbidity and mortality (Neumann et al. 2004).

Prevalence is estimated at 1/53,000 and annual birth incidence at 1/36,000. Pheo is estimated to develop in 10–20% of VHL patients, but depending on the mutation, major phenotype differences can be observed between VHL families.

Classification of VHL subtypes is based on their specific genotype-phenotype correlations, depending on the presence of Pheo. Patients with VHL type 1 have very low risk for Pheo, while type 2 patients often develop Pheo. The mortality due to Pheo in VHL patients is estimated to be 5%. Pheo appears earlier in VHL patients compared to sporadic cases (generally at age 30 years), and the manifestation is often bilateral and multiplex, but malignant cases are rare (Chen et al. 1995; Eisenhofer et al. 2001). Tumor can be extra-adrenal and intra-abdominal, and even extra-abdominal.

Hemangioblastomas are the most frequent tumors in VHL syndrome, developing in 60–80% of VHL patients, generally around age 30 years. The most frequently affected regions are the spinal cord (50%), the cerebellum (37%), and the brainstem (10%). The clinical symptoms are influenced by the location, size, associated edema, and cysts as well. Tumors of the cerebellum are accompanied by headaches, dizziness, nausea, and imbalance and ataxia; brain stem location is associated with hyperesthesia, headaches, dysphagia, and hyperreflexia. Hyperesthesia and pain could also point to spinal cord localization. Although the hemangioblastomas are slowly growing, benign tumors, the subsequent increased pressure in the central nervous system is accountable for major cases of VHL morbidity and mortality.

Angiomas of the retina occur in 50% of the cases. These benign tumors are often recurrent, bilateral, and multiplex. Retinal detachment and blindness regularly develop without definitive therapy (laser coagulation, cryotherapy); therefore, consultations with an ophthalmologist should take place yearly.

Renal cell carcinoma is the second most common lesion in VHL, occurring approximately in 24–70% of the patients. Renal cell carcinoma is often multiplex, bilateral, rapidly progressing tumor with a potential to form metastases early to the regional lymph nodes, the liver, and the brain. Despite these severe manifestations, the disease is usually silent for years, and symptoms (hematuria and pain) appear in advanced stages only.

Pancreas lesions (usually cysts) accompany VHL in 25% of the cases, but autopsy confirms this number is around 70%. Islet cell tumors also appear in 5–10% of the patients. Clinical symptoms are related to the size of the cyst (abdominal discomfort or pain, rarely pancreatitis) (Neumann et al. 1991). Diagnosis can be achieved with ultrasound or CT. The treatment depends on the extension of the cyst. In solitary cases surgical excision is recommended, but if there are no clinical symptoms or signs of malignancy, even conservative therapy is possible with continuous control.

8.2.2 Genetic Background: Function of the VHL Tumor Suppressor Gene

Located in the third chromosome's short arm (3p25 locus), *VHL* tumor suppressor gene's germline mutations are responsible for the von Hippel-Lindau syndrome. According to Knudson's hypothesis (Chap. 1), tumors develop in patients where the wild allele becomes mutated or deleted. *VHL* gene encodes the VHL protein, which forms a stable ubiquitin-ligase complex with Rbx1, Cullin2, and elongin B and C proteins. This complex mediates the function of RNA polymerase II and participates in the ubiquitin-mediated degradation of hypoxia-inducible factor 1 (HIF-1). The prolyl-hydroxylase enzyme serves as a molecular sensor in the presence of oxygen and through hydroxylation degrades the alfa subunit of HIF-1. Under hypoxic conditions or when *VHL* mutated, HIF-1α stabilizes and attaches to HIF-1ß and then translocates to the nucleus where it promotes the transcription of its target genes. The activated genes (VEGF, PDGF, erythropoietin, LDH, and GLUT1 transport) are responsible for the accommodation to hypoxic conditions. This mechanism is called pseudo-hypoxia, and it has also been described in tumors associating with mutations of succinate dehydrogenase subunits encoding genes (*SDHx, discussed later)*. In addition, VHL participates in the regulatory functions of the mitochondria and the cell cycle. According to novel data, VHL is also engaged in the organization of microtubules and in the formation of cilium due to the interaction with the PAR proteins which determine the membrane domains of the polarized epithelial cells. Loss of VHL function results in the false organization of microtubes with the inhibition if ciliogenesis, which results in the disturbance of the cytoskeleton and in the loss of polarization of the epithelial cells (Kaelin Jr 2002).

From genotype-phenotype associations should be highlighted that truncating mutations and large deletions associate with type 1 disease, while missense mutations with type 2 disease. Mutations which disrupt the VHL-HIF protein interaction more often cause renal cell cancer, while mutations in other parts of the gene lead to Pheo. In addition, missense mutations located at the surface of the protein have been found more commonly in Pheo compared to missense mutations located in the deeper protein region (Ong et al. 2007).

8.2.3 Genetic Diagnosis and Genetic Counseling

VHL syndrome is an autosomal dominant disease; therefore, there is 50% chance of an offspring to inherit the disease-related gene alteration from their parents. The whole *VHL* gene needs to be screened in case of VHL syndrome. This requires the bidirectional sequencing of the coding regions and the utilization of the quantitative molecular biological technologies which can detect the heterozygote loss of certain exons. Routine examination for large germline deletions of the *VHL* gene is mandatory, because so-called large deletion can be observed in 15–20% of the VHL patients. Exceptionally sensitive methods are necessary for the detection of germline heterozygote deletions, for example, southern blot hybridization, quantitative real-time PCR, and multiplex ligation probe amplification (Gergics et al. 2009). The clinical manifestation of VHL syndrome varies even between patients with the same mutation, therefore strict clinical and laboratory observation of the pathogenic mutation carriers is highly recommended. The comprehensive and regularly updated VHL mutation database can be found at http://www.umd.be/VHL/.

Pheo is present in 10–20% of VHL patients, but differences in the phenotype can be observed depending on the mutations (Chen et al. 1995). Pheo can be the earliest manifestation of the disease, and it accounts for at least half of the Pheo developed in childhood (Bausch et al. 2014). Malignancy is rare in VHL-associated Pheos, but clinically symptomatic tumors are often developing, and rarely HNPGLs can also be detected. Clinical screening for Pheo in VHL-associated families starts at age 5 years, and annual plasma-free metanephrines or urinary catecholamine and catecholamine metabolites are indicated.

8.3 Neurofibromatosis Type 1 (OMIM 613675)

8.3.1 Prevalence, Phenotype

Neurofibromatosis type 1 (NF-1) or von Recklinghausen disease is an autosomal dominantly inherited hereditary genetic disorder with neurocutaneous abnormalities. Its prevalence is approximately 1: 3–4000 (Bausch et al. 2007).

NF-1 is characterized by neurofibromas on the skin, pigmented "cafe au lait" spots, and the hamartomas of the iris (Lisch nodules) (Otsuka et al. 2001). The disease may be accompanied by nerve optic glioma, Pheo, and carcinoid tumor. Pheo is relatively rare (about 1% of cases) and is expected to occur in older age, but in patients with hypertensive neurofibromatosis, the frequency of Pheo can be as high as 50%. Neurofibromas are benign tumors of the peripheral nerve sheath; they may manifest as cutaneous, subcutaneous, or plexiform lesions. Compression of peripheral nerves, spinal nerves, or spinal cord can cause neurological symptoms. NF1 patients have about 7–12% chance of developing malignant neoplasmic tumors, which often develop from existing subcutaneous or plexiform neurofibromas (in contrast, cutaneous neurofibromas do not transform into malignant form). Café au lait spots can be confirmed in 95% of patients, usually before the age of 30 years. The lesions appear most often in the intertriginous areas first. Occasionally, hypopigmented macules may also appear. Malignant central nervous system tumors, cutaneous hemangiomas, and NF-1-related vasculopathy might also occur.

In terms of differential diagnostics, other syndromes with skin manifestations should be considered (phacomatosis syndromes including Cowden disease, Carney complex, tuberous sclerosis, *discussed in Chaps. 7 and 9 of this book*).

Management of the disease depends on the tumors. Treatment of benign, non-symptomatic neurofibromas is not required. In more severe cases, when neurofibromas develop in the central nervous system and affecting the optic nerve, surgical removal is recommended. Treatment of Pheos is always surgical. The prognosis of NF-1 is good; morbidity and mortality depend on the number of neurofibromas and their subtype. In most cases, regular (yearly) physical examination and ocular examination of patients is sufficient. Rarely, severe malignant tumors can occur (<10% of cases), and NF1 vasculopathy may develop, which includes stenosis of the kidney artery, possibly coarctation of the aorta. In these cases, the morbidity and mortality rates are worse (Bausch et al. 2007).

8.3.2 Genetic Background: Function of the NF1 Protein

NF1 is caused by mutations of the *NF1* tumor suppressor gene, located on the short arm of chromosome 17 (17q11.2). The product of the *NF1* gene is the cytoplasmic-derived neurofibromin protein, which is expressed in large numbers of cells in the central nervous system. Neurofibromin has a role in the signal transduction pathway of the mitogenetic regulatory Ras system. Connecting to the Ras/GTPase-activating protein (GAP), neurofibromin catalyzes the hydrolysis of the activated Ras and thus promotes the formation of inactive GDP-bound Ras, which inhibits cell proliferation. When the neurofibromin function is impaired, MAPKs are activated (Barker et al. 1987).

8.3.3 Genetic Diagnosis and Genetic Counseling

In contrast to other autosomal dominant hereditary syndromes, molecular genetic screening of *NF1* gene was not part of the routine diagnostics before next-generation sequencing era. Nowadays, using comprehensive cancer panels or Pheo/PGL-specific targeted sequencing, the molecular analysis of *NF1* is widely available. Genotype-phenotype correlations are unknown.

The disease has an autosomal dominant hereditary pathway; hence, the offsprings have a 50% chance to inherit the disease-causing mutation from the affected parent. Prenatal testing is also available.

8.4 Hereditary Pheo/PGL Syndromes

This subgroup of hereditary Pheo/PGLs is caused by mutations of the genes encoding the subunits of succinate dehydrogenase (SDH). SDH is composed of four subunits, of which subunits A and B are catalytic subunits and participate in succinate-fumarate hydroxylation. Subunits C and D anchor SDHA and SDHB to the inner mitochondrial membrane. Besides participating in the tricarboxylic acid cycle (TCA), SDH is involved in mitochondrial electron transport chain too. Since the first report showing that the germline mutation of the *SDHD* associated with Pheo/PGLs during the past 18 years, mutations of genes encoding other subunits of *SDH* or mutations of genes encoding other enzymes of TCA have been identified as pathogenetic factors of Pheo/PGL.

The common genetic feature for SDH subunits is that all these genes are nucleus-encoded genes; hence, the disease follows the classical autosomal dominant pattern. Chromosomal localizations and associated phenotypes are listed in Table 8.1.

In familial cases, germline mutations in *SDHB*, *SDHC*, and *SDHD* can be confirmed in about 50–70% of cases. Besides the familial cases, the apparently sporadic cases carry a mutation in one of the *SDHx* genes in 25–30% of the affected patients. Several genotype-phenotype relationships can be observed based on the available literature; however, overlaps between these syndromes are also known.

8.4.1 Paraganglioma Syndrome Type 1 (OMIM 168000)

It was reported in 2000 for the first time that germline mutation of *SDHD* is associated with Pheo/PGL (Baysal et al. 2000). From that time, several reports confirmed that *SDHD* mutations contribute to both intra-abdominal and HNPGLs. The gene is a relatively small gene, encoded by 4 exons. Disease-causing mutations spread all over the gene. Nonsense, frameshift, and missense mutations have been described, but there are more mutations leading to protein breakage. For precise genotype-phenotype associations and for every day clinical genetics practice an online tool, the SDH mutation database (https://databases.lovd.nl/shared/genes/) is available. *SDHD* gene is maternally imprinted which means that only patients inheriting the mutation from the paternal side will be clinically affected (Fig. 8.1).

Based on data obtained in the largest cohort of independent patients with Pheo/PGLs showed that multiple, benign tumors occurred in 74% of *SDHD* mutation carriers. Adrenal Pheos occurred in 53%, extra-adrenal PGLs in 21%, and HNPGLs in 79% of *SDHD* carriers. Age-related penetrance reached 86% by age 50 years for *SDHD* carriers (Neumann et al. 2002).

Table 8.1 Genes and syndromes presenting genetic susceptibility for pheochromocytoma and paraganglioma

Gene (Ref seq.)	Chromosomal localization	Syndrome	Year of gene discovery	Predominant localization of Pheo/PGL tumors	Other manifestations
NF1 NM_000267.3	17q11.2	Neurofibromatosis type 1	1990	Adrenal	Cafe au lait spots Neurofibromas
RET NM_020975.4	10q11.21	Multiple endocrine Neoplasia type 2	1994	Adrenal, freq. bilateral	Medullary thyroid cancer Hyperparathyroidism Neurinoma (MEN2B)
VHL NM_000551.3	3p25.3	von Hippel-Lindau disease	1993	Adrenal, freq. bilateral, extra-adrenal Pheo	Retina angioma Hemangioblastoma Renal cell cancer
SDHD NM_003002.3	11q23.1	PGL1	2000	Head and neck PGL Intra-abdominal Pheo and PGL	C cell hyperplasia and hypercalcemia
SDHC NM_003001.3	1q23.3	PGL3	2001	Head and neck PGL	Gastrointestinal stromal tumor
SDHB NM_003000.2	1p36.13	PGL4	2000	PGL intra-abdominal, malignant	Renal carcinoma, gastrointestinal stromal tumor, leiomyomas
PHD2	1q42.2		2008	PGL	Familial erythrocytosis type 3
KIF1B	1p36.22		2008	Adrenal Pheo	Charcot-Marie-Tooth Disease, Axonal, Type 2a1
SDHAF2/SDH5 NM_017841.2	11q12.2	PGL2	2010	PGL	
TMEM127 NM_017849.3	2q11.2		2010	Adrenal Pheo	
SDHA NM_004168.3	5p15.33	PGL5	2011	PGL	Leigh's syndrome
MAX NM_002382.4	14q23.3		2011	Adrenal Pheo, PGL	
MDH2	7q21.12		2015	Adrenal Pheo, PGL	Epileptic encephalopathy

(continued)

Table 8.1 (continued)

Gene (Ref seq.)	Chromosomal localization	Syndrome	Year of gene discovery	Predominant localization of Pheo/PGL tumors	Other manifestations
FuH	1q43		2014	PGL	Renal cell cancer, leiomyomas
GOT2	16q21		2017	Adrenal Pheo, PGL	
SLC25A11	17p13.2		2018	PGL	

NF1 neurofibromatosis type 1, *RET* rearranged during transfection, *SDHD* succinate dehydrogenase subunit D, *SDHB* succinate dehydrogenase subunit B, *SDHC* succinate dehydrogenase subunit C, *SDHA* succinate dehydrogenase subunit A, *SDHAF2* succinate dehydrogenase assembly factor 2, *PHD2* prolyl-hydroxylase type 2, *KIF1B* kinesin family member 1B, *TMEM127* transmembrane protein 127, *MAX* Myc-associated factor X, *MDH2* malate dehydrogenase type 2, *FH* fumarate hydratase, *GOT2* glutamic-oxaloacetic transaminase 2, *SLC25A11* solute carrier family 25 member 11 (oxoglutarate/malate carrier 2), *VHL* von Hippel-Lindau, *PGL* paraganglioma, *Pheo* pheochromocytoma (adrenal localization), *PGL1-5* paraganglioma syndrome type 1-type 5, *MEN2B* multiple endocrine neoplasia type 2B

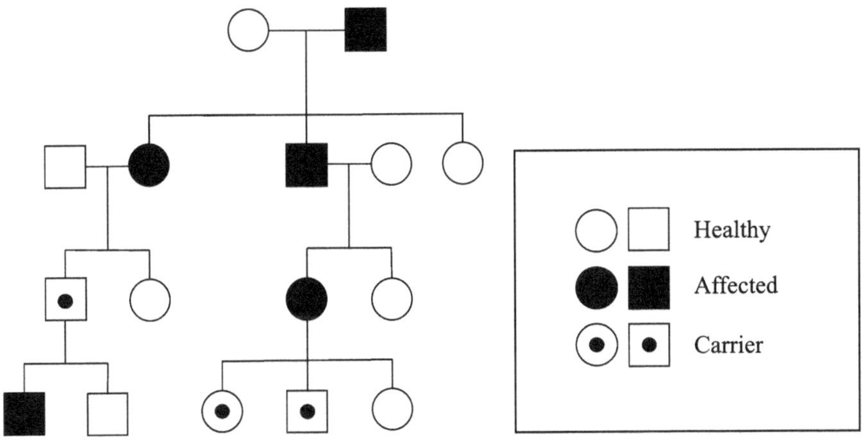

Fig. 8.1 Schematic pedigree showing maternal imprinting in a family with SDHD mutation

8.4.2 Paraganglioma Syndrome Type 2 (OMIM 601650)

The gene responsible for PGL2 is *SDHAF2* (also known as *SDH5)* which encodes a factor necessary for flavination of the SDHA protein. The gene was identified in 2009 (Hao et al. 2009). It represents an extremely rare (<1%) cause for HNPGLs. The inheritance is similar to those described for *SDHD* (autosomal dominant with paternal transmission). Very few genotype-phenotype associations were reported. Based on data obtained on the largest kindred (Kunst et al. 2011), the average age of onset was 33 years, while the penetrance by age 50 years reached 100%. No malignancy was reported. Genetic analysis, therefore, should be offered for patients with HNPGLs who were negative for *SDHD* and *SDHC* mutations, but it should also highlight that the chance to detect any pathogenic variant in *SDHAF2* is low.

8.4.3 Paraganglioma Syndrome Type 3 (OMIM 605373)

SDHC mutation is a rare cause of HNPGLs. It was identified in 2000 (Niemann and Muller 2000), and from then it was reported to account for less than 1% of all HNPGLs and extremely rarely in Pheos or intra-abdominal PGLs. Clinically, the *SDHC*-mutated tumors show benign behavior (Schiavi et al. 2005).

8.4.4 Paraganglioma Syndrome Type 4 (OMIM: 115310)

Germline mutations in the *SDHB* gene can be found in approximately 10% of PHEOs/PGLs (Bjorklund et al. 2016). The overall penetrance is around 50%, but it should be noticed that there are data showing both smaller (21–30%) (Hes et al. 2010; Schiavi et al. 2010; Rijken et al. 2016) and larger (65–100%) (Neumann et al. 2004; Benn et al. 2006; Solis et al. 2009; Ricketts et al. 2010) intervals. This discrepancy can be expected either from the calculation methods used in these studies (inclusion of index cases or just screened individuals, statistical method, etc.) or from populations studied. In many regions, founder mutations have been described which may cause bias in correct determination of the real penetrance (Hensen et al. 2012).

The most important phenotype associated with *SDHB* mutation is malignancy (defined as Pheo/PGL tissues in non-chromaffin tissues) (Gimenez-Roqueplo et al. 2003). Of the 16 Pheo/PGL genes, malignancy was found to associate with *SDHB*, *MAX*, and *FuH* mutations. A recent, multivariate model showed that the presence of metastasis correlated with *SDHB* mutation (OR 5.68 [95% CI 1.79–18.06]) but not with the primary location of the tumor. In *SDHB* carriers, tumors can be found intra-abdominal, intra-adrenal, and also at head and neck regions with an approximately 60%, 20%, and 20%. Malignancy tends to be associated with intra-abdominal, extra-adrenal located tumors.

SDHB mutations have been also found in patients with clear cell renal carcinoma, breast adenocarcinoma, prostate cancer, gastrointestinal stromal tumors, papillary thyroid cancer, and pituitary tumors (Neumann et al. 2004; Ni et al. 2008; Ricketts et al. 2008). Of these tumors, both gastrointestinal stromal tumor and clear cell renal carcinoma are present in the Carney triad caused also by germline *SDHB* mutations (Carney triad consists of gastric leiomyosarcoma, pulmonary chondroma and extra-adrenal PGL). Other associations reported (i.e., pituitary tumors, breast carcinoma, colon tumors) the need for further studies for confirmation and to place these data in clinical practice.

For finding *SDHB* mutation-associated tumors, immunostaining for SDHB protein has been successfully introduced and validated in clinical practice. *SDHB*-associated tumors show completely negative staining. Pheos, PGLs, and renal cell carcinoma specimens confirmed the accuracy of this screening method (Gill et al. 2011; Patocs et al. 2016).

8.4.5 Paraganglioma Syndrome Type 5 (OMIM 600857)

Mutation of SDHA gene causes PGL syndrome type 5. The causative role of this gene was identified in a patient with intra-abdominal PGL (Burnichon et al. 2010). SDHA is a rare cause of Pheo/PGLs; it accounts for <1% of all cases. The penetrance is also low. In addition, the molecular genetic testing of SDHA gene is difficult; this is the largest gene of SDHx genes, and it has three pseudogenes. Based on our experience and also suggested by a recent guideline (Lenders et al. 2014), genetic analysis of *SDHA* is recommended after testing of *SDHB*, *SDHD*, *TMEM127*, and *MAX* for nonsyndromic Pheo and *SDHB*, *SDHD*, and *SDHC* for HNPGLs. Recent practice using next-generation sequencing allows the comprehensive mutation analysis for all cases (Sarkadi et al. 2018; Ben Aim et al. 2019).

Of note, SDHA is a genetic cause of the autosomal recessive inherited mitochondrial complex II deficiency presenting as Leigh syndrome (OMIM: 256000) (Bourgeron et al. 1995).

8.5 Other Genes Associated with Pheo/PGL

In the past decade, another 10 genes were identified by whole exome sequencing as genetic predisposition for Pheo/PGL. Based on data published about the genotype-phenotype association found between genes *SDHA*, *TMEM127*, *MAX*, and *SDHAF2*, it is clear that even their prevalence is rare. Their mutation frequencies were 3.0% for *SDHA*, 2.1% for *TMEM127*, 0,8% for *MAX*, and 0,1 for *SDHAF2* among patients with apparently sporadic Pheo/PGL (Bausch et al. 2017). In addition, the prevalence of the most novel genes (*KIF1B*, *FuH*, *PHD1*, *PHD2*, *HIF2*, *MDH2*, *GOT2*, *SLC25A11*) is largely unknown, but it is expected to be extremely low. Based on their rarity, we do not have special genotype-phenotype correlations. All patients with mutations in one of the *SDHA*, *TMEM127*, *MAX*, and *SDHAF2* genes could have Pheo/PGL all over the body. The earliest age at onset in *SDHA* mutation carriers was 8 years, and extra-adrenal tumors, especially HNPGLs, were found in two third of patients harboring *SDHA* mutations. *MAX* and *TMEM127* mutations were associated mainly with bilateral adrenal Pheos, but HNPGLs were also described. Malignancy occurred in approximately 10% of patients harboring one of the *SDHA*, *MAX*, and *TMEM127* mutations (Bausch et al. 2017). Interestingly, FuH mutation carriers also presented with metastatic Pheo/PGL and with multiple tumors including multiple cutaneous and uterine leiomyomatosis (Castro-Vega et al. 2014). *MDH2* mutation identified with WES associated also with malignant PGL (Cascon et al. 2015). In summary, our knowledge about the genetics of Pheo/PGL extensively increased with the start of using next-generation sequencing in everyday clinical practice. However, it should be noted that the recently described mutations (FuH, MDH2, SLC25A11) were found through systematic screening of large patient cohorts, and their cumulative prevalence is less than 2%, suggesting that these genes are not representing major genetic susceptibility loci for Pheo/PGL. However, these genes also cause autosomal dominantly inherited tumors which should be followed clinically similarly to those associated with earlier identified genes. Therefore, molecular genetic analysis for patients with Pheo/PGL should include these novel genes too (Sarkadi et al. 2018; Ben Aim et al. 2019).

8.6 The Pathomechanism Associated with *SDHx* Mutations

The pathomechanism associated with the abnormal functioning of the SDH protein is unclear. Due to the reduced function of the succinate dehydrogenase enzyme, succinate is accumulated and then translocated into the cytoplasm, where it inhibits the prolyl-hydroxylase enzyme. As a consequence, HIF1 is stabilized and transcription of several genes (hypoxia-sensitive genes: VEGF, PDGF, GLUT1) is enhanced (pathomechanism of pseudo-hypoxia) (Fig. 8.2). This pathomechanism is responsible for tumorigenesis in VHL-associated tumors too. Furthermore, the role of DNA damage due to increased production of reactive oxygen radicals has been implicated with the development of the disease. The other possible pathogenetic processes associating with SDH failure are the activation of ATP synthesis, the increased activation of cellular survival pathways as a result of abnormal mitochondrial function and the impairment of apoptosis. Taken together all biochemical, molecular, and cell biological data, it can be concluded that SDH inactivation leads to the accumulation of its substrate, succinate, which acts as an oncometabolite by inhibiting 2-oxoglutarate-dependent dioxygenases. Of this class of enzymes, inhibition of HIF prolyl-hydroxylases and TET enzymes lead to tumorigenesis through pseudo-hypoxic signaling and DNA hypermethylation (Tretter et al. 2016). Increased succinate to fumarate ratio was demonstrated in *SDHx*-mutated tumors compared to *SDHx* wild type tumors (Lendvai et al. 2014). This mechanism is common for *SDHx* and *VHL*-associated tumors, and it can be differentiated from the second cluster which comprises *RET*-, *NF1*-, *MAX*-, and *TMEM127*-associated tumors. In this latter group, the main pathomechanism is the activation of MAP kinase/AKT/mTOR pathways (Dahia et al. 2005).

8.7 Genetic Diagnosis and Genetic Counseling

The differential diagnosis of the disease aims to exclude the hereditary tumor syndromes. The recent guideline (Lenders et al. 2014) suggests clinical feature-driven molecular genetic testing in centers where NGS-based gene panel or WES analysis is not available. The most challenging situations are cases with bilateral Pheos at young age. In these patients, clinical screening for VHL syndrome is always recommended. By serum calcitonin test, medullary thyroid carcinoma can be excluded. If there is no clinical sign of MEN2 or VHL syndrome and the *VHL* gene mutation screening is negative, genetic testing of *SDHx*, *TMEM127* and *MAX* genes is recommended. In cases of intra-abdominal paragangliomas, the *SDHB* and *SDHD* genes are to be screened for mutation first by direct PCR reaction followed by direct bidirectional DNA sequencing. In the case of head-neck paragangliomas, the *SDHD*, *SDHB*, and *SDHC* genes are to be analyzed first. For comprehensive molecular genetic testing, investigation of heterozygous gene deletion (hemizygosity is common in *SDHD* and *VHL* genes, but can also be found in

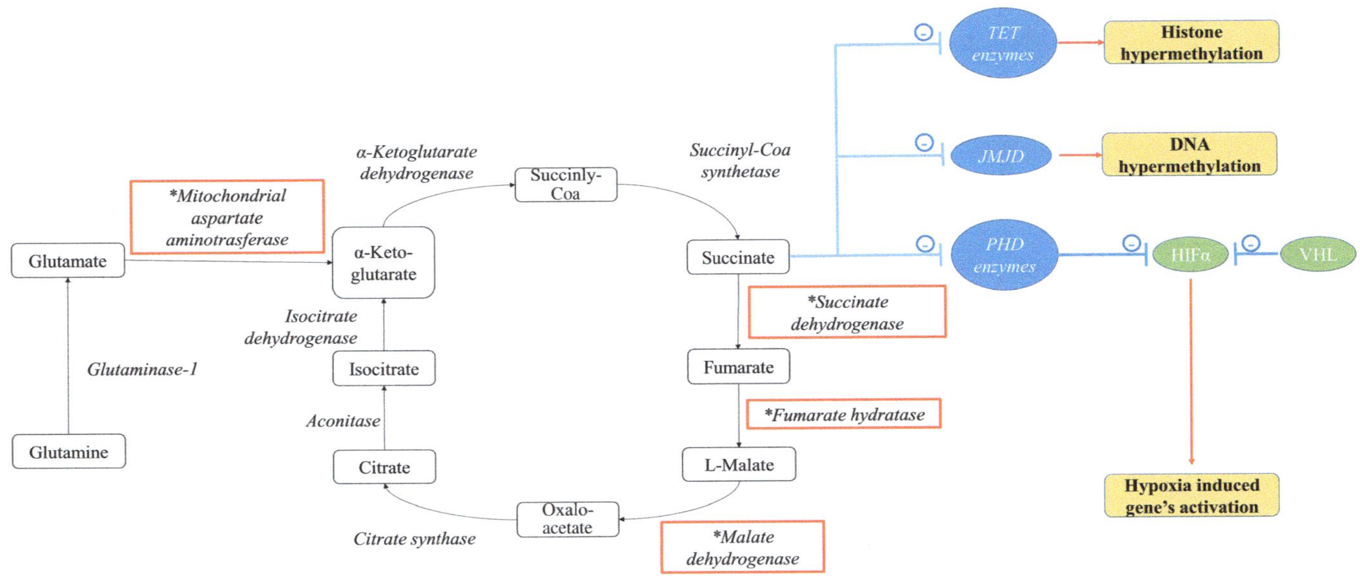

Fig. 8.2 Schematic illustration of the tricarboxylic acid (TCA) cycle and the pathomechanism associated with succinate accumulation. Enzymes are marked with bold letters. Enzymes associated with Pheo/PGL are marked with∗. *PHD* prolyl hydroxylases, *TET* ten-eleven translocation (TET) family of 5-methylcytosine (5mC) hydroxylases, *JMJD* Jumonji C domain-containing histone lysine demethylases, *HIF* hypoxia-induced factor, *VHL* von-Hippel-Lindau protein

SDHB and *SDHC* genes too) should also be carried out using copy number analysis tools in NGS-based techniques, quantitative RT-PCR, and MLPA (further details can be found in Chap. 4).

Followed mutation analysis, gene-specific recommendation and clinical and biochemical surveillance should be started in order to prevent and/or early detect any lesions. In many cases regular systematic whole-body imaging investigation is required. Disease treatment consists of surgical removal of tumors. In the case of hormonally inactive, very slowly growing and non-symptomatic tumors (most often in case of head and neck tumors), conservative treatment is recommended, which consists mainly of monitoring the growth of the tumor. Intra-abdominal paragangliomas should be removed because of the greater risk of malignancy. Malignancy is most at risk for tumors associated with intra-abdominal and *SDHB* mutations. In the case of large tumors causing compression symptoms, when surgical removal is dangerous, irradiation as well as radio-nucleotide treatments can be used.

8.8 Other Rare Disease Accompanied with Pheochromocytoma

The extremely rare disease described below is among the disease group called hamartomatosis or phacomatosis syndromes. These syndromes are characterized by skin malformations. Many of these syndromes, Carney complex, Cowden disease, and Peutz-Jeghers syndrome, associate with various endocrine tumors or endocrine malignancies. These syndromes will be presented in this book in other chapters (Chaps. 8 and 11); only the Sturge-Weber syndrome will be detailed here.

8.8.1 Sturge-Weber Syndrome (OMIM 185300)

The prevalence of Sturge-Weber's syndrome in Europe is estimated to be 1:20,000 to 1:50,000. Symptoms include one-sided naevus flammeus on the face, leptomeningeal angiomatosis with calcification of affected areas, and eye lesions (often causing glaucoma). Neurological symptoms consist of epilepsy and mental retardation. Hemiparesis can also occur. Cranial X-ray and CT scans illustrate the extent of calcification and associated cortical atrophy. In case of drug-resistant epilepsy surgery is required. Genetic background is unknown, the role of somatic mosaicism is assumed (Shirley et al. 2013).

8.9 Conclusions

Pheo/PGLs represent a disease entity with strong genetic background. At least 40% of cases are genetically determined by approximately 16 genes identified to date. This genetic diversity has a major impact on clinical follow-up of the affected patients. Our goals are to provide personalized and adequate clinical follow-up for these patients and their relatives. The post-diagnostic clinical, biochemical and imaging follow-up are determined by the syndrome or gene identified. These syndromes represent a lifelong risk for development of novel tumors. Depending on the gene and even on the mutation detected, specific recommendations have been published and specific recommendations are available. Malignancy, recurrences are the most intruding clinical questions. In these perspectives, *SDHB* is the most important genetic factor for malignant tumors, while *VHL* and *SDHD* mutations prone for development of recurrent tumors. It is also important to note that recurrent tumors are not restricted to the primary localization of the first tumor. In VHL syndrome non-endocrine organs are affected at most, while *SDHx* mutations-associated recurrent tumors affect the contralateral adrenals or extra-adrenal PGLs.

Genetic counseling is mandatory in these syndromes. Pre- and post-testing counseling should be included in the clinical practice. It is important to point out the type of the molecular genetic analysis performed in order to elucidate which genes were tested and potentially other method will be also needed. Nowadays, comprehensive testing using NGS-based technologies is available in many centers, but not in all countries and endocrine centers. In addition, the number of genes identified during the past decade highlights the need for biobanking of DNA samples previously analyzed and showing no mutation. Reanalyzing these samples would increase the number of cases with mutation. However, the usage of these samples requires specific consent form signed by patients. Having in hands a genetic report containing the detected mutation, genetic counseling must also include counseling for risks of both adrenal Pheos and extra-adrenal and HNPGLs.

Acknowledgment The authors acknowledge the financial support of the Higher Education Institutional Excellence Program of the Ministry of Human Capacities in Hungary, within the framework of the Molecular Biology thematic program of the Semmelweis University and Hungarian Scientific Research Grant (OTKA, K125231 to Attila Patócs).

References

Barker D, Wright E, Nguyen K et al (1987) Gene for von Recklinghausen neurofibromatosis is in the pericentromeric region of chromosome 17. Science 236:1100–1102

Bausch B, Borozdin W, Mautner VF et al (2007) Germline NF1 mutational spectra and loss-of-heterozygosity analyses in patients with pheochromocytoma and neurofibromatosis type 1. J Clin Endocrinol Metab 92:2784–2792

Bausch B, Wellner U, Bausch D et al (2014) Long-term prognosis of patients with pediatric pheochromocytoma. Endocr Relat Cancer 21:17–25

Bausch B, Schiavi F, Ni Y et al (2017) Clinical characterization of the pheochromocytoma and paraganglioma susceptibility genes SDHA, TMEM127, MAX, and SDHAF2 for gene-informed prevention. JAMA Oncol 3:1204–1212
Baysal BE, Ferrell RE, Willett-Brozick JE et al (2000) Mutations in SDHD, a mitochondrial complex II gene, in hereditary paraganglioma. Science 287:848–851
Ben Aim L, Pigny P, Castro-Vega LJ et al (2019) Targeted next-generation sequencing detects rare genetic events in pheochromocytoma and paraganglioma. J Med Genet 126(23):1679. https://doi.org/10.1136/jmedgenet-2018-105714
Benn DE, Gimenez-Roqueplo AP, Reilly JR et al (2006) Clinical presentation and penetrance of pheochromocytoma/paraganglioma syndromes. J Clin Endocrinol Metab 91:827–836
Bjorklund P, Pacak K, Crona J (2016) Precision medicine in pheochromocytoma and paraganglioma: current and future concepts. J Intern Med 280:559–573
Bourgeron T, Rustin P, Chretien D et al (1995) Mutation of a nuclear succinate dehydrogenase gene results in mitochondrial respiratory chain deficiency. Nat Genet 11:144–149
Buffet A, Morin A, Castro-Vega LJ, Habarou F, Lussey-Lepoutre C, Letouzé E, Lefebvre H, Guilhem I, Haissaguerre M, Raingeard I, Padilla-Girola M, Tran T, Tchara L, Bertherat J, Amar L, Ottolenghi C, Burnichon N, Gimenez-Roqueplo AP, Favier J (2018) Germline mutations in the mitochondrial 2-oxoglutarate/malate carrier SLC25A11 gene confer a predisposition to metastatic paragangliomas. Cancer Res 78(8):1914–1922
Burnichon N, Briere JJ, Libe R et al (2010) SDHA is a tumor suppressor gene causing paraganglioma. Hum Mol Genet 19:3011–3020
Cascon A, Comino-Mendez I, Curras-Freixes M et al (2015) Whole-exome sequencing identifies MDH2 as a new familial paraganglioma gene. J Natl Cancer Inst 107:djv053
Castro-Vega LJ, Buffet A, De Cubas AA et al (2014) Germline mutations in FH confer predisposition to malignant pheochromocytomas and paragangliomas. Hum Mol Genet 23:2440–2446
Chen F, Kishida T, Yao M et al (1995) Germline mutations in the von Hippel-Lindau disease tumor suppressor gene: correlations with phenotype. Hum Mutat 5:66–75
Dahia PL, Ross KN, Wright ME et al (2005) A HIF1alpha regulatory loop links hypoxia and mitochondrial signals in pheochromocytomas. PLoS Genet 1:72–80
Eisenhofer G, Walther MM, Huynh TT et al (2001) Pheochromocytomas in von Hippel-Lindau syndrome and multiple endocrine neoplasia type 2 display distinct biochemical and clinical phenotypes. J Clin Endocrinol Metab 86:1999–2008
Frank-Raue K, Rybicki LA, Erlic Z et al (2011) Risk profiles and penetrance estimations in multiple endocrine neoplasia type 2A caused by germline RET mutations located in exon 10. Hum Mutat 32:51–58
Gergics P, Patocs A, Toth M et al (2009) Germline VHL gene mutations in Hungarian families with von Hippel-Lindau disease and patients with apparently sporadic unilateral pheochromocytomas. Eur J Endocrinol 161:495–502
Gill AJ, Pachter NS, Clarkson A et al (2011) Renal tumors and hereditary pheochromocytoma-paraganglioma syndrome type 4. N Engl J Med 364:885–886
Gimenez-Roqueplo AP, Favier J, Rustin P et al (2003) Mutations in the SDHB gene are associated with extra-adrenal and/or malignant phaeochromocytomas. Cancer Res 63:5615–5621
Hao HX, Khalimonchuk O, Schraders M et al (2009) SDH5, a gene required for flavination of succinate dehydrogenase, is mutated in paraganglioma. Science 325:1139–1142
Hensen E, Van Duinen N, Jansen J et al (2012) High prevalence of founder mutations of the succinate dehydrogenase genes in the Netherlands. Clin Genet 81:284–288
Hes FJ, Weiss MM, Woortman SA et al (2010) Low penetrance of a SDHB mutation in a large Dutch paraganglioma family. BMC Med Genet 11:92
Kaelin WG Jr (2002) Molecular basis of the VHL hereditary cancer syndrome. Nat Rev Cancer 2:673–682
Kunst HP, Rutten MH, De Monnink JP et al (2011) SDHAF2 (PGL2-SDH5) and hereditary head and neck paraganglioma. Clin Cancer Res 17:247–254
Lenders JW, Duh QY, Eisenhofer G et al (2014) Pheochromocytoma and paraganglioma: an endocrine society clinical practice guideline. J Clin Endocrinol Metab 99:1915–1942

Lendvai N, Pawlosky R, Bullova P et al (2014) Succinate-to-fumarate ratio as a new metabolic marker to detect the presence of SDHB/D-related paraganglioma: initial experimental and ex vivo findings. Endocrinology 155:27–32
Neumann HP, Dinkel E, Brambs H et al (1991) Pancreatic lesions in the von Hippel-Lindau syndrome. Gastroenterology 101:465–471
Neumann HPH, Bausch B, Mcwhinney SR et al (2002) Germ-line mutations in nonsyndromic pheochromocytoma. N Engl J Med 346:1459–1466
Neumann HP, Pawlu C, Peczkowska M et al (2004) Distinct clinical features of paraganglioma syndromes associated with SDHB and SDHD gene mutations. JAMA 292:943–951
Ni Y, Zbuk KM, Sadler T et al (2008) Germline mutations and variants in the succinate dehydrogenase genes in Cowden and Cowden-like syndromes. Am J Hum Genet 83:261–268
Niemann S, Muller U (2000) Mutations in SDHC cause autosomal dominant paraganglioma, type 3. Nat Genet 26:268–270
Ong KR, Woodward ER, Killick P, Lim C, Macdonald F, Maher ER (2007) Genotype-phenotype correlations in von Hippel-Lindau disease. Hum Mutat 28:143–149
Otsuka F, Kawashima T, Imakado S, Usuki Y, Hon-Mura S (2001) Lisch nodules and skin manifestation in neurofibromatosis type 1. Arch Dermatol 137:232–233
Patocs A, Lendvai NK, Butz H et al (2016) Novel SDHB and TMEM127 mutations in patients with pheochromocytoma/paraganglioma syndrome. Pathol Oncol Res 22:673–679
Plouin PF, Amar L, Dekkers OM et al (2016) European Society of Endocrinology Clinical Practice Guideline for long-term follow-up of patients operated on for a phaeochromocytoma or a paraganglioma. Eur J Endocrinol 174:G1–g10
Ricketts C, Woodward ER, Killick P et al (2008) Germline SDHB mutations and familial renal cell carcinoma. J Natl Cancer Inst 100:1260–1262
Ricketts CJ, Forman JR, Rattenberry E et al (2010) Tumor risks and genotype-phenotype-proteotype analysis in 358 patients with germline mutations in SDHB and SDHD. Hum Mutat 31:41–51
Rijken JA, Niemeijer ND, Corssmit EP et al (2016) Low penetrance of paraganglioma and pheochromocytoma in an extended kindred with a germline SDHB exon 3 deletion. Clin Genet 89:128–132
Sarkadi B, Grolmusz VK, Butz H et al (2018) Evolution of molecular genetic methods in the clinical diagnosis of hereditary endocrine tumour syndromes. Orv Hetil 159:285–292
Schiavi F, Boedeker CC, Bausch B et al (2005) Predictors and prevalence of paraganglioma syndrome associated with mutations of the SDHC gene. JAMA 294:2057–2063
Schiavi F, Milne RL, Anda E et al (2010) Are we overestimating the penetrance of mutations in SDHB? Hum Mutat 31:761–762
Shirley MD, Tang H, Gallione CJ et al (2013) Sturge-Weber syndrome and port-wine stains caused by somatic mutation in GNAQ. N Engl J Med 368:1971–1979
Solis DC, Burnichon N, Timmers HJLM et al (2009) Penetrance and clinical consequences of a gross SDHB deletion in a large family. Clin Genet 75:354–363
Tretter L, Patocs A, Chinopoulos C (2016) Succinate, an intermediate in metabolism, signal transduction, ROS, hypoxia, and tumorigenesis. Biochim Biophys Acta 1857:1086–1101

Chapter 9
Diseases Predisposing to Adrenocortical Malignancy (Li–Fraumeni Syndrome, Beckwith–Wiedemann Syndrome, and Carney Complex)

Anne Jouinot and Jérôme Bertherat

Abstract Adrenocortical malignancies can occur in the context of several tumor predisposition syndromes.

The Carney complex (CNC) is responsible for the majority of primary pigmented nodular adrenal diseases and is more rarely associated with adrenocortical carcinoma (ACC). Other core manifestations of CNC include cardiac and cutaneous myxomas, lentiginosis, somatotroph pituitary adenomas, Sertoli tumors, melanocytic schwannoma, and thyroid, breast, and bone tumors. CNC is mostly due to germline inactivating mutations of *PRKAR1A*.

The majority of childhood ACC are related to genetic predisposition. The Beckwith–Wiedemann syndrome (BWS) is an overgrowth and tumor predisposition syndrome due to genetic or epigenetic alterations at the 11p15 locus. Classical tumor spectrum of BWS includes embryonal tumors and childhood ACC. The Li–Fraumeni syndrome (LFS) is a devastating tumor predisposition syndrome, due to germline inactivating mutations of *TP53*, and characterized by a high, various, and early-onset cancer risk. LFS spectrum includes premenopausal breast cancer, soft-tissue sarcoma, osteosarcoma, central nervous system tumor, and ACC, accounting for 50–80% of pediatric cases. Finally, germline predisposition affects up to 10% of adult ACC patients, mostly in part of LFS and Lynch syndrome.

This chapter focuses on the diagnosis, screening, and management of adrenal tumors in part of these tumor predisposition syndromes.

Keywords Carney complex · Beckwith–Wiedemann syndrome · Li–Fraumeni syndrome · primary micronodular adrenal hyperplasia · adrenocortical carcinoma

A. Jouinot · J. Bertherat (✉)
Endocrinology Department, Cochin Hospital, APHP, Paris, France

Institut Cochin, INSERM U1016, CNRS UMR8104, Paris University, Paris, France
e-mail: jerome.bertherat@aphp.fr

P. Igaz, A. Patócs (eds.), *Genetics of Endocrine Diseases and Syndromes*,
Experientia Supplementum 111, https://doi.org/10.1007/978-3-030-25905-1_9

Abbreviations

ACC	Adrenocortical carcinoma
APC	Adenomatous polyposis coli
BRCA2	Breast cancer 2
BWS	Beckwith–Wiedemann Syndrome
cAMP	Cyclic adenosine monophosphate
CDKN1C	Cyclin-dependent kinase inhibitor 1C
CNC	Carney complex
IC	Imprinting center
IGF2	Insulin-like growth factor 2
KCNQ1	Potassium voltage-gated channel subfamily Q member 1
KCNQ1OT1	KCNQ1 overlapping transcript 1
LFS	Li–Fraumeni syndrome
MEN1	Menin 1
MLH1	MutL Homolog 1
MMR	Mismatch repair
MRI	Magnetic resonance imaging
MSH	MutS protein homolog
MUTYH	MutY DNA glycosylase
NF1	Neurofibromin 1
NMD	Nonsense-mediated mRNA decay
PDE	Phosphodiesterases
PKA	Protein kinase A
PMS2	Postmeiotic segregation increased 2
PPNAD	Primary pigmented nodular adrenal disease
PRKACA	Protein kinase cAMP-dependent catalytic subunit alpha
PRKACB	Protein kinase cAMP-dependent catalytic subunit beta
PRKAR1A	Protein kinase cAMP-dependent regulatory subunit type 1 alpha
SDH	Succinate dehydrogenase
TP53	Tumor protein 53
UPD	Uniparental disomy

9.1 Introduction

Adrenocortical tumors can occur in the context of several germline genetic defects (Table 9.1). This chapter focuses on the Carney complex and predispositions to adrenocortical carcinoma (ACC). Historically, childhood ACC has been linked to Li–Fraumeni syndrome and Beckwith–Wiedemann syndrome. More recently, large-scale genomic characterization programs have expanded the number of tumor susceptibility syndromes: new susceptibility genes have been identified and associations with known non-endocrine tumor syndromes have been revealed. Overall, germline predisposition is found in 10% of adult ACC and in up to 80% of childhood ACC. This chapter

Table 9.1 Predispositions to adrenocortical tumors

Adrenocortical tumor	Germline alteration	Syndrome	Predisposition frequency
Adrenocortical carcinoma	11p15, *CDKN1C*	Beckwith–Wiedemann	Rare, childhood onset
	TP53	Li–Fraumeni	50–80% in children, 3–5% in adults
	MLH1, MSH2, MSH6, PMS2	Lynch	3–5%
	MEN1	Multiple endocrine neoplasia type 1	1%
	APC	Familial adenomatous polyposis	Very rare, case reports
	NF1	Neurofibromatosis type 1	Very rare, case reports
	PRKAR1A	Carney complex	Very rare, case reports
	MUTYH	*MUTYH*-associated polyposis	Very rare, case reports
	SDHC, SDHA	Hereditary pheochromocytoma and paraganglioma	Very rare, case reports
	BRCA2	Hereditary breast and ovarian cancer	Very rare, case report
Primary pigmented nodular adrenocortical disease	*PRKAR1A*	Carney complex	80%
	PDE11A, PDE8B, PRKACA, PRKACB		
Primary macronodular adrenal hyperplasia	*ARMC5*		20%
	GNAS	McCune–Albright syndrome	Rare, childhood onset
	MEN1	Multiple endocrine neoplasia type 1	Rare
	FH	Hereditary leiomyomatosis and renal cell carcinoma	Rare
	APC	Familial adenomatous polyposis	Rare

develops several aspects of patient care, from the clinical and molecular diagnosis to the screening and management of adrenal tumors in part of a predisposition syndrome.

9.2 Carney Complex

9.2.1 Definition and Prevalence

The Carney complex (CNC) is a rare tumor predisposition syndrome, which associates endocrine and non-endocrine tumors. The most frequent manifestations of CNC are cutaneous lentigines, myxomas, and ACTH-independent Cushing's syndrome due to primary pigmented nodular adrenocortical disease (PPNAD) (Stratakis et al. 1998). However, the spectrum and severity of manifestations and the age of first tumor onset differ between the patients, even within the same family. CNC is caused in the majority of cases by *PRKAR1A* inactivating mutations (Kirschner et al. 2000).

The prevalence of CNC is still unknown (Lodish and Stratakis 2016), with only several hundreds of patients reported so far (Bertherat et al. 2009). The diagnosis is commonly made in children or young adults, at a median age of 20 years (Stratakis et al. 2001; Bertherat et al. 2009).

9.2.2 Clinical Diagnosis and Indications of Genetic Testing

Since its first description by Carney in 1985 as "the complex of myxomas, spotty pigmentation, and endocrine overactivity" (Carney et al. 1985), various associations of clinical manifestations have been reported. The CNC spectrum has been expended to pituitary adenomas (mostly somatotrophs), thyroid tumors, testicular and ovarian lesions (especially large-cell calcifying Sertoli tumors), melanocytic psammomatous schwannomas, breast ductal adenoma, and osteochondromyxomas. Conversely, PPNAD can be the single manifestation of the disease, named in these cases isolated PPNAD. Isolated lentigines and isolated cardiac myxomas are described as well (Bertherat et al. 2009). Diagnostic criteria have been proposed in 2001 (Stratakis et al. 2001) (Table 9.2). The diagnosis of CNC is established in a proband with either (1) two or more suggestive clinical manifestations or (2) one of these manifestations and an affected first-degree relative or a germline pathogenic variant in *PRKAR1A* on the genetic testing. Therefore, any patient with one manifestation strongly suggestive of CNC, such as PPNAD, should be considered for genetic testing.

9.2.3 Molecular Diagnosis

Germline inactivating mutations in *PRKAR1A* are detected in 70% of patients with CNC and in 80% of those with familial presentation or Cushing's syndrome due to

Table 9.2 Diagnostic criteria for the Carney complex (Stratakis et al. 2001)

Major diagnostic criteria	Frequency (%)
1. Spotty skin pigmentation (lentiginosis) with typical distribution (lips, conjunctiva and inner or outer canthi, vaginal mucosa)	70–77
2. Myxoma (cutaneous and mucosa)[a]	20–32
3. Cardiac myxoma[a]	32–53
4. Breast myxomatosis[a] or fat-suppressed magnetic resonance imaging findings suggestive of this diagnosis	20
5. Primary pigmented adrenocortical disease[a] or paradoxical positive response of urinary glucocorticosteroid excretion to dexamethasone administration during Liddle's test	26–60
6. Acromegaly due to GH-producing adenoma[a]	10–12
7. Large-cell calcifying Sertoli cell tumor[a] or characteristic calcification on testicular ultrasound	33–41
8. Thyroid carcinoma[a] or multiple hypoechoic nodules on thyroid ultrasound in a young patient	5–25
9. Psammomatous melanotic schwannomas[a]	8–10
10. Blue nevus, epithelioid blue nevus[a]	50
11. Breast ductal adenoma[a]	20
12. Osteochondromyxoma[a]	2
Supplementary criteria	
1.Affected first-degree relative	
2. Inactivating mutation of the *PRKAR1A* gene	

The diagnosis of Carney complex is made if the patient exhibits two of the major criteria or one of these and one of the supplementary criteria

[a]*After histological confirmation*

PPNAD (Cazabat et al. 2006; Bertherat et al. 2009). The *PRKAR1A* gene is located at the 17q22–24 locus and encodes the regulatory subunit 1α of the protein kinase A (PKA), a key component of the cAMP signaling pathway (Fig. 9.1). This pathway plays a major role in development, maintenance, and secretory activity of several endocrine glands. *PRKAR1A* is a tumor suppressor gene according to the Knudson theory: one allele is inactivated by a germline mutation and the second allele is inactivated at the somatic level. *PRKAR1A* defects lead to the activation of the cAMP/PKA pathway, which in turn increases cell proliferation and steroidogenesis (Groussin et al. 2002).

Mutations in *PRKAR1A* are spread along the exons and their flanking intronic sequences. Most mutations are considered as "private," identified in only one or few families. De novo mutations are found in 30% of patients and in most sporadic cases (Bertherat et al. 2009). In more than 80% of the mutations, the sequence change (nonsense, frameshift, or splice variants) leads to premature stop codon causing degradation of the mutant mRNA by nonsense-mediated mRNA decay (NMD). In this case, no mutant protein is produced. In the tumor, the loss of the second allele is frequently observed (Kirschner et al. 2000). Rarely, missense mutations, short in-frame insertions/deletions, or splice variants translate into a mutant protein with altered or truncated sequence. This defective mutant protein can exert a dominant-

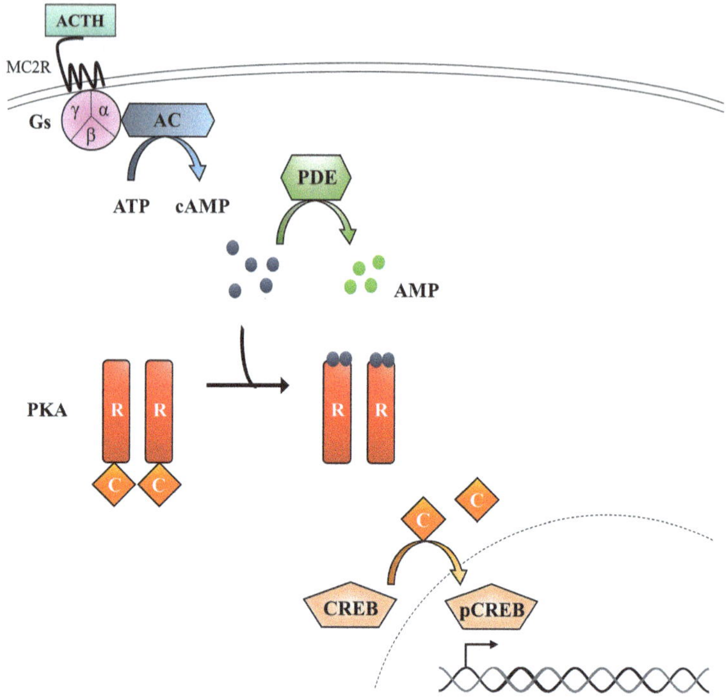

Fig. 9.1 cAMP/PKA signaling pathway in normal adrenal cortex. Adrenocorticotropic hormone (ACTH) stimulates the cAMP pathway after binding to the melanocortin 2 receptor (MC2R), a seven-transmembrane receptor coupled to Gs protein. The activated Gs protein activates the adenylyl cyclase enzyme (AC), which synthetizes cAMP. PKA is a hetero-tetramer formed by 2 regulatory subunits (R) and 2 catalytic subunits (C). The binding of cAMP to the regulatory subunits releases the catalytic subunits. The free catalytic subunits can phosphorylate several targets, including the transcription factor CREB (cAMP response element-binding protein), involved in steroidogenesis. The cAMP is degraded by the phosphodiesterases (PDE), which act as negative regulators of the pathway

negative effect over the wild-type protein. In this case, the somatic allelic loss of the wild-type allele is not always required (Groussin et al. 2002; Horvath et al. 2010).

Some genotype/phenotype correlations have been established (Bertherat et al. 2009). Patients with mutations that escape NMD and lead to a defective mutant protein exhibit a higher number of CNC manifestations. The hotspot mutation c.709 (−7–2)del6 is associated with PPNAD, while the other hotspot mutation c.491-492delTG is associated with cardiac myxomas, lentigines, and thyroid tumors. Exonic mutations are commonly associated with acromegaly, cardiac myxomas, lentigines, and schwannomas. Finally, patients harboring large deletions may present with severe phenotype, possibly as a result of haploinsufficiency of additional neighboring genes (Salpea et al. 2014; Stelmachowska-Banas et al. 2017). At the opposite, patients without *PRKAR1A* mutations show less myxomas and later-onset disease.

In addition to *PRKAR1A*, other genetic alterations in the cAMP/PKA signaling pathway have been reported, including *PDE11A* (Horvath et al. 2006; Libé et al. 2011) and *PDE8B* (Horvath et al. 2008; Rothenbuhler et al. 2012) inactivating germline mutations and *PRKACA* (Beuschlein et al. 2014; Lodish et al. 2015) and *PRKACB* (Forlino et al. 2014) germline duplications. These alterations are mostly associated with isolated PPNAD.

9.2.4 Tumor Spectrum, Management, and Prognosis

The average life expectancy of patients with CNC may be reduced due to cardiac myxomas.

Cardiac myxomas are benign tumors, affecting 30–50% of CNC patients (Stratakis et al. 2001; Bertherat et al. 2009). These tumors can occur at a young age and in any or all cardiac chambers. They can cause severe cardiovascular complications, such as tumor emboli, cardiomyopathy, and arrhythmia. The only definitive treatment is surgery. Recent progress in this area has improved the morbi-mortality of CNC patients (Espiard and Bertherat 2013). Other sites for myxomas include the skin, breast, oropharynx, and female genital tract.

PPNAD is the most frequent endocrine manifestation of the CNC, reported in up to 60% of patients (Bertherat et al. 2009). Isolated PPNAD accounts for 12% of cases (Bertherat et al. 2009). Some patients developed a PPNAD during the first years of life, but the majority are diagnosed during the second and third decade (Stratakis et al. 2001) with a median age of 35 years. After puberty, a female predominance is observed (Bertherat et al. 2009). The usual treatment for patients harboring CS is the bilateral adrenalectomy (Powell et al. 2008). Histopathological examination reveals glands of normal size and weight or slightly enlarged, with multiple small (<10 mm) pigmented nodules around an atrophic cortex (Carney et al. 1985). Other adrenocortical tumors are rarely observed in CNC. Recently, two cases of adrenocortical carcinomas were described in patients affected by CNC. In both cases, a co-secretion of androgens and cortisol and a rapid occurrence of local recurrence and metastasis were observed (Anselmo et al. 2012; Bertherat 2012; Morin et al. 2012).

Other tumors include GH-producing adenomas in 10%, thyroid adenomas in 60%, melanotic psammomatous schwannomas in 10% of CNC patients, testicular tumors—mostly large-cell calcifying Sertoli tumors—in one-third of affected males, and ovarian serous cystadenomas in 14% of affected females.

Malignant tumors are rarely described in CNC: thyroid carcinomas and malignant schwannomas are reported in 3% and 1% of CNC patients, respectively (Stratakis et al. 2001; Bertherat et al. 2009).

Annual screening is recommended for CNC patients and at-risk relatives and includes at least echocardiography, testicular ultrasound, and measurements of urinary free cortisol and IGF-1 levels (Stratakis and Raygada 1993).

9.2.5 Risk of Recurrence and Genetic Counseling

CNC follows an autosomal dominant inheritance. The penetrance is almost complete (>95%) in patients with *PRKAR1A* mutations (Bertherat et al. 2009). After a diagnosis of CNC in an index case, familial genetic testing should be proposed, along with tumor screening in presymptomatic predisposition carriers. In families with CNC where no genetic defect is identified, all at-risk family members are proposed to follow tumor surveillance protocols.

9.3 Beckwith–Wiedemann Syndrome

9.3.1 Definition and Prevalence

Beckwith–Wiedemann syndrome (BWS) is an overgrowth and tumor predisposition syndrome, recovering a great variability of phenotypes. Classical presentations include pre- and postnatal overgrowth, lateralized overgrowth (i.e., hemihypertrophy), macroglossia, visceromegaly, abdominal wall defects with exomphalos, and increased risk of embryonal tumors and adrenocortical cancer (Brioude et al. 2018). BWS is due to genetic or epigenetic alteration of the imprinted 11p15.5 region (Henry et al. 1989; Wilkin et al. 2000).

The diagnosis is commonly made in newborns or infants, with an estimated prevalence of 1 per 10–20,000 births (Mussa et al. 2013; Barisic et al. 2018). Familial presentations represent only 15% of BWS cases. The prevalence is influenced by neither gender nor ethnicity. A five- to tenfold increased risk of BWS is reported with assisted reproductive techniques (Mussa et al. 2017; Cortessis et al. 2018), as for other imprinting disorders.

9.3.2 Clinical Diagnosis and Indications of Genetic Testing

The first description of BWS was made more than 50 years ago (Wiedemann 1964). Several combinations of clinical features have been proposed for the diagnosis (Shuman et al. 1993; Weksberg et al. 2010), with macrosomia, macroglossia, and abdominal wall defects usually considered as major clinical features. However, some patients with 11p15.5 alteration do not display all these features (Ibrahim et al. 2014). Thus, additional definitions were proposed for "incomplete" or "atypical" BWS.

The recent consensus from the European Network for Congenital Imprinting Disorders defines instead the Beckwith–Wiedemann spectrum, which gathers a large range of phenotypes, from some individuals with only one suggestive clinical finding to the classical form of BWS (Brioude et al. 2018). Thus, Beckwith–Wiedemann spectrum encompasses three subsets: (1) classical BWS, (2) lateralized overgrowth syndrome, and (3) patients with 11p15.5 alteration who do not fit into these first two groups. A diagnostic score for Beckwith–Wiedemann spectrum is proposed, with cardinal clinical features scoring each 2 points, and suggestive clinical features scoring each 1 point (Table 9.3). Molecular testing of the 11p15 region is recommended for any patient with a score $\geq$ 2 points. Moreover, a score $\geq$ 4 points is retained for the diagnosis of classical BWS, even without confirmation of 11p15.5 alteration.

Table 9.3 Diagnostic criteria for the genetic testing of Beckwith–Wiedemann spectrum (Brioude et al. 2018)

Cardinal features (2 points per feature)
Macroglossia
Exomphalos
Lateralized overgrowth
Multifocal and/or bilateral Wilms tumor or nephroblastomatosis
Hyperinsulinism (lasting >1 week and requiring escalated treatment)
Pathology findings: adrenal cortex cytomegaly, placental mesenchymal dysplasia, or pancreatic adenomatosis
Suggestive features (1 point per feature)
Birthweight >2 standard deviation scores above the mean
Facial nevus simplex
Polyhydramnios and/or placentomegaly
Ear creases and/or pits
Transient hypoglycemia (lasting <1 week)
Typical Beckwith–Wiedemann tumors (neuroblastoma, rhabdomyosarcoma, unilateral Wilms tumor, hepatoblastoma, adrenocortical carcinoma, or pheochromocytoma)
Nephromegaly and/or hepatomegaly
Umbilical hernia and/or diastasis recti

The diagnosis of the classical Beckwith–Wiedemann syndrome if the patient exhibits a score of ≥4 (this clinical diagnosis does not require the molecular confirmation of an 11p15 anomaly). Genetic testing is indicated in patients with a score of ≥2 (including those with a score of ≥4). Patients with a score of <2 do not meet the criteria for genetic testing

9.3.3 Molecular Diagnosis

BWS is associated with abnormal gene transcription due to molecular alterations within the imprinted 11p15.5 chromosome region. Genomic imprinting is an epigenetic phenomenon where genes are monoallelically expressed in a parent-specific manner. Imprinting centers (IC) are regions that can regulate the expression of imprinted genes in cis over a large distance. IC are characterized by differential DNA methylation of the parental alleles and are also referred to as differentially methylated regions (DMR).

The 11p15.5 region is divided into two functional domains, each harboring an independent IC (Fig. 9.2):

- The telomeric domain contains IC1 (also known as H19/IGF2:IG DMR) and regulates *H19* and *IGF2* expression. This domain is normally unmethylated on the maternal allele and methylated on the paternal allele.
- The centromeric domain contains IC2 (also known as KCNQ1OT1:TSS DMR) and regulates *KCNQ1OT1*, *KCNQ1*, and *CDKN1C* expression. This domain is normally methylated on the maternal allele and unmethylated on the paternal allele.

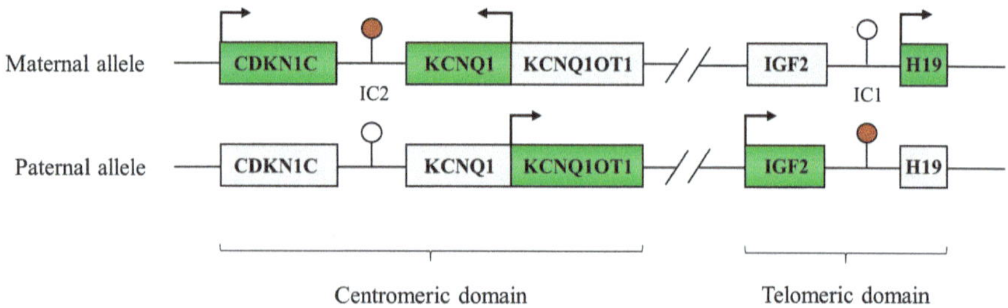

Fig. 9.2 The 11p15 region. The figure depicts the 11p15 locus with the imprinted genes and control regions that are implicated in the pathophysiology of Beckwith–Wiedemann syndrome. The two imprinted centers (IC)—IC1 on the telomeric domain and IC2 on the centromeric domain—are inversely methylated on maternal and paternal allele and result in opposite patterns of gene expression. On the maternal allele, the unmethylation of IC1 is associated with *H19* transcription and *IGF2* repression, and the methylation of IC2 is associated with *CDKNC1* and *KCNQ1* expression and *KCNQ1OT1* repression. Methylation and expression follow opposite pattern on the paternal allele. Red circles indicate methylated imprinting centers. Expressed genes are represented as green boxes and silent genes as gray boxes. The orientation of gene transcription is indicated by black arrows

A molecular defect of the 11p15 region can be found in more than 80% of individuals with BWS (Eggermann et al. 2016). Five distinct mechanisms are described:

- Loss of methylation at IC2 locus on the maternal chromosome in 50% of patients
- Gain of methylation at IC1 locus on the maternal chromosome in 5–10% of patients
- Paternal uniparental disomy (UPD) of 11p15 region in 20% of patients
- *CDKN1C* pathogenic mutation on the maternal allele in 5% of sporadic cases and 40% of familial cases
- Chromosomal alterations in 11p15 (duplications, inversions, translocations) in <5% of patients

These alterations are responsible for *IGF2* overexpression (biallelic instead of only paternal expression), which is a key player of adrenocortical tumorigenesis (Gicquel et al. 1997).

Most sporadic cases of BWS are related to somatic mosaicism (Slatter et al. 1994). Especially, UPD arises from postzygotic somatic recombination in early-stage embryos (Henry et al. 1993). Hence the proportion of affected cells is variable from one tissue to another. Molecular testing of blood samples may not be contributive in case of low level of mosaicism in leukocytes. Therefore, testing other tissues—buccal swabs, skin fibroblasts, or if available hyperplastic tumor tissue—can improve the detection rate of mosaic events.

The distinct molecular groups translate into distinct phenotypes. Segmental UPD of 11p15 is commonly associated with high risk of embryonal tumors and lateralized overgrowth, whereas exomphalos is primarily observed in loss of methylation at IC2 and *CDKN1C* mutations.

9.3.4 Tumor Spectrum, Management, and Prognosis

The prognosis of BWS depends on neonatal period complications and tumor risk.

The morbi-mortality in infants with BWS is mainly due to neonatal complications such as hypoglycemia, major exomphalos, or respiratory obstruction from macroglossia (Smith et al. 2007).

The tumor risk is highest in infants and children under 8 years, whereas adults with BWS do not seem to have an increased risk of tumor development. Embryonal tumors (i.e., Wilms tumor, neuroblastoma, and hepatoblastoma) occur in 8% of children with BWS (Brioude et al. 2013; Mussa et al. 2016). Wilms tumor (also known as nephroblastoma) represents 50% of all tumors, with frequent multifocal and bilateral presentations. Other tumors of the BWS spectrum include hepatoblastoma (15%), neuroblastoma (10%), rhabdomyosarcoma (5%), and ACC (5% of all tumors) (Maas et al. 2016).

The tumor risk and spectrum are strongly related to the genotype. Patients with gain of methylation at IC1 and UPD show the highest risk of tumors, up to 50% (Shuman et al. 2006). Conversely, the tumor risk is only 2–3% in patients with loss of methylation at IC2 (Maas et al. 2016). Patients with gain of methylation at IC1 mostly develop Wilms tumors, whereas patients with *CDKN1C* mutations are rather predisposed to develop other embryonal tumors (Brioude et al. 2013; Maas et al. 2016; Mussa et al. 2016).

Screening using abdominal ultrasound is recommended every 3 months from diagnosis to at least the age of 7 years (Brioude et al. 2013). Treatment strategies and prognosis are the same as in children without BWS. Pediatric tumors are associated with favorable outcomes compared to their adult counterparts, with up to 90% survival in embryonal tumors and 70% in ACC (Porteus et al. 2000; Dehner and Hill 2009).

9.3.5 Risk of Recurrence and Genetic Counseling

The risk of recurrence depends on the underlying molecular defect at the 11p15 region (Cerrato et al. 2008; Baskin et al. 2014). Most cases of BWS are sporadic with a recurrence risk in the family less than 1%. Familial cases account for 15% of BWS and are mostly related to *CDKN1C* mutations, chromosomal alterations in 11p15, and genetic alterations within IC1. These 11p15 alterations are associated with autosomal dominant transmission, with a theoretical 50% risk of inheriting the affected allele. However, the penetrance depends on the sex of the parent from whom the genetic defect is inherited. Thus, the type, size, location, and parental origin of the genetic defect should be taken into consideration for family genetic counseling.

9.4 Li–Fraumeni Syndrome

9.4.1 *Definition and Prevalence*

Li–Fraumeni syndrome (LFS) is an autosomal dominant tumor predisposition syndrome characterized by a high, various, and early-onset cancer risk (Li and Fraumeni 1969; Li et al. 1988). The diagnosis is commonly made in case of familial clustering of childhood cancers, with ACC, soft-tissue sarcoma, central nervous system tumor, and leukemia as the predominant cancer types. LFS is due to germline pathogenic variants in the *TP53* tumor suppressor gene (Malkin et al. 1990).

LFS has an estimated prevalence of 1 per 20,000 births, although a recent analysis of sequencing databases in unselected patients showed a much higher prevalence of germline pathogenic *TP53* variants than the one estimated from family-based studies (de Andrade et al. 2019). The prevalence of LFS is particularly high in southern Brazil, due to a founder germline TP53 mutation (p.R337H), affecting 0.3% of this population (Pinto et al. 2004; Custódio et al. 2013).

9.4.2 *Clinical Diagnosis and Indications of Genetic Testing*

After its first description by Li and Fraumeni in 1969 (Li and Fraumeni 1969), several diagnostic criteria have been proposed for LFS. The classical LFS includes a proband with sarcoma at <45 years, a first-degree relative with any cancer at <45 years, and a first- or second-degree relative with any cancer at <45 years or sarcoma at any age (Li et al. 1988). However, this restricted definition does not include some families with tumor associations suggestive of LFS. Therefore, more flexible definitions, characterized as "Li–Fraumeni-like" syndrome, were proposed (Birch et al. 1994; Eeles 1995).

The definition of LFS has evolved after the discovery of its relation to germline *TP53* mutations in 1990 (Malkin et al. 1990). Enlarged diagnostic criteria were then proposed to cover the different clinical presentations associated with these mutations. The last version of diagnostic criteria, known as revised Chompret's criteria, recommends molecular testing in 4 clinical situations (Chompret et al. 2001; Tinat et al. 2009; Bougeard et al. 2015): (1) familial presentation of LFS tumors, (2) multiple primary tumors, (3) rare cancers suggestive of LFS, and (4) breast cancer before the age of 31 years (Table 9.4). These criteria show excellent sensitivity (82–95%) and acceptable specificity (47–58%) (Gonzalez et al. 2009; Tinat et al. 2009). Among patients matching the Chompret's criteria, 30–35% carry a germline *TP53* mutation (Gonzalez et al. 2009; Tinat et al. 2009).

Table 9.4 Revised Chompret's criteria for the genetic testing of Li–Fraumeni syndrome (LFS) (Bougeard et al. 2015)

1. Familial presentation	Proband with tumor belonging to LFS tumor spectrum[a] before the age of 46 years AND at least one first- or second-degree relative with LFS tumor (except breast cancer if proband has breast cancer) before the age of 56 years or with multiple tumors
2. Multiple primitive tumors	Proband with multiple tumors (except multiple breast tumors), two of which belong to LFS tumor spectrum and first of which occurred before the age of 46 years
3. Rare tumors	Patient with adrenocortical carcinoma, choroid plexus tumor, or rhabdomyosarcoma of embryonal anaplastic subtype, irrespective of family history
4. Early-onset breast cancer	Breast cancer before the age of 31 years

[a]*LFS tumor spectrum includes premenopausal breast cancer, soft-tissue sarcoma, osteosarcoma, central nervous system tumor, and adrenocortical carcinoma*

9.4.3 Molecular Diagnosis

LFS is due to germline mutations in the *TP53* tumor suppressor gene. This gene is also the most frequently mutated gene at a somatic level in sporadic cancers. *TP53* gene encodes the p53 protein, a critical transcription factor that promotes cell cycle arrest, DNA repair, and apoptosis in response to stress signals (Reinhardt and Schumacher 2012). Therefore, p53 is frequently referred to as "the guardian of the genome" (Lane 1992).

TP53 alterations in part of LFS are mostly point mutations, with 70% missense and 20% nonsense or splice mutations (Bouaoun et al. 2016). Although distributed all along the gene, some "hotspot" mutations are described. The most common one is the p.R337H Brazilian mutation in exon 10 (Garritano et al. 2010). De novo mutations are frequent, accounting for up to 20% of LFS diagnoses (Renaux-Petel et al. 2018).

Some genotype–phenotype correlations are reported. On the one hand, missense mutations within the DNA-binding domain can exert a dominant-negative effect on the wild-type p53 protein, or even gain an oncogenic function. These mutations are typically associated with a wide range of early-onset cancers and high penetrance (Bougeard et al. 2015). On the other hand, nonsense mutations or gene deletions result in loss of function and are associated with later onset and lower penetrance. Finally, the p.R337H mutation is associated with a limited spectrum and predisposes primarily to ACC and breast cancer (Mastellaro et al. 2017).

9.4.4 Tumor Spectrum, Management, and Prognosis

The lifetime risk of cancer in LFS is very high: 80% of *TP53* mutation carriers will develop at least one malignancy, and 40% will develop multiple malignancies (Bougeard et al. 2015). The median age of first tumor onset of 27 years (Bougeard et al. 2015) and different patterns of cancer are encountered at the different stages of life (Amadou et al. 2018). During childhood, LFS is dominated by the risk of osteosarcoma (30% of *TP53* mutation carriers), ACC (27%), brain tumors (26%, including choroid plexus carcinoma, medulloblastoma, and glioblastoma), soft-tissue sarcoma (23%, mostly rhabdomyosarcoma), and leukemia (9%)(Bougeard et al. 2015). These tumors are otherwise extremely rare in the general population. Early adult life is associated with an increased risk of breast cancer (80%), soft-tissue sarcomas (27%, mostly leiomyosarcoma, liposarcoma, and fibrohistiocytic tumor), osteosarcoma (6%), lung cancer (8%), and colorectal cancer (5%) (Bougeard et al. 2015). LFS patients typically develop these tumors at an earlier age than that observed in sporadic cases. Conversely, the contribution of LFS to tumor development in late adult life seems rather limited. Only 25% of LFS-related cancers occur after the age of 50 years (Amadou et al. 2018). Prostate cancer (7%) is the most frequent tumor at this time (Bougeard et al. 2015).

Childhood ACC is a signature feature of LFS. *TP53* germline mutations have been observed in 50% of children with apparently sporadic ACC in North America and Europe (Wasserman et al. 2015; Bougeard et al. 2015). In Southern Brazil, the founder p.R337H mutation in exon 10 is observed in up to 90% of pediatric ACC cases (Ribeiro et al. 2001). Overall, 3–10% of LFS children will develop ACC at a median age of 2–3 years (Figueiredo et al. 2006; Bougeard et al. 2015). The frequency of *TP53* germline mutations in ACC decreases with age, reaching less than 5% in adults (Herrmann et al. 2012; Raymond et al. 2013a).

In recent years, several surveillance protocols have been proposed to promote early detection of tumors and reduce cancer morbidity and mortality in LFS. The recent consensus from the American Association for Cancer Research recommends that all patients be offered cancer surveillance based on the "Toronto protocol"(Kratz et al. 2017) (Table 9.5). This intensive screening protocol includes annual whole-body, brain, and breast MRI and has proven benefit on early tumor detection and long-term survival (Villani et al. 2011, 2016). Screening for ACC in childhood should start at birth and include complete physical examination, with particular attention to symptoms of precocious puberty and Cushing's syndrome, and abdominal ultrasound every 3–4 months. Biochemical testing for hormone secretion may be performed every 3–4 months, especially in case of inconclusive ultrasound (Kratz et al. 2017).

Finally, the diagnosis of LFS may impact the therapeutic decisions for ACC patients. Since LFS patients are at risk of radio-induced malignancies (Heymann et al. 2010), adjuvant radiotherapy should be avoid for completely resected ACC.

Table 9.5 Modified "Toronto protocol" for the screening of Li–Fraumeni syndrome tumors (Kratz et al. 2017)

Children (birth to the age of 18 years)
General assessment • Complete physical examination every 3–4 months, including blood pressure, growth curve, Cushing appearance, signs of virilization, and full neurologic assessment • Prompt assessment with primary care physician for any medical concerns
ACC • US of abdomen and pelvis every 3–4 months • In case of unsatisfactory US, blood tests may be performed every 3–4 months: Total testosterone, dehydroepiandrosterone sulfate, and androstenedione
Brain tumor • Annual brain MRI (first MRI with contrast; thereafter without contrast if previous MRI normal)
Soft tissue and bone sarcoma • Annual whole-body MRI
Adults
General assessment • Complete physical examination every 6 months • Prompt assessment with primary care physician for any medical concerns
Breast cancer • Breast awareness and clinical breast examination twice a year from the age of 20 years • Annual breast MRI between 20 and 75 years • Consider risk-reducing bilateral mastectomy
Brain tumor •Annual brain MRI
Soft tissue and bone sarcoma • Annual whole-body MRI and US of abdomen and pelvis
Gastrointestinal cancer • Upper endoscopy and colonoscopy every 2–5 years from the age of 25 years
Melanoma • Annual dermatologic examination

9.4.5 Risk of Recurrence and Family Counseling

LFS shows an autosomal dominant inheritance with generally high penetrance. Therefore, all at-risk relatives of an affected LFS patient should be offered genetic counseling.

In Southern Brazil, considering the particularly high incidence of childhood ACC, a genetic neonatal screening for the p.R337H mutation may be proposed (Custódio et al. 2013).

9.5 Other Tumor Predisposition Syndromes

Besides BWS and LFS, responsible for the majority of childhood tumors, ACC was recently described in part of other tumor susceptibility syndromes.

Among those, Lynch syndrome is of particular therapeutic interest. Lynch syndrome is a dominantly inherited tumor predisposition syndrome, due to germline mutations in DNA mismatch repair genes (MMR) *MLH1*, *MSH2*, *MSH6*, and *PMS2*. This syndrome typically confers an increased risk for colorectal, endometrial, small bowel, and upper tract urothelial cancers (Amsterdam Criteria), but also for sebaceous tumors, ovarian and pancreatic cancers, and ACC. Lynch syndrome accounts for up to 5% of ACC cases (Raymond et al. 2013b; Zheng et al. 2016), which is a similar prevalence to that observed in colorectal and endometrial cancers. As for other Lynch syndrome-related cancers, screening for mismatch repair deficiency in tumor tissue using immunohistochemistry and/or microsatellite analysis can orient toward diagnosis. MMR immunohistochemistry shows the absence of nuclear staining (Raymond et al. 2013b). Microsatellite instability can be detected at the genomic level (Bonneville et al. 2017), but classical microsatellite panels used for colorectal cancer screening were found negative in ACC (Raymond et al. 2013b). Finally, the diagnosis of Lynch syndrome impacts treatment strategies. Lynch tumors are hypermutated and present a large number of neoantigens. These features have been associated with response to immune checkpoints inhibitors (Le et al. 2015), which might represent new therapeutic opportunities for Lynch syndrome-associated ACC.

Other tumor predisposition syndromes each account for less than 1% of ACC and include genes classically responsible for endocrine tumors and hyperplasias—such as *MEN1* (Waldmann et al. 2007) or *SDH* genes (Else et al. 2017)—or for non-endocrine tumors—such as *APC* (Gaujoux et al. 2010), *NF1* (Wagner et al. 2005), *MUTYH* (Pilati et al. 2017), or *BRCA2* (El Ghorayeb et al. 2016) germline mutations.

9.6 Conclusions

CNC predisposes primarily to PPNAD, responsible for severe Cushing's syndrome in children and young adults, and more rarely to ACC. Half of childhood ACC occur in part of tumor predisposition syndromes; LFS and BWS should be evoked in first intention in this population. In adults, germline predisposition affects up to 10% of ACC patients, mostly in part of LFS and Lynch syndrome.

Therefore, every patient with newly diagnosed PNNAD or ACC should be considered for genetic counseling, regardless of the family history.

The diagnosis of a tumor susceptibility syndrome in an index case should initiate appropriate screening for other syndrome-related tumors and familial genetic testing.

References

Amadou A, Waddington Achatz MI, Hainaut P (2018) Revisiting tumor patterns and penetrance in germline TP53 mutation carriers: temporal phases of Li-Fraumeni syndrome. Curr Opin Oncol 30:23–29. https://doi.org/10.1097/CCO.0000000000000423

Anselmo J, Medeiros S, Carneiro V et al (2012) A large family with Carney complex caused by the S147G PRKAR1A mutation shows a unique spectrum of disease including adrenocortical cancer. J Clin Endocrinol Metab 97:351–359. https://doi.org/10.1210/jc.2011-2244

Barisic I, Boban L, Akhmedzhanova D et al (2018) Beckwith Wiedemann syndrome: a population-based study on prevalence, prenatal diagnosis, associated anomalies and survival in Europe. Eur J Med Genet 61:499–507. https://doi.org/10.1016/j.ejmg.2018.05.014

Baskin B, Choufani S, Chen Y-A et al (2014) High frequency of copy number variations (CNVs) in the chromosome 11p15 region in patients with Beckwith-Wiedemann syndrome. Hum Genet 133:321–330. https://doi.org/10.1007/s00439-013-1379-z

Bertherat J (2012) Adrenocortical cancer in Carney complex: a paradigm of endocrine tumor progression or an association of genetic predisposing factors? J Clin Endocrinol Metab 97:387–390. https://doi.org/10.1210/jc.2011-3327

Bertherat J, Horvath A, Groussin L et al (2009) Mutations in regulatory subunit type 1A of cyclic adenosine 5′-monophosphate-dependent protein kinase (PRKAR1A): phenotype analysis in 353 patients and 80 different genotypes. J Clin Endocrinol Metab 94:2085–2091. https://doi.org/10.1210/jc.2008-2333

Beuschlein F, Fassnacht M, Assié G et al (2014) Constitutive activation of PKA catalytic subunit in adrenal Cushing's syndrome. N Engl J Med 370:1019–1028. https://doi.org/10.1056/NEJMoa1310359

Birch JM, Hartley AL, Tricker KJ et al (1994) Prevalence and diversity of constitutional mutations in the p53 gene among 21 Li-Fraumeni families. Cancer Res 54:1298–1304

Bonneville R, Krook MA, Kautto EA et al (2017) Landscape of microsatellite instability across 39 Cancer types. JCO Precis Oncol 2017. https://doi.org/10.1200/PO.17.00073

Bouaoun L, Sonkin D, Ardin M et al (2016) TP53 variations in human cancers: new lessons from the IARC TP53 database and genomics data. Hum Mutat 37:865–876. https://doi.org/10.1002/humu.23035

Bougeard G, Renaux-Petel M, Flaman J-M et al (2015) Revisiting Li-Fraumeni syndrome from TP53 mutation carriers. J Clin Oncol Off J Am Soc Clin Oncol 33:2345–2352. https://doi.org/10.1200/JCO.2014.59.5728

Brioude F, Lacoste A, Netchine I et al (2013) Beckwith-Wiedemann syndrome: growth pattern and tumor risk according to molecular mechanism, and guidelines for tumor surveillance. Horm Res Paediatr 80:457–465. https://doi.org/10.1159/000355544

Brioude F, Kalish JM, Mussa A et al (2018) Expert consensus document: clinical and molecular diagnosis, screening and management of Beckwith-Wiedemann syndrome: an international consensus statement. Nat Rev Endocrinol 14:229–249. https://doi.org/10.1038/nrendo.2017.166

Carney JA, Gordon H, Carpenter PC et al (1985) The complex of myxomas, spotty pigmentation, and endocrine overactivity. Medicine (Baltimore) 64:270–283

Cazabat L, Ragazzon B, Groussin L, Bertherat J (2006) PRKAR1A mutations in primary pigmented nodular adrenocortical disease. Pituitary 9:211–219. https://doi.org/10.1007/s11102-006-0266-1

Cerrato F, Sparago A, Verde G et al (2008) Different mechanisms cause imprinting defects at the IGF2/H19 locus in Beckwith-Wiedemann syndrome and Wilms' tumour. Hum Mol Genet 17:1427–1435. https://doi.org/10.1093/hmg/ddn031

Chompret A, Abel A, Stoppa-Lyonnet D et al (2001) Sensitivity and predictive value of criteria for p53 germline mutation screening. J Med Genet 38:43–47

Cortessis VK, Azadian M, Buxbaum J et al (2018) Comprehensive meta-analysis reveals association between multiple imprinting disorders and conception by assisted reproductive technology. J Assist Reprod Genet 35:943–952. https://doi.org/10.1007/s10815-018-1173-x

Custódio G, Parise GA, Kiesel Filho N et al (2013) Impact of neonatal screening and surveillance for the TP53 R337H mutation on early detection of childhood adrenocortical tumors. J Clin Oncol Off J Am Soc Clin Oncol 31:2619–2626. https://doi.org/10.1200/JCO.2012.46.3711

de Andrade KC, Frone MN, Wegman-Ostrosky T et al (2019) Variable population prevalence estimates of germline TP53 variants: a gnomAD-based analysis. Hum Mutat 40:97–105. https://doi.org/10.1002/humu.23673

Dehner LP, Hill DA (2009) Adrenal cortical neoplasms in children: why so many carcinomas and yet so many survivors? Pediatr Dev Pathol 12:284–291. https://doi.org/10.2350/08-06-0489.1

Eeles RA (1995) Germline mutations in the TP53 gene. Cancer Surv 25:101–124

Eggermann K, Bliek J, Brioude F et al (2016) EMQN best practice guidelines for the molecular genetic testing and reporting of chromosome 11p15 imprinting disorders: Silver-Russell and Beckwith-Wiedemann syndrome. Eur J Hum Genet 24:1377–1387. https://doi.org/10.1038/ejhg.2016.45

El Ghorayeb N, Grunenwald S, Nolet S et al (2016) First case report of an adrenocortical carcinoma caused by a BRCA2 mutation. Medicine (Baltimore) 95:e4756. https://doi.org/10.1097/MD.0000000000004756

Else T, Lerario AM, Everett J et al (2017) Adrenocortical carcinoma and succinate dehydrogenase gene mutations: an observational case series. Eur J Endocrinol 177:439–444. https://doi.org/10.1530/EJE-17-0358

Espiard S, Bertherat J (2013) Carney complex. Front Horm Res 41:50–62. https://doi.org/10.1159/000345669

Figueiredo BC, Sandrini R, Zambetti GP et al (2006) Penetrance of adrenocortical tumours associated with the germline TP53 R337H mutation. J Med Genet 43:91–96. https://doi.org/10.1136/jmg.2004.030551

Forlino A, Vetro A, Garavelli L et al (2014) PRKACB and Carney complex. N Engl J Med 370:1065–1067. https://doi.org/10.1056/NEJMc1309730

Garritano S, Gemignani F, Palmero EI et al (2010) Detailed haplotype analysis at the TP53 locus in p.R337H mutation carriers in the population of southern Brazil: evidence for a founder effect. Hum Mutat 31:143–150. https://doi.org/10.1002/humu.21151

Gaujoux S, Pinson S, Gimenez-Roqueplo A-P et al (2010) Inactivation of the APC gene is constant in adrenocortical tumors from patients with familial adenomatous polyposis but not frequent in sporadic adrenocortical cancers. Clin Cancer Res 16:5133–5141. https://doi.org/10.1158/1078-0432.CCR-10-1497

Gicquel C, Raffin-Sanson ML, Gaston V et al (1997) Structural and functional abnormalities at 11p15 are associated with the malignant phenotype in sporadic adrenocortical tumors: study on a series of 82 tumors. J Clin Endocrinol Metab 82:2559–2565. https://doi.org/10.1210/jcem.82.8.4170

Gonzalez KD, Noltner KA, Buzin CH et al (2009) Beyond Li Fraumeni syndrome: clinical characteristics of families with p53 germline mutations. J Clin Oncol Off J Am Soc Clin Oncol 27:1250–1256. https://doi.org/10.1200/JCO.2008.16.6959

Groussin L, Kirschner LS, Vincent-Dejean C et al (2002) Molecular analysis of the cyclic AMP-dependent protein kinase a (PKA) regulatory subunit 1A (PRKAR1A) gene in patients with Carney complex and primary pigmented nodular adrenocortical disease (PPNAD) reveals novel mutations and clues for pathophysiology: augmented PKA signaling is associated with adrenal tumorigenesis in PPNAD. Am J Hum Genet 71:1433–1442. https://doi.org/10.1086/344579

Henry I, Jeanpierre M, Couillin P et al (1989) Molecular definition of the 11p15.5 region involved in Beckwith-Wiedemann syndrome and probably in predisposition to adrenocortical carcinoma. Hum Genet 81:273–277

Henry I, Puech A, Riesewijk A et al (1993) Somatic mosaicism for partial paternal isodisomy in Wiedemann-Beckwith syndrome: a post-fertilization event. Eur J Hum Genet EJHG 1:19–29

Herrmann LJM, Heinze B, Fassnacht M et al (2012) TP53 germline mutations in adult patients with adrenocortical carcinoma. J Clin Endocrinol Metab 97:E476–E485. https://doi.org/10.1210/jc.2011-1982
Heymann S, Delaloge S, Rahal A et al (2010) Radio-induced malignancies after breast cancer postoperative radiotherapy in patients with Li-Fraumeni syndrome. Radiat Oncol Lond Engl 5:104. https://doi.org/10.1186/1748-717X-5-104
Horvath A, Boikos S, Giatzakis C et al (2006) A genome-wide scan identifies mutations in the gene encoding phosphodiesterase 11A4 (PDE11A) in individuals with adrenocortical hyperplasia. Nat Genet 38:794–800. https://doi.org/10.1038/ng1809
Horvath A, Mericq V, Stratakis CA (2008) Mutation in PDE8B, a cyclic AMP-specific phosphodiesterase in adrenal hyperplasia. N Engl J Med 358:750–752. https://doi.org/10.1056/NEJMc0706182
Horvath A, Bertherat J, Groussin L et al (2010) Mutations and polymorphisms in the gene encoding regulatory subunit type 1-alpha of protein kinase a (PRKAR1A): an update. Hum Mutat 31:369–379. https://doi.org/10.1002/humu.21178
Ibrahim A, Kirby G, Hardy C et al (2014) Methylation analysis and diagnostics of Beckwith-Wiedemann syndrome in 1,000 subjects. Clin Epigenet 6:11. https://doi.org/10.1186/1868-7083-6-11
Kirschner LS, Carney JA, Pack SD et al (2000) Mutations of the gene encoding the protein kinase A type I-alpha regulatory subunit in patients with the Carney complex. Nat Genet 26:89–92. https://doi.org/10.1038/79238
Kratz CP, Achatz MI, Brugières L et al (2017) Cancer screening recommendations for individuals with Li-Fraumeni syndrome. Clin Cancer Res Off J Am Assoc Cancer Res 23:e38–e45. https://doi.org/10.1158/1078-0432.CCR-17-0408
Lane DP (1992) Cancer. p53, guardian of the genome. Nature 358:15–16. https://doi.org/10.1038/358015a0
Le DT, Uram JN, Wang H et al (2015) PD-1 blockade in tumors with mismatch-repair deficiency. N Engl J Med 372:2509–2520. https://doi.org/10.1056/NEJMoa1500596
Li FP, Fraumeni JF (1969) Soft-tissue sarcomas, breast cancer, and other neoplasms. A familial syndrome? Ann Intern Med 71:747–752
Li FP, Fraumeni JF, Mulvihill JJ et al (1988) A cancer family syndrome in twenty-four kindreds. Cancer Res 48:5358–5362
Libé R, Horvath A, Vezzosi D et al (2011) Frequent phosphodiesterase 11A gene (PDE11A) defects in patients with Carney complex (CNC) caused by PRKAR1A mutations: PDE11A may contribute to adrenal and testicular tumors in CNC as a modifier of the phenotype. J Clin Endocrinol Metab 96:E208–E214. https://doi.org/10.1210/jc.2010-1704
Lodish M, Stratakis CA (2016) A genetic and molecular update on adrenocortical causes of Cushing syndrome. Nat Rev Endocrinol 12:255–262. https://doi.org/10.1038/nrendo.2016.24
Lodish MB, Yuan B, Levy I et al (2015) Germline PRKACA amplification causes variable phenotypes that may depend on the extent of the genomic defect: molecular mechanisms and clinical presentations. Eur J Endocrinol 172:803–811. https://doi.org/10.1530/EJE-14-1154
Maas SM, Vansenne F, Kadouch DJM et al (2016) Phenotype, cancer risk, and surveillance in Beckwith-Wiedemann syndrome depending on molecular genetic subgroups. Am J Med Genet A 170:2248–2260. https://doi.org/10.1002/ajmg.a.37801
Malkin D, Li FP, Strong LC et al (1990) Germ line p53 mutations in a familial syndrome of breast cancer, sarcomas, and other neoplasms. Science 250:1233–1238
Mastellaro MJ, Seidinger AL, Kang G et al (2017) Contribution of the TP53 R337H mutation to the cancer burden in southern Brazil: insights from the study of 55 families of children with adrenocortical tumors. Cancer 123:3150–3158. https://doi.org/10.1002/cncr.30703
Morin E, Mete O, Wasserman JD et al (2012) Carney complex with adrenal cortical carcinoma. J Clin Endocrinol Metab 97:E202–E206. https://doi.org/10.1210/jc.2011-2321
Mussa A, Russo S, De Crescenzo A et al (2013) Prevalence of Beckwith-Wiedemann syndrome in north west of Italy. Am J Med Genet A 161A:2481–2486. https://doi.org/10.1002/ajmg.a.36080

Mussa A, Molinatto C, Baldassarre G et al (2016) Cancer risk in Beckwith-Wiedemann syndrome: a systematic review and meta-analysis outlining a novel (Epi)genotype specific histotype targeted screening protocol. J Pediatr 176:142–149.e1. https://doi.org/10.1016/j.jpeds.2016.05.038

Mussa A, Molinatto C, Cerrato F et al (2017) Assisted reproductive techniques and risk of Beckwith-Wiedemann syndrome. Pediatrics 140(1):e20164311. https://doi.org/10.1542/peds.2016-4311

Pilati C, Shinde J, Alexandrov LB et al (2017) Mutational signature analysis identifies MUTYH deficiency in colorectal cancers and adrenocortical carcinomas. J Pathol 242:10–15. https://doi.org/10.1002/path.4880

Pinto EM, Billerbeck AEC, Villares MCBF et al (2004) Founder effect for the highly prevalent R337H mutation of tumor suppressor p53 in Brazilian patients with adrenocortical tumors. Arq Bras Endocrinol Metabol 48:647–650. https://doi.org/10.1590/S0004-27302004000500009

Porteus MH, Narkool P, Neuberg D et al (2000) Characteristics and outcome of children with Beckwith-Wiedemann syndrome and Wilms' tumor: a report from the National Wilms Tumor Study Group. J Clin Oncol 18:2026–2031. https://doi.org/10.1200/JCO.2000.18.10.2026

Powell AC, Stratakis CA, Patronas NJ et al (2008) Operative management of Cushing syndrome secondary to micronodular adrenal hyperplasia. Surgery 143:750–758. https://doi.org/10.1016/j.surg.2008.03.022

Raymond VM, Else T, Everett JN et al (2013a) Prevalence of germline TP53 mutations in a prospective series of unselected patients with adrenocortical carcinoma. J Clin Endocrinol Metab 98:E119–E125. https://doi.org/10.1210/jc.2012-2198

Raymond VM, Everett JN, Furtado LV et al (2013b) Adrenocortical carcinoma is a Lynch syndrome-associated cancer. J Clin Oncol 31:3012–3018. https://doi.org/10.1200/JCO.2012.48.0988

Reinhardt HC, Schumacher B (2012) The p53 network: cellular and systemic DNA damage responses in aging and cancer. Trends Genet TIG 28:128–136. https://doi.org/10.1016/j.tig.2011.12.002

Renaux-Petel M, Charbonnier F, Théry J-C et al (2018) Contribution of de novo and mosaic TP53 mutations to Li-Fraumeni syndrome. J Med Genet 55:173–180. https://doi.org/10.1136/jmedgenet-2017-104976

Ribeiro RC, Sandrini F, Figueiredo B et al (2001) An inherited p53 mutation that contributes in a tissue-specific manner to pediatric adrenal cortical carcinoma. Proc Natl Acad Sci U S A 98:9330–9335. https://doi.org/10.1073/pnas.161479898

Rothenbuhler A, Horvath A, Libé R et al (2012) Identification of novel genetic variants in phosphodiesterase 8B (PDE8B), a cAMP-specific phosphodiesterase highly expressed in the adrenal cortex, in a cohort of patients with adrenal tumours. Clin Endocrinol 77:195–199. https://doi.org/10.1111/j.1365-2265.2012.04366.x

Salpea P, Horvath A, London E et al (2014) Deletions of the PRKAR1A locus at 17q24.2-q24.3 in Carney complex: genotype-phenotype correlations and implications for genetic testing. J Clin Endocrinol Metab 99:E183–E188. https://doi.org/10.1210/jc.2013-3159

Shuman C, Beckwith JB, Weksberg R (1993) Beckwith-Wiedemann syndrome. In: Adam MP, Ardinger HH, Pagon RA et al (eds) GeneReviews®. University of Washington, Seattle (WA)

Shuman C, Smith AC, Steele L et al (2006) Constitutional UPD for chromosome 11p15 in individuals with isolated hemihyperplasia is associated with high tumor risk and occurs following assisted reproductive technologies. Am J Med Genet A 140:1497–1503. https://doi.org/10.1002/ajmg.a.31323

Slatter RE, Elliott M, Welham K et al (1994) Mosaic uniparental disomy in Beckwith-Wiedemann syndrome. J Med Genet 31:749–753

Smith AC, Shuman C, Chitayat D et al (2007) Severe presentation of Beckwith-Wiedemann syndrome associated with high levels of constitutional paternal uniparental disomy for chromosome 11p15. Am J Med Genet A 143A:3010–3015. https://doi.org/10.1002/ajmg.a.32030

Stelmachowska-Banas M, Zgliczynski W, Tutka P et al (2017) Fatal Carney complex in siblings due to De novo large gene deletion. J Clin Endocrinol Metab 102:3924–3927. https://doi.org/10.1210/jc.2017-01045

Stratakis CA, Raygada M (1993) Carney complex. In: Adam MP, Ardinger HH, Pagon RA et al (eds) GeneReviews®. University of Washington, Seattle, Seattle (WA)

Stratakis CA, Kirschner LS, Carney JA (1998) Carney complex: diagnosis and management of the complex of spotty skin pigmentation, myxomas, endocrine overactivity, and schwannomas. Am J Med Genet 80:183–185

Stratakis CA, Kirschner LS, Carney JA (2001) Clinical and molecular features of the Carney complex: diagnostic criteria and recommendations for patient evaluation. J Clin Endocrinol Metab 86:4041–4046. https://doi.org/10.1210/jcem.86.9.7903

Tinat J, Bougeard G, Baert-Desurmont S et al (2009) 2009 version of the Chompret criteria for Li Fraumeni syndrome. J Clin Oncol Off J Am Soc Clin Oncol 27:e108–e109. https://doi.org/10.1200/JCO.2009.22.7967

Villani A, Tabori U, Schiffman J et al (2011) Biochemical and imaging surveillance in germline TP53 mutation carriers with Li-Fraumeni syndrome: a prospective observational study. Lancet Oncol 12:559–567. https://doi.org/10.1016/S1470-2045(11)70119-X

Villani A, Shore A, Wasserman JD et al (2016) Biochemical and imaging surveillance in germline TP53 mutation carriers with Li-Fraumeni syndrome: 11 year follow-up of a prospective observational study. Lancet Oncol 17:1295–1305. https://doi.org/10.1016/S1470-2045(16)30249-2

Wagner AS, Fleitz JM, Kleinschmidt-Demasters BK (2005) Pediatric adrenal cortical carcinoma: brain metastases and relationship to NF-1, case reports and review of the literature. J Neuro-Oncol 75:127–133. https://doi.org/10.1007/s11060-005-0376-z

Waldmann J, Bartsch DK, Kann PH et al (2007) Adrenal involvement in multiple endocrine neoplasia type 1: results of 7 years prospective screening. Langenbeck's Arch Surg 392:437–443. https://doi.org/10.1007/s00423-006-0124-7

Wasserman JD, Novokmet A, Eichler-Jonsson C et al (2015) Prevalence and functional consequence of TP53 mutations in pediatric adrenocortical carcinoma: a children's oncology group study. J Clin Oncol 33:602–609. https://doi.org/10.1200/JCO.2013.52.6863

Weksberg R, Shuman C, Beckwith JB (2010) Beckwith-Wiedemann syndrome. Eur J Hum Genet EJHG 18:8–14. https://doi.org/10.1038/ejhg.2009.106

Wiedemann HR (1964) Familial malformation complex with umbilical hernia and macroglossia – a "new syndrome"? J Genet Hum 13:223–232

Wilkin F, Gagné N, Paquette J et al (2000) Pediatric adrenocortical tumors: molecular events leading to insulin-like growth factor II gene overexpression. J Clin Endocrinol Metab 85:2048–2056. https://doi.org/10.1210/jcem.85.5.6589

Zheng S, Cherniack AD, Dewal N et al (2016) Comprehensive pan-genomic characterization of adrenocortical carcinoma. Cancer Cell 29:723–736. https://doi.org/10.1016/j.ccell.2016.04.002

Chapter 10
Genetics of Pituitary Tumours

Paul Benjamin Loughrey and Márta Korbonits

Abstract Pituitary tumours are relatively common in the general population. Most often they occur sporadically, with somatic mutations accounting for a significant minority of somatotroph and corticotroph adenomas. Pituitary tumours can also develop secondary to germline mutations as part of a complex syndrome or as familial isolated pituitary adenomas. Tumours occurring in a familial setting may present at a younger age and can behave more aggressively with resistance to treatment. This chapter will focus on the genetics and molecular pathogenesis of pituitary tumours.

Keywords Pituitary tumour · Genetics · *AIP* · FIPA · *MEN1* · MEN4 · Carney complex · McCune-Albright syndrome · *DICER1* · X-LAG

List of Abbreviations

ACTH	Adrenocorticotropic hormone
AHR	Aryl hydrocarbon receptor
AIP	Aryl hydrocarbon receptor-interacting protein
bHLHZ	Basic helix-loop-helix leucine zipper
cAMP	Cyclic adenosine monophosphate
CDH23	Cadherin-related 23
CGH	Comparative genomic hybridisation
circRNAs	Circular RNAs
CpG	Cystosine-phosphate-guanine
EGFR	Epidermal growth factor receptor

P. B. Loughrey
Regional Centre for Endocrinology and Diabetes, Royal Victoria Hospital, Belfast, UK

M. Korbonits (✉)
Centre for Endocrinology, William Harvey Research Institute, Barts and The London School of Medicine and Dentistry, Queen Mary University of London, London, UK
e-mail: m.korbonits@qmul.ac.uk

P. Igaz, A. Patócs (eds.), *Genetics of Endocrine Diseases and Syndromes*,
Experientia Supplementum 111, https://doi.org/10.1007/978-3-030-25905-1_10

FGF23	Fibroblast growth factor 23
FIPA	Familial isolated pituitary adenomas
GDP	Guanosine diphosphate
GH	Growth hormone
GHRH	Growth hormone-releasing hormone
GTP	Guanosine triphosphate
GWAS	Genome-wide association studies
HIF1α	Hypoxia-inducible factor 1-α
HSP90	Heat shock protein 90
IGF-1	Insulin-like growth factor 1
lncRNAs	Long non-coding RNAs
MAS	McCune-Albright syndrome
MEN1	Multiple endocrine neoplasia type 1
MEN4	Multiple endocrine neoplasia type 4
MGMT	O^6-methylguanine-DNA methyltransferase
miRNA	MicroRNA
MLLs	Mixed lineage leukaemia interaction proteins
MLPA	Multiplex ligand probe amplification
MRI	Magnetic resonance imaging
mRNA	Messenger ribonucleic acid
NESP55	Neuroendocrine secretory protein 55
NFPA	Non-functioning pituitary adenoma
NF1	Neurofibromatosis type 1
PDE4A4	Phosphodiesterase-4A4
PPAR-α	Peroxisome proliferation-activated receptor-α
PIK3CA	Phosphatidylinositol-4,5-bisphosphate 3-kinase catalytic subunit alpha
PitNET	Pituitary neuroendocrine tumour
PKA	Protein kinase A
POMC	Proopiomelanocortin
PRLR	Prolactin receptor gene
PTEN	Phosphatase and tensin homolog
qRT-PCR	Quantitative reverse transcription polymerase chain reaction
SDH	Succinate dehydrogenase
siRNA	Small interfering RNA
USP8	Ubiquitin specific peptidase 8
USP48	Ubiquitin specific peptidase 48
WES	Whole-exome sequencing
XLαs	Extra-large αs
X-LAG	X-linked acrogigantism syndrome
3Pa	Pituitary adenomas and paragangliomas or phaeochromocytomas
ZAC1	Zinc finger regulator of apoptosis and cell cycle arrest

10.1 Introduction

Pituitary tumours are common and are estimated to have a prevalence of approximately 16.7% (Aflorei and Korbonits 2014; Ezzat et al. 2004). They are also the third most common intracranial tumours (accounting for 10–15% of intracranial neoplasms) behind gliomas and meningiomas (Aflorei and Korbonits 2014; Lim and Korbonits 2018). Despite their prevalence, only approximately 0.1% of pituitary tumours are clinically relevant (Daly et al. 2006b). The term pituitary adenoma is used to refer to a (usually) benign monoclonal growth of the anterior pituitary. Pituitary carcinoma, defined as a tumour with metastasis, is rare and accounts for approximately 0.2% of all pituitary tumours (Heaney 2014), although recent data suggest that there are few, if any, phenotypic differences between pituitary carcinomas and aggressive pituitary tumours, and the name pituitary neuroendocrine tumour (PitNET) has been suggested (Trouillas et al. 2018).

Pituitary adenomas are normally slow growing and may present with local mass effect (headache, visual disturbance), symptoms of a functioning tumour, symptoms of hypopituitarism or a combination of all three. Most pituitary tumours are sporadic (approximately 95%) (Caimari and Korbonits 2016) while hereditary pituitary tumours are rarer (Fig. 10.1). Although hereditary tumours are less common, they may present at an earlier age, be larger and behave in a more aggressive manner resulting in significant morbidity. They can also draw attention to the disease occurring in a family where other family members may benefit from early screening and diagnosis or they can mark the first manifestation of a syndrome of multiple endocrine neoplasia (such as multiple endocrine neoplasia type 1 (MEN1) or Carney complex), making their detection of paramount importance.

Across population studies, the most common pituitary tumours are usually found to be prolactinomas, ranging from 40 to 66% of tumours, followed by non-functioning pituitary adenomas (NFPA) (15–43%), somatotrophinomas (8–16%) and corticotrophinomas (2–6%) (Agustsson et al. 2015; Daly et al. 2006b; Fernandez et al. 2010; Fontana and Gaillard 2009; Gruppetta et al. 2013; Raappana et al. 2010). Thyrotrophinomas are particularly rare and are thought to represent less than 1% of pituitary adenomas.

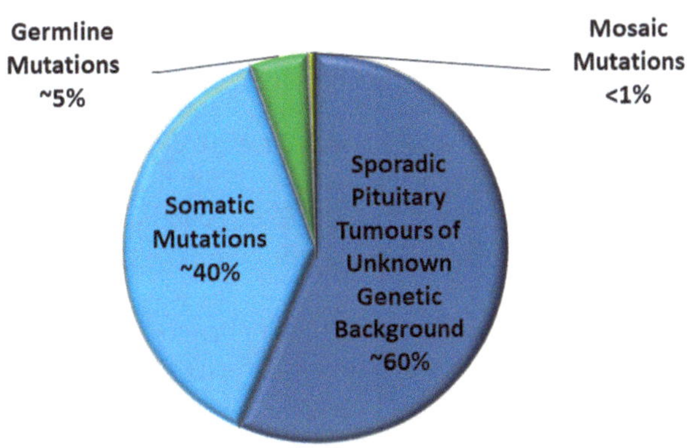

Fig. 10.1 Mutational landscape of pituitary adenomas

10.2 Germline or Mosaic Mutations

Diseases due to germline mutations can be classified as those resulting in pituitary disease only (isolated pituitary disease) and those causing syndromic disease. The former group contains kindreds with germline *AIP* and *GPR101* mutations and possibly other recently described alterations in *CABLES1*, while the latter group contains MEN1, multiple endocrine neoplasia type 4 (MEN4), Carney complex, paraganglioma-related genes (*SDH/MAX*)-related disease and DICER1 syndrome.

10.2.1 Familial Isolated Pituitary Adenomas (FIPA)

10.2.1.1 Aryl Hydrocarbon Receptor-Interacting Protein (*AIP*)

FIPA is defined as more than one family member with a pituitary adenoma without features of syndromes known to be associated with pituitary adenomas (Beckers et al. 2013). It represents approximately 2% of all pituitary adenomas (Daly et al. 2006a) and may be classified as homogeneous when patients in a family have the same tumour type and heterogeneous when patients in a family have varying tumour types (Beckers et al. 2013). *AIP* (OMIM *605555 #102200) mutations account for approximately 20% of FIPA cases (Chahal et al. 2010; Shaid and Korbonits 2017). A small number of FIPA cases may be accounted for by *GPR101* mutations (Gadelha et al. 2017) [see X-linked acrogigantism syndrome (X-LAG) subsection of this review]; however, almost 80% of FIPA is as yet unaccounted for by genetic mutations.

AIP, a gene located on 11q13.2, within a few megabases from the structurally independent *MEN1* gene, consists of 6 exons and codes for the 330 amino-acid 37kd AIP. While it was first described related to the environmental toxin receptor aryl hydrocarbon receptor (AHR) in 1996 (Kuzhandaivelu et al. 1996), *AIP* mutations were not implicated in pituitary tumourigenesis until a large family with pituitary adenoma was identified in Northern Finland in 2006 (Vierimaa et al. 2006), with a founder nonsense *AIP* mutation (Q14Stop), together with some other mutations in independent families. AIP is highly conserved across species (Aflorei et al. 2018) and is expressed in all tissues. In a normal pituitary, AIP expression is restricted to somatotrophs and lactotrophs, whereas in pituitary tumours, AIP is present in all tumour types and is most highly expressed in somatotrophinomas and NFPA (Jaffrain-Rea et al. 2009; Leontiou et al. 2008; Ozfirat and Korbonits 2010).

AIP is a tumour suppressor gene in the pituitary, behaving in an autosomal dominant manner with low 20–23% penetrance (Williams et al. 2012). The exact reasons for this variable penetrance are as yet unclear, but incomplete penetrance is well known in various syndromes with loss-of-function mutations in tumour suppressor genes. Three quarters of the mutations are truncating mutations, and many of the missense mutations reduce the stability of the protein, resulting in reduced protein levels (Hernández-Ramírez et al. 2016). Despite this, immunostaining of pituitary adenomas using the available antibodies did not prove to be useful in identifying patients with *AIP* mutations. Patients with *AIP* mutation characteristically develop their first symptoms under the age of 18 years and are diagnosed a few years later. The tumours usually secrete growth hormone (GH) and/or prolactin (Cazabat et al. 2009; Igreja et al. 2010). *AIP* mutation-positive somatotroph tumours are most commonly sparsely granulated somatotrophinomas and respond poorly to somatostatin analogue therapy (Daly et al. 2010; Shaid and Korbonits 2017). Prolactinomas are the second most common *AIP* mutation-positive tumours, followed by somatomammotrophinoma, NFPAs and extremely rarely thyrotrophinomas and corticotrophinomas (Fig. 10.2) (Korbonits and Kumar 2012). Gigantism occurs in 32% of *AIP* mutations (Beckers et al. 2013), and *AIP* mutations are responsible for 29–50% of those with gigantism (Cuny et al. 2013; Iacovazzo et al. 2016; Rostomyan et al. 2015). While overall more males are identified with *AIP* mutations (Daly et al. 2010), this could be due to a selection bias of patients with gigantism, inevitable due to later puberty and taller stature in males in general; as in large carefully studied families, the gender balance of affected subjects is not skewed (Hernandez-Ramirez et al. 2015).

What Is the Molecular Mechanism Leading to Pituitary Adenomas in Patients with Germline *AIP* Mutations?

AIP is a co-chaperone to heat shock protein 90 (HSP90) (Hernandez-Ramirez et al. 2018; Kazlauskas et al. 2000) and other heat shock proteins. Via these partners, AIP can potentially influence the function of a large number of proteins in various processes such as DNA repair, development and the immune response (Schopf et al. 2017) and interacts with 60% of human protein kinases and 30% of ubiquitin ligases. AHR, a nuclear receptor binding the HSP90-AIP complex, plays a role in toxin metabolism, and a link with environmental pollution has been raised in studies from Italy (Cannavo et al. 2010, 2014, 2016; Ferrau et al. 2018).

AIP mutations may contribute to somatotrophinoma development via altering the cyclic adenosine monophosphate (cAMP) pathway. AIP interacts with phosphodiesterase-4A5/4 (PDE4A5/4A4), an enzyme degrading cAMP (Bolger et al. 2003). While sporadic pituitary adenomas overexpress PDE4A4 and PDE4A8, *AIP* mutation-positive samples show a lack of upregulation of these two enzyme isoforms, suggesting that a functional AIP protein is needed for the upregulation in somatotroph adenomas (Bizzi et al. 2018; Bolger et al. 2016). As the cAMP pathway is well known to be key in somatotroph adenoma genesis, these interesting observations may have important relevance for AIP-related tumourigenesis (Caimari and Korbonits 2016). Another mechanism is via the inhibitory G proteins $G\alpha_{i\text{-}2}$ (Ritvonen et al. 2017; Tuominen et al. 2015), as this protein was found to show reduced expression in *AIP* mutation-positive adenomas. Both the PDE and the inhibitory G protein could contribute to the resistance to somatostatin analogues, in addition to a zinc finger regulator of apoptosis and cell cycle arrest

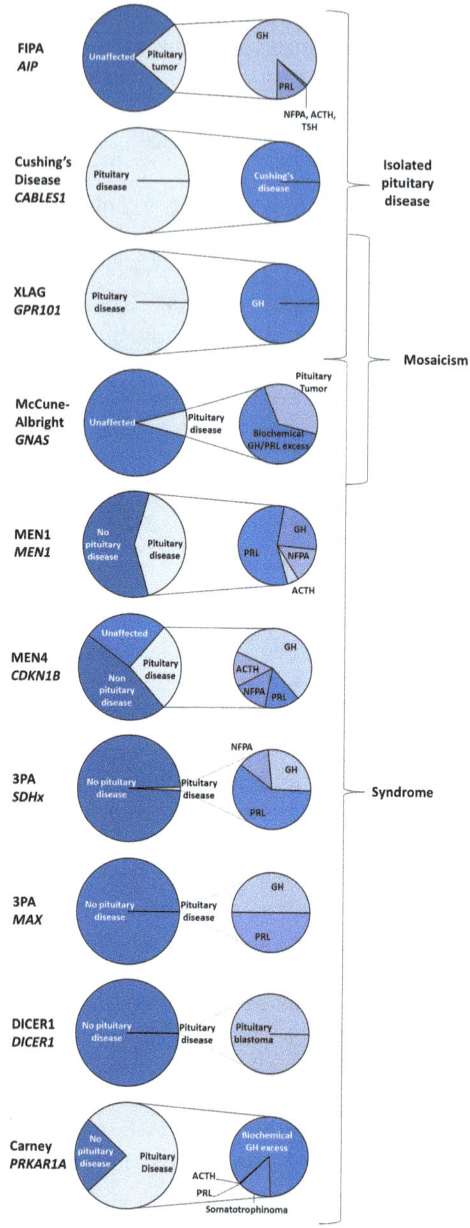

Fig. 10.2 Germline and mosaic mutations associated with pituitary disease [updated from Gadelha et al. (2017), Open Access]. *GH* Growth hormone-secreting tumour, *ACTH* ACTH-secreting tumour, *PRL* Prolactin-secreting tumour

(ZAC1)-related pathway. ZAC1 is an antiproliferative target of somatostatin (Theodoropoulou et al. 2006) and wild-type *AIP* upregulates *ZAC1* expression in GH3 cells while AIP siRNA knockdown reduces ZAC1 mRNA (Chahal et al. 2012; Marques and Korbonits 2017). The ZAC1 pathway may be an additional mechanism accounting for the blunted response to somatostatin analogues in *AIP* mutated tumours (Chahal et al. 2012).

Other binding partners of AIP include PDE2A $G\alpha_{13}$, survivin, thyroid hormone receptor β1, peroxisome proliferation-activated receptor-α (PPAR-α), heat-shock cognate 70, HSPA5, HSPA9, TUBB, TUBB2A, NME1 and SOD1 (Beckers et al. 2013; Hernandez-Ramirez et al. 2018; Nakata et al. 2009; Trivellin and Korbonits 2011); further studies are needed to identify their precise role in pituitary tumourigenesis.

Does AIP Play a Role in Sporadic in Pituitary Adenomas Even When No Germline Mutation Is Present?

No somatic *AIP* mutations have been found to date. However, sporadic pituitary tumours with low AIP protein expression display increased invasiveness (Ibanez-Costa and Korbonits 2017; Jaffrain-Rea et al. 2009; Kasuki Jomori de Pinho et al. 2011; Kasuki et al. 2012; Leontiou et al. 2008).

It is well accepted that disease-causing *AIP* sequence variants lead to loss of function of the protein. Most delete the C-terminal part or the whole protein (truncating mutations), while others (missense, insertion) change the conformation of the protein in a way that leads to rapid proteasomal degradation (Hernández-Ramírez et al. 2016; Salvatori et al. 2017) (Fig. 10.3). Large deletions (whole exome or whole gene) have been identified both in sporadic and simplex cases and should be tested for using multiplex ligand probe amplification (MLPA) or similar methods if Sanger sequencing of *AIP* did not identify a mutation. More recently, panel testing based on next-generation sequencing is becoming the preferred screening method.

There are a few recurring mutations identified in different populations, while founder mutations have also been identified. Recurring mutations (also called hotspots) are often related to methylated CpG (cytosine-phosphate-guanine) sites (Ozfirat and Korbonits 2010), and examples are the c.910C>T, p.R304Stop identified in several countries. Some of the R304Stop mutations also serve as a founder mutation (Italy and Ireland) (Chahal et al. 2011; Occhi et al. 2010; Radian et al. 2017; Williams et al. 2014). The missense variant affecting the same CpG site (c.911G>A, p304Q) has been identified in several FIPA families and sporadic patients, but it has a high minor allele frequency and may represent a polymorphism rather than a disease-causing allele. Other recurring mutations are c.811C>T, p. R271W (Caimari et al. 2018; Daly et al. 2007; De Sousa et al. 2017; Hernandez-Ramirez et al. 2015; Igreja et al. 2010; Jennings et al. 2009; Tichomirowa et al. 2011) and c.241C>T, p.R81∗ (Guaraldi et al. 2012; Leontiou et al. 2008; Toledo et al. 2010; Dutta et al. 2019) changes.

10.2.1.2 X-LAG

X-LAG represents infant-onset gigantism caused by microduplications on the *GPR101* gene (OMIM ∗300393 #300943), either in the germline or in a mosaic form (Daly et al. 2016; Iacovazzo et al. 2016; Rodd et al. 2016; Trivellin et al. 2014). Microduplications cover an approximately 500 Kb region at Xq23.6 and result in

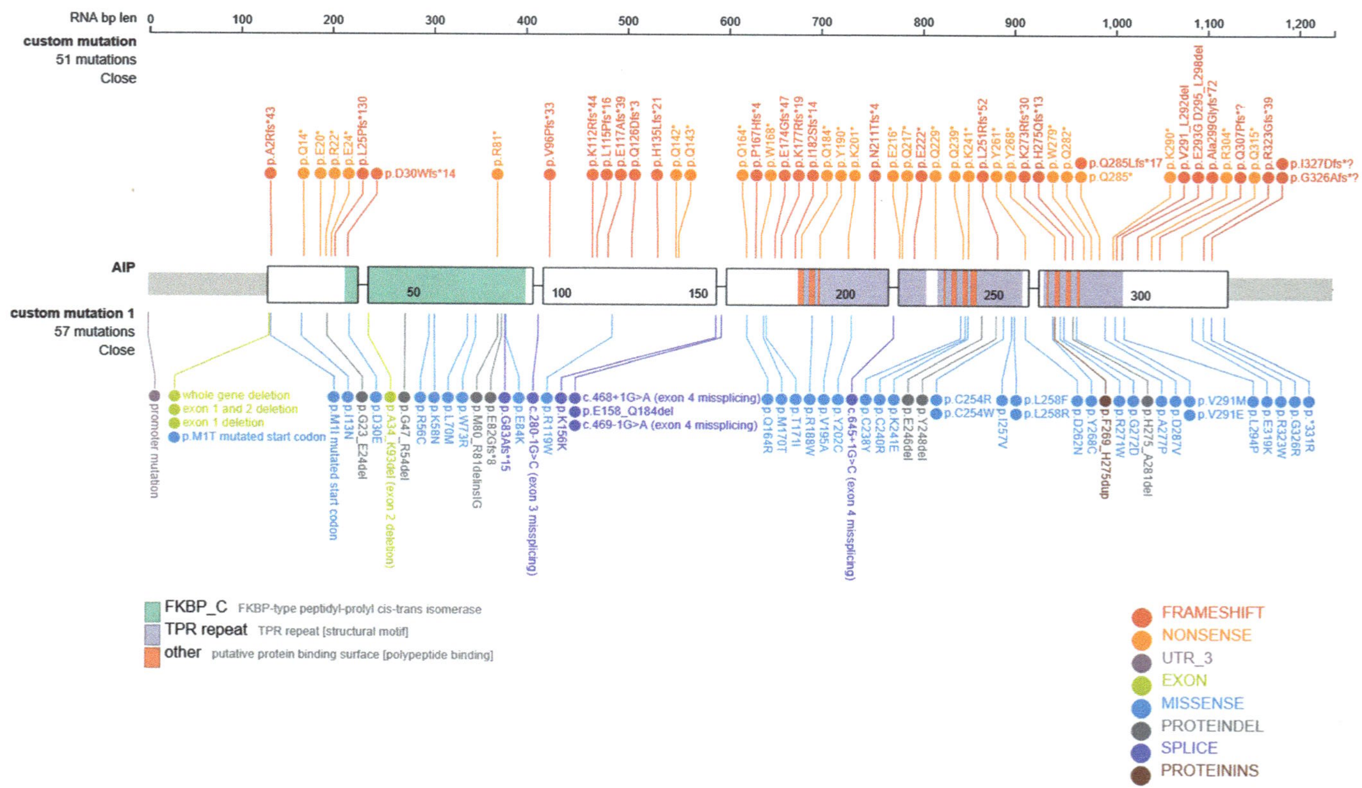

Fig. 10.3 Pathogenic and likely pathogenic *AIP* mutations (classified by authors) identified in patients [37 missense (blue), 26 frameshift (red), 25 nonsense (orange), 7 protein deletion (grey), 7 splice site (purple), 4 large deletions (whole exon or whole gene, green), 1 promoter mutation (plum) and 1 protein insertion (brown)]. Boxes represent exons, numbers represent amino acid numbers, light purple-shaded area represents the tetratricopeptide domains (TPR, conserved palindromic α-helix structures, important for AIP function)

copy number gain of *GPR101* (Beckers et al. 2015). To date, the function of *GPR101* is yet to be fully explained, but it is likely to be involved in the regulation of growth hormone-releasing hormone (GHRH). Interestingly, deletion of *GPR101* was not identified as a cause of GH deficiency in a group of patients with congenital GH deficiency (Castinetti et al. 2016).

Affected individuals are born with normal birth length and weight but as early as 2–3 months of age begin to exhibit rapid growth (Beckers et al. 2015) which may be due to a pituitary tumour or pituitary hyperplasia. With a median age of onset of approximately 1 year old, onset is earlier than other conditions of pituitary gigantism (Beckers et al. 2015). Tumours consist of a mix of densely granulated and sparsely granulated somatotrophs in combination with lactotrophs (Fig. 10.2) (Iacovazzo et al. 2016). Patients will have high levels of GH, insulin-like growth factor 1 (IGF-1) and in ~80% of patients prolactin (Beckers et al. 2015; Iacovazzo and Korbonits 2016). Tumours of affected individuals have upregulated levels of GPR101 (Trivellin et al. 2014).

Although males account for approximately 78% of pituitary gigantism cases, X-LAG is more common in females (approximately 77% of X-LAG cases reported) (Rostomyan et al. 2015), and in male cases, it is usually due to duplication at an early post-zygotic stage resulting in mosaicism (Iacovazzo et al. 2016), unless it is a familial case (Trivellin et al. 2014). X-LAG does not appear to have a particular ethnic preponderance and has been observed in Caucasian European, Southeast Asian, Indian subcontinent, First Nations Canadian and Latino-Afro-Caribbean (Beckers et al. 2015; Iacovazzo et al. 2016).

Macroadenomas appear to be more common than pituitary hyperplasia in this condition (Beckers et al. 2015). In one study, 75% of X-LAG-associated tumours were macroadenomas; all had suprasellar extensions and 25% extended into the cavernous sinus (Iacovazzo et al. 2016). While tumour growth does not seem to be as aggressive as in some *AIP* mutation-positive cases, untreated X-LAG tumours can demonstrate aggressive growth with a patient at age 10 years having developed a $56.2 \times 58.1 \times 45.0$ mm pituitary lesion, optic chiasm compression, bilateral cavernous sinus invasion and encasement of internal carotids with associated hydrocephalus (Naves et al. 2016). It has been speculated that Robert Wadlow, the tallest recorded human in history, had X-LAG (Iacovazzo and Korbonits 2016; Trivellin et al. 2014).

Leukocyte-derived DNA may not demonstrate the presence of duplication in cases of mosaicism; therefore if a phenotype is suggestive of X-LAG or there is high clinical suspicion, it is best to test pituitary or pituitary-derived tissue for duplications (Iacovazzo et al. 2016). This was illustrated by Rodd et al. when a patient negative for microduplication on peripheral blood DNA was found to have microduplication on sampling of pituitary and forearm skin tissue (Rodd et al. 2016). It is also worth noting the small microduplications may not be detected by standard comparative genomic hybridisation (CGH) array and alternative methods such as droplet polymerase chain reaction for *GPR101* or high-density array CGH should be utilised (Iacovazzo et al. 2016).

10.2.1.3 CABLES1

CABLES1 (OMIM *609194) is a glucocorticoid-activated negative regulator of cell cycle in corticotroph cells (Roussel-Gervais et al. 2016). Research to date has found that CABLES1 blocks cell cycle progression in an AtT-20 cell line, and its expression is lost in approximately 55% of corticotroph adenomas (Fig. 10.2) with correlating loss of cyclin-dependent kinase inhibitor 1B (usually known as p27), a cell cycle inhibitor also implicated in MEN4 (Roussel-Gervais et al. 2016). Hernandez-Ramirez et al. found four possible pathogenic missense mutations when screening paediatric and young adult patients with Cushing's disease (Hernandez-Ramirez et al. 2017a). None of them had familial disease. The patients with *CABLES1* variants had macroadenomas; all mutations were missense and none were truncating, which is unusual for a tumour suppressor gene. The role of *CABLES1* in pituitary tumourigenesis requires ongoing research and confirmatory data.

10.2.1.4 Cadherin-Related 23 (*CDH23*)

Recently, germline mutations in the *CDH23* (OMIM *605516 #617540) gene have been suggested as a risk factor for the development of sporadic and familial pituitary tumours (Zhang et al. 2017a). *CDH23* codes for Cadherin-related 23 which is a member of the cadherin superfamily, members of which are involved with cell-to-cell adhesion (Zhang et al. 2017a). Homozygote *CDH23* mutations are associated with deafness and Usher syndrome (Sotomayor et al. 2014), although deafness was not observed in any of the *CDH23*-mutated Chinese pituitary tumour cohort (Zhang et al. 2017a). Similarly, deaf patients are not reported with pituitary adenoma. *CDH23*-mutated pituitary tumours appear to be larger in size and more invasive in their nature and in the sporadic group resulted in tumours of wide-ranging functionality (Zhang et al. 2017a).

10.2.1.5 Prolactin Receptor (*PRLR*)

Recently, in a population of 46 prolactinomas (56% male, 44% female), 6 germline *PRLR* (OMIM *176761) variants were identified. Of these six variants, two were deemed rare and occurred in significantly higher frequency in this study than in the exome aggregation consortium cohort (Gorvin et al. 2018); contrary to this, a similar study of *PRLR* germline variants in 88 patients with prolactinoma did not find an association with this pituitary tumour subtype (Bernard et al. 2016). In other reports, *PRLR* mutations inherited in an autosomal dominant pattern resulting in disruption of the prolactin receptor and familial hyperprolactinaemia have been described with a paradox phenotype (Newey et al. 2013a). On the other hand, compound heterozygosity with inactivating germline variants of *PRLR* (Kobayashi et al. 2018) resulted in hyperprolactinaemia and lack of lactation, representing a classical resistence phenotype. In these cases *PRLR* mutations did not result in any identified abnormality on pituitary magnetic resonance imaging (MRI) (Kobayashi et al. 2018; Newey et al. 2013a).

10.2.2 Syndromic Disease

10.2.2.1 Multiple Endocrine Neoplasia Type 1 (MEN1)

MEN1 is an autosomal dominant syndrome characterised by tumours of the pituitary and parathyroid glands and pancreas. The syndrome was first recognised in 1903 (Erdheim 1903), and in 1954 kindreds with both endocrine and non-endocrine neoplasia were reported (Wermer 1954). The prevalence of MEN1 is approximately 1 in 30,000 (Agarwal et al. 2009; Marini et al. 2006) and shows no gender bias (Agarwal 2017). MEN1 has a high penetrance with 95% of patients manifesting disease by the age of 50 years. The earliest manifestation can be insulinomas, pituitary adenomas or parathyroid tumours.

The overall prevalence of pituitary tumours in MEN1 syndrome is 30–40% (Caimari and Korbonits 2016; de Laat et al. 2015; Goudet et al. 2010; Thakker et al. 2012), while MEN1 accounts for less than 3% of pituitary tumours (Costa and Korbonits 2017; Thakker et al. 2012). Prolactinomas are the most common MEN1-associated pituitary tumours accounting for 50–60% of pituitary tumours in MEN1 (Marini et al. 2006; Thakker 2014). In a French retrospective cohort study of young macroprolactinoma patients, 3/59 (5%) carried a *MEN1* (OMIM *613733 #131100) mutation (Salenave et al. 2015): 25% of MEN1-associated pituitary tumours are somatotrophinomas, 12% are NFPAs and 3% are corticotrophinomas (Marini et al. 2006) (Fig. 10.2). MEN1-associated pituitary tumours tend to occur more commonly in women than men (Goudet et al. 2010) and are generally larger (Gadelha et al. 2017; Schernthaner-Reiter et al. 2016) [macroadenoma in 85% of MEN1 vs. 42% in non-MEN1 (Verges et al. 2002)] and more invasive at presentation (Trouillas et al. 2008). A *MEN1* mutation has been shown to be a significant and independent predictor of resistance to dopamine agonists (Salenave et al. 2015). There is no significantly increased risk of pituitary carcinoma in MEN1 (Beckers et al. 2003); only two MEN1-related pituitary carcinoma cases have been reported (Table 10.1). Parathyroid adenomas (typically occurring before the age of 40) are highly penetrant, affecting approximately 95% of MEN1 patients (Trump et al. 1996), and hyperparathyroidism seems to occur at a higher rate when MEN1 patients also have pituitary adenomas (91.9% vs. 75.9%) (de Laat et al. 2015).

Menin can exist as a component of a histone methyltransferase complex with mixed lineage leukaemia interaction proteins (MLLs) which can regulate transcription (Milne et al. 2005). As part of this complex, it can regulate the cyclin-dependent kinase inhibitors p27 and p18 (Milne et al. 2005). Menin may then have roles in regulation of the cell cycle, and this relationship between menin and p27 may explain the phenotypic similarities between MEN1 and MEN4. The relationship between menin and p27 may also explain the organ-specific effects of *MEN1* mutations as certain tissues rely more on p27-directed regulation of the cell cycle. *Cdkn1b* (coding for p27) knockout mice exhibit gigantism and organ enlargement, including nodular

Table 10.1 Pituitary carcinomas occurring in familial setting

Genetic context	Age at diagnosis	Sex	Details	References
MEN1	28	Male	Thyrotrophinoma	Scheithauer et al. (2009)
MEN1	47	Male	Prolactinoma Ki-67 3% in cervical metastasis	Gordon et al. (2007)
SDHB	53	Female	Clinically non-functioning Ki-67 15% Strong nuclear expression of P53 in 5% of cells	Tufton et al. (2017)
FIPA (*AIP* negative)	57	Male	Prolactinoma Heterogeneous 2-member FIPA kindred	Petrossians et al. (2000)
FIPA (*AIP* negative)	46	Female	Somatotrophinoma Ki-67 17.2% P53 staining positive	Miljic et al. (2017)
MSH2	51	Male	Corticotrophinoma Ki-67 40% P53 staining positive	Bengtsson et al. (2017)

To date, pituitary carcinoma has not been identified in the setting of Carney complex, MAS, X-LAG or *AIP* mutations

pituitary hyperplasia (Fero et al. 1996; Kiyokawa et al. 1996; Nakayama et al. 1996) and spontaneous mutation in this gene results in an MEN1&MEN2 overlap syndrome in rats (Pellegata et al. 2006). Interestingly, one study has found that cyclin-dependent kinase 4 inhibitor C (p18) and menin-insufficient mice ($Cdkn2c^{-/-};Men1^{-/+}$) developed pituitary, parathyroid, thyroid and pancreatic effects via a synergistic effect on Rb kinase activity, while $Cdkn1b^{-/-};Men1^{-/+}$ mice did not exhibit the same synergy (Bai et al. 2007). This suggests that there may be additional pathways involved in menin and p27 interactions.

More recently, the role of microRNAs in experimental models has been investigated. In $Men1^{+/-}$ mouse pituitary tumours miR-15a, miR-16-1 and let-7a miRNAs were significantly downregulated in comparison to wild-type pituitaries (Lines et al. 2018). Knockdown of *MEN1* in HeLa cells and AtT20 mouse pituitary cell line model resulted in decreased expression of miR-15a.

A systematic review of pituitary incidentalomas found that prevalence can be estimated at 22.5% in radiologic studies (Ezzat et al. 2004). Given that MEN1 diagnosis may be fulfilled clinically (without identification of known *MEN1* pathogenic mutation) and many pituitary tumours are detected by pituitary MRI, it is possible that some pituitary tumours in the setting of apparent MEN1 may be phenocopies. This might explain the high incidence of NFPAs in a retrospective study of a MEN1 Dutch cohort (de Laat et al. 2015). Similarly, *AIP* mutation carriers have been identified with small, stable non-functioning pituitary lesions (Hernandez-Ramirez et al. 2015; Korbonits, personal observation). Further studies need to examine these questions in familial pituitary diseases.

The association of *MEN1* and pituitary adenoma is well established. Future clarification of the mechanisms of menin function should assist in establishing the molecular pathology of pituitary tumourigenesis.

10.2.2.2 MEN4

MEN4 is a rare syndrome caused by mutations of *CDKN1B* (OMIM *600778 #610755), located on chromosome 12p13.1 and coding for the cyclin-dependent kinase inhibitor 1B (p27) protein, a 196 amino acid. *CDKN1B* mutations are associated with pituitary adenomas, parathyroid adenomas and pancreatic neuroendocrine tumours; thus this syndrome is phenotypically identical to MEN1. This of course is not surprising as menin regulates p27 which subsequently regulates cell cycle progression by inhibition of cyclin-dependent-kinase-2 complexed with cyclin E, cyclin D and cyclin A (Abbastabar et al. 2018; Alrezk et al. 2017). p27, however, unlike *MEN1*, does not behave like a typical tumour suppressor gene, as it does not adhere to the Knudson two-hit hypothesis (Alrezk et al. 2017). Haploinsufficiency, i.e. only one mutated *CDKN1B*, is sufficient to initiate neoplasia, as illustrated by a $Cdkn1b^{+/-}$ mouse model manifesting pituitary tumours in response to radiation or chemical carcinogens (Fero et al. 1998). Somatic mutations of *CDKN1B* are very rare (Philipp-Staheli et al. 2001).

The novel MEN4 syndrome was initially discovered in rats and was termed MENX (Fritz et al. 2002). It was inherited in a recessive manner in this rodent, in contrast to typical multiple endocrine tumour syndromes in humans (Pellegata et al. 2006). *CDKN1B* was identified using fine mapping and candidate gene screening (Pellegata et al. 2006). In the same paper, Pellegata et al. (2006) described a female patient who presented with a 3 cm somatotrophinoma at age 30 followed by the development of hyperparathyroidism at age 48. Sequencing revealed a heterozygous nonsense mutation at codon 76 resulting in the absence of p27 in tumour cells and the first case of MEN4 described in humans (Pellegata et al. 2006).

As of 2019, only 19 cases of MEN4 have been reported. Seven of these cases have had confirmed or suspected pituitary disease, and all seven were female (Georgitsi et al. 2007; Molatore et al. 2010; Occhi et al. 2013; Pellegata et al. 2006; Sambugaro et al. 2015; Tichomirowa et al. 2012). Of these seven cases, three of the mutations were truncating (Georgitsi et al. 2007; Occhi et al. 2013; Pellegata et al. 2006). Interestingly, it appears that MEN4-associated pituitary tumours are generally less aggressive than those of MEN1 (Alrezk et al. 2017), and in contrast to rats, MEN4 in humans is inherited in an autosomal dominant pattern (Thakker 2014). Pituitary tumour types reported to date are somatotrophinoma (three acromegaly cases, one gigantism), one corticotrophinoma, one NFPA and one suspected prolactinoma (Fig. 10.2).

10.2.2.3 Carney Complex

Carney complex was originally described in 1985 as the classic complex of "myxomas, spotty skin pigmentation and endocrine over-activity" (Carney et al. 1985). The pituitary pathology exhibited in this syndrome varies and can include pituitary hyperplasia, pituitary adenoma or a combination of both (Fig. 10.2). In this review, the focus will be on pituitary manifestations of Carney complex. Carney complex is discussed in more detail in Chap. 9.

Asymptomatic pituitary hyperplasia, biochemical hyperprolactinaemia and rises in GH and IGF-1 are common (75% of Carney complex patients) (Caimari and Korbonits 2016; Correa et al. 2015), while clinically evident acromegaly is rare (10–12%) (Caimari and Korbonits 2016; Correa et al. 2015) (Fig. 10.2). Prolactinomas can develop but are particularly rare (Correa et al. 2015), and two cases of Cushing's disease in association with Carney complex have been described (Hernandez-Ramirez et al. 2017b; Kiefer et al. 2017). The median age of diagnosis of Carney complex is 20 years, and pituitary disease normally presents after the third decade (Boikos and Stratakis 2006). Gigantism has very rarely been reported (Caimari and Korbonits 2016).

Carney complex is inherited as an autosomal dominant syndrome with almost 100% penetrance and may occur as a consequence of a de novo mutation in approximately 30% of patients (Correa et al. 2015; Kaltsas et al. 2000); 57% of the patients are female and the disease does not appear to have any ethnic preponderance (Stratakis et al. 2001). In addition to the 17q22 locus coding for *PRKAR1A* (OMIM ∗188830 #160980) and responsible for 80% of the mutations, *PRKACB* (OMIM ∗176892) amplification has been found in a single case (Forlino et al. 2014), while some families show linkage to 2p16 but the disease-causing gene is still unknown.

Inactivating mutations and large deletions of *PRKAR1A* result in haploinsufficiency of the regulatory (i.e. inhibitory) subunit 1 alpha of protein kinase A (PKA) resulting in constitutional activation of cAMP signalling (Fig. 10.4). Most pathogenic mutations of *PRKAR1A* are base substitutions, small deletions, insertions or rearrangements (Rothenbuhler and Stratakis 2010). Large deletions of *PRKAR1A* result in a more severe disease phenotype (Blyth et al. 2008; Horvath et al. 2008). In a study of 353 patients with *PRKAR1A* mutations, mutations in exons were more often associated with acromegaly (Bertherat et al. 2009), which is thought to be a more slowly progressive disease when occurring in the context of Carney complex (Horvath and Stratakis 2008).

CNC2 (OMIM %605244) is a 10 Mb region located on 2p16 accounting for around 20% of Carney complex families (Kaltsas et al. 2000). These families tend to present at a later stage of life (Correa et al. 2015) with a less severe disease phenotype (Caimari and Korbonits 2016). The exact gene responsible for *CNC2*-associated Carney complex cases is yet to be identified.

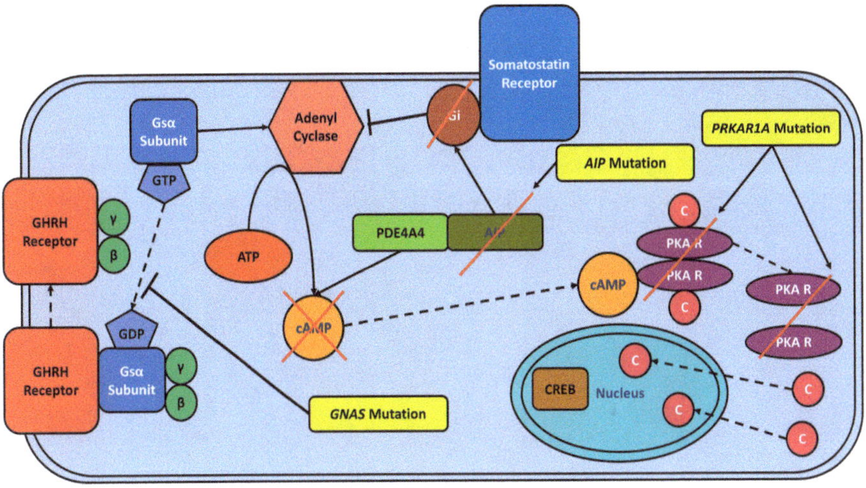

Fig. 10.4 The cAMP pathway in pituitary tumourigenesis. GHRH receptor activation results in the exchange of GDP to GTP. Gsα is subsequently released to activate adenylyl cyclase. At the same time Gsα, via its GTPase activity, exchanges GTP to GDP, therefore ending its own activated state, and dissociates from adenylyl cyclase. *GNAS* mutations (occurring in MAS and sporadic somatotrophinomas) result in a lack of GTP to GDP conversion resulting in uninhibited Gsα and continuous adenylyl cyclase activation. PDE4A4 can degrade cAMP and AIP can bind PDE4A4, but whether this specific interaction results in reduced cAMP levels and lack of AIP to upregulated PDE4A4 activity is still to be shown. Lack of AIP leads to reduced inhibitory G protein (Gi) which may allow enhanced adenylyl cyclase activity and impairment of somatostatin receptor signalling. Mutations of the regulatory subunit (*PRKAR1A*) of protein kinase A (PKA R) result in uninhibited catalytic subunit PKA C (c) which translocates to the nucleus and can phosphorylate targets such as CREB

10.2.2.4 Pituitary Adenomas and Paragangliomas or Phaeochromocytomas (3Pa)

Pituitary adenomas may coexist with paraganglioma or phaeochromocytoma: the 3Pa syndrome. Paragangliomas and phaeochromocytomas occurring in isolation are uncommon with detection rates of approximately 2–5 cases per million population (Eisenhofer et al. 2013; Mazzaglia 2012). *SDHx* mutations are implicated in several neoplasms; however, *SDHx* mutations in pituitary lesions are estimated to account for approximately 0.3% of cases (Gill et al. 2014) and have been described as the least common *SDHx*-associated neoplasm (Gill 2018). Reported cases of pituitary tumours have been NFPAs, somatotrophinomas and prolactinomas (Fig. 10.2) (Denes et al. 2015; O'Toole et al. 2015; Xekouki et al. 2012).

Patients with pituitary adenomas have been described in all *SDH* genes (OMIM *SDHA* ∗600857, *SDHAF2* ∗613019, *SDHB* ∗185470, *SDHC* ∗602413, *SDHD* ∗602690). A unique feature of succinate dehydrogenase (SDH)-related pituitary

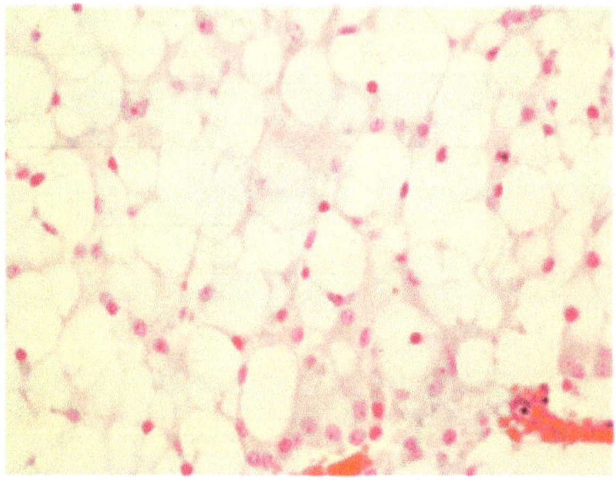

Fig. 10.5 Vacuolated cytoplasm in *SDHB*-mutated pituitary tumour (Tufton et al. 2017, Open Access)

adenomas is intracytoplasmic vacuoles (Fig. 10.5). Although the possibility of large, abnormal mitochondria appear as similar vacuoles in SDH-related kidney tumours, this could not be convincingly proven in pituitary adenomas (Denes et al. 2015). Bi-allelic inactivation of any component of the SDH complex results in negative immunohistochemistry for SDHB (Gill 2018), and this can be used for diagnostic purposes. Loss of heterozygosity due to somatic chromosomal material loss or promoter methylation (*SDHC*) could also represent the "second hit". For pituitary tumours, loss of heterozygosity was confirmed in some of the pituitary adenoma tissues (Denes et al. 2015). In some cases, pituitary tumour staining does not follow this pattern and suggests the possibility that some cases might be coincidental (Papathomas et al. 2014). A patient with *SDHB*-related hormone negative, *SF1*-positive pituitary tumour developed metastasis of the pituitary tumour 9 years after the diagnosis of the macroadenoma, rendering it a pituitary carcinoma (Tufton et al. 2017) (Table 10.1). Interestingly, by 12 months of age *Sdhb*$^{+/-}$ mice develop pituitary hyperplasia and pituitary intranuclear inclusions which have been postulated as an early change leading to pituitary adenoma formation (Xekouki et al. 2015).

In summary, *SDHx* mutations can be associated with pituitary tumours, but the penetrance is very low (Fig. 10.2).

10.2.2.5 MYC-Associated Factor X (*MAX*)

MAX is located on chromosome 14q23.3 and encodes for a transcription factor which is a member of the basic helix-loop-helix leucine zipper (bHLHZ) family (Carroll et al. 2018). MAX may form heterodimers with MYC, MNT and MGA proteins via direct interaction with their bHLHZ domains (Carroll et al. 2018). The resulting heterodimers then bind to E-box sequences in DNA to alter gene expression (Carroll et al. 2018). The binding of heterodimers to E-box sequences is a competitive process, and should MAX heterodimerise with MAD transcription

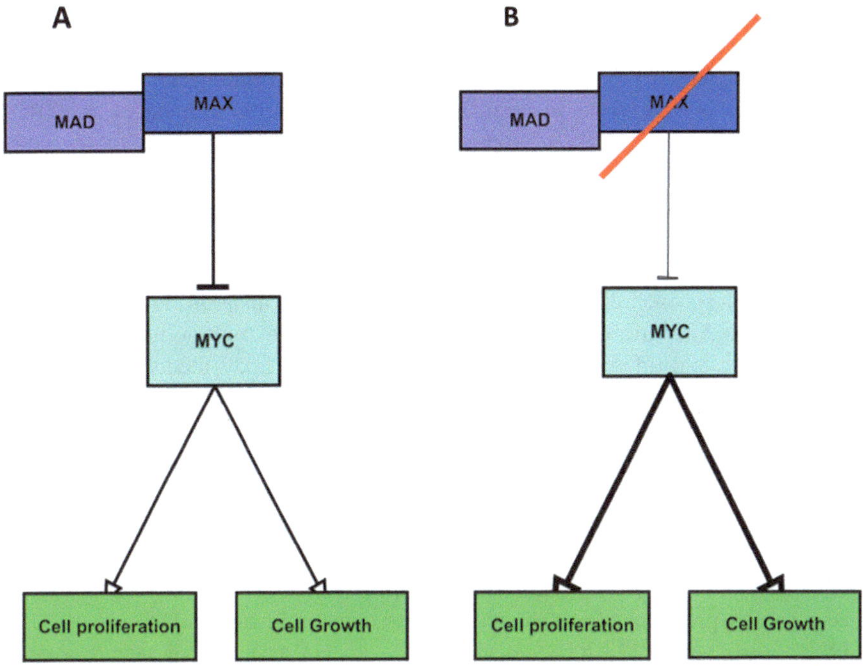

Fig. 10.6 (**a**) Normal heterodimerisation of MAD and MAX resulting in inhibition of MYC with subsequent reduction in cell growth and proliferation. (**b**)Mutation in MAX results in loss of MYC antagonism with subsequent increase in cell growth and proliferation

proteins, the action of the *MYC* oncogene may be antagonised contributing to growth arrest (Dang et al. 1999) (Fig. 10.6), and thus MAX may have a role in tumour suppression.

Germline *MAX* mutations (OMIM ∗154950) have been implicated in renal tumours and small cell lung cancer (Romero et al. 2014), as well as paragangliomas and phaeochromocytomas (Comino-Mendez et al. 2011), while more recently a few cases with large *MAX* deletions were shown to be associated with somatotroph and lactotroph adenomas, including a childhood-onset somatotrophinoma (Daly et al. 2018; Roszko et al. 2017).

10.2.2.6 DICER1

DICER1 syndrome or pleuropulmonary blastoma-familial tumour and dysplasia syndrome occurs secondary to mutations in the *DICER1* gene (OMIM ∗606241) (de Kock et al. 2014) and is inherited in an autosomal dominant manner (Doros et al. 2014; Schultz et al. 2017). *DICER1* is located on 14q32.13, and loss of *Dicer1* is known to result in aberrant growth of the anterior pituitary in a mouse model (Zhang et al. 2010).

MicroRNAs (miRNAs) are non-coding RNAs which post-transcriptionally suppress gene expression (Schultz et al. 2014; Zhang et al. 2010). They have been implicated in pituitary development and pituitary transcription factor 1 expression (which plays a major role in pituitary cell differentiation) (Zhang et al. 2010). DICER1 is an endonuclease of approximately 200 kDa which modifies precursor miRNAs via cleavage to produce mature miRNAs which regulate messenger RNA expression (Krol et al. 2010; Zhang et al. 2010). miRNAs are thought to regulate activity of approximately 50% of protein-coding genes (Krol et al. 2010), and this may explain why *DICER1* mutations may result in such heterogeneous and widespread neoplasia including pleuropulmonary blastoma, ovarian sex cord-stromal tumours, cystic nephroma, thyroid disorders ranging from multinodular goitre, thyroid adenoma and differentiated thyroid cancer, ciliary body medulloepithelioma, botryoid-type embryonal rhabdomyosarcoma of the cervix, nasal chondromesenchymal hamartoma and pineoblastoma (Doros et al. 2014). The different manifestations have different penetrance and typical ages of onsets.

DICER1 mutations are associated with adrenocorticotropic hormone (ACTH)-secreting pituitary blastoma, a rare embryonic tumour first described in 2008 (de Kock et al. 2014; Scheithauer et al. 2008). DICER1-related pituitary disease generally presents before the age of 2 years and presenting features can include III, IV and VI nerve palsies, proptosis, visual disturbance and diabetes insipidus (Doros et al. 2014; Scheithauer et al. 2012, 2008). Lesions may contain a variety of secretory cells, undifferentiated cells and glandular structures and can have high proliferative activity (Scheithauer et al. 2012, 2008). The tumours often show a germline loss-of-function mutation in one allele and a pathogenic somatic variant in another allele (Schultz et al. 2017). Mosaicism for RNase IIIb pathogenic variant is also possible alongside a loss-of-function pathogenic variant to fulfil Knudson's two hits (Schultz et al. 2017). It is thought that this combination of mutations results in a more severe phenotype and can explain "global developmental delay, lung cysts, overgrowth and Wilms tumour" syndrome.

Diagnosis requires identification of heterozygous germline *DICER1* pathogenic variant (Doros et al. 2014). Sequence analysis identifies approximately 65% of probands (Doros et al. 2014), and if sequence analysis is negative, duplication analysis can be considered.

One report exists of a microprolactinoma (6 mm diameter) in a 50-year-old female with a known *DICER1* mutation (Cotton and Ray 2018). This raises the possibility of a causative relationship between *DICER1* mutation and prolactinoma. However, given that DICER1-related pituitary cases are large tumours manifesting before the age of 2 years, there is a significant possibility that this microprolactinoma is not related to the *DICER1* mutation of the patient and represents a phenocopy. No tissue is available for testing for a second hit.

In summary, DICER1 is a novel genetic syndrome which can manifest with pituitary blastoma. The occurrence of *DICER1* mutation and microprolactinoma in a single case likely represents a phenocopy.

10.2.2.7 MSH2

Germline mutations of the mis-match repair gene *MSH2* (OMIM ∗609309) result in Lynch syndrome, a condition predisposing to cancers of multiple organs, particularly the colon. One malignant corticotrophinoma has been reported in association with Lynch syndrome (Table 10.1) (Bengtsson et al. 2017). Examination of the pituitary tumour tissue revealed loss of *MSH2* expression consistent with germline mutation (Bengtsson et al. 2017). A further case of pituitary adenoma alongside glioblastoma multiforme and colorectal polyps has been reported; however, it is unclear whether the pituitary adenoma was as a result of a germline mutation or a phenocopy (Hamilton et al. 1995; Turcot et al. 1959).

10.2.2.8 Neurofibromatosis Type 1 (*NF1*)

Neurofibromatosis is a multisystem genetic disorder inherited in an autosomal dominant manner. While patients with *NF1* mutations (OMIM ∗613113) can have GH excess, this is usually associated with optic gliomas and hypothalamic lesions and not pituitary adenomas (Bizzarri and Bottaro 2015; Hannah-Shmouni et al. 2016; Josefson et al. 2011). Further studies are needed to study the causative relationship between *NF1* mutations and pituitary tumours in the reported cases in the setting of neurofibromatosis (Coire et al. 2010; Hannah-Shmouni et al. 2016; Kurozumi et al. 2002; Smith and Santoreneos 2017).

10.2.2.9 McCune Albright Syndrome (MAS)

MAS is caused by mosaicism for a mutation in *GNAS* (OMIM ∗139320 #174800) (Weinstein et al. 1991). These mutations occur at an early embryonic age resulting in somatic mosaicism of the pituitary gland. The syndrome is characterised by polyostotic fibrous dysplasia, café-au-lait skin lesions and precocious puberty (Horvath and Stratakis 2008; Salpea and Stratakis 2014). Other endocrinopathies include GH excess, gigantism, Cushing's syndrome, thyrotoxicosis and fibroblast growth factor 23 (FGF23)-mediated renal phosphate wasting (Caimari and Korbonits 2016; Horvath and Stratakis 2008; Salpea and Stratakis 2014).

Pathogenic *GNAS* mutations resulting in MAS occur de novo as germline mutations of *GNAS* are incompatible with life (Salpea and Stratakis 2014). MAS develops as a consequence of missense mutations affecting 2 key amino acids, 201 in the majority of the cases [Arg 201 to Cis, His, Ser or Gly (Horvath and Stratakis 2008; Salpea and Stratakis 2014)] or rarely Gln 227 to Arg or Lys (Horvath and Stratakis 2008; Salpea and Stratakis 2014). The equivalent site in other G proteins are known to cause increased function in various other tumour syndromes (O'Hayre et al. 2013). Similarly to *GNAS* mutated sporadic pituitary tumours, relaxation of monoallelic expression is seen in MAS pituitary tumours (Hayward et al. 2001). Patients often have abnormal results on GH axis testing without clear-cut tumour on imaging, with high levels of GH or hyperprolactinaemia in around 21% of patients with MAS (Salpea and Stratakis 2014). Treatment options are limited for these patients, as bone lesions often surround the pituitary fossa, making surgical approach risky and only total anterior hypophysectomy would be curative. There were reports of osteosarcoma in the radiation field of irradiated patients; therefore radiotherapy is advised to be avoided, if possible. Medical therapy with somatostatin analogues and GH receptor antagonists with or without dopamine agonist can often control excess GH and prolactin levels (MAS is discussed in more detail in Chap. 7).

10.3 Somatic Mutations

*10.3.1 GNAS Complex Locus (*GNAS*)*

GNAS [mutated form often referred to as the *gsp* oncogene, (OMIM *139320 #617686)] maps to chromosome 20q13, codes for the ubiquitously expressed stimulatory α subunit of G protein and has been recognised as important in the pathogenesis of somatotrophinomas for almost 30 years (Fig. 10.7) (Spada and Vallar 1992). Heterotrimeric G proteins consist of α, β and γ subunits and are essential for hormonal signalling associated with G-protein-coupled seven transmembrane receptors. Upon ligand binding of the receptor, the G protein binds to the intracellular part of the receptor and then the α subunit dissociates from the β and γ subunits, changes guanosine diphosphate (GDP) binding to guanosine triphosphate (GTP) binding and activates the membrane-bound enzyme adenylyl cyclase. At the same time, it has an intrinsic GTPase activity turning GTP to GDP resulting in dissociation from adenylyl cyclase and termination of the signal (Fig. 10.4). Recurrent mutations in the gene coding for the α subunit *GNAS* at codon 201 and 227 destroy the molecule's GTP hydrolase activity while leaving the adenylyl cyclase activation ability intact. The resulting constitutively active α subunit-adenylyl cyclase complex creates high levels of cAMP (Landis et al. 1989; Lyons et al. 1990; Riminucci et al. 2002; Salpea and Stratakis 2014; Vallar et al. 1987) (Fig. 10.4). Over time, high levels of cAMP result in activation of PKA (Salpea and Stratakis 2014). cAMP may suppress or promote cell proliferation dependent on the cell line in question. The fact that *GNAS* mutations are implicated in somatotroph adenomas suggests that cAMP acts as a somatotroph growth factor (Vitali et al. 2014).

GNAS mutations can contribute to somatotroph adenoma development in a pituitary specific manner, either as a somatic mutation in a pituitary cell resulting in a sporadic somatotrophinomas or as a somatic mutation in embryonic age resulting in mosaicism, as in the case of MAS (Landis et al. 1989; Marques and Korbonits 2017). Mutations of *GNAS* occur in approximately 30–40% of sporadic somatotrophinomas (Hayward et al. 2001; Landis et al. 1989). *GNAS* is normally expressed from the maternal allele (paternally imprinted) in normal pituitary, while relaxation of its monoallelic expression has been found in both *GNAS* mutation

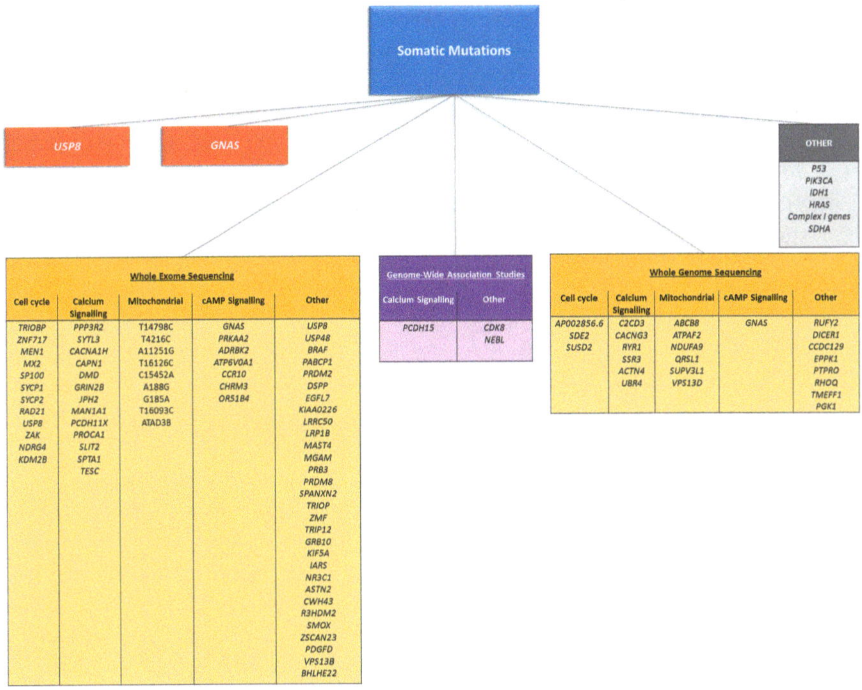

Fig. 10.7 Somatic mutations implicated in pituitary tumourigenesis. While *GNAS* and *USP8* mutations are well established (red boxes), the role of some of the other genes needs further studies and confirmation. Selected gene variants identified in whole-exome sequencing studies (WES) (Bi et al. 2017; Chen et al. 2018; Lan et al. 2016; Newey et al. 2013b; Ronchi et al. 2016; Salomon et al. 2018; Sapkota et al. 2017; Song et al. 2016), genome-wide association studies (GWAS) (Ye et al. 2015) and next-generation sequencing (Nemeth et al. 2019; Valimaki et al. 2015) are listed with reference to possible roles in cell cycle, calcium signalling, cAMP signalling and mitochondrial variants. Other genes implicated in pituitary tumourigenesis via case reports, smaller studies and directed gene studies are listed in the grey box. Many of these genes require further confirmation

negative and positive somatotrophinomas; in *GNAS* mutation-positive adenomas, the mutation is primarily on the maternal allele (Hayward et al. 2001). The *GNAS* locus is complex: this gene also codes for the 55 kDa neuroendocrine secretory protein 55 (NESP55) and extra-large α_s (XLαs) (Hayward et al. 2001); interestingly, imprinting of these other gene products is maintained in somatotrophinomas, suggesting a specific regulatory mechanism for the different transcript of this gene in somatotrophinoma tumourigenesis. The possibility of additional tumourigenic pathways in somatotrophinomas is also supported by the finding that *GNAS* mutation-positive tumours are associated with low copy number alterations, while *GNAS* mutation-negative sporadic somatotroph adenomas are highly heterogeneous and have higher copy number alterations (Hage et al. 2018).

A number of studies have suggested certain clinical parameters linked to *GNAS* mutation-positive tumours, such as older age of onset, smaller tumours (Buchfelder et al. 1999; Larkin et al. 2013; Spada et al. 1990), less-invasive tumours (Buchfelder et al. 1999; Song et al. 2016), higher GH levels (Buchfelder et al. 1999; Larkin et al. 2013) and better response to somatostatin analogues (Buchfelder et al. 1999; Larkin et al. 2013; Song et al. 2016), but results from other studies are variable (Adams et al. 1993, 1995; Harris et al. 1992; Taboada et al. 2009). A recent meta-analysis, based on 8 studies and 310 patients with acromegaly, found that GH response to an acute octreotide suppression test is 9% better in *GNAS* mutation-positive samples compared to negative samples (Efstathiadou et al. 2015).

10.3.2 Ubiquitin Specific Peptidase 8 (USP8)

Corticotroph adenomas are usually sporadic and have rarely been found to occur in the setting of familial syndromes (Albani et al. 2018a; Daniel and Newell-Price 2017). Recently, recurrent somatic mutations have been identified in a significant proportion of corticotroph adenomas affecting the gene *USP8* (OMIM *603158 #219090) (Fig. 10.7) (Ma et al. 2015; Reincke et al. 2015). Mutations of *USP8* result in cleavage of USP8 into a shorter, more active form which ultimately augments epidermal growth factor receptor (EGFR) signalling (Albani et al. 2018a) (Fig. 10.8). Increases in EGFR signalling increase proopiomelanocortin (POMC, the precursor polypeptide of ACTH) transcription and thus increase circulating ACTH (Ballmann et al. 2018). *USP8* mutations are localised to a hotspot region in exon 14 which binds the 14-3-3 family proteins (Albani et al. 2018b). Mutations at this binding site account for approximately 35–62% of Cushing's disease cases (Ma et al. 2015; Reincke et al. 2015), with *USP8* mutations accounting for 20–100% of females and 0–38% of males with corticotroph adenomas (Hayashi et al. 2016; Losa et al. 2018; Ma et al. 2015; Perez-Rivas et al. 2015; Reincke et al. 2015). In paediatric populations *USP8* mutations are implicated in 17.2–31% of corticotrophinomas with a female-to-male ratio 1.8:1 ($n = 42$) (Faucz et al. 2017; Perez-Rivas et al. 2015).

USP8-mutated tumours have higher levels of transcription of *POMC*; however, data on EGFR expression in *USP8*-mutated corticotrophinomas has been conflicting (Hayashi et al. 2016; Ma et al. 2015). One study demonstrated higher levels of EGFR expression in *USP8* mutant tumours (Ma et al. 2015), while another did not find any relationship between EGFR expression and *USP8* mutational status (Hayashi et al. 2016).

A single centre study suggested that *USP8* mutation-positive corticotrophinomas are more likely to achieve surgical remission (defined as requiring postoperative glucocorticoid replacement therapy, normalisation of urinary cortisol levels and suppression of serum cortisol below 18 ng/mL after an overnight low-dose dexamethasone test 5–6 days after surgery) (Losa et al. 2018). Despite this early positive

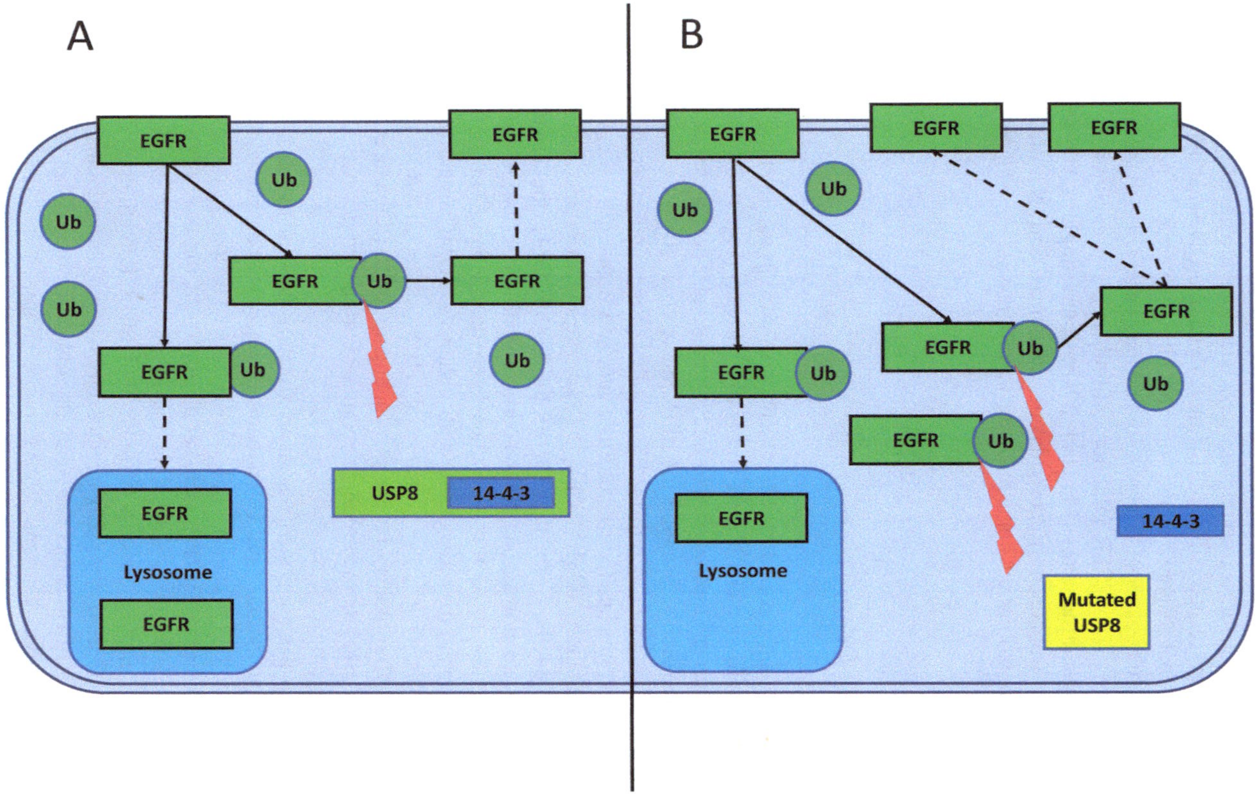

Fig. 10.8 (**a**) Normal deubiquitination and targeting of EGFR for lysosomal degradation. Following internalisation and ubiquitination of EGFR, a proportion of EGFR molecules is deubiquinated by USP8 and recycled to the cell surface. 14-3-3 can bind a specific segment of USP8 which hinders cleavage of USP8 to its activated form. (**b**) Mutations in *USP8* cluster at the 14-3-3 binding site. This results in an inability to bind to 14-3-3 and therefore USP8 can be cleaved to a more active component. This increases deubiquitination of EGFR and recycling to the cell surface with increased EGFR signalling and subsequent ACTH excess

effect on outcome, in the longer term, *USP8* mutations do not seem to exert any effect on 5-year recurrence-free survival (Losa et al. 2018).

USP8 mutations may have implications for sensitivity to medical treatment. *USP8* mutation-positive corticotrophinomas have been found to have higher expression of somatostatin receptor 5 and O^6-methylguanine-DNA-methytransferase (MGMT), meaning that response to the somatostatin receptor 5 ligand pasireotide may be enhanced, while response to temozolomide may be lessened in these tumours (Hayashi et al. 2016). The EGFR inhibitor gefitinib is being explored as a novel therapy for *USP8* mutant tumours (Ma et al. 2015). Interestingly, *USP8* mutations occur at a similar frequency in corticotroph adenomas and Nelson tumours, suggesting these mutations do not contribute to progression to Nelson tumours (Perez-Rivas et al. 2018).

10.3.3 Other Relevant Genes

USP48 (ubiquitin-specific peptidase 48) (OMIM ∗617445) mutations have recently been reported in approximately 27% of corticotrophinomas (Fig. 10.7) (Chen et al. 2018) with similar disease mechanisms to *USP8* mutations. These were not reported in the studies with exome sequencing for 10 (Reincke et al. 2015) or 12 (Ma et al. 2015) corticotroph adenomas. Confirmation by other groups and experimental data are needed to fully appreciate the role of these genetic variants.

While *BRAF* mutations (OMIM ∗164757) are present in craniopharyngiomas (Brastianos et al. 2014; La Corte et al. 2018), the V600E *BRAF* mutation was not found in 37 pituitary adenomas, including 3 corticotrophinomas (Ewing et al. 2007). However, more recently, *BRAF* mutations have been identified in 15 out of 91 *USP8* wild-type corticotrophinomas associated with enhanced POMC transcription and ACTH overproduction (Fig. 10.7) (Chen et al. 2018), although *BRAF* mutations were not reported in the studies with exome sequencing for 10 (Reincke et al. 2015) or 12 (Ma et al. 2015) corticotroph adenomas. Further studies are needed to corroborate these findings.

Gasperre's group has suggested that approximately 60% of the relatively rare oncocytic pituitary adenomas [null cell adenomas, oncocytomas, pituicytomas and spindle cell oncocytomas (Canberk et al. 2014)] have mutations in components of respiratory complex I (Fig. 10.7) (Kurelac et al. 2013). As these result in hypoxia-inducible factor 1-α (HIF1α) destabilisation, this might contribute to the less aggressive phenotype seen in these tumours (Kurelac et al. 2013; Porcelli et al. 2010).

HRAS mutations (OMIM ∗190020) are uncommon in pituitary tumours (Cai et al. 1994) and are more often associated with thyroid carcinoma. They have been implicated in aggressive recurrent prolactinomas (Karga et al. 1992), pituitary spindle cell oncocytoma (Miller et al. 2016) and pituitary carcinoma metastases (Fig. 10.7) (Pei et al. 1994). Although *HRAS* mutations were found in pituitary carcinoma metastases, they were not found in their respective primary lesions (Pei et al. 1994), suggesting this being a late event in tumourigenesis and appears to be indicative of poor prognosis (Sav et al. 2016).

Somatic mutations of the *P53* tumour suppressor gene (OMIM *191170) are uncommon in pituitary tumourigenesis despite P53 immunostaining being regularly reported in pituitary tumour histopathology and is now part of the Trouillas classification (Fig. 10.7) (Trouillas et al. 2013). Somatic *P53* mutations are associated with aggressive pituitary tumours (Kawashima et al. 2009) and 33% of pituitary carcinoma (Tanizaki et al. 2007). They have also been reported as post-radiotherapy phenomena for aggressive pituitary tumours (Pinto et al. 2011). Numbers in these studies are small and so, much like *HRAS*, few conclusions can be drawn with regard to the role of *P53* mutations in pituitary tumourigenesis. A recent study examined the role of a relatively common *P53* single-nucleotide polymorphism rs1042522 with a minor allele frequency of 0.33 (Yagnik et al. 2017). In a group of 42 NFPA patients, they found that carriers of the minor allele (either heterozygous or homozygous) present a decade earlier and have more cavernous sinus invasion. In vitro studies suggest that reduced p21 (cyclin-dependent kinase inhibitor 1A, CDKN1A) expression could be responsible for these effects.

Phosphatidylinositol-4,5-bisphosphate 3-kinase catalytic subunit alpha (*PIK3CA*, OMIM *171834) codes for the p110α catalytic subunit of PI3K, a component of the PI3K/AKT signalling pathway (Shaid and Korbonits 2017). PI3Ks play a role in cell proliferation, adhesion, survival and motility, and *PIK3CA* mutations have been implicated in a range of different cancers (Samuels et al. 2004). Genomic amplifications of *PIK3CA* were found to occur in 20–40% of all pituitary tumour types, and somatic mutations of exons 9 and 20 occur in 9% of invasive adenomas versus 0% of non-invasive lesions (Fig. 10.7) (Lin et al. 2009). Despite this finding, a genotype-phenotype relationship has not been confirmed as a *PIK3CA* variant has been found in a non-invasive microadenoma (Murat et al. 2012). Interestingly, approximately 8.8% of patients with Cowden syndrome harbour *PIK3CA* mutations, but pituitary tumours are *not* associated with this condition (Orloff et al. 2013). Furthermore, none of the exome/whole-genome sequencing studies performed to date have verified the *PIK3CA* data (Lan et al. 2016; Nemeth et al. 2019; Newey et al. 2013b; Ronchi et al. 2016; Sav et al. 2016; Song et al. 2016; Valimaki et al. 2015; Ye et al. 2015), and thus the role of these variants in pituitary tumourigenesis is far from certain.

Pituitary adenomas have been reported in association with Maffucci syndrome, a disease occurring as a result of somatic mosaicism of *IDH1* (OMIM *147700) (Fig. 10.7) or *IDH2* (OMIM *147650) mutations (Hao et al. 2016). Patients classically develop enchondromas and haemangiomas (Hao et al. 2016). Pituitary adenoma has been reported in multiple cases of Maffucci Syndrome (Ono et al. 2012; Ruivo and Antunes 2009), and in some cases *IDH1* mutation has been confirmed in pituitary tumour tissue (Hao et al. 2016; Nejo et al. 2018).

Double-hit inactivating somatic *SDHA* (OMIM *600857) mutations in the absence of germline *SDH* mutations have been described in a macroprolactinoma (Gill et al. 2014). However, numerous other studies performing exome or whole-genome sequencing on pituitary tissue have failed to identify somatic *SDH* mutations (Fig. 10.7) (Bi et al. 2017; Newey et al. 2013b; Sapkota et al. 2017; Song et al. 2016;

Valimaki et al. 2015; Ye et al. 2015), which suggests that these two somatic *SDHA* mutations were non-pathogenic or that this combination of mutations is an exceedingly rare occurrence in pituitary adenoma pathogenesis.

10.3.4 Regulatory RNAs in Pituitary Adenomas

Multiple RNA subtypes have been investigated in the pathogenesis of pituitary tumours with some interesting results.

MicroRNAs (*miRNAs*) are short (19–23 nucleotides) non-coding RNAs which can regulate gene expression and protein synthesis (Li et al. 2014). Interestingly, *DICER1*, one of the key miRNA synthesis regulators, is involved in the development of pituitary blastomas (see separate section for detailed discussion). miRNAs were first studied in pituitary tissue in 2005 (Bottoni et al. 2005). miRNAs generally interact with mRNA to induce degradation of the mRNA or suppress translation of a protein (Wierinckx et al. 2017; Zhang et al. 2017b), and they may act as tumour suppressors or tumour inducers depending on their target. miRNAs have been studied in most types of pituitary adenomas: prolactinomas (Bottoni et al. 2005; Wang et al. 2012), corticotrophinomas (Amaral et al. 2009; Garbicz et al. 2017; Gentilin et al. 2013), NFPA (Butz et al. 2010, 2017; Cheunsuchon et al. 2011; Darvasi et al. 2019; Leone et al. 2014; Song et al. 2018), somatotrophinomas (Butz et al. 2010; D'Angelo et al. 2012; Lee et al. 2017; Leone et al. 2014; Mao et al. 2010; Palumbo et al. 2013; Trivellin et al. 2012) and gonadotroph adenomas (Hou et al. 2018; Leone et al. 2014; Mussnich et al. 2015).

To date much research has centred around miRNAs as predictors of tumour invasiveness and outcomes. There is evidence that miR-15a and miR-16-1 are inversely correlated with somatotrophinoma and prolactinoma size (Bottoni et al. 2005), but not for corticotrophinomas (Amaral et al. 2009). Some miRNAs, such as miRNA-137, miRNA-374a-5p and miRNA-374b-5p, are inversely correlated with NFPA invasiveness (Song et al. 2018); likewise miR-132, miR-15a and miR-16 are inversely correlated with proliferation, invasiveness and migration in pituitary cell lines (Lu et al. 2018; Renjie and Haiqian 2015), while higher levels of miR-16 also correlate with 5-year survival in pituitary tumours (Lu et al. 2018). miR-24, miR-93, miR-34a and miR-126 were significantly under-expressed in invasive pituitary tumours versus non-invasive adenomas (Yu et al. 2017). In a group of 22 macroadenomas and 48 microadenomas of varying cell types, miR-26 was significantly correlated with invasiveness, and this was thought to be via inhibition of *PLAG1* expression (Yu et al. 2016).

Higher levels of the miRNA-106b-5p cluster and its host gene *MCM7* were significantly associated with invasiveness and unfavourable surgical outcome in a cohort of 25 corticotrophinomas (Garbicz et al. 2017). These markers were also markedly upregulated in a sub-group of 5 Crooke's cell adenomas when compared to invasive and non-invasive adenomas in this study (Garbicz et al. 2017). In NFPA, miR-106 was upregulated in metastases of a non-functioning pituitary carcinoma and in 6 atypical NFPA versus 8 typical NFPA as defined by the 2004 World Health Organization classification of pituitary tumours (Zhou et al. 2016). There is evidence miR-106 may promote this invasion and proliferation by targeting phosphatase and tensin homolog (PTEN) through the PI3K/AKT signalling pathway in NFPA (Zhou et al. 2016). There is also evidence of disruption of the PTEN/PI3K/AKT pathway by miR-26b and miR-128 in somatotrophinomas (Palumbo et al. 2013).

More recently, another class of RNA has been studied in pituitary adenoma (Guo et al. 2019; Wang et al. 2018). These *circular RNAs* (*circRNAs*) are a type of RNA in which the 3′ and 5′ ends are joined together, and it is thought that in general their role is to act as a 'sponge' (competitive inhibitor) miRNA (Wang et al. 2018). In a cohort of 10 non-invasive NFPA and 65 invasive NFPA, 154 circRNAs were found to be upregulated and 416 downregulated. Interestingly, this study also examined nine cases of recurrent NFPA, comparing circRNA in tissue before and after recurrence. Ten circRNAs were identified in recurrent tissue which may suggest roles in recurrence (Wang et al. 2018). Similarly, a further 2 circRNAs (hsa_circ_0000066 and hsa_circ_0069707) were found to be significantly associated with progression-free survival in 73 NFPA and may have utility in predicting recurrence (Guo et al. 2019).

Long non-coding RNAs (*lncRNAs*) are longer than 200 nucleotides (Gibb et al. 2011) regulating gene expression via multiple mechanisms including chromatin interactions, histone modification, splicing, transcriptional regulation in the nucleus and interactions with other RNA subtypes within the cytoplasm (Kondo et al. 2017). Recently, a genome-wide expression study identified differential expression of 113 lncRNAs [10 confirmed by real-time quantitative reverse transcription polymerase chain reaction (qRT-PCR)] and 80 mRNAs in NFPAs (Xing et al. 2019). While the function of many of these 113 lncRNAs is unknown, *MEG3* (implicated in other non-pituitary neoplasia) and *ENST00000501583* (associated with hepatocellular carcinoma) were downregulated by 2.5-fold and greater than 4-fold, respectively (Xing et al. 2019). This suggests that these particular lncRNAs may have tumour suppressor roles within the pituitary. These novel findings in pituitary tumourigenesis will no doubt be further explored in the near future.

10.4 Conclusions

There has been a significant change over the last 20 years of our understanding of the genetic background of many tumours, including pituitary tumours. Recurring somatic mutations explain a significant proportion of somatotroph and corticotroph tumours, and germline mutations have been discovered in several isolated or syndromic cases of pituitary tumours. Regulation of gene expression with ever-increasing different molecular mechanisms is likely to play a key role in the majority of the tumours where no DNA alterations can be found. These advances could lead to genetic screening of family members resulting in earlier detection and to novel, personalised genomic medical techniques to optimise management of pituitary tumours.

References

Abbastabar M, Kheyrollah M, Azizian K et al (2018) Multiple functions of p27 in cell cycle, apoptosis, epigenetic modification and transcriptional regulation for the control of cell growth: a double-edged sword protein. DNA Repair (Amst) 69:63–72. https://doi.org/10.1016/j.dnarep.2018.07.008

Adams EF, Brockmeier S, Friedmann E, Roth M, Buchfelder M, Fahlbusch R (1993) Clinical and biochemical characteristics of acromegalic patients harboring gsp-positive and gsp-negative pituitary tumors. Neurosurgery 33:198–203

Adams EF, Lei T, Buchfelder M, Petersen B, Fahlbusch R (1995) Biochemical characteristics of human pituitary somatotropinomas with and without gsp mutations: in vitro cell culture studies. J Clin Endocrinol Metab 80:2077–2081. https://doi.org/10.1210/jcem.80.7.7608258

Aflorei ED, Korbonits M (2014) Epidemiology and etiopathogenesis of pituitary adenomas. J Neuro-Oncol 117:379–394. https://doi.org/10.1007/s11060-013-1354-5

Aflorei ED, Klapholz B, Chen C et al (2018) In vivo bioassay to test the pathogenicity of missense human AIP variants. J Med Genet 55:522–529. https://doi.org/10.1136/jmedgenet-2017-105191

Agarwal SK (2017) The future: genetics advances in MEN1 therapeutic approaches and management strategies. Endocr Relat Cancer 24:T119–t134. https://doi.org/10.1530/erc-17-0199

Agarwal SK, Ozawa A, Mateo CM, Marx SJ (2009) The MEN1 gene and pituitary tumours. Horm Res 71(Suppl 2):131–138. https://doi.org/10.1159/000192450

Agustsson TT, Baldvinsdottir T, Jonasson JG et al (2015) The epidemiology of pituitary adenomas in Iceland, 1955–2012: a nationwide population-based study. Eur J Endocrinol 173:655–664. https://doi.org/10.1530/eje-15-0189

Albani A, Perez-Rivas LG, Reincke M, Theodoropoulou M (2018a) Pathogenesis of Cushing disease: an update on the genetics of corticotropinomas. Endocr Pract 24:907–914. https://doi.org/10.4158/EP-2018-0111

Albani A, Theodoropoulou M, Reincke M (2018b) Genetics of Cushing's disease. Clin Endocrinol 88:3–12. https://doi.org/10.1111/cen.13457

Alrezk R, Hannah-Shmouni F, Stratakis CA (2017) MEN4 and CDKN1B mutations: the latest of the MEN syndromes. Endocr Relat Cancer 24:T195–t208. https://doi.org/10.1530/erc-17-0243

Amaral FC, Torres N, Saggioro F et al (2009) MicroRNAs differentially expressed in ACTH-secreting pituitary tumors. J Clin Endocrinol Metab 94:320–323. https://doi.org/10.1210/jc.2008-1451

Bai F, Pei XH, Nishikawa T, Smith MD, Xiong Y (2007) p18Ink4c, but not p27Kip1, collaborates with Men1 to suppress neuroendocrine organ tumors. Mol Cell Biol 27:1495–1504. https://doi.org/10.1128/mcb.01764-06

Ballmann C, Thiel A, Korah HE et al (2018) USP8 mutations in pituitary Cushing adenomas-targeted analysis by next-generation sequencing. J Endocr Soc 2:266–278. https://doi.org/10.1210/js.2017-00364

Beckers A, Betea D, Valdes Socin H, Stevenaert A (2003) The treatment of sporadic versus MEN1-related pituitary adenomas. J Intern Med 253:599–605

Beckers A, Aaltonen LA, Daly AF, Karhu A (2013) Familial isolated pituitary adenomas (FIPA) and the pituitary adenoma predisposition due to mutations in the aryl hydrocarbon receptor interacting protein (AIP) gene. Endocr Rev 34:239–277. https://doi.org/10.1210/er.2012-1013

Beckers A, Lodish MB, Trivellin G et al (2015) X-linked acrogigantism syndrome: clinical profile and therapeutic responses. Endocr Relat Cancer 22:353–367. https://doi.org/10.1530/erc-15-0038

Bengtsson D, Joost P, Aravidis C et al (2017) Corticotroph pituitary carcinoma in a patient with lynch syndrome (LS) and pituitary tumors in a Nationwide LS cohort. J Clin Endocrinol Metab 102:3928–3932. https://doi.org/10.1210/jc.2017-01401

Bernard V, Bouilly J, Beau I, Broutin I, Chanson P, Young J, Binart N (2016) Germline prolactin receptor mutation is not a major cause of sporadic prolactinoma in humans. Neuroendocrinology 103:738–745. https://doi.org/10.1159/000442981

Bertherat J, Horvath A, Groussin L et al (2009) Mutations in regulatory subunit type 1A of cyclic adenosine 5′-monophosphate-dependent protein kinase (PRKAR1A): phenotype analysis in 353 patients and 80 different genotypes. J Clin Endocrinol Metab 94:2085–2091. https://doi.org/10.1210/jc.2008-2333

Bi WL, Horowitz P, Greenwald NF et al (2017) Landscape of genomic alterations in pituitaryadenomas. Clin Cancer Res 23:1841–1851. https://doi.org/10.1158/1078-0432.Ccr-16-0790

Bizzarri C, Bottaro G (2015) Endocrine implications of neurofibromatosis 1 in childhood. Horm Res Paediatr 83:232–241. https://doi.org/10.1159/000369802

Bizzi MF, Pinheiro SVB, Bolger GB et al (2018) Reduced protein expression of the phosphodiesterases PDE4A4 and PDE4A8 in AIP mutation positive somatotroph adenomas. Mol Cell Endocrinol 476:103–109. https://doi.org/10.1016/j.mce.2018.04.014

Blyth M, Huang S, Maloney V, Crolla JA, Karen Temple I (2008) A 2.3Mb deletion of 17q24.2-q24.3 associated with 'Carney Complex plus'. Eur J Med Genet 51:672–678. https://doi.org/10.1016/j.ejmg.2008.09.002

Boikos SA, Stratakis CA (2006) Carney complex: pathology and molecular genetics. Neuroendocrinology 83:189–199. https://doi.org/10.1159/000095527

Bolger GB, Peden AH, Steele MR et al (2003) Attenuation of the activity of the cAMP-specific phosphodiesterase PDE4A5 by interaction with the immunophilin XAP2. J Biol Chem 278:33351–33363. https://doi.org/10.1074/jbc.M303269200

Bolger GB, Bizzi MF, Pinheiro SV et al (2016) cAMP-specific PDE4 phosphodiesterases and AIP in the pathogenesis of pituitary tumors. Endocr Relat Cancer 23:419–431. https://doi.org/10.1530/erc-15-0205

Bottoni A, Piccin D, Tagliati F, Luchin A, Zatelli MC, degli Uberti EC (2005) miR-15a and miR-16-1 down-regulation in pituitary adenomas. J Cell Physiol 204:280–285. https://doi.org/10.1002/jcp.20282

Brastianos PK, Taylor-Weiner A, Manley PE et al (2014) Exome sequencing identifies BRAF mutations in papillary craniopharyngiomas. Nat Genet 46:161–165. https://doi.org/10.1038/ng.2868

Buchfelder M, Fahlbusch R, Merz T, Symowski H, Adams EF (1999) Clinical correlates in acromegalic patients with pituitary tumors expressing GSP oncogenes. Pituitary 1:181–185

Butz H, Likó I, Czirják S et al (2010) Down-regulation of Wee1 kinase by a specific subset of microRNA in human sporadic pituitary adenomas. J Clin Endocrinol Metab 95:E181–E191. https://doi.org/10.1210/jc.2010-0581

Butz H, Németh K, Czenke D et al (2017) Systematic investigation of expression of G2/M transition genes reveals CDC25 alteration in nonfunctioning pituitary adenomas. Pathol Oncol Res 23:633–641. https://doi.org/10.1007/s12253-016-0163-5

Cai WY, Alexander JM, Hedley-Whyte ET, Scheithauer BW, Jameson JL, Zervas NT, Klibanski A (1994) Ras mutations in human prolactinomas and pituitary carcinomas. J Clin Endocrinol Metab 78:89–93. https://doi.org/10.1210/jcem.78.1.8288721

Caimari F, Korbonits M (2016) Novel genetic causes of pituitary adenomas. Clin Cancer Res 22:5030–5042. https://doi.org/10.1158/1078-0432.Ccr-16-0452

Caimari F, Hernández-Ramírez LC, Dang MN et al (2018) Risk category system to identify pituitary adenoma patients with AIP mutations. J Med Genet 55:254–260. https://doi.org/10.1136/jmedgenet-2017-104957

Canberk S, LiVolsi VA, Baloch Z (2014) Oncocytic lesions of the neuroendocrine system. Adv Anat Pathol 21:69–82. https://doi.org/10.1097/pap.0000000000000011

Cannavo S, Ferraù F, Ragonese M et al (2010) Increased prevalence of acromegaly in a highly polluted area. Eur J Endocrinol 163:509–513. https://doi.org/10.1530/EJE-10-0465

Cannavo S, Ferrau F, Ragonese M et al (2014) Increased frequency of the rs2066853 variant of aryl hydrocarbon receptor gene in patients with acromegaly. Clin Endocrinol 81:249–253. https://doi.org/10.1111/cen.12424
Cannavo S, Ragonese M, Puglisi S et al (2016) Acromegaly is more severe in patients with AHR or AIP gene variants living in highly polluted areas. J Clin Endocrinol Metab 101:1872–1879. https://doi.org/10.1210/jc.2015-4191
Carney JA, Gordon H, Carpenter PC, Shenoy BV, Go VL (1985) The complex of myxomas, spotty pigmentation, and endocrine overactivity. Medicine (Baltimore) 64:270–283
Carroll PA, Freie BW, Mathsyaraja H, Eisenman RN (2018) The MYC transcription factor network: balancing metabolism, proliferation and oncogenesis. Front Med 12:412–425. https://doi.org/10.1007/s11684-018-0650-z
Castinetti F, Daly AF, Stratakis CA et al (2016) GPR101 mutations are not a frequent cause of congenital isolated growth hormone deficiency. Horm Metab Res 48:389–393. https://doi.org/10.1055/s-0042-100733
Cazabat L, Guillaud-Bataille M, Bertherat J, Raffin-Sanson ML (2009) Mutations of the gene for the aryl hydrocarbon receptor-interacting protein in pituitary adenomas. Horm Res 71:132–141. https://doi.org/10.1159/000197869
Chahal HS, Chapple JP, Frohman LA, Grossman AB, Korbonits M (2010) Clinical, genetic and molecular characterization of patients with familial isolated pituitary adenomas (FIPA). Trends Endocrinol Metab 21:419–427. https://doi.org/10.1016/j.tem.2010.02.007
Chahal HS, Stals K, Unterländer M et al (2011) AIP mutation in pituitary adenomas in the 18th century and today. N Engl J Med 364:43–50. https://doi.org/10.1056/NEJMoa1008020
Chahal HS, Trivellin G, Leontiou CA et al (2012) Somatostatin analogs modulate AIP in somatotroph adenomas: the role of the ZAC1 pathway. J Clin Endocrinol Metab 97:E1411–E1420. https://doi.org/10.1210/jc.2012-1111
Chen J, Jian X, Deng S et al (2018) Identification of recurrent USP48 and BRAF mutations in Cushing's disease. Nat Commun 9:3171. https://doi.org/10.1038/s41467-018-05275-5
Cheunsuchon P, Zhou Y, Zhang X et al (2011) Silencing of the imprinted DLK1-MEG3 locus in human clinically nonfunctioning pituitary adenomas. Am J Pathol 179:2120–2130. https://doi.org/10.1016/j.ajpath.2011.07.002
Coire CI, Smyth HS, Rosso D, Horvath E, Kovacs K (2010) A double pituitary adenoma presenting as a prolactin-secreting tumor with partial response to medical therapy. Case report. Endocr Pathol 21:135–138. https://doi.org/10.1007/s12022-009-9104-0
Comino-Mendez I, Gracia-Aznárez FJ, Schiavi F et al (2011) Exome sequencing identifies MAX mutations as a cause of hereditary pheochromocytoma. Nat Genet 43:663–667. https://doi.org/10.1038/ng.861
Correa R, Salpea P, Stratakis CA (2015) Carney complex: an update. Eur J Endocrinol 173:M85–M97. https://doi.org/10.1530/eje-15-0209
Costa MM, Korbonits M (2017) Genetic causes of familial pituitary tumors. In: Reference module in biomedical sciences. Elsevier. https://doi.org/10.1016/B978-0-12-801238-3.64199-5
Cotton E, Ray D (2018) DICER1 mutation and pituitary prolactinoma. Endocrinol Diabetes Metab Case Rep 2018:18-0087. https://doi.org/10.1530/edm-18-0087
Cuny T, Pertuit M, Sahnoun-Fathallah M et al (2013) Genetic analysis in young patients with sporadic pituitary macroadenomas: besides AIP don't forget MEN1 genetic analysis. Eur J Endocrinol 168:533–541. https://doi.org/10.1530/eje-12-0763
D'Angelo D, Palmieri D, Mussnich P et al (2012) Altered microRNA expression profile in human pituitary GH adenomas: down-regulation of miRNA targeting HMGA1, HMGA2, and E2F1. J Clin Endocrinol Metab 97:E1128–E1138. https://doi.org/10.1210/jc.2011-3482
Daly AF, Jaffrain-Rea ML, Ciccarelli A et al (2006a) Clinical characterization of familial isolated pituitary adenomas. J Clin Endocrinol Metab 91:3316–3323. https://doi.org/10.1210/jc.2005-2671

Daly AF, Rixhon M, Adam C, Dempegioti A, Tichomirowa MA, Beckers A (2006b) High prevalence of pituitary adenomas: a cross-sectional study in the province of Liege, Belgium. J Clin Endocrinol Metab 91:4769–4775. https://doi.org/10.1210/jc.2006-1668

Daly AF, Vanbellinghen JF, Khoo SK et al (2007) Aryl hydrocarbon receptor-interacting protein gene mutations in familial isolated pituitary adenomas: analysis in 73 families. J Clin Endocrinol Metab 92:1891–1896

Daly AF, Tichomirowa MA, Petrossians P et al (2010) Clinical characteristics and therapeutic responses in patients with germ-line AIP mutations and pituitary adenomas: an international collaborative study. J Clin Endocrinol Metab 95:E373–E383. https://doi.org/10.1210/jc.2009-2556

Daly AF, Yuan B, Fina F et al (2016) Somatic mosaicism underlies X-linked acrogigantism syndrome in sporadic male subjects. Endocr Relat Cancer 23:221–233. https://doi.org/10.1530/ERC-16-0082

Daly AF, Castermans E, Oudijk L et al (2018) Pheochromocytomas and pituitary adenomas in three patients with MAX exon deletions. Endocr Relat Cancer 25:L37–l42. https://doi.org/10.1530/erc-18-0065

Dang CV, Resar LM, Emison E et al (1999) Function of the c-Myc oncogenic transcription factor. Exp Cell Res 253:63–77. https://doi.org/10.1006/excr.1999.4686

Daniel E, Newell-Price J (2017) Recent advances in understanding Cushing disease: resistance to glucocorticoid negative feedback and somatic USP8 mutations. F1000Res 6:613. https://doi.org/10.12688/f1000research.10968.1

Darvasi O, Szabo PM, Nemeth K et al (2019) Limitations of high throughput methods for miRNA expression profiles in non-functioning pituitary adenomas. Pathol Oncol Res 25:169–182. https://doi.org/10.1007/s12253-017-0330-3

Dutta P, Reddy KS, Rai A, Madugundu AK, Solanki HS, Bhansali A, Radotra BD, Kumar N, Collier D, Iacovazzo D, Gupta P, Raja R, Gowda H, Pandey A, Devgun JS, Korbonits M (2019) Surgery, octreotide, temozolomide, bevacizumab, radiotherapy, and pegvisomant treatment of an AIP mutation-positive child. J Clin Endocrinol Metab 104:3539–3544

de Kock L, Sabbaghian N, Plourde F et al (2014) Pituitary blastoma: a pathognomonic feature of germ-line DICER1 mutations. Acta Neuropathol 128:111–122. https://doi.org/10.1007/s00401-014-1285-z

de Laat JM, Dekkers OM, Pieterman CR et al (2015) Long-term natural course of pituitary tumors in patients with MEN1: results from the DutchMEN1 study group (DMSG). J Clin Endocrinol Metab 100:3288–3296. https://doi.org/10.1210/jc.2015-2015

De Sousa SM, McCabe MJ, Wu K et al (2017) Germline variants in familial pituitary tumour syndrome genes are common in young patients and families with additional endocrine tumours. Eur J Endocrinol 176:635–644. https://doi.org/10.1530/EJE-16-0944

Denes J, Swords F, Rattenberry E et al (2015) Heterogeneous genetic background of the association of pheochromocytoma/paraganglioma and pituitary adenoma: results from a large patient cohort. J Clin Endocrinol Metab 100:E531–E541. https://doi.org/10.1210/jc.2014-3399

Doros L, Schultz KA, Stewart DR et al (2014) DICER1-related disorders. In: Adam MP, Ardinger HH, Pagon RA, Wallace SE, LJH B, Stephens K, Amemiya A (eds) GeneReviews((R)). University of Washington, Seattle, WA

Efstathiadou ZA, Bargiota A, Chrisoulidou A et al (2015) Impact of gsp mutations in somatotroph pituitary adenomas on growth hormone response to somatostatin analogs: a meta-analysis. Pituitary 18:861–867. https://doi.org/10.1007/s11102-015-0662-5

Eisenhofer G, Pacak K, Maher ER, Young WF, de Krijger RR (2013) Pheochromocytoma. Clin Chem 59:466–472. https://doi.org/10.1373/clinchem.2012.182246

Erdheim J (1903) Zur normalen und pathologischen Histologie der Glandula thyreoidea, parathyreoidea und Hypophysis. Beitr Pathol Anat 33:158–236

Ewing I, Pedder-Smith S, Franchi G et al (2007) A mutation and expression analysis of the oncogene BRAF in pituitary adenomas. Clin Endocrinol 66:348–352. https://doi.org/10.1111/j.1365-2265.2006.02735.x

Ezzat S, Asa SL, Couldwell WT, Barr CE, Dodge WE, Vance ML, McCutcheon IE (2004) The prevalence of pituitary adenomas: a systematic review. Cancer 101:613–619. https://doi.org/10.1002/cncr.20412
Faucz FR, Tirosh A, Tatsi C et al (2017) Somatic USP8 gene mutations are a common cause of pediatric Cushing disease. J Clin Endocrinol Metab 102:2836–2843. https://doi.org/10.1210/jc.2017-00161
Fernandez A, Karavitaki N, Wass JA (2010) Prevalence of pituitary adenomas: a community-based, cross-sectional study in Banbury (Oxfordshire, UK). Clin Endocrinol (Oxf) 72:377–382. https://doi.org/10.1111/j.1365-2265.2009.03667.x
Fero ML, Rivkin M, Tasch M et al (1996) A syndrome of multiorgan hyperplasia with features of gigantism, tumorigenesis, and female sterility in p27(Kip1)-deficient mice. Cell 85:733–744
Fero ML, Randel E, Gurley KE, Roberts JM, Kemp CJ (1998) The murine gene p27Kip1 is haplo-insufficient for tumour suppression. Nature 396:177–180. https://doi.org/10.1038/24179
Ferrau F, Romeo PD, Puglisi S et al (2018) GSTP1 gene methylation and AHR rs2066853 variant predict resistance to first generation somatostatin analogs in patients with acromegaly. J Endocrinol Investig. https://doi.org/10.1007/s40618-018-0988-8
Fontana E, Gaillard R (2009) [Epidemiology of pituitary adenoma: results of the first Swiss study]. Rev Med Suisse 5:2172–2174
Forlino A, Vetro A, Garavelli L, Ciccone R, London E, Stratakis CA, Zuffardi O (2014) PRKACB and Carney complex. N Engl J Med 370:1065–1067. https://doi.org/10.1056/NEJMc1309730
Fritz A, Walch A, Piotrowska K et al (2002) Recessive transmission of a multiple endocrine neoplasia syndrome in the rat. Cancer Res 62:3048–3051
Gadelha MR, Kasuki L, Korbonits M (2017) The genetic background of acromegaly. Pituitary 20:10–21. https://doi.org/10.1007/s11102-017-0789-7
Garbicz F, Mehlich D, Rak B et al (2017) Increased expression of the microRNA 106b~25 cluster and its host gene MCM7 in corticotroph pituitary adenomas is associated with tumor invasion and Crooke's cell morphology. Pituitary 20:450–463. https://doi.org/10.1007/s11102-017-0805-y
Gentilin E, Tagliati F, Filieri C et al (2013) miR-26a plays an important role in cell cycle regulation in ACTH-secreting pituitary adenomas by modulating protein kinase Cdelta. Endocrinology 154:1690–1700. https://doi.org/10.1210/en.2012-2070
Georgitsi M, Raitila A, Karhu A et al (2007) Germline CDKN1B/p27Kip1 mutation in multiple endocrine neoplasia. J Clin Endocrinol Metab 92:3321–3325. https://doi.org/10.1210/jc.2006-2843
Gibb EA, Brown CJ, Lam WL (2011) The functional role of long non-coding RNA in human carcinomas. Mol Cancer 10:38. https://doi.org/10.1186/1476-4598-10-38
Gill AJ (2018) Succinate dehydrogenase (SDH)-deficient neoplasia. Histopathology 72:106–116. https://doi.org/10.1111/his.13277
Gill AJ, Toon CW, Clarkson A et al (2014) Succinate dehydrogenase deficiency is rare in pituitary adenomas. Am J Surg Pathol 38:560–566. https://doi.org/10.1097/pas.0000000000000149
Gordon MV, Varma D, McLean CA, Bittar RG, Burgess JR, Topliss DJ (2007) Metastatic prolactinoma presenting as a cervical spinal cord tumour in multiple endocrine neoplasia type one (MEN-1). Clin Endocrinol 66:150–152. https://doi.org/10.1111/j.1365-2265.2006.02697.x
Gorvin CM, Newey PJ, Rogers A et al (2018) Association of prolactin receptor (PRLR) variants with prolactinomas. Hum Mol Genet. https://doi.org/10.1093/hmg/ddy396
Goudet P, Murat A, Binquet C et al (2010) Risk factors and causes of death in MEN1 disease. A GTE (Groupe d'Etude des Tumeurs Endocrines) cohort study among 758 patients. World J Surg 34:249–255. https://doi.org/10.1007/s00268-009-0290-1
Gruppetta M, Mercieca C, Vassallo J (2013) Prevalence and incidence of pituitary adenomas: a population based study in Malta. Pituitary 16:545–553. https://doi.org/10.1007/s11102-012-0454-0
Guaraldi F, Corazzini V, Gallia GL et al (2012) Genetic analysis in a patient presenting with meningioma and familial isolated pituitary adenoma (FIPA) reveals selective involvement of the

R81X mutation of the AIP gene in the pathogenesis of the pituitary tumor. Pituitary 15(Suppl 1):61–67. https://doi.org/10.1007/s11102-012-0391-y
Guo J, Wang Z, Miao Y et al (2019) A two circRNA signature predicts tumour recurrence in clinical nonfunctioning pituitary adenoma. Oncol Rep 41:113–124. https://doi.org/10.3892/or.2018.6851
Hage M, Viengchareun S, Brunet E et al (2018) Genomic alterations and complex subclonal architecture in sporadic GH-secreting pituitary adenomas. J Clin Endocrinol Metab 103:1929–1939. https://doi.org/10.1210/jc.2017-02287
Hamilton SR, Liu B, Parsons RE et al (1995) The molecular basis of Turcot's syndrome. N Engl J Med 332:839–847. https://doi.org/10.1056/nejm199503303321302
Hannah-Shmouni F, Trivellin G, Stratakis CA (2016) Genetics of gigantism and acromegaly. Growth Hormon IGF Res 30-31:37–41. https://doi.org/10.1016/j.ghir.2016.08.002
Hao S, Hong CS, Feng J, Yang C, Chittiboina P, Zhang J, Zhuang Z (2016) Somatic IDH1 mutation in a pituitary adenoma of a patient with Maffucci syndrome. J Neurosurg 124:1562–1567. https://doi.org/10.3171/2015.4.Jns15191
Harris PE, Alexander JM, Bikkal HA, Hsu DW, Hedley-Whyte ET, Klibanski A, Jameson JL (1992) Glycoprotein hormone alpha-subunit production in somatotroph adenomas with and without Gs alpha mutations. J Clin Endocrinol Metab 75:918–923. https://doi.org/10.1210/jcem.75.3.1517386
Hayashi K, Inoshita N, Kawaguchi K et al (2016) The USP8 mutational status may predict drug susceptibility in corticotroph adenomas of Cushing's disease. Eur J Endocrinol 174:213–226. https://doi.org/10.1530/eje-15-0689
Hayward BE, Barlier A, Korbonits M, Grossman AB, Jacquet P, Enjalbert A, Bonthron DT (2001) Imprinting of the G(s)alpha gene GNAS1 in the pathogenesis of acromegaly. J Clin Invest 107: R31–R36. https://doi.org/10.1172/jci11887
Heaney A (2014) Management of aggressive pituitary adenomas and pituitary carcinomas. J Neuro-Oncol 117:459–468. https://doi.org/10.1007/s11060-014-1413-6
Hernandez-Ramirez LC, Gabrovska P, Dénes J et al (2015) Landscape of familial isolated and young-onset pituitary adenomas: prospective diagnosis in AIP mutation carriers. J Clin Endocrinol Metab 100:E1242–E1254. https://doi.org/10.1210/jc.2015-1869
Hernández-Ramírez LC, Martucci F, Morgan RM et al (2016) Rapid proteasomal degradation of mutant proteins is the primary mechanism leading to tumorigenesis in patients with missense AIP mutations. J Clin Endocrinol Metab 101:3144–3154. https://doi.org/10.1210/jc.2016-1307
Hernandez-Ramirez LC, Gam R, Valdés N et al (2017a) Loss-of-function mutations in the CABLES1 gene are a novel cause of Cushing's disease. Endocr Relat Cancer 24:379–392. https://doi.org/10.1530/erc-17-0131
Hernandez-Ramirez LC, Tatsi C, Lodish MB et al (2017b) Corticotropinoma as a component of Carney complex. J Endocr Soc 1:918–925. https://doi.org/10.1210/js.2017-00231
Hernandez-Ramirez LC, Morgan RML, Barry S, D'Acquisto F, Prodromou C, Korbonits M (2018) Multi-chaperone function modulation and association with cytoskeletal proteins are key features of the function of AIP in the pituitary gland. Oncotarget 9:9177–9198. https://doi.org/10.18632/oncotarget.24183
Horvath A, Stratakis CA (2008) Clinical and molecular genetics of acromegaly: MEN1, Carney complex, McCune-Albright syndrome, familial acromegaly and genetic defects in sporadic tumors. Rev Endocr Metab Disord 9:1–11. https://doi.org/10.1007/s11154-007-9066-9
Horvath A, Bossis I, Giatzakis C et al (2008) Large deletions of the PRKAR1A gene in Carney complex. Clin Cancer Res 14:388–395. https://doi.org/10.1158/1078-0432.Ccr-07-1155
Hou Z, Yang J, Wang G, Wang C, Zhang H (2018) Bioinformatic analysis of gene expression profiles of pituitary gonadotroph adenomas. Oncol Lett 15:1655–1663. https://doi.org/10.3892/ol.2017.7505
Iacovazzo D, Korbonits M (2016) Gigantism: X-linked acrogigantism and GPR101 mutations. Growth Horm IGF Res 30–31:64–69. https://doi.org/10.1016/j.ghir.2016.09.007

Iacovazzo D, Caswell R, Bunce B et al (2016) Germline or somatic GPR101 duplication leads to X-linked acrogigantism: a clinico-pathological and genetic study. Acta Neuropathol Commun 4:56. https://doi.org/10.1186/s40478-016-0328-1

Ibanez-Costa A, Korbonits M (2017) AIP and the somatostatin system in pituitary tumours. J Endocrinol 235:R101–R116. https://doi.org/10.1530/joe-17-0254

Igreja S, Chahal HS, King P et al (2010) Characterization of aryl hydrocarbon receptor interacting protein (AIP) mutations in familial isolated pituitary adenoma families. Hum Mutat 31:950–960. https://doi.org/10.1002/humu.21292

Jaffrain-Rea ML, Angelini M, Gargano D et al (2009) Expression of aryl hydrocarbon receptor (AHR) and AHR-interacting protein in pituitary adenomas: pathological and clinical implications. Endocr Relat Cancer 16:1029–1043. https://doi.org/10.1677/erc-09-0094

Jennings JE, Georgitsi M, Holdaway I et al (2009) Aggressive pituitary adenomas occurring in young patients in a large polynesian kindred with a germline R271W mutation in the AIP gene. Eur J Endocrinol 161:799–804

Josefson J, Listernick R, Fangusaro JR, Charrow J, Habiby R (2011) Growth hormone excess in children with neurofibromatosis type 1-associated and sporadic optic pathway tumors. J Pediatr 158:433–436. https://doi.org/10.1016/j.jpeds.2010.09.013

Kaltsas G, Kanakis G, Chrousos G (2000) Carney complex. In: De Groot LJ et al (eds) Endotext. MDText.com, South Dartmouth, MA

Karga HJ, Alexander JM, Hedley-Whyte ET, Klibanski A, Jameson JL (1992) Ras mutations in human pituitary tumors. J Clin Endocrinol Metab 74:914–919. https://doi.org/10.1210/jcem.74.4.1312542

Kasuki Jomori de Pinho L, Vieira Neto L, Armondi Wildemberg LE et al (2011) Low aryl hydrocarbon receptor-interacting protein expression is a better marker of invasiveness in somatotropinomas than Ki-67 and p53. Neuroendocrinology 94:39–48. https://doi.org/10.1159/000322787

Kasuki L, Vieira Neto L, Wildemberg LE, Colli LM, de Castro M, Takiya CM, Gadelha MR (2012) AIP expression in sporadic somatotropinomas is a predictor of the response to octreotide LAR therapy independent of SSTR2 expression. Endocr Relat Cancer 19:L25–L29. https://doi.org/10.1530/erc-12-0020

Kawashima ST, Usui T, Sano T et al (2009) P53 gene mutation in an atypical corticotroph adenoma with Cushing's disease. Clin Endocrinol 70:656–657. https://doi.org/10.1111/j.1365-2265.2008.03404.x

Kazlauskas A, Poellinger L, Pongratz I (2000) The immunophilin-like protein XAP2 regulates ubiquitination and subcellular localization of the dioxin receptor. J Biol Chem 275:41317–41324. https://doi.org/10.1074/jbc.M007765200

Kiefer FW, Winhofer Y, Iacovazzo D et al (2017) PRKAR1A mutation causing pituitary-dependent Cushing disease in a patient with Carney complex. Eur J Endocrinol 177:K7–K12. https://doi.org/10.1530/EJE-17-0227

Kiyokawa H, Kineman RD, Manova-Todorova KO et al (1996) Enhanced growth of mice lacking the cyclin-dependent kinase inhibitor function of p27(Kip1). Cell 85:721–732

Kobayashi T, Usui H, Tanaka H, Shozu M (2018) Variant prolactin receptor in agalactia and hyperprolactinemia. N Engl J Med 379:2230–2236. https://doi.org/10.1056/NEJMoa1805171

Kondo Y, Shinjo K, Katsushima K (2017) Long non-coding RNAs as an epigenetic regulator in human cancers. Cancer Sci 108:1927–1933. https://doi.org/10.1111/cas.13342

Korbonits M, Kumar AV (2012) AIP-related familial isolated pituitary adenomas. In: Adam MP, Ardinger HH, Pagon RA, Wallace SE, Bean LJH, Stephens K, Amemiya A (eds) GeneReviews (R). University of Washington, Seattle, WA

Krol J, Loedige I, Filipowicz W (2010) The widespread regulation of microRNA biogenesis, function and decay. Nat Rev Genet 11:597–610. https://doi.org/10.1038/nrg2843

Kurelac I, MacKay A, Lambros MB et al (2013) Somatic complex I disruptive mitochondrial DNA mutations are modifiers of tumorigenesis that correlate with low genomic instability in pituitary adenomas. Hum Mol Genet 22:226–238. https://doi.org/10.1093/hmg/dds422

Kurozumi K, Tabuchi A, Ono Y, Tamiya T, Ohmoto T, Furuta T, Hamasaki S (2002) [Pituitary adenoma associated with neurofibromatosis type 1: case report]. No Shinkei Geka 30:741–745
Kuzhandaivelu N, Cong YS, Inouye C, Yang WM, Seto E (1996) XAP2, a novel hepatitis B virus X-associated protein that inhibits X transactivation. Nucleic Acids Res 24:4741–4750
La Corte E, Younus I, Pivari F et al (2018) BRAF V600E mutant papillary craniopharyngiomas: a single-institutional case series. Pituitary 21:571–583. https://doi.org/10.1007/s11102-018-0909-z
Lan X, Gao H, Wang F et al (2016) Whole-exome sequencing identifies variants in invasive pituitary adenomas. Oncol Lett 12:2319–2328. https://doi.org/10.3892/ol.2016.5029
Landis CA, Masters SB, Spada A, Pace AM, Bourne HR, Vallar L (1989) GTPase inhibiting mutations activate the alpha chain of Gs and stimulate adenylyl cyclase in human pituitary tumours. Nature 340:692–696. https://doi.org/10.1038/340692a0
Larkin S, Reddy R, Karavitaki N, Cudlip S, Wass J, Ansorge O (2013) Granulation pattern, but not GSP or GHR mutation, is associated with clinical characteristics in somatostatin-naive patients with somatotroph adenomas. Eur J Endocrinol 168:491–499. https://doi.org/10.1530/EJE-12-0864
Lee YJ, Cho JM, Moon JH, Ku CR, Kim J, Kim SH, Lee EJ (2017) Increased miR-338-3p expression correlates with invasiveness of GH-producing pituitary adenomas. Endocrine 58:184–189. https://doi.org/10.1007/s12020-017-1390-6
Leone V, Langella C, D'Angelo D et al (2014) Mir-23b and miR-130b expression is downregulated in pituitary adenomas. Mol Cell Endocrinol 390:1–7. https://doi.org/10.1016/j.mce.2014.03.002
Leontiou CA, Gueorguiev M, van der Spuy J et al (2008) The role of the aryl hydrocarbon receptor-interacting protein gene in familial and sporadic pituitary adenomas. J Clin Endocrinol Metab 93:2390–2401. https://doi.org/10.1210/jc.2007-2611
Li XH, Wang EL, Zhou HM, Yoshimoto K, Qian ZR (2014) MicroRNAs in human pituitary adenomas. Int J Endocrinol 2014:435171. https://doi.org/10.1155/2014/435171
Lim CT, Korbonits M (2018) Update on the clinicopathology of pituitary adenomas. Endocr Pract 24:473–488. https://doi.org/10.4158/EP-2018-0034
Lin Y, Jiang X, Shen Y, Li M, Ma H, Xing M, Lu Y (2009) Frequent mutations and amplifications of the PIK3CA gene in pituitary tumors. Endocr Relat Cancer 16:301–310. https://doi.org/10.1677/erc-08-0167
Lines KE, Newey PJ, Yates CJ et al (2018) MiR-15a/miR-16-1 expression inversely correlates with cyclin D1 levels in Men1 pituitary NETs. J Endocrinol. https://doi.org/10.1530/joe-18-0278
Losa M, Mortini P, Pagnano A, Detomas M, Cassarino MF, Pecori Giraldi F (2018) Clinical characteristics and surgical outcome in USP8-mutated human adrenocorticotropic hormone-secreting pituitary adenomas. Endocrine. https://doi.org/10.1007/s12020-018-1776-0
Lu B, Liu GL, Yu F, Li WJ, Xiang XX, Xiao HZ (2018) MicroRNA16/VEGFR2/p38/NFkappaB signaling pathway regulates cell growth of human pituitary neoplasms. Oncol Rep 39:1235–1244. https://doi.org/10.3892/or.2018.6227
Lyons J, Landis CA, Harsh G et al (1990) Two G protein oncogenes in human endocrine tumors. Science 249:655–659
Ma ZY, Song ZJ, Chen JH et al (2015) Recurrent gain-of-function USP8 mutations in Cushing's disease. Cell Res 25:306–317. https://doi.org/10.1038/cr.2015.20
Mao ZG, He DS, Zhou J et al (2010) Differential expression of microRNAs in GH-secreting pituitary adenomas. Diagn Pathol 5:79. https://doi.org/10.1186/1746-1596-5-79
Marini F, Falchetti A, Del Monte F, Carbonell Sala S, Gozzini A, Luzi E, Brandi ML (2006) Multiple endocrine neoplasia type 1. OrphanetJ Rare Dis 1:38. https://doi.org/10.1186/1750-1172-1-38
Marques P, Korbonits M (2017) Genetic aspects of pituitary adenomas. Endocrinol Metab Clin North Am 46:335–374. https://doi.org/10.1016/j.ecl.2017.01.004
Mazzaglia PJ (2012) Hereditary pheochromocytoma and paraganglioma. J Surg Oncol 106:580–585. https://doi.org/10.1002/jso.23157

Miljic D et al (2017) Changes in pituitary tumour biology and behaviour in FIPA patient with GH secreting aggressive pituitary macro adenoma. Paper presented at the 19th European Congress of Endocrinology, Lisbon
Miller MB, Bi WL, Ramkissoon LA et al (2016) MAPK activation and HRAS mutation identified in pituitary spindle cell oncocytoma. Oncotarget 7:37054–37063. https://doi.org/10.18632/oncotarget.9244
Milne TA, Hughes CM, Lloyd R et al (2005) Menin and MLL cooperatively regulate expression of cyclin-dependent kinase inhibitors. Proc Natl Acad Sci USA 102:749–754. https://doi.org/10.1073/pnas.0408836102
Molatore S, Marinoni I, Lee M et al (2010) A novel germline CDKN1B mutation causing multiple endocrine tumors: clinical, genetic and functional characterization. Hum Mutat 31:E1825–E1835. https://doi.org/10.1002/humu.21354
Murat CB, Braga PB, Fortes MA, Bronstein MD, Correa-Giannella ML, Giorgi RR (2012) Mutation and genomic amplification of the PIK3CA proto-oncogene in pituitary adenomas. Braz J Med Biol Res 45:851–855
Mussnich P, Raverot G, Jaffrain-Rea ML et al (2015) Downregulation of miR-410 targeting the cyclin B1 gene plays a role in pituitary gonadotroph tumors. Cell Cycle 14:2590–2597. https://doi.org/10.1080/15384101.2015.1064207
Nakata A, Urano D, Fujii-Kuriyama Y, Mizuno N, Tago K, Itoh H (2009) G-protein signalling negatively regulates the stability of aryl hydrocarbon receptor. EMBO Rep 10:622–628. https://doi.org/10.1038/embor.2009.35
Nakayama K, Ishida N, Shirane M et al (1996) Mice lacking p27(Kip1) display increased body size, multiple organ hyperplasia, retinal dysplasia, and pituitary tumors. Cell 85:707–720
Naves LA, Daly AF, Dias LA et al (2016) Aggressive tumor growth and clinical evolution in a patient with X-linked acro-gigantism syndrome. Endocrine 51:236–244. https://doi.org/10.1007/s12020-015-0804-6
Nejo T, Tanaka S, Ikemura M et al (2018) Maffucci syndrome complicated by three different central nervous system tumors sharing an IDH1 R132C mutation: case report. J Neurosurg:1–6. https://doi.org/10.3171/2018.6.Jns18729
Nemeth K, Darvasi O, Likó I et al (2019) Next-generation sequencing identifies novel mitochondrial variants in pituitary adenomas. J Endocrinol Investig. https://doi.org/10.1007/s40618-019-1005-6
Newey PJ, Gorvin CM, Thakker RV (2013a) Mutant prolactin receptor and familial hyperprolactinemia. N Engl J Med 369:2012–2020. https://doi.org/10.1056/NEJMoa1307557
Newey PJ, Nesbit MA, Rimmer AJ et al (2013b) Whole-exome sequencing studies of nonfunctioning pituitary adenomas. J Clin Endocrinol Metab 98:E796–E800. https://doi.org/10.1210/jc.2012-4028
O'Hayre M, Vazquez-Prado J, Kufareva I, Stawiski EW, Handel TM, Seshagiri S, Gutkind JS (2013) The emerging mutational landscape of G proteins and G-protein-coupled receptors in cancer. Nat Rev Cancer 13:412–424. https://doi.org/10.1038/nrc3521
O'Toole SM, Denes J, Robledo M, Stratakis CA, Korbonits M (2015) 15 years of paraganglioma: the association of pituitary adenomas and phaeochromocytomas or paragangliomas. Endocr Relat Cancer 22:T105–T122. https://doi.org/10.1530/erc-15-0241
Occhi G, Jaffrain-Rea ML, Trivellin G et al (2010) The R304X mutation of the aryl hydrocarbon receptor interacting protein gene in familial isolated pituitary adenomas: mutational hot-spot or founder effect? J Endocrinol Investig 33:800–805. https://doi.org/10.1007/BF03350345
Occhi G, Regazzo D, Trivellin G et al (2013) A novel mutation in the upstream open reading frame of the CDKN1B gene causes a MEN4 phenotype. PLoS Genet 9:e1003350. https://doi.org/10.1371/journal.pgen.1003350
Ono S, Tanizaki H, Fujisawa A, Tanioka M, Miyachi Y (2012) Maffucci syndrome complicated with meningioma and pituitary adenoma. Eur J Dermatol 22:130–131. https://doi.org/10.1684/ejd.2011.1563

Orloff MS, He X, Peterson C, Chen F, Chen JL, Mester JL, Eng C (2013) Germline PIK3CA and AKT1 mutations in Cowden and Cowden-like syndromes. Am J Hum Genet 92:76–80. https://doi.org/10.1016/j.ajhg.2012.10.021

Ozfirat Z, Korbonits M (2010) AIP gene and familial isolated pituitary adenomas. Mol Cell Endocrinol 326:71–79. https://doi.org/10.1016/j.mce.2010.05.001

Palumbo T, Faucz FR, Azevedo M, Xekouki P, Iliopoulos D, Stratakis CA (2013) Functional screen analysis reveals miR-26b and miR-128 as central regulators of pituitary somatomammotrophic tumor growth through activation of the PTEN-AKT pathway. Oncogene 32:1651–1659. https://doi.org/10.1038/onc.2012.190

Papathomas TG, Gaal J, Corssmit EP et al (2014) Non-pheochromocytoma (PCC)/paraganglioma (PGL) tumors in patients with succinate dehydrogenase-related PCC-PGL syndromes: a clinicopathological and molecular analysis. Eur J Endocrinol 170:1–12. https://doi.org/10.1530/eje-13-0623

Pei L, Melmed S, Scheithauer B, Kovacs K, Prager D (1994) H-ras mutations in human pituitary carcinoma metastases. J Clin Endocrinol Metab 78:842–846. https://doi.org/10.1210/jcem.78.4.8157709

Pellegata NS, Quintanilla-Martinez L, Siggelkow H et al (2006) Germ-line mutations in p27Kip1 cause a multiple endocrine neoplasia syndrome in rats and humans. Proc Natl Acad Sci USA 103:15558–15563. https://doi.org/10.1073/pnas.0603877103

Perez-Rivas LG, Theodoropoulou M, FerraùF et al (2015) The gene of the ubiquitin-specific protease 8 is frequently mutated in adenomas causing Cushing's disease. J Clin Endocrinol Metab 100:E997–E1004. https://doi.org/10.1210/jc.2015-1453

Perez-Rivas LG, Theodoropoulou M, Puar TH et al (2018) Somatic USP8 mutations are frequent events in corticotroph tumor progression causing Nelson's tumor. Eur J Endocrinol 178:59–65. https://doi.org/10.1530/eje-17-0634

Petrossians P, de Herder W, Kwekkeboom D, Lamberigts G, Stevenaert A, Beckers A (2000) Malignant prolactinoma discovered by D2 receptor imaging. J Clin Endocrinol Metab 85:398–401. https://doi.org/10.1210/jcem.85.1.6253

Philipp-Staheli J, Payne SR, Kemp CJ (2001) p27(Kip1): regulation and function of a haploinsufficient tumor suppressor and its misregulation in cancer. Exp Cell Res 264:148–168. https://doi.org/10.1006/excr.2000.5143

Pinto EM, Siqueira SA, Cukier P, Fragoso MC, Lin CJ, de Mendonca BB (2011) Possible role of a radiation-induced p53 mutation in a Nelson's syndrome patient with a fatal outcome. Pituitary 14:400–404. https://doi.org/10.1007/s11102-009-0194-y

Porcelli AM, Ghelli A, Ceccarelli C et al (2010) The genetic and metabolic signature of oncocytic transformation implicates HIF1alpha destabilization. Hum Mol Genet 19:1019–1032. https://doi.org/10.1093/hmg/ddp566

Raappana A, Koivukangas J, Ebeling T, Pirila T (2010) Incidence of pituitary adenomas in Northern Finland in 1992–2007. J Clin Endocrinol Metab 95:4268–4275. https://doi.org/10.1210/jc.2010-0537

Radian S, Diekmann Y, Gabrovska P et al (2017) Increased population risk of AIP-related acromegaly and gigantism in Ireland. Hum Mutat 38:78–85. https://doi.org/10.1002/humu.23121

Reincke M, Sbiera S, Hayakawa A et al (2015) Mutations in the deubiquitinase gene USP8 cause Cushing's disease. Nat Genet 47:31–38. https://doi.org/10.1038/ng.3166

Renjie W, Haiqian L (2015) MiR-132, miR-15a and miR-16 synergistically inhibit pituitary tumor cell proliferation, invasion and migration by targeting Sox5. Cancer Lett 356:568–578. https://doi.org/10.1016/j.canlet.2014.10.003

Riminucci M, Collins MT, Lala R, Corsi A, Matarazzo P, Gehron Robey P, Bianco P (2002) An R201H activating mutation of the GNAS1 (Gsalpha) gene in a corticotroph pituitary adenoma. Mol Pathol 55:58–60

Ritvonen E, Pitkänen E, Karppinen A et al (2017) Impact of AIP and inhibitory G protein alpha 2 proteins on clinical features of sporadic GH-secreting pituitary adenomas. Eur J Endocrinol 176:243–252. https://doi.org/10.1530/eje-16-0620

Rodd C, Millette M, Iacovazzo D et al (2016) Somatic GPR101 duplication causing X-linked acrogigantism (XLAG)-diagnosis and management. J Clin Endocrinol Metab 101:1927–1930. https://doi.org/10.1210/jc.2015-4366

Romero OA, Torres-Diz M, Pros E et al (2014) MAX inactivation in small cell lung cancer disrupts MYC-SWI/SNF programs and is synthetic lethal with BRG1. Cancer Discov 4:292–303. https://doi.org/10.1158/2159-8290.Cd-13-0799

Ronchi CL, Peverelli E, Herterich S et al (2016) Landscape of somatic mutations in sporadic GH-secreting pituitary adenomas. Eur J Endocrinol 174:363–372. https://doi.org/10.1530/eje-15-1064

Rostomyan L, Daly AF, Petrossians P et al (2015) Clinical and genetic characterization of pituitary gigantism: an international collaborative study in 208 patients. Endocr Relat Cancer 22:745–757. https://doi.org/10.1530/erc-15-0320

Roszko KL, Blouch E, Blake M et al (2017) Case report of a prolactinoma in a patient with a novel MAX mutation and bilateral pheochromocytomas. J Endocr Soc 1:1401–1407. https://doi.org/10.1210/js.2017-00135

Rothenbuhler A, Stratakis CA (2010) Clinical and molecular genetics of Carney complex. Best Pract Res Clin Endocrinol Metab 24:389–399. https://doi.org/10.1016/j.beem.2010.03.003

Roussel-Gervais A, Couture C, Langlais D et al (2016) The Cables1 gene in glucocorticoid regulation of pituitary corticotrope growth and Cushing disease. J Clin Endocrinol Metab 101:513–522. https://doi.org/10.1210/jc.2015-3324

Ruivo J, Antunes JL (2009) Maffucci syndrome associated with a pituitary adenoma and a probable brainstem tumor. J Neurosurg 110:363–368. https://doi.org/10.3171/2008.8.Jns08150

Salenave S, Ancelle D, Bahougne T et al (2015) Macroprolactinomas in children and adolescents: factors associated with the response to treatment in 77 patients. J Clin Endocrinol Metab 100:1177–1186. https://doi.org/10.1210/jc.2014-3670

Salomon MP, Wang X, Marzese DM et al (2018) The epigenomic landscape of pituitary adenomas reveals specific alterations and differentiates among acromegaly, Cushing's disease and endocrine-inactive subtypes. Clin Cancer Res 24:4126–4136. https://doi.org/10.1158/1078-0432.Ccr-17-2206

Salpea P, Stratakis CA (2014) Carney complex and McCune Albright syndrome: an overview of clinical manifestations and human molecular genetics. Mol Cell Endocrinol 386:85–91. https://doi.org/10.1016/j.mce.2013.08.022

Salvatori R, Radian S, Diekmann Y et al (2017) In-frame seven amino-acid duplication in AIP arose over the last 3000 years, disrupts protein interaction and stability and is associated with gigantism. Eur J Endocrinol 177:257–266. https://doi.org/10.1530/EJE-17-0293

Sambugaro S, Di Ruvo M, Ambrosio MR et al (2015) Early onset acromegaly associated with a novel deletion in CDKN1B 5′UTR region. Endocrine 49:58–64. https://doi.org/10.1007/s12020-015-0540-y

Samuels Y, Wang Z, Bardelli A et al (2004) High frequency of mutations of the PIK3CA gene in human cancers. Science 304:554. https://doi.org/10.1126/science.1096502

Sapkota S, Horiguchi K, Tosaka M, Yamada S, Yamada M (2017) Whole-exome sequencing study of thyrotropin-secreting pituitary adenomas. J Clin Endocrinol Metab 102:566–575. https://doi.org/10.1210/jc.2016-2261

Sav A, Rotondo F, Syro LV, Di Ieva A, Cusimano MD, Kovacs K (2016) Biomarkers of pituitary carcinomas. Expert Rev Endocrinol Metab 11:253–261. https://doi.org/10.1080/17446651.2016.1179110

Scheithauer BW, Horvath E, Abel TW et al (2008) Pituitary blastoma. Acta Neuropathol 116:657–666. https://doi.org/10.1007/s00401-008-0388-9

Scheithauer BW, Kovacs K, Nose V et al (2009) Multiple endocrine neoplasia type 1-associated thyrotropin-producing pituitary carcinoma: report of a probable de novo example. Hum Pathol 40:270–278. https://doi.org/10.1016/j.humpath.2008.06.013

Scheithauer BW et al (2012) Pituitary blastoma: a unique embryonal tumor. Pituitary 15:365–373. https://doi.org/10.1007/s11102-011-0328-x

Schernthaner-Reiter MH, Trivellin G, Stratakis CA (2016) MEN1, MEN4, and Carney complex: pathology and molecular genetics. Neuroendocrinology 103:18–31. https://doi.org/10.1159/000371819

Schopf FH, Biebl MM, Buchner J (2017) The HSP90 chaperone machinery. Nat Rev Mol Cell Biol 18:345–360. https://doi.org/10.1038/nrm.2017.20

Schultz KA, Yang J, Doros L et al (2014) DICER1-pleuropulmonary blastoma familial tumor predisposition syndrome: a unique constellation of neoplastic conditions. Pathol Case Rev 19:90–100. https://doi.org/10.1097/pcr.0000000000000027

Schultz KAP, Rednam SP, Kamihara J et al (2017) PTEN, DICER1, FH, and their associated tumor susceptibility syndromes: clinical features, genetics, and surveillance recommendations in childhood. Clin Cancer Res 23:e76–e82. https://doi.org/10.1158/1078-0432.Ccr-17-0629

Shaid M, Korbonits M (2017) Genetics of pituitary adenomas. Neurol India 65:577–587. https://doi.org/10.4103/neuroindia.NI_330_17

Smith N, Santoreneos S (2017) Non-functioning pituitary macroadenoma in a child with neurofibromatosis type 1. ANZ J Surg 87:E220–E221. https://doi.org/10.1111/ans.13108

Song ZJ, Reitman ZJ, Ma ZY et al (2016) The genome-wide mutational landscape of pituitary adenomas. Cell Res 26:1255–1259. https://doi.org/10.1038/cr.2016.114

Song W, Qian L, Jing G et al (2018) Aberrant expression of the sFRP and WIF1 genes in invasive non-functioning pituitary adenomas. Mol Cell Endocrinol 474:168–175. https://doi.org/10.1016/j.mce.2018.03.005

Sotomayor M, Gaudet R, Corey DP (2014) Sorting out a promiscuous superfamily: towards cadherin connectomics. Trends Cell Biol 24:524–536. https://doi.org/10.1016/j.tcb.2014.03.007

Spada A, Vallar L (1992) G-protein oncogenes in acromegaly. Horm Res 38:90–93. https://doi.org/10.1159/000182498

Spada A, Arosio M, Bochicchio D, Bazzoni N, Vallar L, Bassetti M, Faglia G (1990) Clinical, biochemical, and morphological correlates in patients bearing growth hormone-secreting pituitary tumors with or without constitutively active adenylyl cyclase. J Clin Endocrinol Metab 71:1421–1426. https://doi.org/10.1210/jcem-71-6-1421

Stratakis CA, Kirschner LS, Carney JA (2001) Clinical and molecular features of the Carney complex: diagnostic criteria and recommendations for patient evaluation. J Clin Endocrinol Metab 86:4041–4046. https://doi.org/10.1210/jcem.86.9.7903

Taboada GF, Tabet AL, Naves LA, de Carvalho DP, Gadelha MR (2009) Prevalence of gsp oncogene in somatotropinomas and clinically non-functioning pituitary adenomas: our experience. Pituitary 12:165–169. https://doi.org/10.1007/s11102-008-0136-0

Tanizaki Y, Jin L, Scheithauer BW, Kovacs K, Roncaroli F, Lloyd RV (2007) P53 gene mutations in pituitary carcinomas. Endocr Pathol 18:217–222. https://doi.org/10.1007/s12022-007-9006-y

Thakker RV (2014) Multiple endocrine neoplasia type 1 (MEN1) and type 4 (MEN4). Mol Cell Endocrinol 386:2–15. https://doi.org/10.1016/j.mce.2013.08.002

Thakker RV, Newey PJ, Walls GV et al (2012) Clinical practice guidelines for multiple endocrine neoplasia type 1 (MEN1). J Clin Endocrinol Metab 97:2990–3011. https://doi.org/10.1210/jc.2012-1230

Theodoropoulou M, Zhang J, Laupheimer S et al (2006) Octreotide, a somatostatin analogue, mediates its antiproliferative action in pituitary tumor cells by altering phosphatidylinositol 3-kinase signaling and inducing Zac1 expression. Cancer Res 66:1576–1582. https://doi.org/10.1158/0008-5472.CAN-05-1189

Tichomirowa MA, Barlier A, Daly AF et al (2011) High prevalence of AIP gene mutations following focused screening in young patients with sporadic pituitary macroadenomas. Eur J Endocrinol 165:509–515. https://doi.org/10.1530/EJE-11-0304
Tichomirowa MA, Lee M, Barlier A et al (2012) Cyclin-dependent kinase inhibitor 1B (CDKN1B) gene variants in AIP mutation-negative familial isolated pituitary adenoma kindreds. Endocr Relat Cancer 19:233–241. https://doi.org/10.1530/erc-11-0362
Toledo RA, Mendonca BB, Fragoso MC et al (2010) Isolated familial somatotropinoma: 11q13-loh and gene/protein expression analysis suggests a possible involvement of AIP also in non-pituitary tumorigenesis. Clinics (Sao Paulo) 65:407–415. https://doi.org/10.1590/S1807-59322010000400010
Trivellin G, Korbonits M (2011) AIP and its interacting partners. J Endocrinol 210:137–155. https://doi.org/10.1530/joe-11-0054
Trivellin G, Butz H, Delhove J et al (2012) MicroRNA miR-107 is overexpressed in pituitary adenomas and inhibits the expression of aryl hydrocarbon receptor-interacting protein in vitro. Am J Physiol Endocrinol Metab 303:E708–E719. https://doi.org/10.1152/ajpendo.00546.2011
Trivellin G, Daly AF, Faucz FR et al (2014) Gigantism and acromegaly due to Xq26 microduplications and GPR101 mutation. N Engl J Med 371:2363–2374. https://doi.org/10.1056/NEJMoa1408028
Trouillas J, Labat-Moleur F, Sturm N et al (2008) Pituitary tumors and hyperplasia in multiple endocrine neoplasia type 1 syndrome (MEN1): a case-control study in a series of 77 patients versus 2509 non-MEN1 patients. Am J Surg Pathol 32:534–543. https://doi.org/10.1097/PAS.0b013e31815ade45
Trouillas J, Roy P, Sturm N et al (2013) A new prognostic clinicopathological classification of pituitary adenomas: a multicentric case-control study of 410 patients with 8 years post-operative follow-up. Acta Neuropathol 126:123–135. https://doi.org/10.1007/s00401-013-1084-y
Trouillas J, Burman P, McCormack A, Petersenn S, Popovic V, Dekkers O, Raverot G (2018) Aggressive pituitary tumours and carcinomas: two sides of the same coin? Eur J Endocrinol 178: C7–C9. https://doi.org/10.1530/EJE-18-0250
Trump D, Farren B, Wooding C et al (1996) Clinical studies of multiple endocrine neoplasia type 1 (MEN1). QJM 89:653–669
Tufton N, Roncaroli F, Hadjidemetriou I et al (2017) Pituitary carcinoma in a patient with an SDHB mutation. Endocr Pathol 28:320–325. https://doi.org/10.1007/s12022-017-9474-7
Tuominen I, Heliövaara E, Raitila A et al (2015) AIP inactivation leads to pituitary tumorigenesis through defective Galphai-cAMP signaling. Oncogene 34:1174–1184. https://doi.org/10.1038/onc.2014.50
Turcot J, Despres JP, St Pierre F (1959) Malignant tumors of the central nervous system associated with familial polyposis of the colon: report of two cases. Dis Colon Rectum 2:465–468
Valimaki N, Demir H, Pitkänen E et al (2015) Whole-genome sequencing of growth hormone (GH)-secreting pituitary adenomas. J Clin Endocrinol Metab 100:3918–3927. https://doi.org/10.1210/jc.2015-3129
Vallar L, Spada A, Giannattasio G (1987) Altered Gs and adenylate cyclase activity in human GH-secreting pituitary adenomas. Nature 330:566–568. https://doi.org/10.1038/330566a0
Verges B, Boureille F, Goudet P et al (2002) Pituitary disease in MEN type 1 (MEN1): data from the France-Belgium MEN1 multicenter study. J Clin Endocrinol Metab 87:457–465. https://doi.org/10.1210/jcem.87.2.8145
Vierimaa O, Georgitsi M, Lehtonen R et al (2006) Pituitary adenoma predisposition caused by germline mutations in the AIP gene. Science 312:1228–1230. https://doi.org/10.1126/science.1126100
Vitali E, Peverelli E, Giardino E et al (2014) Cyclic adenosine 3′-5′-monophosphate (cAMP) exerts proliferative and anti-proliferative effects in pituitary cells of different types by activating both cAMP-dependent protein kinase A (PKA) and exchange proteins directly activated by cAMP (Epac). Mol Cell Endocrinol 383:193–202. https://doi.org/10.1016/j.mce.2013.12.006

Wang C, Su Z, Sanai N et al (2012) microRNA expression profile and differentially-expressed genes in prolactinomas following bromocriptine treatment. Oncol Rep 27:1312–1320. https://doi.org/10.3892/or.2012.1690

Wang J, Wang D, Wan D et al (2018) Circular RNA in invasive and recurrent clinical nonfunctioning pituitary adenomas: expression profiles and bioinformatic analysis. World Neurosurg 117:e371–e386. https://doi.org/10.1016/j.wneu.2018.06.038

Weinstein LS, Shenker A, Gejman PV, Merino MJ, Friedman E, Spiegel AM (1991) Activating mutations of the stimulatory G protein in the McCune-Albright syndrome. N Engl J Med 325:1688–1695. https://doi.org/10.1056/NEJM199112123252403

Wermer P (1954) Genetic aspects of adenomatosis of endocrine glands. Am J Med 16:363–371

Wierinckx A, Roche M, Legras-Lachuer C, Trouillas J, Raverot G, Lachuer J (2017) MicroRNAs in pituitary tumors. Mol Cell Endocrinol 456:51–61. https://doi.org/10.1016/j.mce.2017.01.021

Williams F, Hunter S, Bradley L, Morrison P, Chahal HS, Korbonits M, Atkinson AB (2012) Results and challenges of genetic testing in a large familial isolated pituitary adenoma (FIPA) kindred with an R304X AIP mutation. Endocrine Abstracts 28:P245

Williams F, Hunter S, Bradley L et al (2014) Clinical experience in the screening and management of a large kindred with familial isolated pituitary adenoma due to an aryl hydrocarbon receptor interacting protein (AIP) mutation. J Clin Endocrinol Metab 99:1122–1131. https://doi.org/10.1210/jc.2013-2868

Xekouki P, Pacak K, Almeida M et al (2012) Succinate dehydrogenase (SDH) D subunit (SDHD) inactivation in a growth-hormone-producing pituitary tumor: a new association for SDH? J Clin Endocrinol Metab 97:E357–E366. https://doi.org/10.1210/jc.2011-1179

Xekouki P, Szarek E, Bullova P et al (2015) Pituitary adenoma with paraganglioma/pheochromocytoma (3PAs) and succinate dehydrogenase defects in humans and mice. J Clin Endocrinol Metab 100:E710–E719. https://doi.org/10.1210/jc.2014-4297

Xing W, Qi Z, Huang C et al (2019) Genome-wide identification of lncRNAs and mRNAs differentially expressed in non-functioning pituitary adenoma and construction of an lncRNA-mRNA co-expression network. Biol Open 8. https://doi.org/10.1242/bio.037127

Yagnik G, Jahangiri A, Chen R, Wagner JR, Aghi MK (2017) Role of a p53 polymorphism in the development of nonfunctional pituitary adenomas. Mol Cell Endocrinol 446:81–90. https://doi.org/10.1016/j.mce.2017.02.017

Ye Z, Li Z, Wang Y et al (2015) Common variants at 10p12.31, 10q21.1 and 13q12.13 are associated with sporadic pituitary adenoma. Nat Genet 47:793–797. https://doi.org/10.1038/ng.3322

Yu C, Li J, Sun F, Cui J, Fang H, Sui G (2016) Expression and clinical significance of miR-26a and pleomorphic adenoma gene 1 (PLAG1) in invasive pituitary adenoma. Med Sci Monit 22:5101–5108

Yu G, Wang H, Yu S et al (2017) Study on miRNAs' expression for the invasion of pituitary adenomas. Turk Neurosurg. https://doi.org/10.5137/1019-5149.Jtn.20760-17.1

Zhang Z, Florez S, Gutierrez-Hartmann A, Martin JF, Amendt BA (2010) MicroRNAs regulate pituitary development, and microRNA 26b specifically targets lymphoid enhancer factor 1 (Lef-1), which modulates pituitary transcription factor 1 (Pit-1) expression. J Biol Chem 285:34718–34728. https://doi.org/10.1074/jbc.M110.126441

Zhang Q, Peng C, Song J et al (2017a) Germline mutations in CDH23, encoding cadherin-related 23, are associated with both familial and sporadic pituitary adenomas. Am J Hum Genet 100:817–823. https://doi.org/10.1016/j.ajhg.2017.03.011

Zhang T, Yang Z, Gao H (2017b) Advancements in the study of miRNA regulation during the cell cycle in human pituitary adenomas. J Neurooncol 134:253–258. https://doi.org/10.1007/s11060-017-2518-5

Zhou K, Zhang T, Fan Y, Serick, Du G, Wu P, Geng D (2016) MicroRNA-106b promotes pituitary tumor cell proliferation and invasion through PI3K/AKT signaling pathway by targeting PTEN. Tumour Biol 37:13469–13477. https://doi.org/10.1007/s13277-016-5155-2

Chapter 11
Timeline of Advances in Genetics of Primary Aldosteronism

Lucie S. Meyer, Martin Reincke, and Tracy Ann Williams

Abstract The overwhelming majority of cases of primary aldosteronism (PA) occur sporadically due to a unilateral aldosterone-producing adenoma (APA) or bilateral idiopathic adrenal hyperplasia. Familial forms of PA are rare with four subtypes defined to date (familial hyperaldosteronism types I–IV). The molecular basis of familial hyperaldosteronism type I (FH type I or glucocorticoid-remediable aldosteronism) was established in 1992; two decades later the genetic variant causing FH type III was identified and germline mutations causing FH type IV and FH type II were determined soon after. Effective diagnostic protocols and methods to detect the overactive gland in unilateral PA by adrenal venous sampling followed by laparoscopic adrenalectomy have made available APAs for scientific studies. In rapid succession, following the widespread use of next-generation sequencing, recurrent somatic driver mutations in APAs were identified in genes encoding ion channels and transporters. The development of highly specific monoclonal antibodies against key enzymes in adrenal steroidogenesis has unveiled the heterogeneous features of the diseased adrenal in PA and helped reveal the high proportion of APAs with driver mutations. We discuss what is known about the genetics of PA that has led to a clearer understanding of the disease pathophysiology.

Keywords Primary aldosteronism · Aldosterone-producing adenoma · Bilateral adrenal hyperplasia · Familial hyperaldosteronism · PASNA

L. S. Meyer · M. Reincke
Medizinische Klinik und Poliklinik IV, Klinikum der Universität München, Ludwig-Maximilians-Universität München, Munich, Germany

T. A. Williams (✉)
Medizinische Klinik und Poliklinik IV, Klinikum der Universität München, Ludwig-Maximilians-Universität München, Munich, Germany

Division of Internal Medicine and Hypertension, Department of Medical Sciences, University of Turin, Turin, Italy
e-mail: Tracy.Williams@med.uni-muenchen.de

P. Igaz, A. Patócs (eds.), *Genetics of Endocrine Diseases and Syndromes*,
Experientia Supplementum 111, https://doi.org/10.1007/978-3-030-25905-1_11

List of Abbreviations

ACTH	Adrenocorticotropic hormone
APA	Aldosterone-producing adenoma
APCC	Aldosterone-producing cell cluster
ARR	Aldosterone-to-renin ratio
ATP	Adenosine triphosphate
AVS	Adrenal venous sampling
BAH	Bilateral adrenal hyperplasia
$Ca_v1.3$	Calcium voltage-gated channel subunit alpha 1D
$Ca_v3.2$	Calcium voltage-gated channel subunit alpha 1H
ClC-2	Chloride channel protein 2
ENS@T	European Network for the Study of Adrenal Tumours
FH	Familial hyperaldosteronism
GIRK1-4	G protein-activated inwardly rectifying potassium channel 1-4
GRA	Glucocorticoid-remediable aldosteronism
HAC15 cell	Human adrenocortical cells
HEK cells	Human embryonic kidney cells
MRA	Mineralocorticoid receptor antagonists
NCI H295R cell line	Human adrenocortical cell line
NGS	Next-generation sequencing
PA	Primary aldosteronism
pAATLs	Potential APCC-to-APA-transitional lesions
PASNA	Primary aldosteronism with seizures and neurologic abnormalities
PMCA	Plasma membrane Ca^{2+}-ATPase
SFRP2	Secreted frizzled related protein 2
SSCP	Single-strand conformation polymorphism
TASK1	Potassium two-pore domain channel subfamily K member 3
TM	Transmembrane
zF	Zona fasciculata
zG	Zona glomerulosa
zR	Zona reticularis

11.1 Introduction

Aldosterone was first isolated by Grundy et al. (1952) from extracts of beef adrenals. The development of a sensitive bioassay for mineralocorticoid activity (Simpson and Tait 1952) helped monitor the purification of aldosterone from large quantities of beef adrenals, and the crystal structure of aldosterone was resolved shortly thereafter (Simpson et al. 1953, 1954). The index case of primary aldosteronism (PA) was discovered by Jerome Conn in a 34-year-old female in 1954 and reported in the literature the following year (Conn 1955) (Fig. 11.1). The patient came to medical attention because of intermittent spasms, severe muscular weakness, and paralysis. High blood pressure, low plasma potassium, high plasma sodium concentrations, and alkalosis led to the suspicion of mineralocorticoid excess as the cause. The patient agreed to intensive metabolic investigations (which lasted for almost 8 months) which established 4–30 times the level of mineralocorticoid activity in the patient's urine compared with the normal range (Conn 1955; Chalmers 1960). Conn recommended surgical exploration of the adrenals which revealed a right cortical adenoma 4 cm in diameter. Unilateral adrenalectomy resulted in dramatic improvement within 14 days with resolution of electrolyte abnormalities and normalization of blood pressure and minimal urinary mineralocorticoid activity (Conn 1955).

PA would subsequently be considered as a rare disease, and this view prevailed until the widespread application of the screening test (ARR, aldosterone-to-renin ratio) to include normokalemic patients with hypertension in addition to those with hypokalemia (Gordon et al. 1993, 1994; Stowasser 2001) which led to a 5- to 15-fold increase in the diagnosis of PA (Mulatero et al. 2004). The majority of patients with PA are normokalemic (Stowasser 2001; Mulatero et al. 2004); hypokalemia is observed in 9–37% of cases (Mulatero et al. 2004), although the method of blood withdrawal may mask hypokalemia (Stowasser and Gordon 2016).

The prevalence of PA in the general population with hypertension is estimated as 5–15% (Gordon et al. 1994; Rossi et al. 2006; Monticone et al. 2017a), increasing with the severity of hypertension (Calhoun et al. 2002; Mosso et al. 2003; Monticone et al. 2017a) and rising to 20% in patients with resistant hypertension (Calhoun et al. 2002). Therefore, although more individuals are being diagnosed with PA through wider screening, it is nonetheless underdiagnosed because the syndrome has no easily distinguishable phenotype and is not widely recognized by general practitioners (Mulatero et al. 2016) who have little knowledge of, or do not adhere to, the Endocrine Society clinical practice guideline (Funder et al. 2016).

Several studies have reported the higher prevalence of cardiovascular and cerebrovascular morbidity and mortality in patients with PA relative to patients with primary hypertension with matched cardiovascular risk profiles (Sechi et al. 2006; Mulatero et al. 2013; Savard et al. 2013; Monticone et al. 2018b). These reports demonstrate the importance of an early diagnosis and appropriate treatment to mitigate the increased risk associated with the disorder. PA comprises unilateral and bilateral forms which are specifically treatable and thus must be accurately differentiated. Unilateral PA is usually treated by unilateral adrenalectomy (to remove the source of aldosterone excess); bilateral PA is mainly treated pharmacologically with mineralocorticoid receptor antagonists (MRA) (Funder et al. 2016; Young 2019).

Adrenal venous sampling (AVS) is the recommended method by the Endocrine Society guideline to differentiate unilateral from bilateral forms (Funder et al. 2016). AVS has improved sensitivity over nonfunctional imaging methods (Kempers et al. 2009; Mathur et al. 2010; Williams et al. 2018) although specific imaging and biochemical characteristics may accurately predict unilateral PA in young individuals (Umakoshi et al. 2018; Williams et al. 2018). Surgical treatment of unilateral PA

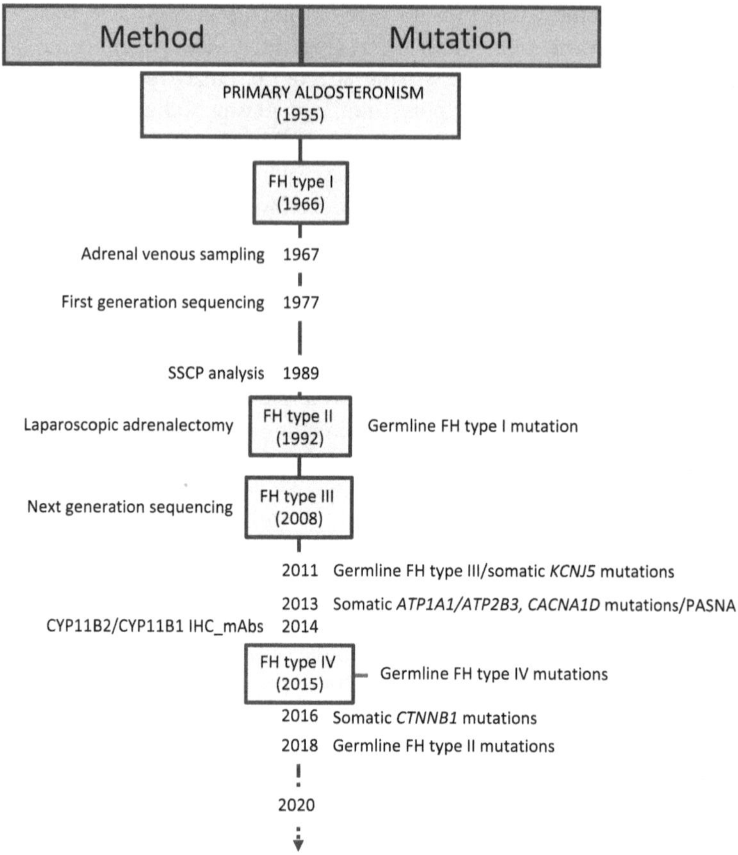

First description	Reference	Identification of driver mutation
PA (APA)	Conn 1955	Choi 2011 Beuschlein 2013 Azizan 2013 Scholl 2013 Åkerström 2016
FH type I	Sutherland 1966	Lifton 1992
FH type II	Stowasser 1992	Scholl 2018 Fernandes-Rosa 2018
FH type III	Geller 2008*	Choi 2011
FH type IV	Scholl 2015	Scholl 2015
PASNA	Scholl 2013	Scholl 2013

Method	Reference
Adrenal venous sampling	Melby 1967
Laparoscopic adrenalectomy	Gagner 1992
First generation sequencing	Sanger 1977
SSCP analysis	Orita 1989
Next generation sequencing	Wheeler 2008
CYP11B2/CYP11B1 mAbs	Gomez-Sanchez 2014

Fig. 11.1 Timeline of breakthrough discoveries in the genetics in primary aldosteronism. The first description of each familial form of PA is shown in boxes with the relative year of publication, associated causative mutations are indicated on the right, and innovative methods contributing to major insights into the genetics and pathophysiology of PA are on the left. References are shown in the table. FH, familial hyperaldosteronism; SSCP, single-strand conformation polymorphism

should resolve the excess aldosterone secretion in all patients. Persistence of aldosteronism after adrenalectomy may indicate that the initial diagnosis was incorrect, with the patient having bilateral rather than unilateral disease (Williams et al. 2017; Yang et al. 2018). Resolution of hypertension is achieved in less than half of patients with significant clinical benefits obtained in the majority of surgically treated patients for unilateral PA (Williams et al. 2017; Burrello et al. 2019). Medically treated patients display similar cardiovascular outcomes as patients with primary hypertension if the MRA dosage is titrated to increase plasma renin activity ≥1 μg/L/h (Hundemer et al. 2018).

PA describes a group of disorders which comprise sporadic and familial forms. Sporadic PA is commonly caused by unilateral aldosterone-producing adenomas (APA) or bilateral adrenal hyperplasia (BAH), less often by unilateral adrenal hyperplasia (Åkerström et al. 2012) and very rarely by an aldosterone-producing carcinoma. There are four familial forms recognized to date (familial hyperaldosteronism types I–IV) that are autosomal dominant traits accounting for less than 5% of all diagnosed cases of PA (Perez-Rivas et al. 2018; Young 2019, Figure 1, Table). Somatic APA mutations have been described in genes encoding ion channels (*KCNJ5, CACNA1D*) and ion transporters (*ATP1A1*, *ATP2B3*) and these mutations are thought to specifically drive aldosterone excess (Prada et al. 2017; Monticone et al. 2018a), whereas mutations in *CTNNB1* (Åkerström et al. 2016) and the rare somatic mutations associated with APA (*PRKACA*, *GNAS*) are also found in cortisol-producing adenomas and are likely to play a role in cell proliferation (Zennaro et al. 2017) (Fig. 11.1).

The role of genetics in the pathophysiology of PA has become increasingly clear with the identification of somatic and germline mutations that drive constitutive aldosterone production in sporadic APA and familial PA marking a milestone in our understanding of this common form of endocrine hypertension.

11.2 Germline Mutations Causing Primary Aldosteronism

11.2.1 Chimeric 11β-Hydroxylase/Aldosterone Synthase (CYP11B1/CYP11B2) *Gene in Familial Hyperaldosteronism Type I*

The first inherited form of PA, later referred to as familial hyperaldosteronism type I (FH type I), was described in 1966 by Sutherland and coworkers in a father and his son characterized with benign hypertension, potassium deficiency, increased aldosterone secretion, and suppressed renin plasma activity (Sutherland et al. 1966, Figure 1). Adrenal exploration did not find a tumor but revealed an enlarged left adrenal which was surgically removed. Macroscopically the resected gland (weighing 7 g) showed multiple nodules of 0.1–0.4 cm diameter which were microscopically composed of mainly clear zF (zona fasciculata) cells. Hypertension persisted postsurgery, but subsequent examination of the son revealed an increase in serum potassium concentrations in response to dexamethasone. Because of this, a controlled study on the father was initiated which demonstrated clearly the increase of serum potassium and the reduction of serum sodium concentrations and blood pressure in response to dexamethasone (Sutherland et al. 1966). Sutherland realized he had described a form of hyperaldosteronism distinct from the original case described by Conn (1955), and the syndrome was subsequently referred to as glucocorticoid-remediable aldosteronism (GRA) and successively as FH type I (Sutherland et al. 1966).

In 1992, Lifton and coworkers defined the molecular basis of FH type I. They demonstrated that a gene duplication arising from the unequal crossing-over of the closely linked *CYP11B1* and *CYP11B2* genes (encoding the 95% identical cytochrome P450 enzymes 11ß-hydroxylase and aldosterone synthase, respectively) results in fusion of regulatory sequences of *CYP11B1* (comprising the adrenocorticotropic hormone [ACTH]-responsive promoter) with coding sequences of *CYP11B2* (encoding aldosterone synthase) (Lifton et al. 1992a). The site of crossing-over occurs at regions of greatest sequence identity between *CYP11B1* and *CYP11B2* with variable positions described between the start of intron 2 to intron 4 (especially the intron 2 to exon 3 junction and exon 4–intron 4 region) (Lifton et al. 1992b; MacConnachie et al. 1998; Carvajal et al. 2011).

CYP11B1 is normally expressed in the zF, regulated by ACTH, and CYP11B2 in the zona glomerulosa (zG), regulated by angiotensin II and K^+ (Miller and Auchus 2011; Stowasser and Gordon 2016). The chimeric *CYP11B1/CYP11B2* gene encodes aldosterone synthase regulated by ACTH, thus explaining the ectopic expression of aldosterone synthase in the zF and the decreased production of aldosterone by glucocorticoids (such as dexamethasone) via suppression of ACTH secretion (Fig. 11.2) (Lifton et al. 1992a). The abnormal colocalization of aldosterone synthase with 17 α-hydroxylase (CYP17A1) and cortisol in the zF can account for the elevated production of the two "hybrid steroids" 18-hydroxycortisol and 18-oxocortisol (Ulick and Chu 1982; Gomez-Sanchez et al. 1984; Lenders et al. 2018).

The Endocrine Society guideline recommends genetic testing for FH type I in all patients with early-onset (<20 years of age) PA and for those with a family history of the disease (Funder et al. 2016). Instead of measurement of hybrid steroids or glucocorticoid response, diagnosis is usually now made by the highly specific and sensitive PCR amplification of a large fragment of the chimeric gene (Stowasser et al. 1997). FH type I symptoms range from mild to severe with an increased risk of cerebrovascular complications, hemorrhagic stroke, and intercranial aneurysms (Litchfield et al. 1998; Mulatero et al. 2002). FH type I is treated with low-dose glucocorticoids with additional administration of MRAs if required (Funder et al. 2016) (Table 11.1).

11.2.2 ClC-2 (CLCN2) Chloride Channel Mutations in Familial Hyperaldosteronism Type II

Familial hyperaldosteronism type II (FH type II) was first described by Gordon et al. as a familial form with a clinically distinct phenotype from FH type I (Gordon et al.

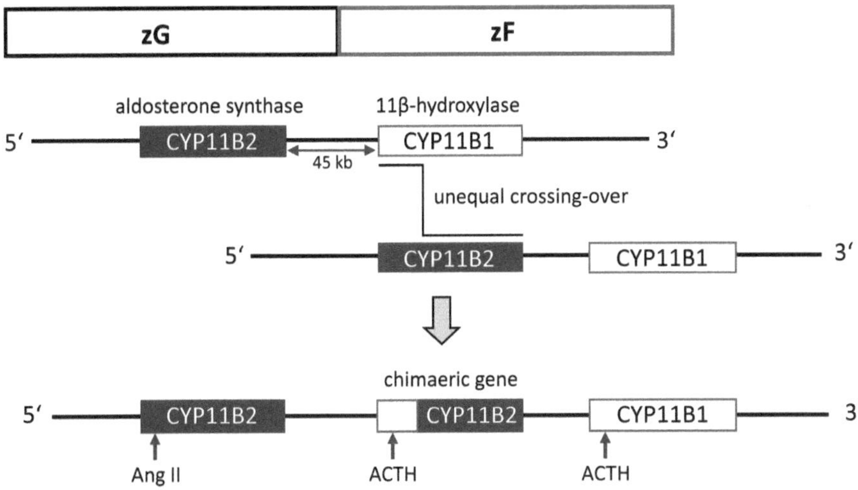

Fig. 11.2 A *CYP11B2/CYP11B1* chimeric gene causes FH type I. FH type I is caused by a gene duplication arising from an unequal crossing-over between the highly homologous *CYP11B2* and *CYP11B1* genes. The point of crossing-over occurs between intron 2 and intron 4 (Lifton et al. 1992b). The resulting chimeric gene has the ACTH-responsive promoter of *CYP11B1* driving the ectopic expression of aldosterone synthase in the zona fasciculata (zF) instead of the zona glomerulosa (zG)

1991) (Fig. 11.1). Genetic linkage to chromosome region 7p22 was suspected (Lafferty et al. 2000), but no causative mutations were identified despite next-generation sequencing (NGS) of the entire linked locus (Stowasser and Gordon 2016). In 2018, Scholl et al. performed exome sequencing of 3 individuals diagnosed with FH type II from a multiplex family originally described by Stowasser et al. (1992) and (Scholl et al. (2018). A heterozygous missense mutation in the *CLCN2* gene was identified encoding p.Arg172Gln in ClC-2, a voltage-gated chloride channel. Additional members of the kindred were identified carrying the same variant; 7 of the 8 mutant ClC-2-Arg172Gln carriers had elevated ARRs but one carrier was normotensive and did not have an elevated ARR, indicating incomplete penetrance (Scholl et al. 2018) (Fig. 11.1).

Exome analysis of 35 unrelated individuals with an extreme phenotype with early-onset PA by the age of 10 years also identified the ClC-2-Arg172Gln variant in one individual in addition to two further missense mutations, p.Met22Lys (occurring de novo) and p.Tyr26Asn, and an in frame deletion, p.Lys362del. Exome analysis of an additional 45 unrelated individuals with early-onset PA by the age of 20 years identified another variant in ClC-2 (p.Ser865Arg) and two further independent occurrences of p.Arg172Gln (one de novo) (Scholl et al. 2018). Thus, in all, Scholl identified 5 novel variants in ClC-2 comprising p.Arg172Gln (4 independent occurrences), p.Met22Lys, p.Tyr26Asn, p.Lys362del, and Ser865Arg from 81 probands with early-onset PA. Because the first missense ClC-2 variant was discovered in the original family described with FH type II by Stowasser et al.

Table 11.1 Target genes for germline and somatic mutations in primary aldosteronism

Diagnosis	Target Gene	Affected Protein	Chromosome	OMIM Gene/ locus	OMIM Phenotype	Mutation Type	Prevalence	Phenotype	Treatment
FH type I	*CYP11B1/ CYP11B2*	Aldosterone synthase (cytochrome P450 enzyme)	8q24.3	*610613.0002	#103900	Germline Heterozygous AD	Rare	Abnormal expression of aldosterone synthase in zF Elevated hybrid steroid production Usually severe, early-onset, associated with stroke at young age	Dexamethasone MRA
FH type II	*CLCN2*	ClC-2 (voltage-gated Cl^- channel)	3q27.1	*600570	#605635	Germline Heterozygous AD	Extremely rare	Variable clinical phenotype Usually severe, early-onset	Unilateral ADX MRA
FH type III	*KCNJ5*	GIRK4 (inwardly rectifying K^+ channel)	11q24.3	*600734	#613677	Germline Heterozygous AD	Extremely rare	Usually severe, early-onset	Bilateral ADX MRA
FH type IV	*CACNA1H*	$Ca_v3.2$ (T-type Ca^{2+} channel)	16p13.3	*607904	#617027	Germline Heterozygous AD	Extremely rare	Variable clinical phenotype Usually severe, early-onset	Unilateral ADX MRA CCB
PASNA	*CACNA1D*	$Ca_v1.3$ (L-type Ca^{2+} channel)	3p21.1	*114206	#615474	Germline Heterozygous AD	Extremely rare	Severe neurological abnormalities	MRA CCB
APA	*KCNJ5*	GIRK4 (inwardly rectifying K^+ channel)	11q24.3	–	–	Sporadic Heterozygous	35–80% of APA	Variable clinical phenotype	Unilateral ADX

APA	*CACNA1D*	$Ca_v1.3$ (L-type Ca^{2+} channel)	3p21.1	–	–	Sporadic Heterozygous	10% of APA	Variable clinical phenotype	Unilateral ADX
APA	*ATP1A1*	Na^+/K^+-ATPase 1	1p13.1	–	–	Sporadic Heterozygous	5% of APA	Variable clinical phenotype	Unilateral ADX
APA	*ATP2B3*	Ca^{2+}-ATPase 3	Xq28	–	–	Sporadic Heterozygous	1–3% of APA	Variable clinical phenotype	Unilateral ADX

AD, autosomal dominant; ADX, adrenalectomy; APA, aldosterone-producing adenoma; CCB, calcium channel blocker; FH, familial hyperaldosteronism; MRA, mineralocorticoid receptor antagonist; OMIM, online Mendelian inheritance in man; PASNA, primary aldosteronism with severe neurological abnormalities; zF, zona fasciculata

(1992), this form of PA caused by ClC-2 mutations is referred to as FH type II (Scholl et al. 2018).

ClC-2 is present in several tissues and ClC-2 immunohistochemistry demonstrated strong localized immunostaining to the zG cells of the human adrenal cortex consistent with a role in aldosterone production (Scholl et al. 2018). Patch-clamp electrophysiology recordings using human embryonic kidney cells (HEK 293T cells) expressing either wild-type or a mutated ClC-2 channel demonstrated that variants cause a shift in voltage activation resulting in a higher open probability than the wild-type channel. In zG cells, the gating changes observed with the ClC-2 mutants would be predicted to cause increased chloride efflux at resting potential (Scholl et al. 2018), and in human NCI H295R adrenocortical cells, expression of ClC-2 mutants caused a significant increase in *CYP11B2* gene (encoding aldosterone synthase) expression (Scholl et al. 2018).

Fernandes-Rosa et al. (2018) identified a de novo mutation in *CLCN2*, distinct from those described by Scholl et al. (2018) encoding ClC-2-Gly24Asp in a nine-year-old patient diagnosed with PA (Fernandes-Rosa et al. 2018) (Fig. 11.1). Patch-clamp analysis of zG cells in mouse adrenal gland slices (from *Clcn2*$^{-/-}$ versus *Clcn2*$^{+/+}$ mice) demonstrated the pivotal role of ClC-2 in mediating chloride currents in glomerulosa cells. Electrophysiological recordings of *Xenopus* oocytes expressing either wild-type ClC-2 or ClC-2-Gly24Asp showed that the mutation caused a strong increase in chloride conductance at resting potentials and expression in human adrenocortical cells increased aldosterone synthase expression. The reports of Scholl et al. (2018) and Fernandes-Rosa et al. (2018) were the first to establish a function for an anion channel in aldosterone biosynthesis, primary aldosteronism, and hypertension (Fernandes-Rosa et al. 2018; Scholl et al. 2018).

11.2.3 GIRK4 (KCNJ5) Potassium Channel Mutations in Familial Hyperaldosteronism Type III

The index case of FH type III was reported in 1959 in a 10-year-old boy with a history of frequent headaches (since the age of 3 years), polydipsia, polyuria, and enuresis (Therien et al. 1959; Geller et al. 2008). Severe hypertension, hypokalemia, metabolic alkalosis, elevated urinary aldosterone, and low urinary sodium concentrations led to the diagnosis of PA. Bilateral adrenalectomy normalized blood pressure 16 days after surgery. Adrenal pathology showed bilateral enlargement (right, 8 g; left, 8.96 g) and massive cortical hyperplasia with focal nodules of the zF. At 1 year after surgery, the patient was normotensive, cured of headaches, polyuria, polydipsia, and enuresis, and received maintenance steroid replacement therapy with satisfactory outcome (Therien et al. 1959; Geller et al. 2008).

The index case subsequently had 2 daughters who presented with severe hypertension aged 7 and 4 years (Geller et al. 2008) (Fig. 11.1). Both were markedly hypokalemic with elevated serum aldosterone concentrations despite suppressed plasma renin activity. Dexamethasone failed to suppress serum aldosterone levels or improve blood pressure levels. The young patients were lost to follow-up but presented again aged 18 and 15 years with severe hypertension, despite multiple antihypertensive medications, hypokalemia, and exceptionally high urinary concentrations of 18-oxocortisol and 18-hydroxycortisol. As observed 10 years earlier, dexamethasone did not improve blood pressure and failed to suppress both serum aldosterone concentrations (which were doubled) and cortisol levels after a 1-week trial (0.5 mg dexamethasone twice daily) (Geller et al. 2008). Bilateral adrenalectomy normalized blood pressure and serum potassium levels within 2 weeks. Pathologic examination noted bilateral enlargement and massive diffuse hyperplasia of the zF with no evidence of nodularity.

Pedigree analysis indicated autosomal dominant transmission of the trait with the father of the index case, who died aged 36 years of severe hypertension and heart failure, the presumed source of the causative mutation (Geller et al. 2008). Geller et al. attempted to identify variants in affected individuals of the kindred by single-strand conformation polymorphism (SSCP) and direct DNA sequence analysis of candidate genes but could not pinpoint a disease-causing mutation (Geller et al. 2008). Despite this, a new hereditary form of PA with a distinct phenotype had been described and was designated FH type III (Mulatero 2008).

Shortly after Geller's description (2008), advances in DNA sequencing technology helped uncover the genetic basis of FH type III. As discussed later, exome sequencing of APAs identified somatic mutations in the *KCNJ5* gene which encodes the G protein-activated inwardly rectifying K^+ channel (GIRK4) (Choi et al. 2011). Thus, subsequent direct sequencing of *KCNJ5* in the 3 affected individuals in the kindred described by Geller et al. (2008) found a heterozygous mutation encoding a GIRK4-p.Thr158Ala variant (Choi et al. 2011) (Fig. 11.1). This was followed shortly after by the identification of other kindreds with FH type III carrying GIRK4 mutations (p.Gly151Glu or p.Gly151Arg) (Mulatero et al. 2012b; Scholl et al. 2012) with contrasting clinical phenotypes. GIRK4-Gly151Arg carriers in the two kindreds described by Scholl et al. (2012) had severe progressive aldosteronism and bilateral hyperplasia requiring bilateral adrenalectomy to control blood pressure. In contrast, hypertension of GIRK4-p.Gly151Glu carriers was controlled with spironolactone, and adrenal imaging showed no evidence of hyperplasia. Electrophysiology recordings in vitro demonstrated the more extreme effect of p. Gly151Glu which caused greater Na^+ ion conductance and increased cell lethality than p.Gly151Arg (Scholl et al. 2012). The increased cell death induced by p. Gly151Glu can account for the limited adrenocortical mass and the milder aldosteronism of patients carrying this variant compared with patients with p.Gly151Arg.

A characteristic feature of adrenal zG cells is the high negative potential (−80 mV), determined primarily by K^+ conductance (Spat and Hunyady 2004) which appears to be mediated in humans by the two-pore domain "leak" K^+ channel TASK1 (Nogueira et al. 2010). GIRK4 is highly expressed in the zG and exists as homo-tetramers or as hetero-tetramers with GIRK subunits (GIRK1, GIRK2, GIRK3) depending on cell type and tissue (Gomez-Sanchez and Oki 2014). Expression of the GIRK4-Gly151Arg and GIRK4-Thr158Ala mutant channels in HEK

293T (human embryonic kidney 293T) cells demonstrated that the mutations cause a loss of channel selectivity for K^+ and an influx of Na^+ into the cells (Choi et al. 2011). This effect was much milder for p.Thr158Ala than p.Gly151Arg, and a later study by Scholl et al. (2012) demonstrated the more profound effect of p.Gly151Glu on Na^+ influx than p.Gly151Arg. In zG cells, Na^+ influx would cause depolarization of the cell membrane and opening of voltage-gated Ca^{2+} channels and trigger Ca^{2+} signaling-mediated activation of *CYP11B2* transcription and aldosterone biosynthesis (Clyne et al. 1996; Spat and Hunyady 2004; Choi et al. 2011). The direct demonstration for an effect of a GIRK4 mutation on aldosterone production came from Oki et al. (2012) by transduction of human adrenocortical HAC15 cells with a lentivirus carrying mutated *KCNJ5* encoding GIRK4-Thr158Ala which produced a 5.3-fold increase in aldosterone production under basal conditions relative to wild type (Oki et al. 2012).

At least 12 families with FH type III have been described with 6 different mutations (Monticone et al. 2017b). The residue usually mutated in FH type III is Gly151 of the GlyTyrGly signature sequence for the selectivity filter of potassium channels (Heginbotham et al. 1992). Patients with FH type III exhibit variable clinical features but are mostly early onset with severe forms of the disease (Table 11.1).

11.2.4 $Ca_v3.2$ (*CACNA1H*) Calcium Channel Mutations in Familial Hyperaldosteronism Type IV

Scholl et al. (2015b) identified five individuals of 40 unrelated patients with early-onset PA (by age 10 years) carrying a heterozygous variant in the *CACNA1H* gene encoding a gain-of-function $Ca_v3.2$-Met1549Val mutation (Scholl et al. 2015b). The mutation carriers had similar clinical phenotypes with severe early-onset hypertension, elevated ARRs, and no evidence of an adrenal mass or hyperplasia at imaging. Because FH type III was defined at this point by mutations in GIRK4, $Ca_v3.2$ variants classify a new familial form of PA, FH type IV (Fig. 11.1; Table 11.1).

$Ca_v3.2$ is a member of the T-type α1-subunit family of the low-voltage-gated calcium channels and comprises the pore-forming subunit for Ca^{2+} import. The p. Met1549Val mutation occurs within a Met-Phe-Val conserved motif that regulates channel inactivation (Marksteiner et al. 2001). Shortly after Scholl's report (2015), a patient with a de novo $Ca_v3.2$-Met1549Ile mutation with PA diagnosed aged 2 months (who later had an additional diagnosis of multiplex developmental disorder) was also described (Daniil et al. 2016).

Expression of $Ca_v3.2$-Met1549Val in HEK 293T cells and electrophysiology recordings reported a slightly reduced activation followed by a tenfold slower channel inactivation. Further, the mutated channels displayed a shift of channel activation at less depolarizing potentials. Thus, Ca^{2+} influx is mediated by the mutant channel at lower membrane potentials and the channel pore remains open for longer resulting in increased Ca^{2+} influx (Scholl et al. 2015b). Expression of $Ca_v3.2$-Met1549Val in human adrenocortical cells (HAC15 and NCI H295R cells) resulted in a sevenfold increase in aldosterone production compared with control cells (empty vector transfected cells), thereby formally demonstrating the effect of the mutation on increased aldosterone production (Reimer et al. 2016).

Three other $Ca_v3.2$ germline mutations were also described by Daniil et al. (2016) (p.Ser196Leu, p.Pro2083Leu, and p.Val1951Glu). These mutations, lying outside of the Met-Phe-Val signature motif, were all identified in patients diagnosed with PA at >35 years and presented with variable phenotypes. The p.Val1951Glu mutation was identified in a patient diagnosed with a unilateral adrenal nodule at imaging who was successfully treated by unilateral adrenalectomy (Daniil et al. 2016).

11.2.5 *$Ca_v1.3$ (CACNA1D) Calcium Channel Mutations in PASNA Syndrome*

The identification of somatic mutations in *CACNA1D* in APA, as discussed later, prompted Scholl et al. (2013) to search for germline variants in the same gene in 100 patients diagnosed with early-onset PA. Hotspot regions for mutations in *CACNA1D* were sequenced; 2 individuals with de novo germline heterozygous mutations encoding $Ca_v1.3$-Gly403Asp or $Ca_v1.3$-Ile770Met heterozygous mutations were identified (Scholl et al. 2013) (Fig. 11.1).

Both patients displayed severe hypertension (diagnosed in one case at birth and in the other at age 5 years) with elevated ARRs, but the clinical phenotype of both patients diverged from other early-onset forms of PA because additional serious neurologic abnormalities were evident with seizures and cerebral palsy, and thus, the condition was called primary aldosteronism with seizures and neurologic abnormalities (PASNA) (Scholl et al. 2013) (Fig. 11.1).

CACNA1D encodes $Ca_v1.3$, the pore-forming α-subunit of a voltage-gated L-type Ca^{2+} channel, the second most abundantly expressed Ca^{2+} channel in adrenal zG cells after $Ca_v3.2$ (Scholl et al. 2013). $Ca_v1.3$ is activated at large depolarizing potentials, in contrast to $Ca_v3.2$ which is activated by small changes in membrane potential. Electrophysiology studies of transiently expressed mutated or wild-type $Ca_v1.3$ demonstrated that p.Gly403Asp and p.Ile770Met shift the voltage dependence of channel activation to more hyperpolarized potentials which is likely to cause increased Ca^{2+} influx in zG cells, the stimulus for aldosterone biosynthesis (Scholl et al. 2013). The pore-forming α1-subunit of $Ca_v1.3$ comprises 4 homologous transmembrane (TM) repeat domains (repeat I-IV) which are each composed of 6 transmembrane segments. The p.Gly403Asp and p.Ile770Met missense mutations are each situated in S6 segments of homologous repeat domains I and II, respectively, suggesting a potential role for S6 in mediating pore gating (Scholl et al. 2013).

$Ca_v1.3$ is highly expressed in the brain and the neurological phenotype of PASNA is likely due to abnormal neuronal Ca^{2+} signaling. Indeed, at least seven

$Ca_V1.3$ mutations associated with autism spectrum disorders and epilepsy have also been identified (Pinggera and Striessnig 2016; Pinggera et al. 2017). Of these, three are located within a S6 segment (p.Val401Leu and p.Gly407Arg in TM repeat I; p. Ala749Gly in TM repeat II) but do not appear to be also associated with PA, although close monitoring of these carriers with biochemical assessment for PA would be recommended (Pinggera et al. 2017).

11.3 Somatic Variants Associated with Primary Aldosteronism

The discovery of somatic mutations in APAs was a major discovery in understanding the pathophysiology of these tumors. When mutation analysis is performed by NGS and targeted to regions of the adenoma specifically expressing aldosterone synthase, the proportion of APAs carrying a mutation in a target gene (*KCNJ5, CACNA1D, ATP1A1, ATP2B3, or CTNNB1*) reaches almost 90% (Nanba et al. 2018) (Fig. 11.1). The first somatic missense mutations associated with APA were identified by Choi in *KCNJ5* and reported together with the germline variant causing FH type III (Choi et al. 2011). Somatic APA *ATP1A1, ATP2B3*, and *CACNA1D* variants were reported 3 years later (Azizan et al. 2013; Beuschlein et al. 2013; Scholl et al. 2013) with the description of mutations in *CTNNB1* following shortly thereafter (Åkerström et al. 2016) (Fig. 11.1).

11.3.1 Somatic Variants in the K^+ Channel GIRK4 (KCNJ5)

Using exome sequencing, Choi et al. (2011) identified somatic mutations in *KCNJ5* encoding GIRK4-p.Gly151Arg or p.Leu168Arg missense mutations in 8 of 22 APAs (Choi et al. 2011). The p.Gly151Arg mutation was subsequently described as a germline hereditary mutation in a family with FH type III (Scholl et al. 2012) and the p.Thr158Ala mutation as a somatic mutation (albeit rarely) (Mulatero et al. 2012b). At least 17 different somatic APA-GIRK4 mutations have been identified which are usually located in or near the selectivity filter for K^+, but the majority of these are rare occurrences with the p.Gly151Arg and p.Leu168Arg missense mutations prevailing by far (Scholl et al. 2015a; Prada et al. 2017; Zennaro et al. 2018).

The high frequency of somatic *KCNJ5* variants in APAs found by Choi et al. (2011) was confirmed by 2 large multicenter studies the following year (Åkerström et al. 2012; Boulkroun et al. 2012). In one study, a prevalence of 34% was found in a cohort of 380 APAs collected through ENS@T (European Network for the Study of Adrenal Tumours, http://www.ensat.org) and reported the increased representation of *KCNJ5* mutations in women compared with men (49% versus 19%, $P < 0.001$) and an association of *KCNJ5* mutation status with younger patients and higher presurgical plasma aldosterone concentrations (Boulkroun et al. 2012). In the second study, GIRK4-p.Gly151Arg or p.Leu168Arg mutations were identified in APAs ($n = 339$) at a prevalence of 47% and were absent in 9 cases of unilateral hyperplasia (Åkerström et al. 2012). This report also noted the marked increased prevalence of *KCNJ5* mutations in women compared with men (63% versus 24%).

A later meta-analysis grouped data from 13 studies with 1636 patients diagnosed with an APA and reported the association of somatic *KCNJ5* mutations with a more pronounced hyperaldosteronism, younger age, women, and larger tumors (Lenzini et al. 2015). East Asian populations (60–80%) (Lenzini et al. 2015; Wang et al. 2015; Wu et al. 2015; Zheng et al. 2015) consistently report a higher incidence of APA *KCNJ5* mutations than Western populations (35–50%) (Åkerström et al. 2012; Boulkroun et al. 2012; Lenzini et al. 2015) which is potentially explained by a bias for surgical treatment of patients with a more severe phenotype driven by an APA with a *KCNJ5* mutation. There may be a referral bias for patients with unilateral PA over bilateral PA in centers in Japan because in a nationwide study, 86% of patients with PA were diagnosed with an APA versus 14% with BAH (Miyake et al. 2014) in contrast to around 30% of patients with unilateral PA in Western nations (Schirpenbach and Reincke 2007).

11.3.2 Somatic Mutations in the Ca^{2+} Channel $Ca_v1.3$ (CACNA1D)

Somatic variants in the Ca^{2+} channel $Ca_v1.3$, encoded by *CACNA1D*, are the second most frequent mutation associated with sporadic APAs with a prevalence of 9.3% (Fernandes-Rosa et al. 2014) (Fig. 11.1). Unlike APAs harboring *KCNJ5* mutations, which occur more often in the young and in women, APAs with somatic *CACNA1D* mutations are more prevalent in older patients and in men (Fernandes-Rosa et al. 2014). There are at least 31 known somatic APA mutations involving 25 amino acid residues (Prada et al. 2017) widely distributed throughout $Ca_v1.3$. These missense mutations may affect conserved sites in the pore-forming region, the voltage sensor, and a cytoplasmic linker of the voltage sensor with the pore (Azizan et al. 2013; Scholl et al. 2013). $Ca_v1.3$ variants have been shown to shift the voltage-dependent opening of the channel pore to more negative potentials and impair channel inactivation (Azizan et al. 2013; Scholl et al. 2013). In zG cells, these effects result in an increase in intracellular Ca^{2+} concentration and stimulation of *CYP11B2* gene transcription and aldosterone production.

APAs carrying *CACNA1D* mutations generally have a small diameter, often less than 1 cm (Azizan et al. 2013; Fernandes-Rosa et al. 2014), and are reported to comprise predominantly zG-like cells (although the number of adenomas with *CACNA1D* mutations assessed for histopathology is small and not all studies agree) (Azizan et al. 2013; Monticone et al. 2015; Scholl et al. 2015a). The small size of APA with *CACNA1D* mutations suggests they are more likely to be overlooked by nonfunctional imaging. Indeed, a much higher frequency of *CACNA1D* mutations was found in CYP11B2-positive adrenocortical micronodules from cross-sectional image negative adrenals surgically removed from patients diagnosed with unilateral PA (Yamazaki et al. 2017). Moreover, Ca^{2+} channel blockers are commonly used antihypertensive medications which could potentially mask cases of PA caused by APA with *CACNA1D* mutations.

11.3.3 Somatic Mutations in a Na^+/K^+-ATPase 1 (ATP1A1) and a Ca^{2+}-ATPase 3 (ATP2B3)

The Na^+/K^+- and Ca^{2+}-ATPases belong to the P-type ATPases (subclass P_2), a large family of active transporters characterized by the formation of phosphorylated enzyme intermediate (hence the name P type) in the pump mechanism for the temporary conservation of energy from ATP (Palmgren and Nissen 2011). Somatic variants in the Na^+/K^+-ATPase subunit α-1 (encoded by *ATP1A1*) and Ca^{2+}-ATPase 3 (encoded by *ATP2B3*) are found in 5% and 1–3% of APAs, respectively (Beuschlein et al. 2013; Fernandes-Rosa et al. 2014; Williams et al. 2014; Åkerström et al. 2015) (Fig. 11.1). Germline variants have been identified in both *ATP1A1* and *ATP2B3*, but no association with PA has been reported (Lassuthova et al. 2018; Schlingmann et al. 2018; Zanni et al. 2012).

The Na^+/K^+-ATPase is composed of a large catalytic α-subunit (which itself comprises multiple subunits) and a smaller β-subunit. The α-subunit functions in ATP hydrolysis coupled to Na^+ and K^+ exchange across the plasma membrane (3 Na^+ are exchanged outward for 2 K^+ inward against respective concentration gradients for the hydrolysis of 1 ATP); the role of the β-subunit is not well defined. Beuschlein et al. (2013) and Azizan et al. (2013) described missense mutations (p. Leu104Arg or p.Val332Gly) and an in-frame deletion (p.Phe100_Leu104del) in the α1-subunit (*ATP1A1*, a component of the α-subunit) of the Na^+/K^+-ATPase. The variants were situated in domains M1, M4, and M9 of the 10 transmembrane-domain (M1-M10) α1-subunit. M1 and M4 play a pivotal role in the binding and gating of K^+, and mutations of residues in these domains can disturb K^+ binding and impair pump function (Beuschlein et al. 2013; Williams et al. 2014), in contrast to alterations in M9 which may alter Na^+ binding (Fernandes-Rosa et al. 2017). The Na^+/K^+-ATPase p.Leu104Arg and p.Val332Gly mutations were shown to cause loss of pump activity and a strong reduction in K^+ binding (Beuschlein et al. 2013). Electrophysiology recordings of ex vivo primary cultures of adenoma cells with an *ATP1A1* or an *ATP2B3* mutation compared with cells from adjacent cortex without a mutation showed higher levels of membrane depolarization in the mutated cells (Beuschlein et al. 2013). Since the first reports of *ATP1A1* mutations, several other somatic *ATP1A1* mutations in APA have been reported (Williams et al. 2014; Åkerström et al. 2015; Kitamoto et al. 2016; Nishimoto et al. 2016b).

Plasma membrane Ca^{2+}-ATPase (PMCA) is a high Ca^{2+} affinity, low transport capacity pump which extrudes Ca^{2+} out of the cell to maintain intracellular Ca^{2+}

homeostasis (Brini and Carafoli 2011). Several isoforms and splice variants of Ca^{2+}-ATPase are known and a number of somatic APA mutations, mainly deletions, have been identified in Ca^{2+}-ATPase encoded by variants in *ATP2B3* (encoding Ca^{2+}-ATPase isoform 3).

The first somatic variants in *ATP2B3* associated with APA were reported by Beuschlein et al. (2013). Different in-frame deletions (c.1272_1277delGCTGGT and c.1273_1278delCTGGTC) causing the same deletion (p.Leu425_Val426del) of amino acids highly conserved across the P-type ATPases in the M4 transmembrane helix were discovered. The Ca^{2+}-ATPase Leu425_Val426del mutation is predicted to cause a major distortion of the Ca^{2+} binding site and an impaired ability to pump Ca^{2+} out of the cell resulting in increased intracellular Ca^{2+} concentrations (Beuschlein et al. 2013). A later study compared the electrophysiology of HEK 293 T cells and human adrenocortical cells expressing the mutated Ca^{2+} ATPase and the wild-type pump and confirmed the predicted reduced capacity to export Ca^{2+} and impaired pump function and further demonstrated an increased expression of CYP11B2 and aldosterone production in adrenal cells expressing Ca^{2+}-ATPase Leu425_Val426del (Tauber et al. 2016). Since the initial discovery of the Ca^{2+}-ATPase Leu425_Val426del variants, several groups have likewise reported deletion mutations in this ATPase, occurring within a restricted region from p.Thr423 to p. Leu433 (Åkerström et al. 2015; Scholl et al. 2015a; Kitamoto et al. 2016).

11.3.4 Somatic Mutations in β-Catenin (CTNNB1)

β-catenin plays a key role in the canonical WNT pathway that is crucial for embryonic development and tissue homeostasis. In the presence of the signal protein WNT, β-catenin accumulates in the cell and migrates to the nucleus to act as co-receptor for activating WNT responsive genes. In the absence of WNT, β-catenin is degraded via the ubiquitin-proteosome pathway (MacDonald et al. 2009). Activating somatic mutations have been described in *CTNNB1*, encoding β-catenin, in around 30% of nonfunctioning adenomas, cortisol-producing adenomas, and adrenocortical carcinomas (Tissier et al. 2005). The mutations were generally point mutations in exon 3, resulting in alteration of p.Ser45, a phosphorylation site within a signature motif for glycogen synthase kinase-3β. Tumors with these mutations always showed abnormal β-catenin accumulation within cells (in the cytoplasm and nucleus) indicating constitutive β-catenin activation. Evidence for constitutive activation of WNT/β-catenin signaling has also been reported in APAs (33 of 47, 70%). The deregulated WNT signaling is likely caused by decreased expression of the WNT inhibitor SFRP2 (secreted frizzled related protein 2) (Berthon et al. 2014). Somatic *CTNNB1* mutations in APAs have been reported albeit at a lower frequency than for other adrenocortical adenomas with a prevalence of 2–5% (Scholl et al. 2015a; Åkerström et al. 2016), and thus additional factors account for the high proportion of tumors with constitutive WNT/β-catenin signaling (Berthon et al. 2014) (Fig. 11.1).

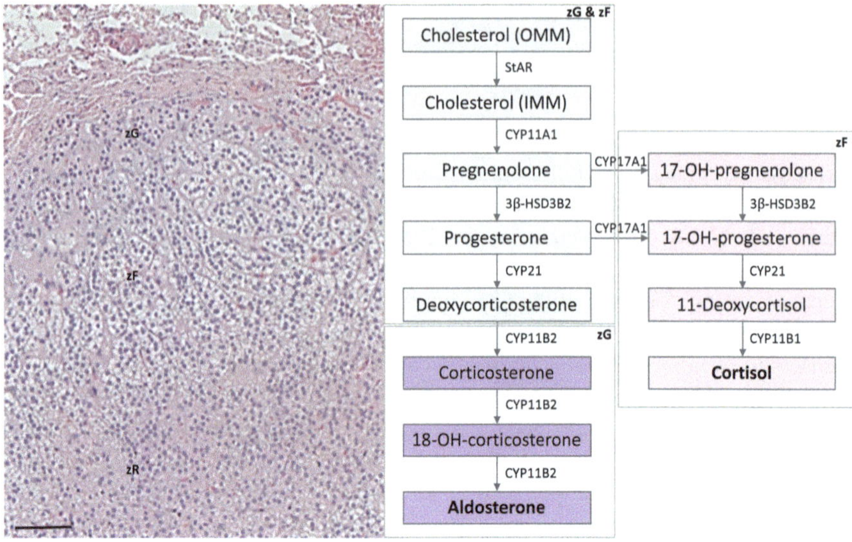

Fig. 11.3 Adrenocortical zonation and steroidogenesis. Hematoxylin and eosin (H&E) staining of a normal human adrenal (left panel) showing the histology of the three cortical zones and schematic overview of steroidogenesis in the zG and zF (right panel). OMM, outer mitochondrial membrane; IMM, inner mitochondrial membrane; CYP11A1, cholesterol side-chain cleavage enzyme; CYP17A1, 17α-hydroxylase; 3β-HSD3B2, 3β-hydroxysteroid dehydrogenase; CYP21, 21-hydroxylase; CYP11B2, aldosterone synthase; CYP11B1, 11β hydroxylase; zG, zona glomerulosa; zF, zona fasciculata; zR, zona reticularis. Scale bar = 100 μm

11.4 Adrenal Histopathology in Primary Aldosteronism

Most of the enzymes involved in aldosterone biosynthesis are expressed in both the zG and the zF, but the restricted synthesis of aldosterone to the zG and of cortisol to the zF (referred to as functional zonation) (Fig. 11.3) is determined by the expression of the terminal enzymes for aldosterone biosynthesis (aldosterone synthase, CYP11B2) and cortisol synthesis (11β hydroxylase, CYP11B1) in the respective functional zones. CYP11B2 and CYP11B1 are 95% identical at the amino acid levels (Lifton et al. 1992a, b). Despite this high level of identity, polyclonal antibodies were developed to CYP11B2 and CYP11B1 and used in immunohistochemistry to describe the presence of nests of CYP11B2 expressing cells beneath the capsule which the authors called aldosterone-producing cell clusters (APCCs) (Nishimoto et al. 2010) (Fig. 11.4). In 2014, specific monoclonal antibodies against CYP11B2 and CYP11B1 were developed for high amplification immunohistochemistry and immunofluorescence (Gomez-Sanchez et al. 2014) (Figs. 11.1, 11.4, and 11.5). Celso Gomez-Sanchez subsequently made the antibodies freely available upon request to a high number of research groups with commercial availability from Sigma-Millipore for clinical applications (a requirement in some countries). These were followed shortly after by the development, also by Gomez-Sanchez, of

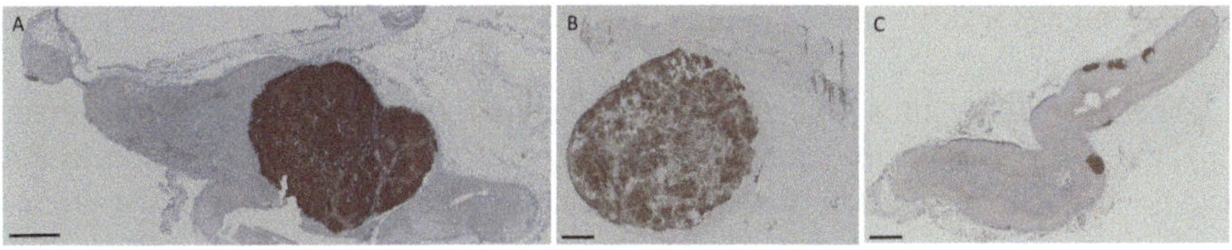

Fig. 11.4 CYP11B2 immunohistochemistry of human adrenals. CYP11B2 immunohistochemistry of adrenals resected from patients diagnosed with unilateral PA demonstrates the heterogeneity of CYP11B2 expression and the distinct histopathologic feature referred to as aldosterone-producing cell cluster (APCC). Panel A, an APA with strong homogeneous CYP11B2 expression; Panel B, an APA with strong but highly heterogeneous CYP11B2 expression; Panel C, an adrenal showing multiple APCCs. Immunohistochemistry was performed using a specific mouse monoclonal antibody against CYP11B2, a kind gift from Prof Celso E Gomez-Sanchez, University of Mississippi Medical Center, Jackson, MS, USA

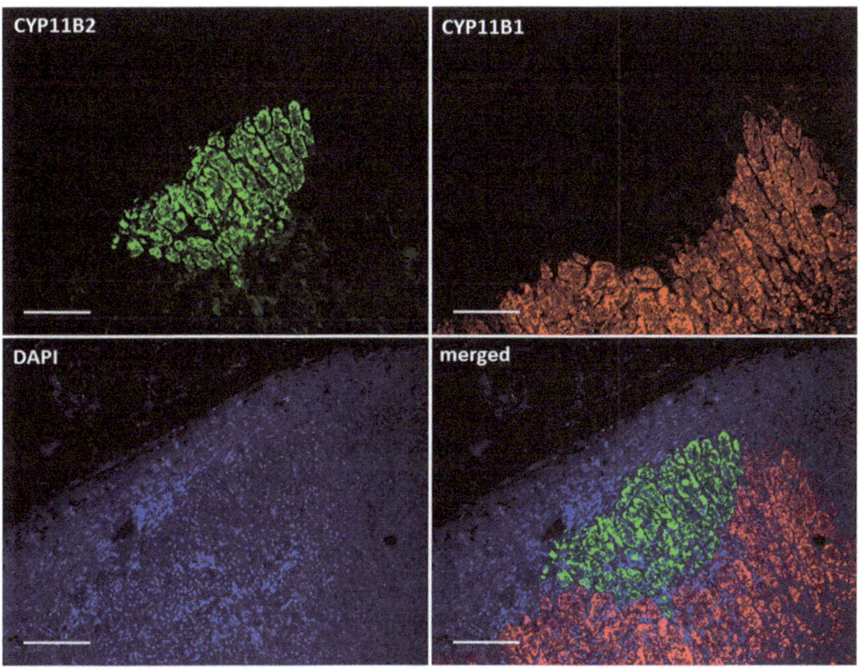

Fig. 11.5 Double immunofluorescence staining of an aldosterone-producing cell cluster. Double immunofluorescence staining of an aldosterone-producing cell cluster from a normal human adrenal using monoclonal mouse CYP11B2 and rat CYP11B1 antibodies and donkey Alexa Fluor 488 anti-mouse and Alexa Fluor 594 anti-rat secondary antibodies. Cell nuclei are stained with DAPI. Scale bars = 200 μm. Monoclonal antibodies to CYP11B2 and CYP11B1 were a kind gift from Prof Celso E Gomez-Sanchez, University of Mississippi Medical Center, Jackson, MS, USA

another highly specific monoclonal antibody against 17α-hydroxylase (CYP17A1) (Nakamura et al. 2016).

The availability of specific monoclonal antibodies against key steroidogenic enzymes has revealed the complex heterogeneity of the diseased adrenal in PA and has had a tremendous impact on understanding the histopathology of the adrenal under normal and diseased states (Nakamura et al. 2014, 2016; Fernandes-Rosa et al. 2015a, 2015b; Monticone et al. 2015; Gomez-Sanchez et al. 2017a; Gomez-Sanchez et al. 2017b; Omata et al. 2017b, 2018; Meyer et al. 2018; Seccia et al. 2018) (Fig. 11.1). APAs display CYP11B2 expression of variable intensity which can be homogeneous or heterogeneous (Fig. 11.4). A clear adenoma with CYP11B2 expression will often have APCCs and hyperplasia in the adjacent zG (Boulkroun et al. 2010; Nanba et al. 2013).

The majority of APAs comprise predominantly clear, lipid-laden zF-like cells, and as far back as 1992, Gordon et al. reported that these APAs were ACTH sensitive and responsible for production of the hybrid steroids 18-oxocortisol and 18-hydroxycortisol (Gordon et al. 1992). They also noted angiotensin II-responsive APAs with a distinct morphologic composition comprising around 20% of zG-like cells in patients who do not produce hybrid steroids. The morphologic difference was proposed to have an underlying genetic basis, a thesis which preceded Choi's discovery of somatic APA *KCNJ5* mutations by almost 10 years (Gordon et al. 1992). Evidence supporting a genetic basis for morphologic heterogeneity in APA was first obtained by Azizan et al. (2012) with the demonstration that APAs with *KCNJ5* mutations comprise predominantly zF cells with higher *CYP17A1* expression than APAs without *KCNJ5* mutations (Azizan et al. 2012), and several groups have supported this finding (Dekkers et al. 2014; Åkerström et al. 2015; Monticone et al. 2015; Scholl et al. 2015a; Yamazaki et al. 2018) also reporting higher CYP11B1 and CYP17A1 expression by immunohistochemistry (Monticone et al. 2015; Inoue et al. 2018). As well as the zF-like morphologic phenotype of adrenals carrying a *KCNJ5* mutation, they also appear to have a distinctive transcriptome signature (Åkerström et al. 2015).

Increased hybrid steroid concentrations have been consistently reported in patients with PA relative to normotensive individuals or patients with primary hypertension, but this is limited to patients with an APA and not to those with BAH (Ulick et al. 1993; Yamakita et al. 1994; Stowasser et al. 1996; Mosso et al. 2001; Mulatero et al. 2012a; Satoh et al. 2015; Eisenhofer et al. 2016). As mentioned above, Gordon et al. (1992) reported the production of hybrid steroids by ACTH-responsive APAs with zF-like cells which fits well with the later finding of increased production of 18-hydroxycortisol and 18-oxocortisol only in patients with an APA carrying *KCNJ5* mutations (Williams et al. 2016). The reason for the increased production of the hybrid steroids in APA with *KCNJ5* mutations is likely due to colocalization of CYP11B2 and CYP17A1 (with the latter necessary to supply the required precursor metabolites) (Gomez-Sanchez and Williams 2018). Thus, co-expression of CYP11B2 and CYP17A1 by immunofluorescence should identify cells with the potential to produce hybrid steroids (Nakamura et al. 2016; Gomez-Sanchez et al. 2017b; Gomez-Sanchez and Williams 2018). Accordingly, an aberrant co-expression of CYP17A1 with CYP11B2 was observed in many cells by immunofluorescence in two siblings with FH type III (and only few cells showed co-expression of CYP11B1 and CYP11B2) explaining the abnormally high production of 18-oxocortisol in these individuals (Gomez-Sanchez et al. 2017b).

11.5 The Pathophysiological Role of Aldosterone-Producing Cell Clusters

APCCs were first identified as distinct nests of CYP11B2-positive cells located beneath the adrenal capsule (Nishimoto et al. 2010). The cell clusters extend into the zF and display strong immunostaining for CYP11B2 but are negative for CYP11B1 and CYP17A1 immunostaining (Boulkroun et al. 2010; Omata et al. 2017a) (Figs. 11.4 and 11.5). The zG adjacent to an APA frequently displays APCCs when it would be expected that high aldosterone production by the tumor would suppress CYP11B2 in the peri-tumoral tissue. NGS of APCCs demonstrated that they carry known driver mutations for aldosterone excess (in *CACNA1D* and in *ATP1A1* and *ATP2B3* but very rarely in *KCNJ5*) even when found in normal adrenals (Nanba et al. 2013; Nishimoto et al. 2015; Nanba et al. 2017).

Continuous CYP11B2 expression in the zG of the young (<12 years) progressively changes to a discontinuous expression with aging associated with an accumulation of APCCs (Nishimoto et al. 2016a; Nanba et al. 2017). Any pathophysiological relevance of these observations is unclear, but age-related abnormal aldosterone physiology has been inferred from a cohort of normal individuals with a positive association of the ARR and autonomous aldosteronism with increasing age (Nanba et al. 2017).

CYP11B2 immunohistochemistry of 15 adrenals of patients with bilateral PA suggested that an increase in number or size of APCCs with somatic mutations may underlie the constitutive aldosterone production in these cases (Omata et al. 2018). In a different study design, Meyer et al. (2018) compared the histopathology of 43 adrenals from patients diagnosed with unilateral PA with postsurgical persistent aldosteronism (absent or partial biochemical success) (Williams et al. 2017) with that of 52 adrenals from age- and sex-matched patients with biochemical cure (complete biochemical success) (Meyer et al. 2018). The persistence of aldosteronism after unilateral adrenalectomy indicates that the diagnosis was incorrect and the underlying disorder was likely bilateral PA with asymmetrical aldosterone production and thus a different phenotype from the study of Omata et al. (2018). Meyer et al. reported a higher prevalence of adrenals with evidence of hyperplasia and a lower prevalence of solitary functional adenomas in adrenals from patients with persistent aldosteronism after surgery (and likely bilateral PA with asymmetrical aldosterone production) compared with patients with age- and sex-matched adrenals who were biochemically cured indicating a role for CYP11B2 immunohistochemistry to identify patients requiring close postsurgical follow-up (Meyer et al. 2018; Volpe et al. 2019).

11.6 Pathogenesis of Aldosterone-Producing Adenomas

In the initial paper by Choi et al. (2011), Ca^{2+} influx caused by somatic APA *KCNJ5* mutations was proposed to account for both enhanced cell proliferation and aldosterone production because Ca^{2+} has an established role in both functions (Berridge 1995; Clyne et al. 1996). However, the expression of a mutation causing FH type III and sporadic PA (GIRK-Thr158Ala) (Choi et al. 2011; Mulatero et al. 2012b) in adrenocortical cells resulted in enhanced aldosterone production but not an increase in cell proliferation (Oki et al. 2012). However, APAs are slow-growing tumors, developing over very many years, and proliferative effects of mutations may not be easily observable using cell culture systems.

APCCs have been proposed as a potential origin of APAs transitioning via a histopathologic structure referred to as pAATLs (potential APCC-to-APA-transitional lesions) (Nishimoto et al. 2016b). pAATLs are reported to comprise an outer subcapsular portion like an APCC with an inner micro-APA-like portion with a different somatic aldosterone-driver mutation (Nishimoto et al. 2016b). An alternative (or additional) model is an analogy to the two-hit model first proposed by Knudson in 1971 (Knudson 1971); a tumor would develop only in the presence of two mutations (an inherited mutation and an incurred second mutation or two sporadic mutations incurred after conception). In PA, two sequential events would be required, one mutation or hit triggering cell proliferation and a second hit driving aldosterone excess (Zennaro et al. 2018).

11.7 Conclusions

The timeline of discoveries in the genetics of PA spans just over 25 years from the molecular basis of FH type I (GRA) (Lifton et al. 1992a) to the genetic cause of FH type II (Scholl et al. 2018; Fernandes-Rosa et al. 2018) with germline mutations causing FH type III, FH type IV, and PASNA and recurrent somatic mutations in target genes in APAs discovered in the interim (Choi et al. 2011; Scholl et al. 2013, 2015a, b). These studies were enabled by breakthrough advances in molecular techniques especially from the application of NGS methods. Improvements in the clinical management of PA have been made with the development of AVS (Melby et al. 1967) to precisely differentiate surgically treatable PA (unilateral PA) from medically treated forms (bilateral PA) and with the use of laparoscopic adrenalectomy (Gagner et al. 1992). Immunohistochemistry using specific CYP11B2 and CYP11B1 monoclonal antibodies has unveiled the complex and diverse features of the diseased adrenal in PA, revealed previously unknown histopathologic features, and may help define which patients have an increased likelihood of persistent aldosteronism (Meyer et al. 2018; Volpe et al. 2019). Targeted NGS to areas of the adrenal showing specific expression of aldosterone synthase has revealed the high prevalence of the somatic mutations in APA and provided insights into potential roles of APCCs (Nanba et al. 2018; Omata et al. 2018). Advances in the bioanalysis of liquid biopsies by mass spectrometry-based steroid measurements suggest the high potential of employing this approach in future diagnostic protocols in PA (Baron et al. 2018; Guo et al. 2018) including possible selection of patients with an APA, with a distinct genotype-associated peripheral plasma steroid profile, for surgical management (Eisenhofer et al. 2016; Williams et al. 2016; Yang et al. 2019). In a novel approach, selective inhibitors of the mutated GIRK4 channel have been identified that may block the detrimental effects of Na^+ influx and membrane depolarization caused by *KCNJ5* mutations (Scholl et al. 2017). Such compounds (macrolide antibiotics and macrolide derivatives without antibiotic activity) could potentially be useful in a noninvasive diagnostic strategy and to treat patients with APAs carrying *KCNJ5* mutations (Scholl et al. 2017). The progress made in uncovering the underlying genetic causes of PA may translate to future applications for the clinical management of patients with PA.

Acknowledgments The work of M. Reincke is supported by the European Research Council (ERC) under the European Union's Horizon 2020 research and innovation programme (grant agreement No [694913]). M Reincke and TA Williams are supported by the Deutsche Forschungsgemeinschaft (DFG, German Research Foundation) Projektnummer: 314061271 – TRR 205. M. Reincke is additionally supported by DFG grant RE 752/20-1 and by the Else Kröner-Fresenius Stiftung in support of the German Conns Registry-Else-Kröner Hyperaldosteronism Registry (2013_A182 and 2015_A171).

References

Åkerström T, Crona J, Delgado Verdugo A et al (2012) Comprehensive re-sequencing of adrenal aldosterone producing lesions reveal three somatic mutations near the KCNJ5 potassium channel selectivity filter. PLoS One 7(7):e41926. https://doi.org/10.1371/journal.pone.0041926

Åkerström T, Willenberg HS, Cupisti K et al (2015) Novel somatic mutations and distinct molecular signature in aldosterone-producing adenomas. Endocr Relat Cancer 22(5):735–744. https://doi.org/10.1530/erc-15-0321

Åkerström T, Maharjan R, Sven Willenberg H et al (2016) Activating mutations in CTNNB1 in aldosterone producing adenomas. Sci Rep 6:19546. https://doi.org/10.1038/srep19546

Azizan EA, Lam BY, Newhouse SJ et al (2012) Microarray, qPCR, and KCNJ5 sequencing of aldosterone-producing adenomas reveal differences in genotype and phenotype between zona glomerulosa- and zona fasciculata-like tumors. J Clin Endocrinol Metab 97(5):E819–E829. https://doi.org/10.1210/jc.2011-2965

Azizan EA, Poulsen H, Tuluc P et al (2013) Somatic mutations in ATP1A1 and CACNA1D underlie a common subtype of adrenal hypertension. Nat Genet 45(9):1055–1060. https://doi.org/10.1038/ng.2716

Baron S, Amar L, Faucon AL et al (2018) Criteria for diagnosing primary aldosteronism on the basis of liquid chromatography-tandem mass spectrometry determinations of plasma

aldosterone concentration. J Hypertens 36(7):1592–1601. https://doi.org/10.1097/hjh.0000000000001735
Berridge MJ (1995) Calcium signalling and cell proliferation. BioEssays 17(6):491–500. https://doi.org/10.1002/bies.950170605
Berthon A, Drelon C, Ragazzon B et al (2014) WNT/beta-catenin signalling is activated in aldosterone-producing adenomas and controls aldosterone production. Hum Mol Genet 23 (4):889–905. https://doi.org/10.1093/hmg/ddt484
Beuschlein F, Boulkroun S, Osswald A et al (2013) Somatic mutations in ATP1A1 and ATP2B3 lead to aldosterone-producing adenomas and secondary hypertension. Nat Genet 45 (4):440–444., 444e1-2. https://doi.org/10.1038/ng.2550
Boulkroun S, Samson-Couterie B, Dzib JF et al (2010) Adrenal cortex remodeling and functional zona glomerulosa hyperplasia in primary aldosteronism. Hypertension 56(5):885–892. https://doi.org/10.1161/hypertensionaha.110.158543
Boulkroun S, Beuschlein F, Rossi GP et al (2012) Prevalence, clinical, and molecular correlates of KCNJ5 mutations in primary aldosteronism. Hypertension 59(3):592–598. https://doi.org/10.1161/hypertensionaha.111.186478
Brini M, Carafoli E (2011) The plasma membrane Ca(2)+ ATPase and the plasma membrane sodium calcium exchanger cooperate in the regulation of cell calcium. Cold Spring Harb Perspect Biol 3(2):a004168. https://doi.org/10.1101/cshperspect.a004168
Burrello J, Burrello A, Stowasser M et al (2019) The primary aldosteronism surgical outcome score for the prediction of clinical outcomes after adrenalectomy for unilateral primary aldosteronism. Ann Surg. https://doi.org/10.1097/SLA.0000000000003200
Calhoun DA, Nishizaka MK, Zaman MA, Thakkar RB, Weissmann P (2002) Hyperaldosteronism among black and white subjects with resistant hypertension. Hypertension 40(6):892–896
Carvajal CA, Stehr CB, Gonzalez PA et al (2011) A de novo unequal cross-over mutation between CYP11B1 and CYP11B2 genes causes familial hyperaldosteronism type I. J Endocrinol Investig 34(2):140–144. https://doi.org/10.3275/717110.1007/bf03347044
Chalmers TM (1960) Conn's syndrome. Postgrad Med J 36:198–200
Choi M, Scholl UI, Yue P et al (2011) K+ channel mutations in adrenal aldosterone-producing adenomas and hereditary hypertension. Science (New York, NY) 331(6018):768–772. https://doi.org/10.1126/science.1198785
Clyne CD, White PC, Rainey WE (1996) Calcium regulates human CYP11B2 transcription. Endocr Res 22(4):485–492
Conn JW (1955) Presidential address. I. Painting background. II. Primary aldosteronism, a new clinical syndrome. J Lab Clin Med 45(1):3–17
Daniil G, Fernandes-Rosa FL, Chemin J et al (2016) CACNA1H mutations are associated with different forms of primary aldosteronism. EBioMedicine 13:225–236. https://doi.org/10.1016/j.ebiom.2016.10.002
Dekkers T, ter Meer M, Lenders JW et al (2014) Adrenal nodularity and somatic mutations in primary aldosteronism: one node is the culprit? J Clin Endocrinol Metab 99(7):E1341–E1351. https://doi.org/10.1210/jc.2013-4255
Eisenhofer G, Dekkers T, Peitzsch M et al (2016) Mass spectrometry-based adrenal and peripheral venous steroid profiling for subtyping primary aldosteronism. Clin Chem 62(3):514–524. https://doi.org/10.1373/clinchem.2015.251199
Fernandes-Rosa FL, Williams TA, Riester A et al (2014) Genetic spectrum and clinical correlates of somatic mutations in aldosterone-producing adenoma. Hypertension 64(2):354–361. https://doi.org/10.1161/hypertensionaha.114.03419
Fernandes-Rosa FL, Amar L, Tissier F et al (2015a) Functional histopathological markers of aldosterone producing adenoma and somatic KCNJ5 mutations. Mol Cell Endocrinol 408:220–226. https://doi.org/10.1016/j.mce.2015.01.020
Fernandes-Rosa FL, Giscos-Douriez I, Amar L et al (2015b) Different somatic mutations in multinodular adrenals with aldosterone-producing adenoma. Hypertension 66(5):1014–1022. https://doi.org/10.1161/hypertensionaha.115.05993

Fernandes-Rosa FL, Boulkroun S, Zennaro MC (2017) Somatic and inherited mutations in primary aldosteronism. J Mol Endocrinol 59(1):R47–r63. https://doi.org/10.1530/jme-17-0035
Fernandes-Rosa FL, Daniil G, Orozco IJ et al (2018) A gain-of-function mutation in the CLCN2 chloride channel gene causes primary aldosteronism. Nat Genet 50(3):355–361. https://doi.org/10.1038/s41588-018-0053-8
Funder JW, Carey RM, Mantero F et al (2016) The management of primary aldosteronism: case detection, diagnosis, and treatment: an Endocrine Society clinical practice guideline. J Clin Endocrinol Metab 101(5):1889–1916. https://doi.org/10.1210/jc.2015-4061
Gagner M, Lacroix A, Bolte E (1992) Laparoscopic adrenalectomy in Cushing's syndrome and pheochromocytoma. New Engl J Med 327(14):1033. https://doi.org/10.1056/nejm199210013271417
Geller DS, Zhang J, Wisgerhof MV, Shackleton C, Kashgarian M, Lifton RP (2008) A novel form of human Mendelian hypertension featuring nonglucocorticoid-remediable aldosteronism. J Clin Endocrinol Metab 93(8):3117–3123. https://doi.org/10.1210/jc.2008-0594
Gomez-Sanchez CE, Oki K (2014) Minireview: Potassium channels and aldosterone dysregulation: is primary aldosteronism a potassium channelopathy? Endocrinology 155(1):47–55. https://doi.org/10.1210/en.2013-1733
Gomez-Sanchez CE, Williams TA (2018) Visualizing adrenal steroids in primary aldosteronism. Hypertension 72(6):1269–1271. https://doi.org/10.1161/hypertensionaha.118.11369
Gomez-Sanchez CE, Montgomery M, Ganguly A et al (1984) Elevated urinary excretion of 18-oxocortisol in glucocorticoid-suppressible aldosteronism. J Clin Endocrinol Metab 59 (5):1022–1024. https://doi.org/10.1210/jcem-59-5-1022
Gomez-Sanchez CE, Qi X, Velarde-Miranda C et al (2014) Development of monoclonal antibodies against human CYP11B1 and CYP11B2. Mol Cell Endocrinol 383(1–2):111–117. https://doi.org/10.1016/j.mce.2013.11.022
Gomez-Sanchez CE, Kuppusamy M, Reincke M, Williams TA (2017a) Disordered CYP11B2 expression in primary aldosteronism. Horm Metab Res 49(12):957–962. https://doi.org/10.1055/s-0043-122238
Gomez-Sanchez CE, Qi X, Gomez-Sanchez EP, Sasano H, Bohlen MO, Wisgerhof M (2017b) Disordered zonal and cellular CYP11B2 enzyme expression in familial hyperaldosteronism type 3. Mol Cell Endocrinol 439:74–80. https://doi.org/10.1016/j.mce.2016.10.025
Gordon RD, Stowasser M, Tunny TJ, Klemm SA, Finn WL, Krek AL (1991) Clinical and pathological diversity of primary aldosteronism, including a new familial variety. Clin Exp Pharm Physiol 18(5):283–286
Gordon RD, Klemm SA, Tunny TJ, Stowasser M (1992) Primary aldosteronism: hypertension with a genetic basis. Lancet 340(8812):159–161
Gordon RD, Ziesak MD, Tunny TJ, Stowasser M, Klemm SA (1993) Evidence that primary aldosteronism may not be uncommon: 12% incidence among antihypertensive drug trial volunteers. Clin Exp Pharm Physiol 20(5):296–298
Gordon RD, Stowasser M, Tunny TJ, Klemm SA, Rutherford JC (1994) High incidence of primary aldosteronism in 199 patients referred with hypertension. Clin Exp Pharm Physiol 21 (4):315–318
Grundy HM, Simpson SA, Tait JF (1952) Isolation of a highly active mineralocorticoid from beef adrenal extract. Nature 169(4306):795–796
Guo Z, Poglitsch M, McWhinney BC et al (2018) Aldosterone LC-MS/MS assay-specific threshold values in screening and confirmatory testing for primary aldosteronism. J Clin Endocrinol Metab 103(11):3965–3973. https://doi.org/10.1210/jc.2018-01041
Heginbotham L, Abramson T, MacKinnon R (1992) A functional connection between the pores of distantly related ion channels as revealed by mutant K+ channels. Science (New York, NY) 258 (5085):1152–1155
Hundemer GL, Curhan GC, Yozamp N, Wang M, Vaidya A (2018) Cardiometabolic outcomes and mortality in medically treated primary aldosteronism: a retrospective cohort study. Lancet Diabetes Endocrinol 6(1):51–59. https://doi.org/10.1016/s2213-8587(17)30367-4

Inoue K, Yamazaki Y, Kitamoto T et al (2018) Aldosterone suppression by dexamethasone in patients with KCNJ5-mutated aldosterone-producing adenoma. J Clin Endocrinol Metab 103 (9):3477–3485. https://doi.org/10.1210/jc.2018-00738
Kempers MJ, Lenders JW, van Outheusden L et al (2009) Systematic review: diagnostic procedures to differentiate unilateral from bilateral adrenal abnormality in primary aldosteronism. Ann Intern Med 151(5):329–337
Kitamoto T, Suematsu S, Yamazaki Y et al (2016) Clinical and steroidogenic characteristics of aldosterone-producing adenomas with ATPase or CACNA1D gene mutations. J Clin Endocrinol Metab 101(2):494–503. https://doi.org/10.1210/jc.2015-3284
Knudson AG Jr (1971) Mutation and cancer: statistical study of retinoblastoma. Proc Natl Acad Sci U S A 68(4):820–823
Lafferty AR, Torpy DJ, Stowasser M et al (2000) A novel genetic locus for low renin hypertension: familial hyperaldosteronism type II maps to chromosome 7 (7p22). J Med Genet 37 (11):831–835
Lassuthova P, Rebelo AP, Ravenscroft G et al (2018) Mutations in ATP1A1 cause dominant Charcot-Marie-tooth type 2. Am J Hum Genet 102:505–514. https://doi.org/10.1016/j.ajhg.2018.01.023.
Lenders JWM, Williams TA, Reincke M, Gomez-Sanchez CE (2018) DIAGNOSIS OF ENDOCRINE DISEASE: 18-Oxocortisol and 18-hydroxycortisol: is there clinical utility of these steroids? Eur J Endocrinol 178(1):R1–R9. https://doi.org/10.1530/eje-17-0563
Lenzini L, Rossitto G, Maiolino G, Letizia C, Funder JW, Rossi GP (2015) A meta-analysis of somatic KCNJ5 K(+) channel mutations in 1636 patients with an aldosterone-producing adenoma. J Clin Endocrinol Metab 100(8):E1089–E1095. https://doi.org/10.1210/jc.2015-2149
Lifton RP, Dluhy RG, Powers M et al (1992a) A chimaeric 11 beta-hydroxylase/aldosterone synthase gene causes glucocorticoid-remediable aldosteronism and human hypertension. Nature 355(6357):262–265. https://doi.org/10.1038/355262a0
Lifton RP, Dluhy RG, Powers M et al (1992b) Hereditary hypertension caused by chimaeric gene duplications and ectopic expression of aldosterone synthase. Nat Genet 2:66–74. https://doi.org/10.1038/ng0992-66
Litchfield WR, Anderson BF, Weiss RJ, Lifton RP, Dluhy RG (1998) Intracranial aneurysm and hemorrhagic stroke in glucocorticoid-remediable aldosteronism. Hypertension 31(1 Pt 2):445–450
MacConnachie AA, Kelly KF, McNamara A et al (1998) Rapid diagnosis and identification of cross-over sites in patients with glucocorticoid remediable aldosteronism. J Clin Endocrinol Metab 83(12):4328–4331. https://doi.org/10.1210/jcem.83.12.5309
MacDonald BT, Tamai K, He X (2009) Wnt/beta-catenin signaling: components, mechanisms, and diseases. Dev Cell 17(1):9–26. https://doi.org/10.1016/j.devcel.2009.06.016
Marksteiner R, Schurr P, Berjukow S, Margreiter E, Perez-Reyes E, Hering S (2001) Inactivation determinants in segment IIIS6 of Ca(v)3.1. J Physiol 537(Pt 1):27–34
Mathur A, Kemp CD, Dutta U et al (2010) Consequences of adrenal venous sampling in primary hyperaldosteronism and predictors of unilateral adrenal disease. J Am Coll Surg 211 (3):384–390. https://doi.org/10.1016/j.jamcollsurg.2010.05.006
Melby JC, Spark RF, Dale SL, Egdahl RH, Kahn PC (1967) Diagnosis and localization of aldosterone-producing adenomas by adrenal-vein catheterization. New Engl J Med 277 (20):1050–1056. https://doi.org/10.1056/nejm196711162772002
Meyer LS, Wang X, Susnik E et al (2018) Immunohistopathology and steroid profiles associated with biochemical outcomes after adrenalectomy for unilateral primary aldosteronism. Hypertension 72(3):650–657. https://doi.org/10.1161/hypertensionaha.118.11465
Miller WL, Auchus RJ (2011) The molecular biology, biochemistry, and physiology of human steroidogenesis and its disorders. Endocr Rev 32(1):81–151. https://doi.org/10.1210/er.2010-0013
Miyake Y, Tanaka K, Nishikawa T et al (2014) Prognosis of primary aldosteronism in Japan: results from a nationwide epidemiological study. Endocr J 61(1):35–40

Monticone S, Castellano I, Versace K et al (2015) Immunohistochemical, genetic and clinical characterization of sporadic aldosterone-producing adenomas. Mol Cell Endocrinol 411:146–154. https://doi.org/10.1016/j.mce.2015.04.022
Monticone S, Burrello J, Tizzani D et al (2017a) Prevalence and clinical manifestations of primary aldosteronism encountered in primary care practice. J Am Coll Cardiol 69(14):1811–1820. https://doi.org/10.1016/j.jacc.2017.01.052
Monticone S, Tetti M, Burrello J et al (2017b) Familial hyperaldosteronism type III. J Hum Hypertens 31(12):776–781. https://doi.org/10.1038/jhh.2017.34
Monticone S, Buffolo F, Tetti M, Veglio F, Pasini B, Mulatero P (2018a) GENETICS IN ENDOCRINOLOGY: the expanding genetic horizon of primary aldosteronism. Eur J Endocrinol 178(3):R101–r111. https://doi.org/10.1530/eje-17-0946
Monticone S, D'Ascenzo F, Moretti C et al (2018b) Cardiovascular events and target organ damage in primary aldosteronism compared with essential hypertension: a systematic review and meta-analysis. Lancet Diabetes Endocrinol 6(1):41–50. https://doi.org/10.1016/s2213-8587(17)30319-4
Mosso L, Gomez-Sanchez CE, Foecking MF, Fardella C (2001) Serum 18-hydroxycortisol in primary aldosteronism, hypertension, and normotensives. Hypertension 38(3 Pt 2):688–691
Mosso L, Carvajal C, Gonzalez A et al (2003) Primary aldosteronism and hypertensive disease. Hypertension 42(2):161–165. https://doi.org/10.1161/01.Hyp.0000079505.25750.11
Mulatero P (2008) A new form of hereditary primary aldosteronism: familial hyperaldosteronism type III. J Clin Endocrinol Metab 93(8):2972–2974. https://doi.org/10.1210/jc.2008-1241
Mulatero P, di Cella SM, Williams TA et al (2002) Glucocorticoid remediable aldosteronism: low morbidity and mortality in a four-generation Italian pedigree. J Clin Endocrinol Metab 87 (7):3187–3191. https://doi.org/10.1210/jcem.87.7.8647
Mulatero P, Stowasser M, Loh KC et al (2004) Increased diagnosis of primary aldosteronism, including surgically correctable forms, in centers from five continents. J Clin Endocrinol Metab 89(3):1045–1050. https://doi.org/10.1210/jc.2003-031337
Mulatero P, di Cella SM, Monticone S et al (2012a) 18-hydroxycorticosterone, 18-hydroxycortisol, and 18-oxocortisol in the diagnosis of primary aldosteronism and its subtypes. J Clin Endocrinol Metab 97(3):881–889. https://doi.org/10.1210/jc.2011-2384
Mulatero P, Tauber P, Zennaro MC et al (2012b) KCNJ5 mutations in European families with nonglucocorticoid remediable familial hyperaldosteronism. Hypertension 59(2):235–240. https://doi.org/10.1161/hypertensionaha.111.183996
Mulatero P, Monticone S, Bertello C, Viola A et al (2013) Long-term cardio- and cerebrovascular events in patients with primary aldosteronism. J Clin Endocrinol Metab 98(12):4826–4833. https://doi.org/10.1210/jc.2013-2805
Mulatero P, Monticone S, Burrello J, Veglio F, Williams TA, Funder J (2016) Guidelines for primary aldosteronism: uptake by primary care physicians in Europe. J Hypertens 34 (11):2253–2257. https://doi.org/10.1097/hjh.0000000000001088
Nakamura Y, Maekawa T, Felizola SJ et al (2014) Adrenal CYP11B1/2 expression in primary aldosteronism: immunohistochemical analysis using novel monoclonal antibodies. Mol Cell Endocrinol 392(1–2):73–79. https://doi.org/10.1016/j.mce.2014.05.002
Nakamura Y, Kitada M, Satoh F et al (2016) Intratumoral heterogeneity of steroidogenesis in aldosterone-producing adenoma revealed by intensive double- and triple-immunostaining for CYP11B2/B1 and CYP17. Mol Cell Endocrinol 422:57–63. https://doi.org/10.1016/j.mce.2015.11.014
Nanba K, Tsuiki M, Sawai K et al (2013) Histopathological diagnosis of primary aldosteronism using CYP11B2 immunohistochemistry. J Clin Endocrinol Metab 98(4):1567–1574. https://doi.org/10.1210/jc.2012-3726
Nanba K, Vaidya A, Williams GH, Zheng I, Else T, Rainey WE (2017) Age-related autonomous aldosteronism. Circulation 136(4):347–355. https://doi.org/10.1161/circulationaha.117.028201
Nanba K, Omata K, Else T et al (2018) Targeted molecular characterization of aldosterone-producing adenomas in white Americans. J Clin Endocrinol Metab 103(10):3869–3876. https://doi.org/10.1210/jc.2018-01004

Nishimoto K, Nakagawa K, Li D et al (2010) Adrenocortical zonation in humans under normal and pathological conditions. J Clin Endocrinol Metab 95(5):2296–2305. https://doi.org/10.1210/jc.2009-2010

Nishimoto K, Tomlins SA, Kuick R et al (2015) Aldosterone-stimulating somatic gene mutations are common in normal adrenal glands. Proc Natl Acad Sci U S A 112(33):E4591–E4599. https://doi.org/10.1073/pnas.1505529112

Nishimoto K, Seki T, Hayashi Y et al (2016a) Human adrenocortical remodeling leading to aldosterone-producing cell cluster generation. Int J Endocrinol 2016:7834356. https://doi.org/10.1155/2016/7834356

Nishimoto K, Seki T, Kurihara I et al (2016b) Case report: nodule development from subcapsular aldosterone-producing cell clusters causes hyperaldosteronism. J Clin Endocrinol Metab 101(1):6–9. https://doi.org/10.1210/jc.2015-3285

Nogueira EF, Gerry D, Mantero F, Mariniello B, Rainey WE (2010) The role of TASK1 in aldosterone production and its expression in normal adrenal and aldosterone-producing adenomas. Clin Endocrinol 73(1):22–29. https://doi.org/10.1111/j.1365-2265.2009.03738.x

Oki K, Plonczynski MW, Luis Lam M, Gomez-Sanchez EP, Gomez-Sanchez CE (2012) Potassium channel mutant KCNJ5 T158A expression in HAC-15 cells increases aldosterone synthesis. Endocrinology 153(4):1774–1782. https://doi.org/10.1210/en.2011-1733

Omata K, Tomlins SA, Rainey WE (2017a) Aldosterone-producing cell clusters in normal and pathological states. Horm Metab Res 49(12):951–956. https://doi.org/10.1055/s-0043-122394

Omata K, Yamazaki Y, Nakamura Y et al (2017b) Genetic and histopathologic intertumor heterogeneity in primary aldosteronism. J Clin Endocrinol Metab 102(6):1792–1796. https://doi.org/10.1210/jc.2016-4007

Omata K, Satoh F, Morimoto R et al (2018) Cellular and genetic causes of idiopathic hyperaldosteronism. Hypertension 72(4):874–880. https://doi.org/10.1161/hypertensionaha.118.11086

Orita M, Iwahana H, Kanazawa H et al (1989) Detection of polymorphisms of human DNA by gel electrophoresis as single-strand conformation polymorphisms. Proc Natl Acad Sci U S A 86(8):2766–2770

Palmgren MG, Nissen P (2011) P-type ATPases. Annu Rev Biophys 40:243–266. https://doi.org/10.1146/annurev.biophys.093008.131331

Perez-Rivas LG, Williams TA, Reincke M (2018) Inherited forms of primary hyperaldosteronism: new genes, new phenotypes and proposition of a new classification. Exp Clin Endocrinol 127(2–03):93–99. https://doi.org/10.1055/a-0713-0629

Pinggera A, Striessnig J (2016) Cav 1.3 (CACNA1D) L-type Ca(2+) channel dysfunction in CNS disorders. J Physiol 594(20):5839–5849. https://doi.org/10.1113/jp270672

Pinggera A, Mackenroth L, Rump A et al (2017) New gain-of-function mutation shows CACNA1D as recurrently mutated gene in autism spectrum disorders and epilepsy. Hum Mol Genet 26(15):2923–2932. https://doi.org/10.1093/hmg/ddx175

Prada ETA, Burrello J, Reincke M, Williams TA (2017) Old and new concepts in the molecular pathogenesis of primary aldosteronism. Hypertension 70(5):875–881. https://doi.org/10.1161/hypertensionaha.117.10111

Reimer EN, Walenda G, Seidel E, Scholl UI (2016) CACNA1H(M1549V) mutant calcium channel causes autonomous aldosterone production in HAC15 cells and is inhibited by mibefradil. Endocrinology 157(8):3016–3022. https://doi.org/10.1210/en.2016-1170

Rossi GP, Bernini G, Caliumi C et al (2006) A prospective study of the prevalence of primary aldosteronism in 1,125 hypertensive patients. J Am Coll Cardiol 48(11):2293–2300. https://doi.org/10.1016/j.jacc.2006.07.059

Sanger F, Nicklen S, Coulson AR (1977) DNA sequencing with chain-terminating inhibitors. Proc Natl Acad Sci U S A 74(12):5463–5467

Satoh F, Morimoto R, Ono Y et al (2015) Measurement of peripheral plasma 18-oxocortisol can discriminate unilateral adenoma from bilateral diseases in patients with primary aldosteronism. Hypertension 65(5):1096–1102. https://doi.org/10.1161/hypertensionaha.114.04453

Savard S, Amar L, Plouin PF, Steichen O (2013) Cardiovascular complications associated with primary aldosteronism: a controlled cross-sectional study. Hypertension 62(2):331–336. https://doi.org/10.1161/hypertensionaha.113.01060

Schirpenbach C, Reincke M (2007) Primary aldosteronism: current knowledge and controversies in Conn's syndrome. Nat Clin Pract Endocrinol Metab 3(3):220–227. https://doi.org/10.1038/ncpendmet0430

Schlingmann KP, Bandulik S, Mammen C et al (2018) Germline de novo mutations in atp1a1 cause renal hypomagnesemia, refractory seizures, and intellectual disability. Am J Hum Genet 103 (5):808–816. https://doi.org/10.1016/j.ajhg.2018.10.004

Scholl UI, Nelson-Williams C, Yue P et al (2012) Hypertension with or without adrenal hyperplasia due to different inherited mutations in the potassium channel KCNJ5. Proc Natl Acad Sci U S A 109(7):2533–2538. https://doi.org/10.1073/pnas.1121407109

Scholl UI, Goh G, Stolting G et al (2013) Somatic and germline CACNA1D calcium channel mutations in aldosterone-producing adenomas and primary aldosteronism. Nat Genet 45 (9):1050–1054. https://doi.org/10.1038/ng.2695

Scholl UI, Healy JM, Thiel A et al (2015a) Novel somatic mutations in primary hyperaldosteronism are related to the clinical, radiological and pathological phenotype. Clin Endocrinol 83 (6):779–789. https://doi.org/10.1111/cen.12873

Scholl UI, Stolting G, Nelson-Williams C, et al. (2015b) Recurrent gain of function mutation in calcium channel CACNA1H causes early-onset hypertension with primary aldosteronism. eLife 4:e06315. doi:https://doi.org/10.7554/eLife.06315

Scholl UI, Abriola L, Zhang C et al (2017) Macrolides selectively inhibit mutant KCNJ5 potassium channels that cause aldosterone-producing adenoma. J Clin Invest 12(7):2739–2750. https://doi.org/10.1172/jci91733

Scholl UI, Stolting G, Schewe J et al (2018) CLCN2 chloride channel mutations in familial hyperaldosteronism type II. Nat Genet 50(3):349–354. https://doi.org/10.1038/s41588-018-0048-5

Seccia TM, Caroccia B, Gomez-Sanchez EP, Gomez-Sanchez CE, Rossi GP (2018) The biology of normal zona glomerulosa and aldosterone-producing adenoma: pathological implications. Endocr Rev 39(6):1029–1056. https://doi.org/10.1210/er.2018-00060

Sechi LA, Novello M, Lapenna R et al (2006) Long-term renal outcomes in patients with primary aldosteronism. JAMA 295(22):2638–2645. https://doi.org/10.1001/jama.295.22.2638

Simpson SA, Tait JF (1952) A quantitative method for the bioassay of the effect of adrenal cortical steroids on mineral metabolism. Endocrinology 50(2):150–161. https://doi.org/10.1210/endo-50-2-150

Simpson SA, Tait JF, Wettstein A, Neher R, Von Euw J, Reichstein T (1953) Isolierung eines neuen kristallisierten Hormons aus Nebennieren mit besonders hoher Wirksamkeit auf den Mineralstoffwechsel. Experientia 9(9):333–335

Simpson SA, Tait JF, Wettstein A et al (1954) Aldosteron. Isolierung und Eigenschaften. Über Bestandteile der Nebennierenrinde und verwandte Stoffe. 91. Mitteilung. Helv Chim Acta 37 (4):1163–1200. https://doi.org/10.1002/hlca.19540370423

Spat A, Hunyady L (2004) Control of aldosterone secretion: a model for convergence in cellular signaling pathways. Phys Rev 84(2):489–539. https://doi.org/10.1152/physrev.00030.2003

Stowasser M (2001) Primary aldosteronism: rare bird or common cause of secondary hypertension? Curr Hypertens Rep 3(3):230–239

Stowasser M, Gordon RD (2016) Primary aldosteronism: changing definitions and new concepts of physiology and pathophysiology both inside and outside the kidney. Phys Rev 96 (4):1327–1384. https://doi.org/10.1152/physrev.00026.2015

Stowasser M, Gordon RD, Tunny TJ, Klemm SA, Finn WL, Krek AL (1992) Familial hyperaldosteronism type II: five families with a new variety of primary aldosteronism. Clin Exp Pharm Physiol 19(5):319–322

Stowasser M, Bachmann AW, Tunny TJ, Gordon RD (1996) Production of 18-oxo-cortisol in subtypes of primary aldosteronism. Clin Exp Pharm Physiol 23(6–7):591–593

Stowasser M, Gartside MG, Gordon RD (1997) A PCR-based method of screening individuals of all ages, from neonates to the elderly, for familial hyperaldosteronism type I. Aust NZ J Med 27 (6):685–690

Sutherland DJ, Ruse JL, Laidlaw JC (1966) Hypertension, increased aldosterone secretion and low plasma renin activity relieved by dexamethasone. Can Med Assoc J 95(22):1109–1119

Tauber P, Aichinger B, Christ C et al (2016) Cellular pathophysiology of an adrenal adenoma-associated mutant of the plasma membrane Ca(2+)-ATPase ATP2B3. Endocrinology 157 (6):2489–2499. https://doi.org/10.1210/en.2015-2029

Therien B, Mellinger RC, Caldwell JR, Howard PJ (1959) Primary aldosteronism due to adrenal hyperplasia; occurrence in a boy aged 10 years. AMA J Dis Child 98(1):90–99

Tissier F, Cavard C, Groussin L et al (2005) Mutations of beta-catenin in adrenocortical tumors: activation of the Wnt signaling pathway is a frequent event in both benign and malignant adrenocortical tumors. Cancer Res 65(17):7622–7627. https://doi.org/10.1158/0008-5472.Can-05-0593

Ulick S, Chu MD (1982) Hypersecretion of a new corticosteroid, 18-hydroxycortisol in two types of adrenocortical hypertension. Clin Exp Hypertens Part A 4(9–10):1771–1777

Ulick S, Blumenfeld JD, Atlas SA, Wang JZ, Vaughan ED Jr (1993) The unique steroidogenesis of the aldosteronoma in the differential diagnosis of primary aldosteronism. J Clin Endocrinol Metab 76(4):873–878. https://doi.org/10.1210/jcem.76.4.8473399

Umakoshi H, Ogasawara T, Takeda Y et al (2018) Accuracy of adrenal computed tomography in predicting the unilateral subtype in young patients with hypokalaemia and elevation of aldosterone in primary aldosteronism. Clin Endocrinol 88(5):645–651. https://doi.org/10.1111/cen.13582

Volpe C, Hamberger B, Zedenius J, Juhlin CC (2019) Impact of immunohistochemistry on the diagnosis and management of primary aldosteronism: an important tool for improved patient follow-up. Scand J Surg. https://doi.org/10.1177/1457496918822622

Wang B, Li X, Zhang X et al (2015) Prevalence and characterization of somatic mutations in Chinese aldosterone- aldosterone-producing adenoma patients. Medicine (Baltimore) 94(16): e708. https://doi.org/10.1097/MD.0000000000000708

Wheeler DA, Srinivasan M, Egholm M et al (2008) The complete genome of an individual by massively parallel DNA sequencing. Nature 452(7189):872–876. https://doi.org/10.1038/nature06884

Williams TA, Monticone S, Schack VR et al (2014) Somatic ATP1A1, ATP2B3, and KCNJ5 mutations in aldosterone-producing adenomas. Hypertension 63(1):188–195. https://doi.org/10.1161/hypertensionaha.113.01733

Williams TA, Peitzsch M, Dietz AS et al (2016) Genotype-specific steroid profiles associated with aldosterone-producing adenomas. Hypertension 67(1):139–145. https://doi.org/10.1161/hypertensionaha.115.06186

Williams TA, Lenders JWM, Mulatero P et al (2017) Outcomes after adrenalectomy for unilateral primary aldosteronism: an international consensus on outcome measures and analysis of remission rates in an international cohort. Lancet Diabetes Endocrinol 5(9):689–699. https://doi.org/10.1016/s2213-8587(17)30135-3

Williams TA, Burrello J, Sechi LA et al (2018) Computed tomography and adrenal venous sampling in the diagnosis of unilateral primary aldosteronism. Hypertension 72(3):641–649. https://doi.org/10.1161/hypertensionaha.118.11382

Wu VC, Huang KH, Peng KY et al (2015) Prevalence and clinical correlates of somatic mutation in aldosterone producing adenoma-Taiwanese population. Sci Rep 5:11396. https://doi.org/10.1038/srep11396

Yamakita N, Mune T, Morita H, Yasuda K, Miura K, Gomez-Sanchez CE (1994) Plasma 18-oxocortisol levels in the patients with adrenocortical disorders. Clin Endocrinol 40 (5):583–587

Yamazaki Y, Nakamura Y, Omata K et al (2017) Histopathological classification of cross-sectional image-negative hyperaldosteronism. J Clin Endocrinol Metab 102(4):1182–1192. https://doi.org/10.1210/jc.2016-2986

Yamazaki Y, Omata K, Tezuka Y et al (2018) Tumor cell subtypes based on the intracellular hormonal activity in KCNJ5-mutated aldosterone-producing adenoma. Hypertension 72 (3):632–640. https://doi.org/10.1161/hypertensionaha.118.10907

Yang Y, Reincke M, Williams TA (2018) Treatment of unilateral pa by adrenalectomy: potential reasons for incomplete biochemical cure. Exp Clin Endocrinol 127(2–03):100–108. https://doi.org/10.1055/a-0662-6081

Yang Y, Burrello J, Burrello A et al (2019) Classification of microadenomas in patients with primary aldosteronism by steroid profiling. J Steroid Biochem Mol Biol 189:274–282. pii: S0960-0760(18)30479-5. https://doi.org/10.1016/j.jsbmb.2019.01.008

Young WF Jr (2019) Diagnosis and treatment of primary aldosteronism: practical clinical perspectives. J Intern Med 285(2):126–148. https://doi.org/10.1111/joim.12831

Zanni G, Cali T, Kalscheuer VM et al (2012) Mutation of plasma membrane Ca(2+) ATPase isoform 3 in a family with X-linked congenital cerebellar ataxia impairs Ca(2+) homeostasis. Proc Natl Acad Sci U S A 109:14514–14519. https://doi.org/10.1073/pnas.1207488109

Zennaro MC, Boulkroun S, Fernandes-Rosa F (2017) Genetic causes of functional adrenocortical adenomas. Endocr Rev 38(6):516–537. https://doi.org/10.1210/er.2017-00189

Zennaro MC, Fernandes-Rosa FL, Boulkroun S (2018) Overview of aldosterone-related genetic syndromes and recent advances. Curr Opin Endocrinol Diab Obes 25(3):147–154. https://doi.org/10.1097/med.0000000000000409

Zheng FF, Zhu LM, Nie AF et al (2015) Clinical characteristics of somatic mutations in Chinese patients with aldosterone-producing adenoma. Hypertension 65(3):622–628. https://doi.org/10.1161/hypertensionaha.114.03346

Chapter 12
Congenital Adrenal Hyperplasia

Dóra Török

Abstract Congenital adrenal hyperplasia (CAH) is a group of seven autosomal recessively inherited disorders of various enzymes participating in adrenal steroid hormone synthesis. Patients present with various symptoms depending on the nature and severity of the enzymatic block. More than 95% of all CAH patients suffer from 21-hydroxylase deficiency. The genetic background is well characterized for all CAH subtypes. Characterization of their genetic background has provided important pathophysiologic understanding of steroid biosynthesis disorders. Genotyping is important for confirming diagnosis, determining prognostic factors, and for genetic counseling for family planning and may reveal new therapeutic approaches.

Keywords Congenital adrenal hyperplasia · Adrenal insufficiency · 21-hydroxylase deficiency · Steroid biosynthesis

List of Abbreviations

11-OHD	11β-hydroxylase deficiency
17-OHD	17α-hydroxylase deficiency
17-OHP	17-hydroxyprogesterone
21-OHD	21-hydroxylase deficiency
ACTH	Adrenocorticotropic hormone
CAH	Congenital adrenal hyperplasia
CNV	Copy number variation
CRH	Corticotropin-releasing hormone
DOC	11-deoxycorticosterone
HLA	Human leukocyte antigen
HSD3B2	3β-hydroxysteroid dehydrogenase type 2 deficiency
LC-MS	Liquid Chromatography-Mass Spectrometry

D. Török (✉)
2nd Department of Pediatrics, Semmelweis University, Budapest, Hungary
e-mail: torok.dora@med.semmelweis-univ.hu

P. Igaz, A. Patócs (eds.), *Genetics of Endocrine Diseases and Syndromes*, Experientia Supplementum 111, https://doi.org/10.1007/978-3-030-25905-1_12

MHC	Major histocompatibility complex
MLPA	Multiplex ligation-dependent probe amplification
NCCAH	Non-classic CAH
OMIM	Online Mendelian Inheritance in Man
PCR	Polymerase chain reaction
POR	Cytochrome P450 oxidoreductase
SCC	Side-chain cleavage enzyme
StAR	Steroidogenic acute regulatory protein
SV, SV-CAH	Classic simple virilizing CAH
SW, SW-CAH	Classic salt-wasting CAH

12.1 Background

Congenital adrenal hyperplasia (CAH) is a group of autosomal recessively inherited disorders of various enzymes participating in adrenal glucocorticoid synthesis (Fig. 12.1). The clinical picture is variable based on the affected enzymes, but adrenal insufficiency due to impaired cortisol synthesis is a common feature. Low cortisol levels lead to the overproduction of corticotropin-releasing hormone (CRH) in the hypothalamus and consequently adrenocorticotropic hormone (ACTH) in the pituitary, resulting in hyperplasia of the adrenal glands and accumulations of steroid precursors proximal from the blocked enzyme. The accumulated precursors may shunt to alternative biosynthetic pathways; these atypical steroids may be able to bind to steroid receptors with variable affinity and activation ability. This translates to a large spectrum of clinical consequences, including adrenal insufficiency, fluid and electrolyte abnormalities, disordered sex development, infertility, pubertal and growth abnormalities, hypertension, and increased metabolic risk in adulthood. The actual clinical features and severity depend on the nature and severity of the enzymatic defect.

More than 95% of all CAH cases are caused by a 21-hydroxylase deficiency (21-OHD). 21-OHD is classified into three subgroups, the classic salt wasting (SW, SW-CAH), the classic simple virilizing (SV, SV-CAH) and non-classic (NCCAH, or late onset). The second most frequent type, the 11β-hydroxylase deficiency (11-OHD) accounts for approximately the remaining 5% of cases. 11-OHD is classified into classic and non-classic subgroups. Less common forms of CAH are 3β-hydroxysteroid dehydrogenase type 2 deficiency (HSD3B2), 17α-hydroxylase deficiency (17-OHD), congenital lipoid adrenal hyperplasia, side-chain cleavage enzyme deficiency (SCC), and cytochrome P450 oxidoreductase deficiency (POR). These forms are usually sporadic, and are more commonly found in small, isolated populations (Table 12.1).

The front-line diagnosis of the different CAH forms is based on clinical presentation and biochemical features. The measurement of the precursor before the enzymatic block is usually diagnostic, like 17-hydroxyprogesterone (17-OHP) for 21-OHD.

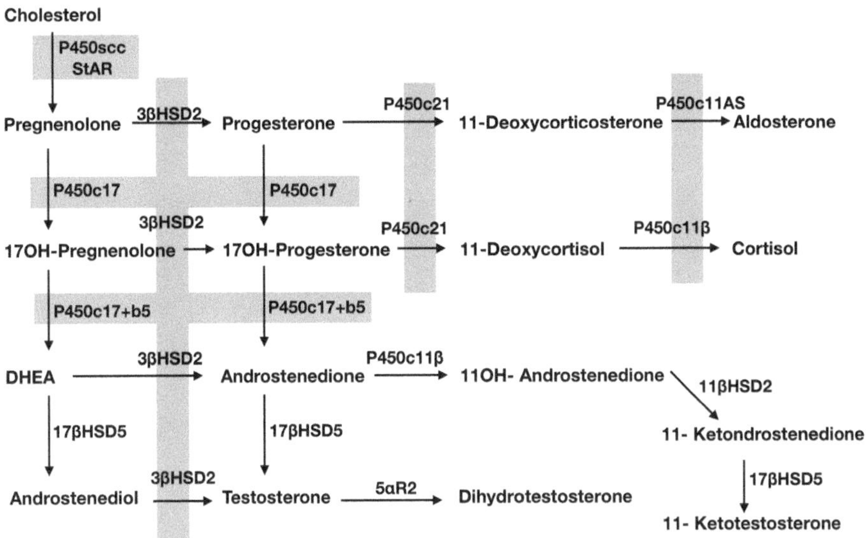

Fig. 12.1 Schematic representation of steroid biosynthesis. Gray boxes indicate specific enzymes affected in different types of CAH. P450scc: cholesterol side-chain cleavage enzyme, StAR: steroid acute regulatory protein, 3βHSD2: 3β-hydroxysteroid dehydrogenase type 2, P450c21: 21-hydroxylase, P450c11AS: aldosterone synthase, P450c17: 17α-hydroxylase, P450c11β: 11-β-hydroxylase, b5: cytochrome b5, 11βHSD2: 11β-hydroxysteroid dehydrogenase type 2, 17βHSD5:17β-hydroxysteroid dehydrogenase type 5, 5αR2: 5α-reductase type 2

ACTH-stimulation increases the sensitivity of biochemical testing. However, biochemical methods are unable to identify heterozygous carriers. Genotyping is essential for confirming the diagnosis, identifying heterozygotes, genetic counseling, and provides prognostic information on disease severity. Genetic studies provided insight into pathophysiology, genotype–phenotype relationships, and characterization of some unique chromosomal areas.

12.2 Genetic Forms of Congenital Adrenal Hyperplasia

12.2.1 21-Hydroxylase Deficiency

21-OHD (Online Mendelian Inheritance in Man (OMIM 201910)) is the most common form of CAH, responsible for approximately 95% of cases. Although 21-OHD clinically represents a continuous spectrum, it is classified into classic SW, classic SV, and non-classic forms. The classic forms are characterized by virilization of the external genitalia in newborn girls and precocious puberty in both sexes due to androgen overproduction, and adrenal insufficiency. Approximately 75% of all classic CAH cases have the severe SW form and lack both cortisol and aldosterone. In the absence of neonatal screening, the SW form presents with a

Table 12.1 Main characteristics of different types of CAH

Type of CAH	Gene	Elevated metabolite	Clinical manifestation	Substitution therapy
21-OHD	*CYP21A2*	17-OHP, 21-deoxycortisol, androstenedione	SW-CAH: Virilized genitalia, neonatal salt wasting SV-CAH: Virilized genitalia NCCAH: Precocious pubarche, hirsutism, female infertility	Glucocorticoids ± mineralocorticoids
11-OHD	*CYP11B1*	DOC, 11-deoxycortisol, androstenedione	Classic: Virilized genitalia, hypertension, hypokalemia Non-classic: Precocious pubarche, hirsutism, female infertility	Glucocorticoids
17-OHD	*CYP17A1*	DOC, corticosterone, progesterone	Phenotypic female, absence of sexual characteristics, hypertension, hypokalemia	Glucocorticoids
HSD3B2	*HSD3B2*	17OH-pregnenolone, DHEA, renin	Classic: Ambiguous genitalia, neonatal salt wasting Non-classic: Precocious pubarche, hirsutism, female infertility	Glucocorticoids + mineralocorticoids
POR	*POR*	Pregnenolone, progesterone, 17-OHP, DOC, corticosterone	Ambiguous genitalia, skeletal malformations	Glucocorticoids + mineralocorticoids
Lipoid	*StAR*	Renin	Classic: Phenotypic female, neonatal salt wasting Non-classic: Adrenal insufficiency, variable genitalia and gonadal function	Glucocorticoids + mineralocorticoids
SCC	*CYP11A1*	Renin	Classic: Phenotypic female, neonatal salt wasting Non-classic: Adrenal insufficiency, variable genitalia and gonadal function	Glucocorticoids + mineralocorticoids

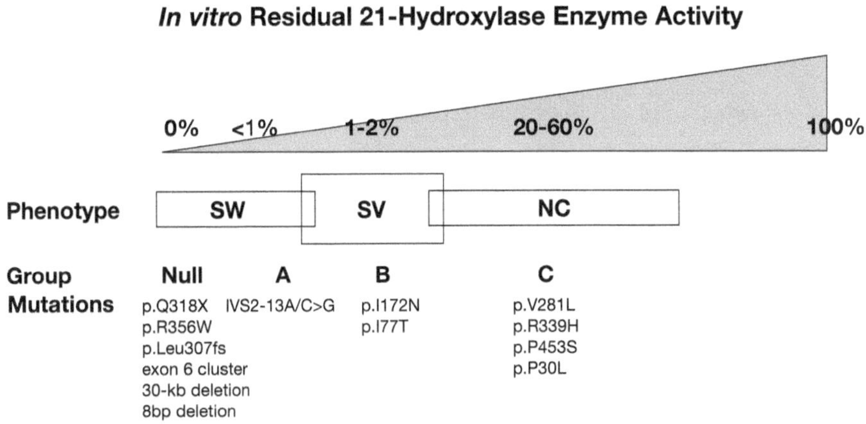

Fig. 12.2 Residual in vitro 21-hydroxylase activity of common *CYP21A2* mutations

life-threatening salt-wasting crisis in the neonatal period. Patients with SV form may escape salt wasting because of some residual 21-hydroxylase activity and small amounts of aldosterone production (Fig. 12.2). Girls with classic CAH (both SW and SV) are born with virilized genitalia, which makes early diagnosis possible even without neonatal screening; however, boys can only be diagnosed when salt-wasting crisis happens or later when early signs of hyperandrogenism become visible. NCCAH manifests later in childhood or even in adulthood with precocious pubarche in both sexes or with symptoms similar to polycystic ovary syndrome, subfertility. NCCAH patients, especially males, are often asymptomatic (El-Maouche et al. 2017).

CYP21A2 (other nomenclature *P450c21B*, *CYP21*, *CYP21B*) encodes 21-hydroxylase, a cytochrome P450 type II enzyme of 495 amino acids, mainly expressed in the adrenal cortex. *CYP21A1P*, a nonfunctional duplicated pseudogene is located 30 kb apart from *CYP21A2* in the human leukocyte antigen (HLA) class III region in the major histocompatibility (MHC) locus on the short arm of chromosome 6 (6p21.3). The gene and the pseudogene are approximately 98% homologous. The pseudogene is inactive because of approximately 11 deleterious mutations in its coding region (Fig. 12.3).

Both *CYP21A2* and its pseudogene are arranged in tandem repeat with the gene of the fourth component of complement C4 (*C4A* and *C4B* genes) (Fig. 12.3). The region is flanked by centromeric tenascin (*TNXA* and *TNXB*) and telomeric RP (*RP1* and *RP2*) genes. The unique structure of the region was probably formed by an ancestral duplication of a 30-kb region containing the *CYP21A2* and *C4* genes. The frequency of genomic recombination in this region is very high due to the strong homology. *RP1* encodes a serine/threonine nuclear protein kinase, *C4* encodes the fourth component of the complement system, *TNXB* encodes tenascin-X extracellular matrix protein. *RP1*, *CYP21A2*, *TNXB* all have corresponding highly homologous, inactive pseudogenes (*RP2*, *CYP21A1P*, *TNXA*). The RCCX module (*RP*, *C4*, *CYP21*, *TNX*) forms a bimodular structure on most chromosomes (*RP1-C4-CYP21A1P-TNXA-RP2-C4-CYP21A2-TNXB*), *CYP21A1P* gene being in the

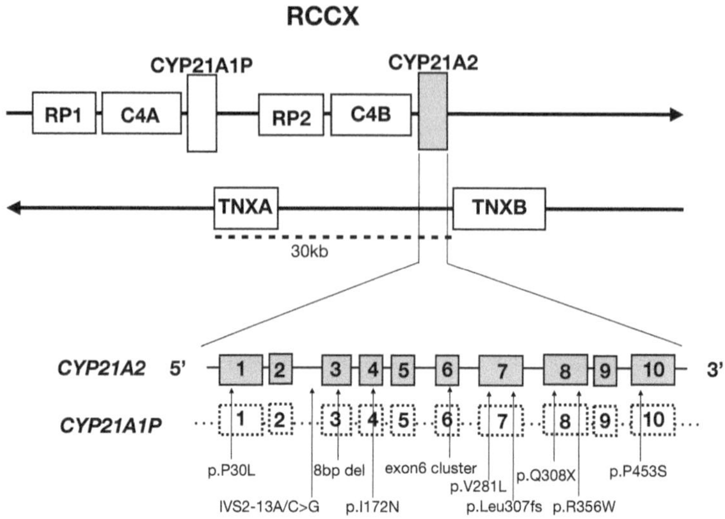

Fig. 12.3 The localization of *CYP21A2* and *CYP21A1P* in the MHC region. There is a high degree of homology between *CYP21A2* and its pseudogene. The mutations in the pseudogene are marked by arrows

telomeric position and *CYP21A2* gene in the centromeric position. Mono-modular and tri-modular haplotypes are also possible. Copy number variations (CNV) of *C4*, *CYP21* and *TNX* are common, and in CAH CNV has the ability to modify the severity of the disease. Also, detection of CNVs might raise diagnostic challenges (Doleschall et al. 2017).

Recombinations frequently occur because of high degree of homology between *CYP21A2* and its pseudogene. Most disease-causing mutations of *CYP21A2* are pseudogene-derived via gene conversion, which transfers the deleterious pseudogene mutations to the active gene. Chimeric genes are frequently formed due to large deletions. During meiosis, misalignment can result in a 30-kb deletion, which produces nonfunctioning *CYP21A1P/CYP21A2* chimeric genes. Different types of chimeras exist depending on the break points: nine different *CYP21A1P/CYP21A2* chimeras (CH) have been reported so far (CH1–9) (Fig. 12.4).

De novo mutations cause approximately 1–2% of cases. These de novo mutations result in unusual haplotypes and large genetic variation, which is present in 1:10^3–10^5 sperm cells. Uniparental disomy of chromosome 6 is a rare cause of CAH (Hannah-Shmouni et al. 2017; Simonetti et al. 2018).

12.2.1.1 Genotype–Phenotype Correlations in 21-Hydroxylase Deficiency

21-OHD phenotypically represents a continuous spectrum with an incomplete genotype–phenotype correlation of approximately 90%. Most patients are

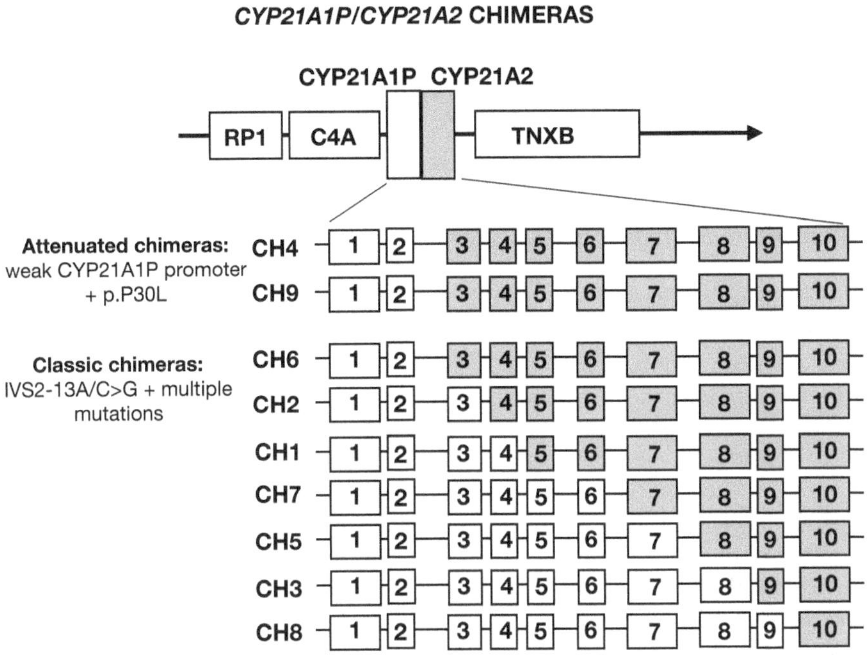

Fig. 12.4 Chimera junction sites. During meiosis, misalignment can result in a 30-kb deletion, which produces nonfunctioning *CYP21A1P/CYP21A2* chimeric genes. Different types of chimeras exist depending on the break points, and nine different *CYP21A1P/CYP21A2* chimeras (CH) have been reported so far (CH1–9). Attenuated chimeras are associated with milder phenotype

compound heterozygotes harboring two different mutations, and the phenotype is usually defined by the less severe mutation with the more residual enzyme activity. The strongest phenotypic variation is seen in SV, while SW and NCCAH phenotypes are more predictable. Classic CAH is diagnosed via neonatal screening in most countries; the male:female ratio is equal. However, there is a female predominance in NCCAH, because males are usually asymptomatic. Long-term health outcomes of classic CAH, e.g., metabolic syndrome, cardiovascular risk, and osteoporosis, are poorly predictable based on the genotype; these are most likely treatment-related comorbidities.

CYP21A2 mutations affect 21-hydroxylase enzyme activity differently in in vitro settings (Fig. 12.3). Based on the remaining in vitro enzyme activity, the mutations are classified into four subgroups, null, A, B, and C. Deletions or nonsense mutations affect critical enzyme functions, such as enzyme stability, heme binding or anchoring and result in complete loss of activity (null) and SW phenotype. Missense mutations affect the transmembrane region or conserved hydrophobic patches and allow 1–2% residual enzyme activity. Missense mutations are found mostly in SV patients. Point mutations p.V281L, p.P453S, p.P30L affect oxidoreductase interactions, salt-bridge and hydrogen-bonding networks, and allow 20–60% residual enzyme activity. Missense mutations are usually associated with NCCAH phenotype, and significant phenotype variability has been reported for p.P30L.

Large deletions form two types of CYP21A1P/CYP21A2 chimeras: classic and attenuated chimeras. In classic chimeras, the deletion totally inactivates CYP21A2 gene and classic chimeras are associated with zero 21-hydroxylase activity and SW phenotype. Most of the chimeras are of the classic type. The classic CYP21A1P/CYP21A2 chimeras contain the IVS2-13A/C>G mutation and sometimes other pseudogene mutations too (Hannah-Shmouni et al. 2017). In attenuated chimeras, some 21-hydroxylase activity is preserved, because the junction site is upstream of the pseudogene mutation IVS2-13A/C>G within intron 2. CH-4 and CH-9 attenuated chimeras have been described so far, and SV and NCCAH phenotypes have been reported. Approximately 96% of large deletions are classic chimeras and 4% are attenuated chimeras (Hannah-Shmouni et al. 2017).

Subtle variations in transcriptional regulation or downstream protein translation may modify genotype–phenotype concordance in all mutation groups. Genotype–phenotype concordance is high in p.V281L, p.Q318X, p.R356W, and 8 bp deletions. Approximately, a quarter of CAH patients who carry p.I172N mutation SW present with SW phenotype and the rest with SV phenotype. Similarly, intron 2 IVS2-13A/C>G splicing mutation can be associated with both SW and SV forms. It is noteworthy that if CAH is diagnosed early via newborn screening and treatment is introduced in the first days of life, it might be challenging to differentiate SW and SV on a clinical basis.

CNVs may lead to misinterpretation of genotypes. p.Q318X is sometimes associated with CYP21A2 duplication, therefore the mutated allele coexists with a normal CYP21A2-like gene within the RCCX module on the same chromosome. Since the normal gene is expressed, 21-hydroxylase enzyme activity is not diminished, this situation is not considered as a mutated allele but as a genetic variant.

Compound heterozygotes carry two different mutations within the two CYP21A2 alleles. These two mutations are often from different subgroups with different severities. In this case, the phenotype is usually determined by the less severe mutation with the more residual enzyme activity. However, significant variations in the genotype–phenotype correlation occur.

In addition to genetic variations within the RCCX module, several other factors modify the genotype–phenotype correlation. Some of these affect steroid action, sodium-electrolyte homeostasis, androgen receptor sensitivity (CAG repeats), RNA splicing factors, P450 oxidoreductase polymorphisms, glucocorticoid receptor sensitivity, or extra-adrenal 21-hydroxylase activity. The genotype–phenotype relationships require further research (Narasimhan and Khattab 2019).

12.2.1.2 Congenital Adrenal Hyperplasia-Tenascin-X-Syndrome

Deletions that cause a chimera truncating the *TNXB* gene cause both CAH and hypermobility-type Ehlers-Danlos syndrome (Fig. 12.5). Tenascin X is an extracellular matrix protein coded by the *TNXB* gene. This combined syndrome is called

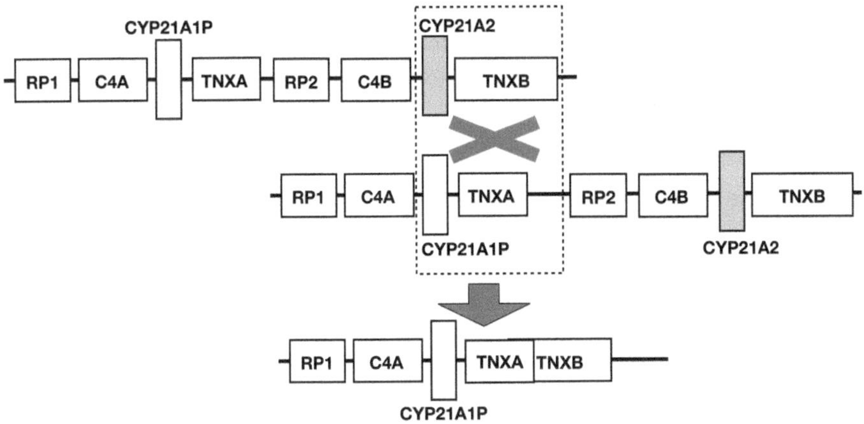

Fig. 12.5 CAH-X chimera. Misalignments during meiosis causing deletions that result in a chimera truncating the *TNXB* gene and deleting the active *CYP21A2* gene cause both CAH and hypermobility-type Ehlers-Danlos syndrome

CAH-X syndrome. According to population studies, approximately one-tenth of all CAH patients have CAH-X syndrome.

Three types of chimeras have been described in association with CAH-X (CAH-X CH-1, CAH-X CH-2, CAH-X CH-3). CAH-X CH-1 is caused by a 120 kb deletion in exon 35 of *TNXB* and results in haploinsufficiency and reduced tenascin-X synthesis, CAH-X CH-2 is caused by the c.12174C>G variant in exon 40 of TNXB, which causes a dominant negative effect due to loss of a critical disulfide bond in the tenascin-X fibrinogen-like domain (Miller and Merke 2018), and CAH-X CH-3 is caused by a cluster of three variants with dominant negative effects.

The clinical presentation of CAH-X patients is different for CAH. In addition to symptoms of SW-CAH, i.e., salt wasting, virilization, adrenal insufficiency, etc., they present with joint hypermobility, joint pain, joint dislocations, midline defects, or major structural cardiac abnormalities (Miller and Merke 2018).

12.2.1.3 Incidence

The worldwide incidence of classic CAH is 1:13–16,000 live births based on large-scale results from newborn screening programs. However, the prevalence in certain populations can be very different. The carrier rate of classic CAH is approximately 2%. NCCAH is very common; the prevalence is estimated to 1:1000 individuals. In certain ethnic groups, there are predominant haplotypes, which may have resulted from an ancient founder effect, unequal crossing over, or gene conversion from the pseudogene. For example, the p.V281L mutation is very frequent among the Ashkenazi Jewish population of New York, a large gene deletion is observed in Native Americans, the

IVS2-13A/C>G and p.V281L are frequent in the Middle European population. IVS2-13A/C>G is also predominant among Yupik Inuits in western Alaska and Iranians. In Finland, half of all CAH cases are caused by one of the three most common haplotypes (El-Maouche et al. 2017).

12.2.1.4 Molecular Analysis of *CYP21A2*

Genetic diagnosis of 21-OHD is challenging because of the complexity of its genomic region. There may be more than one RCCX modules on the same chromosome or more than one mutation in one allele and mutations in the pseudogene also have to be differentiated from mutations of CYP21A2. Therefore, molecular diagnostic approaches should be performed in certified laboratories with adequate quality controls and experience. Molecular genetic findings should be interpreted together with hormonal results and clinical presentation. Genotyping of the parents may be helpful in differentiating *cis* or *trans* configuration. Targeted site-directed mutation analysis of the 12 most common mutations fails to detect mutations in approximately 10% of cases, therefore whole coding region sequencing is recommended. Sequencing is especially important in cases of genotype–phenotype discordance.

The *CYP21A2* gene (Fig. 12.3) consists of ten exons. Real-time polymerase chain reaction (PCR) and multiplex ligation-dependent probe amplification (MLPA) are used for detecting large gene deletions and duplications. A long-range PCR protocol is used for sequencing the whole *CYP21A2* gene and part of the *TNXB* gene. The forward primer is common for both *CYP21A2* and the pseudogene, but the reverse primer anneals a nonhomologous part of the *TNXB* gene, therefore *CYP21A2* and *CYP21A1P* mutations can be differentiated accurately. Junction sites for chimeras can also be detected. Whole-gene sequencing can detect new mutations in addition to the common mutations, and reveal *TNXA/TNXB* mutations, too (Doleschall et al. 2017).

There are limitations of PCR-based techniques. Allele dropout is a general problem in PCR-based Sanger sequencing. Analysis of parental samples may overcome this problem and confirm homozygosity. The routinely used long-range PCR amplicon is unable to detect the *CYP21A2* duplication; another specific long-range PCR is needed. MLPA is not able to distinguish all attenuated chimeras for classic chimeras. Thus, an experienced laboratory using multiple techniques is optimal for CAH diagnostics (Hannah-Shmouni et al. 2017; Audi et al. 2018).

12.2.1.5 Neonatal Screening

All neonatal screening programs should include screening for 21-OHD since it is a potentially life-threatening condition that can be prevented effectively by means of neonatal screening. The first-tier method of screening is measurement of 17-OHP in blood spot samples; however, verification is required. Immunoassays result in relatively high false positive rate. As a second-tier measurement, liquid chromatography-tandem mass spectrometry (LC-MS/MS) or ACTH-stimulation test are preferred over genotyping unless an index case with identified mutations is known in the family. The newborn with positive screening results should be referred to a pediatric endocrinology expert immediately.

As a verification second-tier test the blood spot samples from the screening can be used either for dot blotting, ligation detection assays, real-time quantitative PCR, full sequencing, or minisequencing. Since more than 90% of patients carry one of the most frequent mutations, if none of these is detected, the patient may be considered healthy; however, if at least one is detected, further evaluation is required. Testing of parental samples may be useful. However, genetic studies may be costlier and more time-consuming than LC-MS/MS (Speiser et al. 2018).

12.2.1.6 Prenatal Diagnosis and Therapy

Prenatal diagnosis of 21-OHD is not recommended routinely. This is an invasive approach, using fetal DNA obtained by amniocentesis or chorionic villus sampling. Prenatal therapy is considered experimental and should be carried out only through ethically approved research protocols. The primary goal of prenatal therapy is suppression of fetal excess androgen synthesis in female fetuses to prevent virilization by maternal steroid therapy that effectively crosses the placenta, e.g., dexamethasone. However, in such case early, noninvasive determination of fetal sex allows cessation of unnecessary treatment of male fetuses. Screening for Y-chromosomal DNA in maternal blood is possible from the seventh week of gestation. However, there have been some concerns regarding the safety of prenatal dexamethasone therapy, and therefore it is not routinely recommended. Other than research setting, preconception counseling, genetic testing of parents, and risk determination are recommended instead of amniocentesis or chorionic villus sampling, since knowing the genetic status of the fetus does not have immediate therapeutic consequences. Close monitoring and early biochemical screening of the newborn is recommended. However, the risks of prenatal therapy may outweigh benefits (Speiser et al. 2018).

12.2.2 11β-Hydroxylase Deficiency

11β-hydroxylase deficiency (OMIM 202010) is responsible for approximately 5% of all CAH cases with an overall incidence of 1 in 100–200,000 live births, mostly explained by the p.R448H founder mutation. The highest prevalence is among Moroccan Jews (1:5–7000). 11-OHD is caused by mutations in the 11β-hydroxylase gene (*CYP11B1*), a P450 type I mitochondrial enzyme, catalyzing the conversion of 11-deoxycortisol to cortisol and 11-deoxycorticosterone (DOC) to corticosterone (Fig. 12.1). Defect of *CYP11B1* results in stop of cortisol and aldosterone biosynthesis, but mineralocorticoid deficiency does not occur, because elevated DOC and possibly other metabolites have significant mineralocorticoid activity and cause severe salt retention and hypertension. Severe glucocorticoid deficiency does not occur either, because excess corticosterone has some glucocorticoid activity. Hyperandrogenism occurs because precursors are shunted into the androgen synthesis pathway. 11-OHD is classified into classic and non-classic form. Classic 11-OHD patients present with virilization of the external genitalia of newborn girls, and with precocious pubarche and hypertension in both sexes. The non-classic form usually presents later in life.

The *CYP11B1* gene is located on chromosome 8q24.3, consists of 9 exons, and is 40-kb apart from the aldosterone synthase (*CYP11B2*) gene. More than 50 *CYP11B1* mutations have been described, most of them are missense or nonsense mutations, while splice-site mutations, small deletions and insertions, and complex rearrangements have also been reported. A variety of milder mutations result in non-classic 11-OHD. Unequal crossing-over between *CYP11B1* and the highly homologous *CYP11B2* results in a chimera that is under the control of angiotensin II and potassium, rather than ACTH, resulting in familial hyperaldosteronism type 1 (glucocorticoid-remediable aldosteronism), which is not considered a type of CAH (Khattab et al. 2017) (see Chap. 11).

12.2.3 17α-Hydroxylase Deficiency

17α-hydroxylase deficiency (17-OHD) (OMIM 202110) is caused by defective mutation in *CYP17A1* gene and is responsible for approximately 1% of all CAH cases. The CYP17A1 enzyme is a microsomal P450 type II enzyme with dual enzymatic activity: 17-α hydroxylation of pregnenolone and progesterone and the conversion of 17-hydroxypregnenolone to dehydroepiandrosterone and of 17-OHP to androstenedione through the 17,20 lyase reaction. Therefore, 17-OHD impairs both adrenal and gonadal function by glucocorticoid and sex steroid deficiency in both sexes. Patients do not experience mineralocorticoid or glucocorticoid deficiency, because corticosterone and DOC have significant glucocorticoid and mineralocorticoid activity respectively; on the contrary, symptoms of mineralocorticoid excess develop, such as hypertension and severe hypokalemia. Patients with severe 17-OHD present as phenotypic females regardless of chromosomal sex (both 46,XX and 46,XY) with hypertension, hypokalemia, and sexual infantilism. Patients with partial 17-OHD may present as undervirilized males (46,XY), neonates with ambiguous genitalia. Isolated 17,20 lyase deficiency is a rare disorder, caused by amino acid substitutions located within the area of the enzyme that interacts with the electron-donor redox partner, P450 oxidoreductase (POR). This defect causes impaired sex steroid biosynthesis only and is not considered a type of CAH. Male patients may present with undervirilization and later gynecomastia, while female patients present with delayed pubarche and oligomenorrhea.

The *CYP17A1* gene consists of 8 exons and is located on chromosome 10 (10q24.32). The CYP17A1 enzyme is 508 amino acids long. More than 70 inactivating mutations have been described. Usually, sequencing the whole coding region is necessary for genetic diagnostics. In some populations there is a higher incidence of 17-OHD, such as Canadian Mennonites, Dutch Frieslanders, Japanese, East Asians, and Brazilian, most likely due to a founder effect (Auchus 2017).

12.2.4 3β-Hydroxysteroid Dehydrogenase Type 2 Deficiency

3β-hydroxysteroid dehydrogenase type 2 (HSD3B2) deficiency (OMIM 201810) is rare with unknown incidence. The enzyme has two isoforms, type 1 and type 2, each coded by different genes on chromosome 1 (1p12), *HSD3B1* and *HSD3B2*. Both genes consist of 4 exons. *HSD3B1* is expressed in the placenta and peripheral tissues, while *HSD3B2* is expressed in the gonads and adrenal glands. *HSD3B2* catalyzes the conversion of pregnenolone, 17-hydroxypregnenolone, and dehydroepiandrosterone to progesterone, 17-OHP, and androstenedione, respectively. Both gonadal and adrenal steroid syntheses are affected. Depending on the severity of the enzyme deficiency, both affected males and females may be born with ambiguous genitalia. The existence of a mild, non-classic form was suggested based on biochemical findings, but genetic studies did not confirm the presence of such mutations (Al Alawi et al. 2019).

12.2.5 P450 Oxidoreductase Deficiency

POR deficiency (OMIM 613571) is rare with unknown incidence. The *POR* gene is located on the long arm of chromosome 7 (7q11.23), 32.9 kb long and consists of 15 exons. POR is an electron donor of CYP17A1, CYP19A1 (aromatase), and CYP21A2; therefore, POR deficiency biochemically presents as a combined CYP17A1 and CYP17A2 deficiency. Both sexes present with sexual ambiguity. Reduced CYP19A1 activity leads to androgen accumulation in the placenta, leading to the virilization of the female fetus and even the mother. Adrenal insufficiency is present.

Skeletal, especially craniofacial malformations may occur. The clinical presentation overlaps with Antley-Bixler syndrome (OMIM 201750), characterized by craniosynostosis and radiohumeral synostosis. Patients with mild-to-moderate malformations are usually compound heterozygotes for missense mutations, while patients with severe malformation harbor a major loss-of-function mutation. POR inactivating mutations are missense, frameshift, and splice-site mutations. The most frequent point mutation in Caucasians is p.A287P, while p.R457H is frequent in Japan. More than 20 mutations have been described so far. If the mutation affects the 17-hydroxylase interacting region of POR, biochemically POR deficiency can present as apparent 17,20 lyase deficiency (Miller 2018).

12.2.6 Lipoid Congenital Adrenal Hyperplasia

Lipoid CAH (OMIM 201710) is rare with unknown incidence, most common in Japanese, Korean, and Palestinian Arab populations. Lipoid CAH is caused by a mutation in the steroidogenic acute regulatory protein (StAR) that facilitates cholesterol transfer in the mitochondria, the rate-limiting step of steroid hormone biosynthesis. The defect severely affects both adrenal and gonadal steroidogenesis. In classic lipoid CAH, there is a near total loss of all steroid hormones. Due to StAR-dependent damage in steroid biosynthesis, accumulation of toxic cholesterol esters occur, leading to cellular damage and secondary loss of StAR-independent steroid synthesis.

The gene encoding StAR is located on chromosome 8 (8p11.23). The clinical presentation is a severe salt-wasting crisis due to glucocorticoid and mineralocorticoid deficiency in a phenotypic female in the neonatal period. If not diagnosed early the outcome is often fatal. Several mutations have been described in exons 5, 6, and 7. A milder form of lipoid CAH is caused by mutations with 20–30% of residual StAR activity. Most patients carry the p.R188C *StAR* mutation. A non-classic lipoid CAH has also been described (Miller 2018).

12.2.7 Cholesterol Side-Chain Cleavage Enzyme Deficiency

Mutations in the *CYP11A1* gene cause SCC deficiency (OMIM 118485). SCC deficiency is an extremely rare form of CAH; altogether 28 patients have been reported, most of them from Eastern Turkey. Phenotype is variable, possibly due to variable effect of mutations on the enzyme activity (Miller 2018).

12.3 Genetic Counseling

All forms of CAH are inherited in an autosomal recessive manner. Genotype and phenotype correlations are strong, and children within the same family usually have similar disease severity. Genetic counseling is recommended for families of known CAH patients, CAH patients entering puberty, or NCCAH patients upon diagnosis. The focus of the genetic counseling is the risk of having an affected child. CAH carriers usually do not have symptoms. If both parents are carriers, there is a 25% probability that each subsequent siblings of the index case will have CAH and 50% probability that each will be a heterozygous carrier. The genetic risk is same for males and females; however, clinical severity (i.e., need for genitoplasty surgery in affected girls) may be different.

Prenatal diagnosis from amniocentesis or chorion villous samples is not recommended outside of a research setting, since the risk of sampling outweighs the possible benefit. Prenatal dexamethasone therapy is able to prevent the virilization of external genitalia for female fetuses; however, there are controversies. Unaffected fetuses are also treated for a short period, which may have negative emotional and cognitive consequences. Currently, there are no standardized evidence-based protocols for prenatal therapy for CAH (Dörr et al. 2015).

The incidence of classical 21OHD in the general population is 1:10–20,000, with a carrier rate of 1:50–71, median 1:60. The chance that a patient with CAH will have a child with classic CAH is 1:120 [chance of having a carrier partner (0.016) × 0.5]. Two-thirds of NCCAH patients are compound heterozygotes with one mild and one severely affected allele. The chance that an NCCAH patient will have a child with classic CAH is 1:360 (chance of having a carrier partner × chance of NCCAH patient being compound heterozygote × 0.25 = 0.016 × 0.666 × 0.25). Interestingly, this risk may be actually higher, as a retrospective study found 2.5% risk of NCCAH women having classic CAH children. Hormonal testing, even with ACTH stimulation, does not identify carriers accurately, and genetic testing is mandatory to identify carriers.

Counseling should be provided by an experienced clinical genetic counselor. The clinical prognosis is preferably discussed with a multidisciplinary group of experts, involving pediatric surgeon, gynecologist, and endocrinologist.

There are some special points that should be addressed. Genetic testing, due to the complex nature of the affected gene regions, might miss mutant alleles. The sensitivity is better if there is a known index case in the family. The optimal timing of genetic counseling is before conception. The genetic testing of the partner of the proband or both parents of the index case is recommended for accurate risk determination. Testing of other family members, especially children, is not recommended routinely. Genetic testing of underaged related family members without clinical symptoms may be prohibited by law in some countries. The impact of a positive result on the families, their attitude toward risks and treatment should be discussed in detail (Speiser et al. 2018).

References

Al Alawi AM, Nordenström A, Falhammar H (2019) Clinical perspectives in congenital adrenal hyperplasia due to 3β-hydroxysteroid dehydrogenase type 2 deficiency. Endocrine 63 (3):407–421. https://doi.org/10.1007/s12020-018-01835-3

Auchus RJ (2017) Steroid 17-hydroxylase and 17,20-lyase deficiencies, genetic and pharmacologic. J Steroid Biochem Mol Biol 165(Pt A):71–78. https://doi.org/10.1016/j.jsbmb.2016.02.002

Audi L, Ahmed SF, Krone N et al (2018) GENETICS IN ENDOCRINOLOGY: approaches to molecular genetic diagnosis in the management of differences/disorders of sex development (DSD): position paper of EU COST Action BM 1303 'DSDnet'. Eur J Endocrinol 179(4):R197–R206. https://doi.org/10.1530/EJE-18-0256

Doleschall M, Luczay A, Koncz K et al (2017) A unique haplotype of RCCX copy number variation: from the clinics of congenital adrenal hyperplasia to evolutionary genetics. Eur J Hum Genet 25(6):702–710. https://doi.org/10.1038/ejhg.2017.38

Dörr HG, Binder G, Reisch N et al (2015) Experts' opinion on the prenatal therapy of congenital adrenal hyperplasia (CAH) due to 21-hydroxylase deficiency—guideline of DGKED in cooperation with DGGG (S1-level, AWMF registry no. 174/013, July 2015). Geburtshilfe Frauenheilkd 75(12):1232–1238. https://doi.org/10.1055/s-0041-109717

El-Maouche D, Arlt W, Merke DP (2017) Congenital adrenal hyperplasia. Lancet 390 (10108):2194–2210. https://doi.org/10.1016/S0140-6736(17)31431-9

Hannah-Shmouni F, Chen W, Merke DP (2017) Genetics of congenital adrenal hyperplasia. Endocrinol Metab Clin N Am 46(2):435–458. https://doi.org/10.1016/j.ecl.2017.01.008

Khattab A, Haider S, Kumar A et al (2017) Clinical, genetic, and structural basis of congenital adrenal hyperplasia due to 11β-hydroxylase deficiency. Proc Natl Acad Sci USA 114(10): E1933–E1940. https://doi.org/10.1073/pnas.1621082114

Miller WL (2018) MECHANISMS IN ENDOCRINOLOGY: rare defects in adrenal steroidogenesis. Eur J Endocrinol 179(3):R125–R141. https://doi.org/10.1530/EJE-18-0279

Miller WL, Merke DP (2018) Tenascin-X, congenital adrenal hyperplasia, and the CAH-X syndrome. Horm Res Paediatr 89(5):352–361. https://doi.org/10.1159/000481911

Narasimhan ML, Khattab A (2019) Genetics of congenital adrenal hyperplasia and genotype-phenotype correlation. Fertil Steril 111(1):24–29. https://doi.org/10.1016/j.fertnstert.2018.11.007

Simonetti L, Bruque CD, Fernández CS et al (2018) CYP21A2 mutation update: comprehensive analysis of databases and published genetic variants. Hum Mutat 39(1):5–22. https://doi.org/10.1002/humu.23351

Speiser PW, Arlt W, Auchus RJ et al (2018) Congenital adrenal hyperplasia due to steroid 21-hydroxylase deficiency: an Endocrine Society clinical practice guideline. J Clin Endocrinol Metab 103(11):4043–4088. https://doi.org/10.1210/jc.2018-01865

Part IV
Endocrine Diseases Inherited as Monogenic Traits: Monogenic Diseases Predisposing to Hormone Deficiency, Infertility and Diabetes Mellitus

Chapter 13
Pituitary Transcription Factor Mutations Leading to Hypopituitarism

Peter Gergics

Abstract Congenital pituitary hormone deficiency is a disabling condition. It is part of a spectrum of disorders including craniofacial midline developmental defects ranging from holoprosencephaly through septo-optic dysplasia to combined and isolated pituitary hormone deficiency. The first genes discovered in the human disease were based on mouse models of dwarfism due to mutations in transcription factor genes. High-throughput DNA sequencing technologies enabled clinicians and researchers to find novel genetic causes of hypopituitarism for the more than three quarters of patients without a known genetic diagnosis to date. Transcription factor (TF) genes are at the forefront of the functional analysis of novel variants of unknown significance due to the relative ease in in vitro testing in a research lab. Genetic testing in hypopituitarism is of high importance to the individual and their family to predict phenotype composition, disease progression and to avoid life-threatening complications such as secondary adrenal insufficiency.

This chapter aims to highlight our current understanding about (1) the contribution of TF genes to pituitary development (2) the diversity of inheritance and phenotype features in combined and select isolated pituitary hormone deficiency and (3) provide an initial assessment on how to approach variants of unknown significance in human hypopituitarism. Our better understanding on how transcription factor gene variants lead to hypopituitarism is a meaningful step to plan advanced therapies to specific genetic changes in the future.

Keywords Pituitary hormone deficiency · Transcription factor · Inheritance · Genetic testing · Variants of unknown significance

P. Gergics (✉)
Department of Human Genetics, University of Michigan, Ann Arbor, MI, USA
e-mail: gergicsp@med.umich.edu

P. Igaz, A. Patócs (eds.), *Genetics of Endocrine Diseases and Syndromes*, Experientia Supplementum 111, https://doi.org/10.1007/978-3-030-25905-1_13

List of Abbreviations

ACTH	Adrenocorticotropic hormone
AL	Anterior lobe of pituitary
Bmp	Bone morphogenetic protein
CGA	Choriogonadotropin alpha subunit
CNS	Central nervous system
CPHD	Combined pituitary hormone deficiency
Fgf	Fibroblast growth factor
FSH	Follicle-stimulating hormone
GH	Growth hormone
GHD	Growth hormone deficiency
GR	Glucocorticoid receptor
HH	Hypogonadotropic hypogonadism
IAD	Isolated ACTH deficiency
IGHD	Isolated growth hormone deficiency
IL	Intermediate lobe of pituitary
LH	Luteinizing hormone
MSH-α	Melanocyte-stimulating hormone, alpha
ONH	Optic nerve hypoplasia
PC(SK)	Proprotein convertase (subtilisin/kexin)
PL	Posterior lobe of pituitary
POMC	Pro-opiomelanocortin
PRL	Prolactin
RAR	Retinoic acid receptor
Shh	Sonic hedgehog
TF	Transcription factor
TR	Thyroid hormone receptor
TSH	Thyroid-stimulating hormone
VUS	Variants of unknown significance
WES	Whole exome sequencing
Wnt	Wingless-type MMTV integration site family/beta-catenin

13.1 Introduction

13.1.1 Incidence and Diagnosis of Human Hypopituitarism

Hypopituitarism affects around 1 in 4000 live births (Castinetti et al. 2012, 2008a; Regal et al. 2001). Combined pituitary hormone deficiency (CPHD) is defined by the deficiency of GH (growth hormone) and at least one more hormone of TSH, ACTH, LH, FSH, PRL (thyroid-stimulating hormone, adrenocorticotropic hormone, luteinizing hormone, follicle-stimulating hormone, and prolactin, respectively). The incidence of CPHD is estimated to be 1:8000 according to the Genetics Home Reference at the National Institutes of Health (ghr.nlm.nih.gov). The most common pituitary hormone deficient is GH in 1:4000–1:10,000 individuals (Alatzoglou and Dattani 2010), while other isolated pituitary hormone deficiencies are rare. Congenital hypothyroidism has an incidence of 1:3000 (Grosse and Van Vliet 2011), isolated hypogonadotropic hypogonadism (isolated HH) has an incidence under 1:10,000 and is frequently associated with anosmia/hyposmia (Hayes et al. 1998; Seminara et al. 2000). The incidence of congenital isolated ACTH (corticotrope) deficiency (IAD) is largely unknown (Patti et al. 2018). Overall, this places hypopituitarism in the upper end of rare diseases (Richter et al. 2015).

Genetic factors substantially influence height, and short stature is a common cause for referrals to endocrinologists (Pfäffle 2006). The diagnosis of pituitary hormone deficiency is based on guidelines by professional organizations and medical institutes (Ergin et al. 2015). We refer to these for specific details regarding the clinical diagnosis of growth hormone deficiency (GHD) in children (Chinoy and Murray 2016), GHD in adults (Molitch et al. 2011), congenital HH (Boehm et al. 2015) and congenital central hypothyroidism (Leger et al. 2014). Guidelines are not yet established for isolated ACTH deficiency (IAD) (Andrioli et al. 2006) or PRL deficiency in particular. The focus of this chapter is to explore the non-acquired/genetic causes with special attention to transcription factor (TF) genes.

Transcription factors are widely recognized as regulators of pituitary development. Mouse models provided the fundamental evidence for their role in pituitary development; however, not all of the orthologous human genes turned out to be involved in human pituitary disease. An extensive list of TFs involved in vertebrate pituitary development is provided in Table 13.1 [TF classification is based on http://tfclass.bioinf.med.uni-goettingen.de (Wingender et al. 2015)].

Around 2000 TFs are known today. Nearly a third of them are known to have functions during development. They are classified based on protein domains and about 80% of all TFs have C2H2-zinc-finger, homeodomain or helix-loop-helix motifs (Vaquerizas et al. 2009). Most of the genes currently known in the pathogenesis of human isolated growth hormone deficiency (IGHD) or CPHD are TFs discussed in this review. Genes predominantly involved in HH are discussed elsewhere (Maione et al. 2018). Also, those genes that are involved in signaling (*BMP4, CDON, FGF8, FGFR1, GPR161, HHIP, IGSF1, PROKR2, SHH, WDR11*), RNA processing (*EIF2B5, HNRNPU, POLR3A, RBM28, RNPC3*), and other processes (*CHD7, IFT72, 52KCNQ1, PNPLA6, ZSWIM6*) (Di Iorgi et al. 2016; Fang et al. 2016b; Norppa et al. 2018; Tommiska et al. 2017) are not the focus of this review.

Table 13.1 Transcription factors in pituitary development

TF superclass	TF class and family	Human gene	Full name	Human chromosomal localization
Helix-turn-helix	HD-LIM-type	*LHX3* *LHX4* *ISL1*	LIM homeobox 3 LIM homeobox 4 ISL LIM homeobox 1	9q34.3 1q25.2 5q11.1
	HD-NK	*NKX2–1*	NK2 homeobox 1	14q13.3
	HD-paired	*PAX6*	Paired box 6	11p13
	HD-paired-related	*PROP1* *HESX1* *OTX2* *PITX2* *PITX1*	PROP paired-like homeobox 1 Homeobox, ES cell expressed 1 Orthodenticle homeobox 2 Paired-like homeodomain 2 Paired-like homeodomain 1	5q35.3 3p14.3 14q22.3 4q25 5q31.1
	HD-POU	*POU1F1*	POU class 1 homeobox 1	3p11.2
	HD-SINE	*SIX3* *SIX6*	Sine oculis homeobox homolog 3 Sine oculis homeobox homolog 6	2p21 14q23.1
	HD-TALE type-PKNOX	*TGIF1*	TGFB-induced factor homeobox 1	18p11.31
	HD-VAX	*VAX1*	Ventral anterior homeobox 1	10q25.3
	Forkhead and winged helix	*FOXA2* *FOXL2* *FOXO1*	Forkhead box A2 Forkhead box L2 Forkhead box O1	20p11.21 3q22.3 13q14.11
Helix-loop-helix	Per-Arnt-Sim (PAS)-ARNT	*ARNT2*	Aryl-hydrocarbon receptor nuclear translocator 2	15q25.1
Basic helix-loop-helix (bHLH)	MyoD-ASC-related	*ASCL1*	Achaete-scute family bHLH transcription factor 1	12q23.2
	Tal-related-Neurogenin-ATO	*NEUROD1* *NEUROD4*	Neuronal differentiation 1 Neuronal differentiation 4	2q31.3 12q13.2
All alpha helical	HMG-SOX-related-group B	*SOX2* *SOX3*	SRY (sex determining region Y)-box 2 SRY (sex determining region Y)-box 3	3q26.33 Xq27.1
	HMG-TCF-related	*TCF7L1*	Transcription factor 7-like 1	2p11.2
Basic leucine zipper	CEBP related-PAR	*TEF*	Thyrotrophic embryonic factor	22q13.2

(continued)

Table 13.1 (continued)

TF superclass	TF class and family	Human gene	Full name	Human chromosomal localization
Zn-finger (ZnF)	C2H2-ZnF-three-ZnF-Kruppel-related-EGR	*EGR1*	Early growth response 1	5q31.2
	C2H2-ZnF-more than three adjacent ZnF	*GLI2* *GLI3* *ZIC2*	GLI family zinc finger 2 GLI family zinc finger 3 ZIC family member 2	2q14.2 7p14.1 13q32.3
	C2H2-ZnF-multiple dispersed ZnF	*INSM1*	Insulinoma-associated 1	20p11.23
	C4-ZnF-FTZF1-related	*NR5A1*	Nuclear receptor subfamily 5, group A, member 1	9q33.3
	C4-ZnF-GATA-double	*GATA2*	GATA binding protein 2	3q21.3
Immunoglobulin fold	RHR-NFKB-related	*NFKB2*	Nuclear factor of kappa light polypeptide gene enhancer in B-cells 2 (p49/p100)	10q24.32
	T-box-Brachyury-related	*TBX19*	T-box 19	1q24.2

CEBP CCAAT/enhancer-binding protein beta, *HD* homeodomain, *LIM* Lin-11, Isl-1, Mec-3, *HMG* high mobility group, *FTZF1* Fushi tarazu transcription factor-1, *GATA* ability to bind to GATA nucleotide sequence, *NK* homologous to the naked cuticle or 93D/E gene cluster in Drosophila, *PAR* proline and acidic amino acid-rich, *PKNOX* Pre-B-Cell Leukemia Homeobox (PBX)/Knotted 1 Homeobox 1, *POU* Pit1, OCT1/2 unc-86, *RHR* Rel homology region, *SINE* sine oculis, *TALE* Three Amino acid Loop Extension, *TGFB* Transforming growth factor beta, *ZIC* zinc finger protein of the cerebellum

13.1.2 Why Does Genetic Diagnosis Matter in Hypopituitarism?

About 15% of CPHD cases have mutations in *PROP1, POU1F1, LHX3, LHX4,* or *HESX1* but systematic screens have not been done for all genes implicated in the disorder (De Rienzo et al. 2015; Fang et al. 2016b). Genetic diagnosis in hypopituitarism has consequences for disease progression and family screening. The international GENHYPOPIT network—with more than 1200 patients (Brue 2018)—reported that only ~25% of their GHD patients were diagnosed neonatally, 32% during puberty, and about 10% well into adulthood (Brue et al. 2017). Pituitary hormone deficiency can evolve over the course of time; therefore, intermittent screening for new hormone deficiency is warranted. For example, IGHD diagnosed in childhood can evolve to

CPHD with TSH and LH deficiency in young adulthood, and with ACTH deficiency later in adulthood (>30 year) (Brue et al. 2017; Coya et al. 2007; Halasz et al. 2006). While some gene deficiencies present with a consistent phenotype (*PROP1*, *POU1F1*), incomplete penetrance and variable expressivity pose a challenge in predicting pituitary disease progression and extra-pituitary manifestations (i.e., *LHX4*, *GLI2*). The size of the pituitary is often smaller than normal in patients with hypopituitarism; however, patients with *PROP1* variants may exhibit pituitary hyperplasia and apparent dynamic changes in the organ size (waxing and waning) (Obermannova et al. 2011; Turton et al. 2005a). The diagnosis of *PROP1* variants in these cases can prevent invasive procedures and spontaneous regression can be anticipated (Dattani 2005). Additionally, the rationale for genetic testing of close family members is quintessential to prevent serious/life-threatening conditions such as secondary adrenal insufficiency (Pekic et al. 2011).

13.1.3 Genetic Diagnostics in Hypopituitarism

Endocrinologists and medical geneticists typically share the responsibility of establishing the genetic diagnosis in hypopituitarism. There is no "state of the art" hypopituitarism-specific genetic diagnostics guideline published by a medical society to date. Family history is the most essential component in the analysis. To identify the genetic origin for hypopituitarism it is important to consider several genetic models: (1) large families with multiple affected individuals suggesting a dominant inheritance; (2) consanguineous families where the odds for recessive disorders is increased; or (3) trios with an affected child with at least one unaffected parent, suggesting incompletely penetrant dominant, recessive, or de novo variants in the proband. In addition, people from the Iberian Peninsula or Lithuania have a higher probability of carrying one of the two founder mutations of *PROP1* (Dusatkova et al. 2016).

The technology used to detect genetic changes includes single gene Sanger sequencing, panel sequencing of the most well-established genes, or next-generation sequencing technologies to assess coding regions genome-wide (Whole Exome Sequencing—WES). Single gene sequencing revealed that around 11% of CPHD patients had variants in *PROP1*, whereas *POU1F1*, *LHX4*, *LHX3*, and *HESX1* were around 1% each, respectively (Fang et al. 2016b). In most diseases the overall genetic diagnosis "solve rate" of WES is ~30% and that would be an excellent progress from the current 15% at best with traditional methods (Trujillano et al. 2017). Papers reporting on results with whole genome sequencing are scarce in hypopituitarism. Only a few publications provide insight into the incidence of larger, chromosomal changes. Copy number variations account for ~8% of the congenital hypopituitarism cases (Correa et al. 2018; Dateki et al. 2010a; Takagi et al. 2015). Recently, a targeted version of WES using the principle of molecular inversion probes was reported to screen 51 patients for 30 known and 37 candidate genes, which has excellent perspectives in screening and identifying more novel variants (Perez Millan et al. 2018).

13.2 Pituitary Gland Structure, Function, and Development

13.2.1 The Structure of the Pituitary: "One Gland Above All"

The pituitary is the major neuroendocrine gland serving as a key hub between the central nervous system (CNS) and the majority of endocrine organs. The mammalian pituitary can be divided into three lobes: anterior (AL), intermediate (IL), and posterior (PL). The AL and IL are derived from the evaginating oral ectoderm (Rathke's cleft) and ensphere both the stalk and the anterolateral aspect of the PL. The IL is rudimentary in humans and a common site for cystic lesions (Rathke's cleft cysts). A fine mesh of a portal vessel system in the anterior lobe allows direct communication from the hypothalamus to the pituitary through blood flow. The axon terminals are surrounded by glial-like cell types (pituicytes) and form the posterior lobe (PL) (Goto et al. 2015).

13.2.2 The Basic Function of the Pituitary

Pituitary function is essential in growth, fertility, lactation, stress response, and general homeostasis. The anterior lobe has five major cell types producing six major hormones: somatotrophs (producing GH); lactotrophs (PRL); melano-corticotropes (POMC) and its cleavage products: ACTH, α-MSH; thyrotrophs (TSH); and gonadotrophs (LH, FSH). TSH, FSH, and LH are heterodimers of the choriogonadotropin alpha subunit (CGA) and specific beta subunits TSHB, FSHB, and LHB, respectively. The proportion of these cell types is unequal in the adult pituitary such as ~40% are somatotrophs, ~40% lactotrophs, ~10% gonadotrophs, 10% corticotropes, and only 5% are thyrotropes (Kulig et al. 1998). While these make up the majority of resident cells in the AL, there is a fraction that is hormone negative and includes non-differentiated stem cells, progenitor cells, folliculostellate cells, endothelial cells, pericytes, and mesenchymal cells. Defects leading to the loss of predominant cell types can frequently result in a hypoplastic AL (Gangat and Radovick 2017). The PL contains the axon terminals of hypothalamic neurons in the supraoptic and paraventricular nuclei producing arginine-vasopressin (AVP) and oxytocin (OXT). While AVP and OXT are stored in the terminals they are surrounded by a subset of glial-like cells (Goto et al. 2015). Single cell sequencing technologies did not reveal a new major physiological cell type so far but a better resolution of known cell types important in critical stages of development, adaptation to stimuli and neoplasia are highly anticipated (Cheung et al. 2018).

13.3 Lessons from Mouse Pituitary Development to Human Hypopituitarism

13.3.1 Early Patterning of the Pituitary Primordium

Spatiotemporal expression of TFs in the ventral diencephalon and the oral ectoderm results in the formation of the AL/IL/PL between mouse E9 and E12 days. In addition to a severe pituitary abnormality, a wide spectrum of features is present when specific TFs are disrupted. Defects in *Pitx2, Isl1, Nkx2.1* result in complex anomalies involving the CNS, the eyes, and multiple non-ectodermal organs such as the heart and the thyroid. *Hesx1, Vax1, Pax6, Otx2, Six3, Six6* deficient mice present with CNS, eye, and other malformations predominantly in the head region (McCabe and Dattani 2014). Others show CNS abnormalities and disorders affecting the ventral motor neurons [*Lhx3/Lhx4*, (Gergics et al. 2015)], segmental bone formation [*Gli2*, (Haddad-Tovolli et al. 2015)] or the gonads [*Sox3*, (Rizzoti et al. 2004)]. *Sox2* is essential in the specification of all pituitary hormone producing and folliculostellate cells and is considered as a signature pituitary stem cell marker (Fauquier et al. 2008). *Sox2/Sox9* co-expressing cells are regarded as committed progenitor cells in the pituitary (Rizzoti et al. 2013).

Pituitary organogenesis and hormone cell specification are outlined in Figs. 13.1 and 13.2.

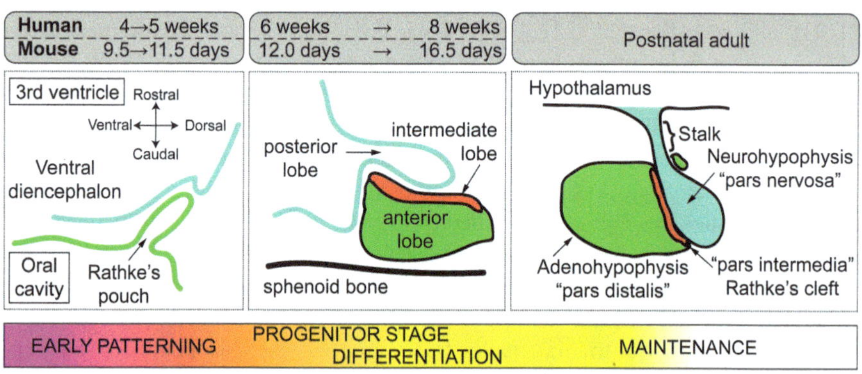

Fig. 13.1 Schematic development of the pituitary in the mouse and human in the midsagittal plane. By mouse embryonic day E16.5, the organ reaches its final shape. Several signaling pathways regulate pituitary development. A continuous Shh expression gets interrupted by Wnt signaling from the diencephalon at E9.5 and the Rathke's pouch protrudes from the rooftop of the oral cavity. These events result in altered expressions of *Bmps* and *Fgfs* and define the pituitary organizer domain of the ventral diencephalon [references within Osmundsen et al. (2017)]. Fgf and Notch signaling orchestrate the evagination of the hypothalamic floor plate of the third ventricle to form the infundibulum and the subsequent PL (Goto et al. 2015)

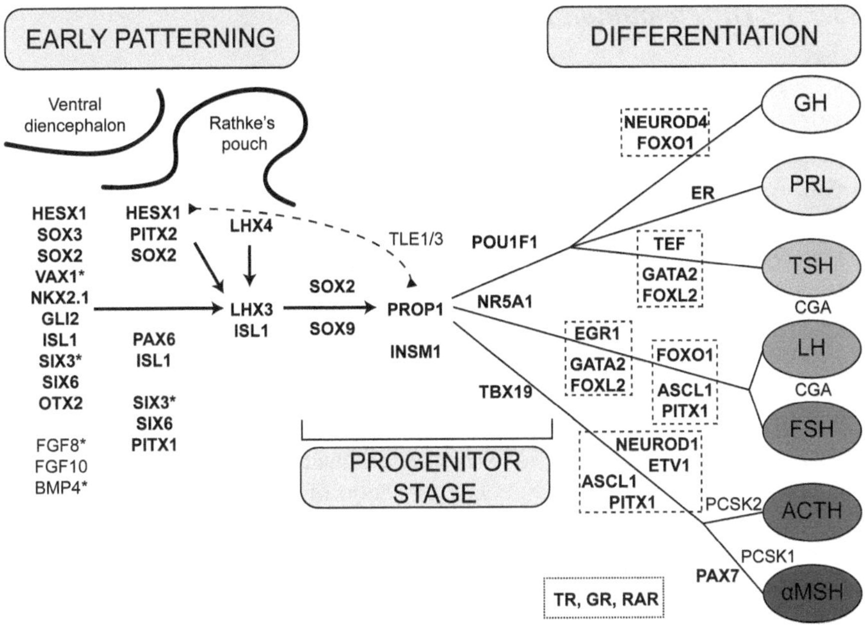

Fig. 13.2 Involvement of transcription factors in the development hormone producing cells in the pituitary anterior lobe. Multiple transcription factors (TFs) participate in the specification of pituitary hormone producing cells. Details of the three main phases of pituitary development are described in the main text. Asterisk: Supernumerary pituitary gland formation is noted in the—Bmp inhibitor—*Noggin*$^{-/-}$ (Davis and Camper 2007), *Tg(Cga-Fgf8)Rsd* (Treier et al. 2001), *Six3*$^{+/-}$ *Hesx1*$^{cre/+}$ (Gaston-Massuet et al. 2008), and *Vax1*$^{-/-}$ mice (Bharti et al. 2011). In the differentiation phase certain TFs are needed for multiple lineages. For example, *Gata2* is a major factor in the transcriptional regulation of *Cga*, *Tshb*, *Lhb* (Dasen et al. 1999). An array of steroid/retinoid/thyroid hormone receptor stimulation is also needed for physiological pituitary hormone expression. Solid arrows mark upstream/downstream relation between factors but do not necessarily mark direct regulation. Dotted curve represents repressive relationship. Acronyms in bold are TFs and correspond to the Table 13.1

13.3.2 Progenitor Cell Determination

Prop1 (Prophet of Pit1) is a key pituitary-specific TF (Sornson et al. 1996). All pituitary hormone producing cell types go through a *Prop1* expressing progenitor stage (Davis et al. 2016). Its main downstream target *Pou1f1* is a lineage determining factor for somatolactotrophs and most thyrotrophs (Li et al. 1990). *Insm1* is key in the differentiation of multiple neuroendocrine cell types. In the absence of *Insm1*, the *Sox2/Sox9+* pituitary stem/progenitor cell pool is maintained, lineage-specific transcription factors (*Pou1f1, Tbx19, NeuroD1, Nr5a1*) are moderately expressed, but all GH, TSH, LH/FSH cells are missing, and PRL, ACTH, and αMSH cell numbers are drastically reduced (Welcker et al. 2013).

13.3.3 Differentiation Phase

The *POU1F1* Lineage (Somatolactotrophs and Thyrotrophs)
Pou1f1 (formerly *Pit-1*) is a signature pituitary transcription factor that directly regulates the transcription of *Gh*, *Prl*, *Tshb*, and *Cga* (Gordon et al. 1993; Li et al. 1990). A cluster of thyrotrophs in the rostral tip develops independently of *Pou1f1* (Lin et al. 1994). Notable significant other factors for this lineage are: *Neurod4* (Ando et al. 2018), *Foxo1* (Kapali et al. 2016) for somatotrophs, the estrogen receptor for lactotrophs (Day et al. 1990), and thyrotroph embryonic factor (TEF) for thyrotrophs (Drolet et al. 1991).

Gonadotroph and Melanocorticotroph Lineages
Nr5a1 (previously known as *Sf1*) is a hallmark TF for gonadotroph commitment (Zhao et al. 2001). *Egr1* is expressed predominantly in gonadotrophs (Man et al. 2014). *Tbx19* (previously known as *Tpit*) is a signature TF of melanocorticotrope commitment and in the transcriptional regulation of POMC (Budry et al. 2011). *Pax7* is a pioneer transcription factor acting as a selector to melanotrope over corticotrope faith through chromatin remodeling (Budry et al. 2012). The expression of specific proprotein convertases (PC or PCSK) is key in the differential cleavage of POMC (Marcinkiewicz et al. 1993).

13.4 Human Gene Variants in Pituitary Hormone Deficiency

13.4.1 Interpretation of Novel Genes/Variants in the Era of Whole Exome/Genome Sequencing

The discovery of specific genes in hypopituitarism started in the 1990s with *Pou1f1* about 60 years after the discovery of the Snell dwarf (*Pou1f1*$^{dw/dw}$) (Li et al. 1990). A dozen other genes such as *PROP1, HESX1, LHX3, LHX4* were described in human hypopituitarism in the next two decades. Thanks to the Human Genome Project and the availability of Sanger sequencing, genetic testing improved for patients with hypopituitarism. Single gene sequencing was amenable as long as a limited number of candidate genes needed to be screened. As the number of candidate genes increased, automated panel sequencing took over (Klee et al. 2011).

The rise of next-generation sequencing technologies from around 2007 changed the landscape dramatically and dozens of novel candidate genes and variants were identified in a decade (Warr et al. 2015). This flipped the order such that the candidate genes and variants were found in the human first and then functional studies in cell lines and vertebrate model organisms were implemented to discern the pathogenicity and disease mechanism. In this new era, the most difficult task is to evaluate the many novel genes and variants with unknown significance (VUS).

Analyzing VUS in patients with hypopituitarism is of utmost importance since less than 15% of hypopituitarism patients have a genetic diagnosis (De Rienzo et al. 2015; Fang et al. 2016b). Professional organizations such as the American College of Medical Genetics (ACMG), the Association for Molecular Pathology (AMP) (Richards et al. 2015), ClinGen Sequence Variant Interpretation (SVI) Working Group (ClinGen SVI WG) (Strande et al. 2017) in the USA, or the Association for Clinical Genomic Science in the UK developed recommendations for variant interpretation. This effort is ongoing and expanding to develop some disease-specific guidelines as well. These recommendations classify VUS based on evidence of (1) known physiological expression and function, (2) changes in these when the variant is present, as well as on (3) animal and in vitro model systems and rescue experiments corresponding to the human disease.

Initial evaluation of VUS includes the assessment of the (1) probability for loss of intolerance (pLI) of the gene; (2) frequency of the VUS in a matched population [e.g., Genome Aggregation Database (gnomAD), gnomad.broadinstitute.org (Lek et al. 2016)]; (3) protein structure and function prediction combined with evolutionary conservation [e.g. Combined Annotation Dependent Depletion (CADD), cadd.gs.washington.edu, (Rentzsch et al. 2019)].

A more detailed analysis includes investigation of (4) spatial and temporal expression of the mRNA/protein especially in the disease-affected tissues (postnatally, e.g., Genotype-Tissue Expression (GTEx) project, gtexportal.org/home/, Tabula Muris, tabula-muris.ds.czbiohub.org (Schaum et al. 2018), The Human Protein Atlas www.proteinatlas.org/humanproteome/tissue) or embryonic ages (Brinkmeier et al. 2009; Ma et al. 2009) (5) knockout vertebrate models (e.g., Mouse Genome Informatics: www.informatics.jax.org/phenotypes.shtml, The Zebrafish Information Network zfin.org).

These surveys can support the role of a VUS but further (6) in vitro and (7) in vivo vertebrate studies are necessary to elevate the level of proof for pathogenicity. The in vitro studies need to demonstrate the biological difference between the wild type and the variant protein. The more elegant approach uses cultured native cells from healthy and affected individuals, or immortalized or engineered cells such as induced pluripotent stem cells (iPS) or CRISPR-edited cells (Strande et al. 2017). Established in vitro assays are excellent to use if they are available, but many times there is no available assay and the validation of a new one can be tedious. In vivo studies still pose the greatest bottleneck in the analysis as time to generate a mouse carrying the orthologous VUS can be at least 6 months. Other model systems like the Zebrafish are excellent for knock-down and rescue experiments in a shorter time frame (Davis et al. 2014).

13.4.2 TF Gene Variants in Patients with Hypopituitarism

13.4.2.1 TF Gene Variants in Patients with Combined Pituitary Hormone Deficiency and Isolated Growth Hormone Deficiency

This chapter has two comprehensive goals for clinicians and researchers who encounter patients with hypopituitarism: (1) to describe the landscape of genetic and phenotypic heterogeneity in hypopituitarism and (2) to create a resource for the first steps of in vitro testing for VUS in select hypopituitarism genes based on published scenarios.

Phenotypic Heterogeneity in Hypopituitarism
The majority of human genes tested in patients with CPHD, IGHD, IAD to date are TFs, which are illustrated in Tables 13.2, 13.3, and 13.4. We aimed to collect information on the genetics and common phenotypic features of around 300 probands and families. Due to space limitations of this chapter not all original references could be cited.

An Approach to Perform In Vitro Testing of VUS in TF Genes
One can achieve a detailed analysis on a computer for a small set of novel genes/variants in a shorter time; however, the next step is frequently to start in vitro testing. A generalized view of active TFs is that they localize to the nucleus, bind to specific promoter/enhancer DNA sequences with partner proteins, and change the mRNA expression of target genes (Vaquerizas et al. 2009). Loss of function (nonsense and select frame shift) variants may require little to no testing if the gene is sensitive to haploinsufficiency indicated by dominant inheritance and a high pLI score (Lek et al. 2016) (Tables 13.2 and 13.4).

Depending on the affected functional domain in the TF, the assessment can include the following by overexpressing the TF from a plasmid DNA in cell culture: (1) quantitative assessment of protein expression by Western blot; (2) subcellular localization of the green fluorescence protein tagged TF, (3) protein-DNA binding assays such as electrophoretic mobility shift assay (EMSA) where the TF binds to specific DNA sequences, (4) transactivation reporter assays, and (5) protein–protein binding by co-immunoprecipitation.

PROP1

Patients with *PROP1* variants present with a highly consistent phenotype: GH, TSH, and more than two-thirds of the cases have ACTH, FSH/LH, PRL deficiency. Typically, they present with AL hypoplasia, 1:10 patients have AL hyperplasia, and PL is intact. Waxing and waning of the pituitary size over time is common (Obermannova et al. 2011; Turton et al. 2005a). Patients carry homozygous or compound heterozygous variants. About three-quarters of variants are missense/nonsense while one-quarter are splicing or large deletions (Fang et al. 2016b; Madeira et al. 2017). Two founder mutations are well known: c. 301-302delAG from the Iberian Peninsula

Table 13.2 Heredity and pituitary hormone deficiency in patients with CPHD/IGHD and pathogenic variants in prevalent pituitary transcription factor genes by 2019[a]

			Inheritance				Deficient hormone other than GH in CPHD			
Gene	pLI	Number of index cases[a]	Typical	Rare	IGHD	CPHD	TSH	ACTH	FSH LH	PRL
PROP1	0.094	>60	R	–	None	+++++	+++++	++++	+++++	++++
POU1F1	0.036	~40	R	D (5)	+	+++++	+++++	None	None	+++++
LHX3	0.007	~30	R	DIP (2)	None	+++++	+++++	++	+++	++++
LHX4	0.018	~30	DIP	R (1)	+	+++++	+++++	++++	+++	+
HESX1	0.001	>20	D	R (6)	++	++++	+++++	+++++	+++	++
OTX2	0.939	~10	D	R (1)[b]	+++	+++	+++++	+++	+++	+
GLI2	0.990	>50	DIP	–	++	++++	+++++	+++++	++++	Rare
GLI3	1.000	~20	D	–	+++++	Rare	Rare	Rare	Rare	Rare

pLI probability for loss of function intolerance (Source: https://gnomad.broadinstitute.org). A pLI $\geq$ 0.9 suggests extreme intolerance to loss of function variants. pLI $\leq$ 0.1 are tolerant. Those genes with a low pLI have a propensity to tolerate damages to one allele and both alleles need to be disrupted for dysfunction. This can be seen with cases of recessive inheritance when carrying homozygous or compound heterozygous variants

Proportion of published cases/families: $\geq$80%: +++++; 79–60%: ++++; 59–40%: +++; 39–20%: ++; 19–10%: +; <10%: rare; CPHD is defined as GHD plus one more pituitary hormone deficient. *R* recessive, *D* dominant, *DIP* dominant with incomplete penetrance, *(N)* of published probands with nontypical inheritance

[a]Assessment of CPHD/IGHD patients is based on literature review (1990-early 2019), Human Gene Mutation Database Professional (www.biobase-international.com) (Qiagen, Germantown, MD) and Online Mendelian Inheritance in Man (www.omim.org McKusick-Nathans Institute of Genetic Medicine at Johns Hopkins University School of Medicine, Baltimore MD, & National Center for Biotechnology Information, Bethesda, MD)

[b]Evidence for causality is low in Catania et al. (2019)

Table 13.3 Pituitary and extra-pituitary morphological features in patients with CPHD/IGHD and pituitary transcription factor gene variants

Gene	Incidence					
	Pituitary AL					
	Hypoplasia	Hyperplasia	EPP	PSIS	CNS	Other
PROP1[a]	+++++[b]	+	ND	ND	ND	Various minor features
POU1F1[a]	+++++	Rare	ND	ND	ND	Various minor features
LHX3	+++	+	ND	ND	Rare	Limited neck rotation, enlarged fontanel, hearing impairment, frontal bossing (all +++++)
LHX4	++++	Rare	++++	ND	Chiari I. (+)	Underdeveloped sella (++), thin stalk (+), micropenis (+)
HESX1	+++	ND	+++	Rare	SOD (+), ONH (+)	Various minor features
OTX2	+++	ND	++++	++	Chiari I. (+)	Micro/anophtalmia (++++), ONH (++), facial and genital defects (+)
GLI2	++++	ND	+++	+	HPE-like (++)	Postaxial polydactyly (++), cleft lip and palate (+)
GLI3	++[c]	ND	ND	ND	See other	PHS or subPHS (all)

Assessment and grading are identical to Table 14.2. Note that pituitary size/morphology can be normal

AL anterior lobe, *EPP* ectopic posterior pituitary, *PSIS* pituitary stalk interruption syndrome, *CNS* central nervous system, *ND* not described, *SOD* septo-optic dysplasia, *ONH* optic nerve hypoplasia, *HPE* holoprosencephaly

[a]See details for PSIS/CNS in (Brue et al. 2017). Incidence cannot be established

[b]Waxing and waning of pituitary size was described in Turton et al. (2005b) and Obermannova et al. (2011)

[c]"Pituitary agenesis" was described

(Cogan et al. 1998; Dusatkova et al. 2016) and c. 296-297delGA from Lithuania (Navardauskaite et al. 2014). Functional testing includes binding to/transactivation on the PRDQ9 sequence (Kelberman et al. 2009). While the pituitary phenotype is extremely consistent there are two reports of stating extra-pituitary features: (1) two patients with pituitary stalk interruption syndrome (PSIS) and four with heart/kidney malformations and deafness were described from the GENHYPOPIT network in consanguineous patients with *PROP1* and *POU1F1* variants (Brue et al. 2017); (2) one CPHD patient was described with ectopic posterior pituitary (EPP) who carried a heterozygous c.301_302delAG, which is inconsistent with the recessive inheritance (Avbelj Stefanija et al. 2015). However, it is possible that these individuals had additional genetic or environmental causes of the atypical features.

Table 13.4 Probability for loss of function intolerance in transcription factor genes in CPHD/IGHD patients with few or no published cases

Gene	pLI	Gene	pLI	Gene	pLI
PAX6	1	*ISL1*	0.896	***SOX3***	0.475
NFKB2	1	*PITX1*	0.892	***NKX2–1***	0.378
FOXO1	0.997	*FOXL2*	0.88	***TCF7L1***	0.36
FOXP3	0.994	*VAX1*	0.784	*EGR1*	0.327
ARNT2	0.991	*NEUROD1*	0.772	*INSM1*	0.269
NR5A1	0.991	***FOXA2***	0.742	*NEUROD4*	0.097
GATA2	0.981	***SOX2***	0.735	***TGIF1***	0.01
PITX2	0.979	*ASCL1*	0.697	*TBX19*	0
ZIC2	0.974	*TEF*	0.615		
SIX3	0.951	***SIX6***	0.554		

Genes with few published CPHD/IGHD cases are in bold. Cases with IAD are underlined

POU1F1

Patients with *POU1F1* variants show the most consistent manifestation of all CPHD patients with GH, TSH, PRL deficiency and no other hormones being affected, AL hypoplasia, and PL placed normally. Typical inheritance is recessive (homozygous and compound heterozygous), although there are some examples of dominant inheritance. There are two published families with IGHD carrying a heterozygous p.P76L (Sobrier et al. 2016) or a homozygous p.E230K (Gat-Yablonski et al. 2002). Functional testing is performed by transactivation on the *Gh*, *Prl* and *Tshb* promoters (Hendriks-Stegeman et al. 2001; Turton et al. 2005b), altered promoter/enhancer autoregulation (Vallette-Kasic et al. 2001), exon trapping of splice variants (Inoue et al. 2012; Takagi et al. 2017; Turton et al. 2012).

POU1F1 variants with dominant inheritance have an incomplete penetrance and reveal mechanisms other than roles as a transcriptional regulator on the known promoters. The most common dominant variant p.R271W was shown as a dominant negative transcriptional repressor as well as amino acid R271 binding to MATR3 and SATB1 in the nuclear matrix enabling features in chromatin remodeling (Cohen et al. 2006; Pellegrini et al. 2006; Skowronska-Krawczyk et al. 2014). POU1F1 p.P76L presented with IGHD, and the variant protein exhibited increased interaction with ELK1, PITX1, and LHX3a and with the enhancer region of *GH1* (Sobrier et al. 2015). Splice variants revealed either complete skipping of exon 2 (c.142+3A>G and c.214+1G>T) (Inoue et al. 2012; Turton et al. 2012) or splicing into the longer beta isoform of POU1F1 possessing repressor activities in vitro (c.143-83A>G) (Takagi et al. 2017). The variant p.K216E has an increased (not decreased!) activation of *Gh* and *Prl* and drastically reduced retinoic acid dependent autoactivation of the *Pou1f1* enhancer (Cohen et al. 1999).

LHX3

The typical hypopituitarism patient with homozygous *LHX3* variants presents with GH and TSH deficiency, two-thirds with LH/FSH and PRL deficiency while only a third of them have ACTH deficiency (Bechtold-Dalla Pozza et al. 2012). Less than half of the patients have abnormal pituitary size, with AL hypoplasia and eutopic PL. Additional features are fairly common, such as limited neck rotation (not present in *Lhx3*$^{-/-}$ mice), enlarged fontanels, hearing impairment, frontal bossing or more rarely thinning of the corpus callosum and dolichocephaly (Bonfig et al. 2011; Jullien et al. 2018; Kristrom et al. 2009; Rajab et al. 2008; Ramzan et al. 2017).

One family was published with a generation of two miscarriages, one child with compound heterozygous *LHX3* p.C118Y & c.252-3 C>G variants with CPHD and limited neck rotation while members of this family carrying the c.252-3 C>G splice variant had a high incidence of limited neck rotation (Sobrier et al. 2012). Another heterozygous variant also showed CPHD but no other distinctive features and the phenotype was incompletely penetrant (Jullien et al. 2018).

Variants are tested by using the activator LHX3A isoform for transactivation and DNA binding on *Cga, Gh, Prl, Tshb* promoters (Bechtold-Dalla Pozza et al. 2012; Rajab et al. 2008). Heterozygous variants are typically tested for dominant negative effects on the same promoters together with POU1F1 interaction (Jullien et al. 2018; Sobrier et al. 2012).

LHX4

These patients typically present with dominant inheritance and incomplete penetrance. GH, TSH deficiency is high while more than half of the cases have ACTH and less than half of them have gonadotroph deficiency and PRL deficiency is rare. AP hypoplasia and EPP are typical, underdeveloped sella is common. Rare features include Chiari I malformation and thin stalk (Castinetti et al. 2008b; Cohen et al. 2017; Dateki et al. 2010a; Machinis et al. 2001; Pfaeffle et al. 2008; Rochette et al. 2015). There are two examples of IGHD described (Cohen et al. 2017; Gucev et al. 2016).

Functional testing is typically carried out on the same promoters as with LHX3 or on the *Pou1f1* and *Fshb* promoters. Haploinsufficiency appears to be the typical mode of dominant action (same references as in previous paragraph and Fuxman Bass et al. 2015).

The only patient with a homozygous allele (p.T126 M) described so far presented with the features of a typical heterozygous *LHX4* patient (CPHD, AP aplasia, EPP, sella defect) but also with midfacial hypoplasia, small upturned nose with depressed nasal bridge, low-set crumpled ears and death during the first postnatal week (Gregory et al. 2015b). Homozygosity mapping and high conservation of amino acid 126 suggested pathogenicity. Transactivation ability of p.T126 M alone on the *Prl* promoter was not different; however, the interaction with POU1F1 was significantly reduced on the reporter construct.

HESX1

Less than two dozen *HESX1* families with hypopituitarism were described to date. Thus far, those with recessive inheritance are all CPHD (Fang et al. 2016a; Reynaud et al. 2011; Sobrier et al. 2006), while heterozygous *HESX1* patients can be IGHD (Cohen et al. 2003; McNay et al. 2007; Vivenza et al. 2011) or CPHD (Corneli et al. 2008; Coya et al. 2007; Reynaud et al. 2012; Tajima et al. 2003; Takagi et al. 2016; Thomas et al. 2001). The variants identified so far are predominantly missense. The onset of hormone deficiency is typically early and frequently evolving from IGHD to CPHD (Coya et al. 2007; Reynaud et al. 2011). GH, TSH, ACTH deficiency is very high while FSH/LH and PRL deficiency is gradually fewer. AL hypoplasia and EPP are common and rare features can include variable penetrance of PSIS, thin stalk, septo-optic dysplasia (SOD), and optic nerve hypoplasia (ONH). *HESX1* is a well-characterized gene in SOD (Dattani et al. 1998). Only a few SOD cases are reported to have hypopituitarism (Cohen et al. 2003; Coya et al. 2007; Thomas et al. 2001). Functional testing of variants includes testing HESX1's ability to repress activation caused by PROP1 on a multimerized paired HD binding site (P3E4) reporter, binding to DNA (Cohen et al. 2003; Fang et al. 2016a; McNay et al. 2007; Reynaud et al. 2012; Sobrier et al. 2006; Takagi et al. 2016).

SOX2

Individuals with *SOX2* variants present with anophtalmia, intellectual disability, and growth delay/short stature. Hypopituitarism is frequently not assessed (Schilter et al. 2013) and is reviewed in the works by Bakrania et al. (Bakrania et al. 2007) and Schneider et al. (Schneider et al. 2009). Information is limited to less than 20 cases that present with isolated HH (Bakrania et al. 2007; Errichiello et al. 2018; Kelberman et al. 2006; Sato et al. 2007; Takagi et al. 2014b), IGHD (Kelberman et al. 2006; Schilter et al. 2013; Schneider et al. 2009), and a few with CPHD (Blackburn et al. 2018; Kelberman et al. 2006; Macchiaroli et al. 2014; Schneider et al. 2009). They often have bilateral/unilateral anophtalmia (missing in *Sox2*-null mice), but other features including ONH, EPP, learning disability are occasionally present. Inheritance is dominant and in patients with hypopituitarism most variants are de novo frame shifts. Functional testing of variants involves transactivation of the *Hesx1* promoter and binding to consensus SOX DNA binding sites (Kelberman et al. 2006; Takagi et al. 2014b). The role of *Sox2* in pituitary tumors requires further investigation.

SOX3

The Xq26–27 chromosomal region of *SOX3* was first implicated in a large family with X-linked mental retardation (XLMR) and IGHD in 1996 (Laumonnier et al. 2002). Very few families were described to date and most of them have CPHD: GH and TSH deficiencies, occasional LH/FSH deficiency and rarely ACTH or PRL (Alatzoglou et al. 2011; Bauters et al. 2014; Izumi et al. 2014; Takagi et al. 2014a; Woods et al. 2005). In these hemizygous males, most genetic changes are small, in-frame deletions and insertions affecting polyalanine tracts (Alatzoglou et al. 2011; Izumi et al. 2014; Laumonnier et al. 2002). There are two examples of CPHD with complete *SOX3* duplications (Bauters et al. 2014; Woods et al. 2005). Larger chromosomal duplications can result in XX sex reversal (Sutton et al. 2011). The single missense variant example (p.R5Q) had CPHD and a central incisor (Alatzoglou et al. 2011). EPP is occasionally reported (Woods et al. 2005).

The polyalanine tract changes result in perinuclear/cytoplasmic aggregates, impair the ability to transactivate via consensus SOX DNA binding sites, and have a reduced propensity to inhibit Wnt/Ctnnb/TCF mediated transcription (Alatzoglou et al. 2011; Takagi et al. 2014a; Woods et al. 2005).

OTX2

Families with *OTX2* variants present with an autosomal dominant inheritance and incomplete penetrance. Incomplete penetrance and variable expressivity are well demonstrated in *Otx2*$^{-/-}$ mice in a genetic background specific manner (Hide et al. 2002). Patients with heterozygous *OTX2* variants can present with ocular only, or ocular with hypopituitarism phenotypes, while cases of hypopituitarism-only cases are rare (Diaczok et al. 2008). The ocular phenotype is anophtalmia/microphtalmia typically involving both eyes (Gerth-Kahlert et al. 2013 from Ragge and Wyatt). In the cases with ocular and pituitary phenotypes, the same ocular phenotypes were observed as well as optic nerve hypoplasia/dysplasia/aplasia (ONH) (Dateki et al. 2008; Gorbenko Del Blanco et al. 2012; Prasov et al. 2012; Schilter et al. 2011; Tajima et al. 2009). IGHD is almost as common as CPHD (Ashkenazi-Hoffnung et al. 2010; Dateki et al. 2008; Delahaye et al. 2012; Henderson et al. 2009; Lonero et al. 2016). Less than two dozen hypopituitarism cases are described, and they typically present with CPHD (GH, TSH, and fewer ACTH and FSH/LH and rarely PRL deficiency), EPP, and five of them had PSIS (all ONH and IGHD references and Diaczok et al. 2008; Shimada et al. 2016; Takagi et al. 2015; Vincent et al. 2014). The one published recessive CPHD case with an *OTX2* variant is only based on in silico prediction and segregation (Catania et al. 2019). Missense, nonsense, frame shift variants and large deletions are all common with *OTX2*. Although some reviews suggest that variants in the N-terminal region of the protein are associated with ocular features and in the C-terminal with pituitary involvement, we believe there are not enough cases with hypopituitarism to support this idea (Gorbenko Del Blanco et al. 2012; Schilter et al. 2011). In vitro variant testing is performed with single or multimerized consensus bicoid binding sites and transactivation is carried out on native promoters of *Hesx1, Pou1f1* as well (Dateki et al. 2008, 2010b; Diaczok et al. 2008; Gorbenko Del Blanco et al. 2012; Shimada et al. 2016; Tajima et al. 2009). Knock-down of the endogenous zebrafish mRNA in combination with other genes resulted in a complex eye, head, and mandible phenotype comparable to the human otocephaly-dysgnatia complex (Chassaing et al. 2012).

GLI2 and *ZIC2*

Patients with *GLI2* variants typically show autosomal dominant inheritance with incomplete penetrance (Babu et al. 2019; Bear et al. 2014; Flemming et al. 2013; Franca et al. 2013; Juanes et al. 2016; Roessler et al. 2005; Shirakawa et al. 2018; Simm et al. 2018; Zwaveling-Soonawala et al. 2018). CPHD (GH, TSH, ACTH most of the time, LH/FSH frequently, PRL rarely deficient) is the most common while IGHD is infrequent (Bear et al. 2014; Gregory et al. 2015a; Juanes et al. 2016; Roessler et al. 2005; Shirakawa et al. 2018). Most patients have hypoplastic AL, about half of the patients have EPP, and a few have absent PP/PSIS. About 10% of the patients have postaxial polydactyly and/or HPE-like features. While most variants are unique to the family the allele affected by both p.M1352V and p.D1520N variants was described by multiple authors in CPHD (Flemming et al. 2013; Franca et al. 2013; Zwaveling-Soonawala et al. 2018). Most variants described are missense. Functional assessment includes binding to a consensus GLI-site in the *PTCH1* promoter. Transactivation studies test variants either on the octamerized GLI-binding site from the enhancer of *Hnf3b* (*Foxa2*) or on the single GLI-binding site from the promoter of keratin 17. The variant testing includes two steps on these reporter constructs: (1) Testing the mutated full-length GLI2 alone and (2) testing the mutated full-length GLI2 together with a *GLI2* cDNA construct missing the N-terminal (1–328) repressor domain (ΔN-GLI2). The ΔN-GLI2 acts a potent activator on these reporter constructs and co-transfection of the mutant + ΔN-GLI2 can demonstrate a dominant negative effect. Embryonic sarcoma cell line (C3H10T1/2) was used to demonstrate osteogenic differentiation upon transfection with normal *GLI2*. In vivo assays were demonstrated with frog eggs where injection of normal *GLI2* results in secondary tail formation (Babu et al. 2019; Flemming et al. 2013; Roessler et al. 2005).

ZIC2 is a common HPE gene and a member of the GLI TF subfamily. A heterozygous p.Gln364Leufs∗2 variant was described in a child with alobar HPE, complex facial/dental features, and the involvement of both the AL/PL with subsequent CPHD (GH, TSH) and central diabetes insipidus (Tasdemir et al. 2014).

GLI3

Heterozygous variants in *GLI3* are known to cause Greig cephalopolysyndactyly and Pallister–Hall syndrome (PHS). A clear genotype–phenotype correlation exists where variants affecting the middle-third of the open reading frame (nucleotides 1998–3481) can be found in PHS only. PHS is characterized by the presence of major criteria such as hypothalamic hamartoma and mesaxial polydactyly plus several minor features (bifid epiglottis, IGHD, CPHD, genital hypoplasia, imperforate anus, and small nails) (Demurger et al. 2015; Johnston et al. 2005; Kang et al. 1997). A sub-PHS is diagnosed when one major criterion is present with at least one minor criterion. Most published cases with hypopituitarism or pituitary agenesis are in patients with PHS and to lesser extent with sub-PHS. Almost all patients have IGHD, several of the minor features and adrenal and renal agenesis (Demurger et al. 2015; Johnston et al. 2005). Very few cases were described with CPHD (Li et al. 2015; Narumi et al. 2010). Detailed imaging of the pituitary region is not available. Functional testing is similar to *GLI2*.

TF Genes with Limited Evidence in Hypopituitarism

FOXA2

A few patients with heterozygous *FOXA2* variants were described so far. They share the features of CPHD (GH, TSH, ACTH), and have a high incidence of hyperinsulinemia, hypoplastic/absent AL, EPP and have a range of minor features such as single central incisor, dysmorphic facial features, biliary tract abnormalities, heart defects, and neurodevelopmental delay (Boda et al. 2018; Giri et al. 2017; Tsai et al. 2015; Vajravelu et al. 2018). These patients have either missense or large deletions affecting 20p11.21. *FOXA2* is expressed in multiple tissues corresponding to the phenotype spectrum (Giri et al. 2017). Transactivation can be tested on the human *GLUT2* (phGT2–294), *ABCC8, KCNJ11, HADH, SHH, GLI2,* and *NKX2–2* promoter reporters (Giri et al. 2017; Vajravelu et al. 2018).

ARNT2

ARNT2 is part of the protein complex that includes the aryl hydrocarbon receptor-interacting protein (AIP), widely studied in specific groups of pituitary adenomas (Raitila et al. 2010; Rostomyan et al. 2017) and cancer (Bogeas et al. 2018). *ARNT2* is highly expressed in the mouse and human CNS, retina, kidney, lung, and the pituitary (Webb et al. 2013). A recessive *ARNT2* c.1373_1374dupTC variant was identified in a large family with CPHD, kidney, urogenital tract, eye, and CNS anomalies (postnatal microcephaly, frontotemporal hypoplasia, seizures) (Webb et al. 2013). This variant resulted in a frame shift and nonsense mediated decay of the transcript.

PAX6

PAX6 patients typically present with aniridia and microphtalmia (Lim et al. 2017). Few patients were described with borderline GHD, HH, central hypothyroidism or low cortisol levels (Hergott-Faure et al. 2012; Shimo et al. 2014; Solomon et al. 2009). *PAX6* heterozygous variants were described in two cases of IGHD (Takagi et al. 2015). One of them presented with cleft palate, optic disc cupping, AL hypoplasia, and EPP and had a 310 kb deletion of the *PAX6* enhancer. The other case with a missense p.N116S had AL hypoplasia. Functional analysis included showing normal protein expression, subcellular localization, binding to a consensus *PAX6* binding element from the promoter of CD19 (Mishra et al. 2002) as well as transactivation on a hexamer *PAX6* consensus binding element where only the latter showed significant impairment.

TGIF1

TGIF1 is highly expressed in the liver, kidney, gonads, forebrain, and several other tissues including the pituitary during development and postnatally (Hu et al. 2011). TGIF1 acts as a repressor in retinoid X receptor (RXR) mediated transcription in a TGFB/SMAD-dependent manner (Bartholin et al. 2006; Bertolino et al. 1995). Patients with heterozygous variants in *TGIF1* typically present with variable degrees of midline defects ranging from a single central incisor to HPE (Dubourg et al. 2004; El-Jaick et al. 2007). A pool of 30 patients with CPHD were screened, and only one patient had a *TGIF1* variant (p.Q267X). This individual had CPHD (GH, TSH, LH/FSH), AL hypoplasia, and a single central incisor. No functional studies were carried out (Tatsi et al. 2013). The repressor effect of TGIF1 is typically demonstrated in the context of retinoic acid activating on a promoter construct of *RBP2* (DR1-TATA-luc) or TGFB activating a promoter construct of *MMP1* (3-TP-lux). TGIF1 co-immunoprecipitated with RXRA and SMAD3 (El-Jaick et al. 2007). Another patient with a complex CNS phenotype with pituitary hypoplasia and single central incisor had a chromosomal rearrangement affecting *TGIF1* (Kantaputra et al. 2006).

PITX2

Heterozygous *PITX2* variants are one cause of Axenfeld-Rieger syndrome (ARS) characterized by the defects of the eye anterior segment, hypodontia (including single central incisor), maxillary hypoplasia, umbilical protrusion, and heart defects in humans (Franco et al. 2017; Seifi and Walter 2018; Semina et al. 1996). No *PITX2* variants have yet been discovered in patients with hypopituitarism. A few papers studying *PITX2* variants are clear on the lack of hypopituitarism and the presence of ARS with the patient variants studied (Quentien et al. 2011), while others have no more indication of pituitary involvement than a flattened sella turcica (Idrees et al. 2006) and some actually state the lack of *PITX2* variants (Lowry et al. 2007). Mouse mutants heterozygous for *Pitx2* loss of function alleles do not have hypopituitarism.

NKX2–1, TCF7L1, INSM1, SIX3, *and* SIX6

A large chromosomal deletion involving *NKX2–1* (and *MBIP, NKX2.8, PAX9, SLC25A1*) was described in a patient with pituitary stalk duplication and exaggerated response to TRH stimulation (Accornero et al. 2010). So far, one nonsense variant of *NKX2–1* was implicated in one family with IGHD and HH (Balicza et al. 2018). Heterozygous missense variants in the Wnt signaling repressor *TCF7L1* were described in two patients with IGHD and SOD-like features (Gaston-Massuet et al.

2016). There are very few variants reported in *INSM1*; however, it appears to be a very specific marker for neuroendocrine differentiation in primary lung cancer (Mukhopadhyay et al. 2019). HPE and micro/anophtalmia is prevalent in patients with *SIX3* or *SIX6* variants but there is no clear evidence for pathogenicity in human hypopituitarism thus far (Gallardo et al. 1999; Martinez-Frias et al. 2014; Rauchman et al. 2001).

13.4.2.2 Select Genetic Causes of Isolated Pituitary Hormone Deficiency

Isolated ACTH Deficiency (IAD)

Genetic causes for IAD include two established genes: *TBX19* and *POMC*. Pathogenic *TBX19* TF variants result in recessive, neonatal onset ACTH deficiency, and they represent about two-thirds of the patients with IAD (Couture et al. 2012; Metherell et al. 2004; Pulichino et al. 2003). Patients present with severe hypoglycemia and high mortality unless promptly treated with hydrocortisone (Abali et al. 2019; Couture et al. 2012; Vallette-Kasic et al. 2005). Recessive mutations were described in *POMC* resulting in a protein translation defect with red hair pigmentation, severe, early onset obesity, and secondary adrenal insufficiency (Aslan et al. 2014; Krude et al. 1998). The mechanism of corticotrope deficiency remains elusive and likely indirect in patients with heterozygous, de novo *NFKB2* TF mutations who present with IAD, hypogammaglobulinemia similar to common variable immunodeficiency (CVID), alopecia, lymphocyte and NK-cell defects, and trachyonychia (Brue et al. 2014; Chen et al. 2013; Lougaris et al. 2015).

Isolated TSH Deficiency (ITD)

While congenital hypothyroidism has an incidence 1:3000 congenital central hypothyroidism (isolated thyrotroph deficiency) is extremely rare (<1:20,000) (Grosse and Van Vliet 2011; van Tijn et al. 2005). Variants in *TSHB* and *TRHR* are the longest known causes (Collu et al. 1997; Hayashizaki et al. 1989). Variants in *TSHB* typically affect the "seat belt" region where TSHB binds CGA in a tightly regulated process to form biologically active TSH (Matzuk et al. 1988; Nicholas et al. 2017). The mechanism by which heterozygous *TRHR* variants lead to TSH deficiency is not completely understood (Collu et al. 1997). The cause of isolated TSH deficiency can be clarified with TRH stimulation testing. *TSHB* defects preserve the secretory response of CGA and PRL (Bonomi et al. 2001). The response is blunted if *TRHR* is defective (Collu et al. 1997).

Recently, an X-linked cause of TSH deficiency was described in men carrying variants in *IGSF1*. They present with PRL deficiency and macroorchidism, but no GHD (Asakura et al. 2015; Hughes et al. 2016; Joustra et al. 2016; Nakamura et al. 2013; Sun et al. 2012; Tajima et al. 2013; Tenenbaum-Rakover et al. 2016). *TBLX1* is the newest member of genes in isolated congenital central hypothyroidism (Heinen et al. 2016).

Isolated Growth Hormone Deficiency (IGHD)

Typical genetic causes for IGHD remain to be those in *GHRHR*, *GH1* while defects in *SOX3*, *HESX1 GLI3*, *OTX2* are rare (Alatzoglou and Dattani 2010; Demurger et al. 2015). Overall, *GHRH* and *GH1* defects are recessive (type I GHD) but a non-insignificant pool of patients shows autosomal-dominant or X-linked inheritance (Alatzoglou and Dattani 2012). *SOX3*, *GLI3*, and *OTX2* were discussed previously.

Isolated LH/FSH Deficiency

Currently more than 30 genes are implicated in congenital HH with or without anosmia. This is a huge increase since 2000, when only four well-established congenital HH genes were known: *KAL1*, *GNRHR*, *DAX1*, and *PCSK1* (Seminara et al. 2000). An extensive review was recently published (Maione et al. 2018).

13.5 Concluding Remarks

Current diagnostic opportunities have enabled physicians to establish the clinical diagnosis of pituitary hormone deficiency with high confidence. Advancements in DNA sequencing technology provided an incredible pool of novel candidate genes and variants to test for the clinician and the researcher. We have just begun to understand the functional consequences of changes in the coding region of the genome. According to the Genetics Home Reference at the NIH, the coding information is only 1% of our genome. Improving of the understanding of large copy number variations as well as the "meaning" of the noncoding genome will be driven by the progression of whole genome sequencing technology and bioinformatics analysis. Currently, the treatment of pituitary hormone deficiency consists of replacement of growth hormone and end organ hormones such as thyroid hormone or steroid hormones. Creating artificial endocrine organs is at its dawn. Gene therapy for specific genetic defects is at its very early stages for non-pituitary diseases. Improving our understanding on how genetic defects in the most common TF genes lead to disease such as hypopituitarism is fundamental in this progress.

Acknowledgments This work was supported by the grant entitled "Cell specific expression in the pituitary gland" awarded to Sally A Camper (PI) by the National Institutes of Health (R01 HD034283) with Peter Gergics as co-investigator on this grant. The author apologizes to other colleagues whose work was not cited due to space limitations. The author would like to thank Sally A. Camper for her careful review and feedback on the manuscript, to the members of her lab collecting information on specific genes/variants, and to his family for their continued support toward his research productivity.

References

Abali ZY, Yesil G, Kirkgoz T et al (2019) Evaluation of growth and puberty in a child with a novel TBX19 gene mutation and review of the literature. Hormones (Athens). https://doi.org/10.1007/s42000-019-00096-7

Accornero S, Danesino C, Bastianello S, D'Errico I, Guala A, Chiovato L (2010) Duplication of the pituitary stalk in a patient with a heterozygous deletion of chromosome 14 harboring the thyroid transcription factor-1 gene. J Clin Endocrinol Metab 95:3595–3596. https://doi.org/10.1210/jc.2010-0621

Alatzoglou KS, Dattani MT (2010) Genetic causes and treatment of isolated growth hormone deficiency-an update. Nat Rev Endocrinol 6:562–576. https://doi.org/10.1038/nrendo.2010.147

Alatzoglou KS, Dattani MT (2012) Phenotype-genotype correlations in congenital isolated growth hormone deficiency (IGHD). Indian J Pediatr 79:99–106. https://doi.org/10.1007/s12098-011-0614-7

Alatzoglou KS, Kelberman D, Cowell CT et al (2011) Increased transactivation associated with SOX3 polyalanine tract deletion in a patient with hypopituitarism. J Clin Endocrinol Metab 96: E685–E690. https://doi.org/10.1210/jc.2010-1239

Ando M, Goto M, Hojo M et al (2018) The proneural bHLH genes Mash1, Math3 and NeuroD are required for pituitary development. J Mol Endocrinol 61:127–138. https://doi.org/10.1530/JME-18-0090

Andrioli M, Pecori Giraldi F, Cavagnini F (2006) Isolated corticotrophin deficiency. Pituitary 9:289–295. https://doi.org/10.1007/s11102-006-0408-5

Asakura Y, Abe K, Muroya K et al (2015) Combined growth hormone and thyroid-stimulating hormone deficiency in a Japanese patient with a novel frameshift mutation in IGSF1. Horm Res Paediatr 84:349–354. https://doi.org/10.1159/000438672

Ashkenazi-Hoffnung L, Lebenthal Y, Wyatt AW (2010) A novel loss-of-function mutation in OTX2 in a patient with anophthalmia and isolated growth hormone deficiency. Hum Genet 127:721–729. https://doi.org/10.1007/s00439-010-0820-9

Aslan IR, Ranadive SA, Valle I, Kollipara S, Noble JA, Vaisse C (2014) The melanocortin system and insulin resistance in humans: insights from a patient with complete POMC deficiency and type 1 diabetes mellitus. Int J Obes 38:148–151. https://doi.org/10.1038/ijo.2013.53

Avbelj Stefanija M, Kotnik P, Bratanič N et al (2015) Novel mutations in HESX1 and PROP1 genes in combined pituitary hormone deficiency. Horm Res Paediatr 84:153–158. https://doi.org/10.1159/000433468

Babu D, Fanelli A, Mellone S et al (2019) Novel GLI2 mutations identified in patients with Combined Pituitary Hormone Deficiency (CPHD): evidence for a pathogenic effect by functional characterization. Clin Endocrinol 90:449–456. https://doi.org/10.1111/cen.13914

Bakrania P, Robinson DO, Bunyan DJ et al (2007) SOX2 anophthalmia syndrome: 12 new cases demonstrating broader phenotype and high frequency of large gene deletions. Br J Ophthalmol 91:1471–1476. https://doi.org/10.1136/bjo.2007.117929

Balicza P, Grosz Z, Molnár V et al (2018) NKX2-1 new mutation associated with myoclonus, dystonia, and pituitary involvement. Front Genet 9:335. https://doi.org/10.3389/fgene.2018.00335

Bartholin L, Powers SE, Melhuish TA, Lasse S, Weinstein M, Wotton D (2006) TGIF inhibits retinoid signaling. Mol Cell Biol 26:990–1001. https://doi.org/10.1128/MCB.26.3.990-1001.2006

Bauters M, Frints SG, Van Esch H et al (2014) Evidence for increased SOX3 dosage as a risk factor for X-linked hypopituitarism and neural tube defects. Am J Med Genet A 164a:1947–1952. https://doi.org/10.1002/ajmg.a.36580

Bear KA, Solomon BD, Antonini S et al (2014) Pathogenic mutations in GLI2 cause a specific phenotype that is distinct from holoprosencephaly. J Med Genet 51:413–418. https://doi.org/10.1136/jmedgenet-2013-102249

Bechtold-Dalla Pozza S, Hiedl S, Roeb J et al (2012) A recessive mutation resulting in a disabling amino acid substitution (T194R) in the LHX3 homeodomain causes combined pituitary hormone deficiency. Horm Res Paediatr 77:41–51. https://doi.org/10.1159/000335929

Bertolino E, Reimund B, Wildt-Perinic D, Clerc RG (1995) A novel homeobox protein which recognizes a TGT core and functionally interferes with a retinoid-responsive motif. J Biol Chem 270:31178–31188. https://doi.org/10.1074/jbc.270.52.31178

Bharti K, Gasper M, Bertuzzi S, Arnheiter H (2011) Lack of the ventral anterior homeodomain transcription factor VAX1 leads to induction of a second pituitary. Development 138:873–878. https://doi.org/10.1242/dev.056465

Blackburn PR, Chacon-Camacho OF, Ortiz-González XR et al (2018) Extension of the mutational and clinical spectrum of SOX2 related disorders: description of six new cases and a novel association with suprasellar teratoma. Am J Med Genet A 176:2710–2719. https://doi.org/10.1002/ajmg.a.40644

Boda H, Miyata M, Inagaki H, Shinkai Y, Kato T, Yoshikawa T, Kurahashi H (2018) FOXA2 gene mutation in a patient with congenital complex pituitary hormone deficiency. Eur J Med Genet. https://doi.org/10.1016/j.ejmg.2018.11.004

Boehm U, Bouloux PM, Dattani MT et al (2015) Expert consensus document: European Consensus Statement on congenital hypogonadotropic hypogonadism—pathogenesis, diagnosis and treatment. Nat Rev Endocrinol 11:547–564. https://doi.org/10.1038/nrendo.2015.112

Bogeas A, Morvan-Dubois G, El-Habr EA et al (2018) Changes in chromatin state reveal ARNT2 at a node of a tumorigenic transcription factor signature driving glioblastoma cell aggressiveness. Acta Neuropathol 135:267–283. https://doi.org/10.1007/s00401-017-1783-x

Bonfig W, Krude H, Schmidt H (2011) A novel mutation of LHX3 is associated with combined pituitary hormone deficiency including ACTH deficiency, sensorineural hearing loss, and short neck-a case report and review of the literature. Eur J Pediatr 170:1017–1021. https://doi.org/10.1007/s00431-011-1393-x

Bonomi M, Proverbio MC, Weber G, Chiumello G, Beck-Peccoz P, Persani L (2001) Hyperplastic pituitary gland, high serum glycoprotein hormone alpha-subunit, and variable circulating thyrotropin (TSH) levels as hallmark of central hypothyroidism due to mutations of the TSH beta gene. J Clin Endocrinol Metab 86:1600–1604. https://doi.org/10.1210/jcem.86.4.7411

Brinkmeier ML, Davis SW, Carninci P et al (2009) Discovery of transcriptional regulators and signaling pathways in the developing pituitary gland by bioinformatic and genomic approaches. Genomics 93:449–460. https://doi.org/10.1016/j.ygeno.2008.11.010

Brue T (2018) Lessons from screening of genetic causes of hypopituitarism in session S54—"New developments of pituitary disease", session 54 edn. In: The Endocrine Society's 100th Annual Meeting and Expo (ENDO 2018), Chicago, IL

Brue T, Quentien MH, Khetchoumian K et al (2014) Mutations in NFKB2 and potential genetic heterogeneity in patients with DAVID syndrome, having variable endocrine and immune deficiencies. BMC Med Genet 15:139. https://doi.org/10.1186/s12881-014-0139-9

Brue T, Saveanu A, Jullien N et al (2017) Lessons from monogenic causes of growth hormone deficiency. Ann Endocrinol (Paris) 78:77–79. https://doi.org/10.1016/j.ando.2017.04.001

Budry L, Couture C, Balsalobre A, Drouin J (2011) The Ets factor Etv1 interacts with Tpit protein for pituitary pro-opiomelanocortin (POMC) gene transcription. J Biol Chem 286:25387–25396. https://doi.org/10.1074/jbc.M110.202788

Budry L, Balsalobre A, Gauthier Y et al (2012) The selector gene Pax7 dictates alternate pituitary cell fates through its pioneer action on chromatin remodeling. Genes Dev 26:2299–2310. https://doi.org/10.1101/gad.200436.112

Castinetti F, Reynaud R, Saveanu A et al (2008a) [Clinical and genetic aspects of combined pituitary hormone deficiencies]. Ann Endocrinol (Paris) 69:7–17. https://doi.org/10.1016/j.ando.2008.01.001

Castinetti F, Saveanu A, Reynaud R et al (2008b) A novel dysfunctional LHX4 mutation with high phenotypical variability in patients with hypopituitarism. J Clin Endocrinol Metab 93:2790–2799. https://doi.org/10.1210/jc.2007-2389

Castinetti F, Reynaud R, Saveanu A, Barlier A, Brue T (2012) Genetic causes of combined pituitary hormone deficiencies in humans. Ann Endocrinol (Paris) 73:53–55. https://doi.org/10.1016/j.ando.2012.03.025

Catania A, Legati A, Peverelli L et al (2019) Homozygous variant in OTX2 and possible genetic modifiers identified in a patient with combined pituitary hormone deficiency, ocular involvement, myopathy, ataxia, and mitochondrial impairment. Am J Med Genet A 179(5):827–831. https://doi.org/10.1002/ajmg.a.61092

Chassaing N, Sorrentino S, Davis EE et al (2012) OTX2 mutations contribute to the otocephaly-dysgnathia complex. J Med Genet 49:373–379. https://doi.org/10.1136/jmedgenet-2012-100892

Chen K, Coonrod EM, Kumánovics A et al (2013) Germline mutations in NFKB2 implicate the noncanonical NF-kappaB pathway in the pathogenesis of common variable immunodeficiency. Am J Hum Genet 93:812–824. https://doi.org/10.1016/j.ajhg.2013.09.009

Cheung LYM, George AS, McGee SR, Daly AZ, Brinkmeier ML, Ellsworth BS, Camper SA (2018) Single-cell RNA sequencing reveals novel markers of male pituitary stem cells and hormone-producing cell types. Endocrinology 159:3910–3924. https://doi.org/10.1210/en.2018-00750

Chinoy A, Murray PG (2016) Diagnosis of growth hormone deficiency in the paediatric and transitional age. Best Pract Res Clin Endocrinol Metab 30:737–747. https://doi.org/10.1016/j.beem.2016.11.002

Cogan JD, Wu W, Phillips JA 3rd et al (1998) The PROP1 2-base pair deletion is a common cause of combined pituitary hormone deficiency. J Clin Endocrinol Metab 83:3346–3349. https://doi.org/10.1210/jcem.83.9.5142

Cohen LE, Zanger K, Brue T, Wondisford FE, Radovick S (1999) Defective retinoic acid regulation of the Pit-1 gene enhancer: a novel mechanism of combined pituitary hormone deficiency. Mol Endocrinol 13:476–484. https://doi.org/10.1210/mend.13.3.0251

Cohen RN, Cohen LE, Botero D, Yu C, Sagar A, Jurkiewicz M, Radovick S (2003) Enhanced repression by HESX1 as a cause of hypopituitarism and septooptic dysplasia. J Clin Endocrinol Metab 88:4832–4839. https://doi.org/10.1210/jc.2002-021868

Cohen RN, Brue T, Naik K, Houlihan CA, Wondisford FE, Radovick S (2006) The role of CBP/p300 interactions and Pit-1 dimerization in the pathophysiological mechanism of combined pituitary hormone deficiency. J Clin Endocrinol Metab 91:239–247. https://doi.org/10.1210/jc.2005-1211

Cohen E, Maghnie M, Collot N et al (2017) Contribution of LHX4 mutations to pituitary deficits in a cohort of 417 unrelated patients. J Clin Endocrinol Metab 102:290–301. https://doi.org/10.1210/jc.2016-3158

Collu R, Tang J, Castagné J et al (1997) A novel mechanism for isolated central hypothyroidism: inactivating mutations in the thyrotropin-releasing hormone receptor gene. J Clin Endocrinol Metab 82:1561–1565. https://doi.org/10.1210/jcem.82.5.3918

Corneli G, Vivenza D, Prodam F et al (2008) Heterozygous mutation of HESX1 causing hypopituitarism and multiple anatomical malformations without features of septo-optic dysplasia. J Endocrinol Investig 31:689–693. https://doi.org/10.1007/bf03346416

Correa FA, Jorge AA, Nakaguma M et al (2018) Pathogenic copy number variants in patients with congenital hypopituitarism associated with complex phenotypes. Clin Endocrinol 88:425–431. https://doi.org/10.1111/cen.13535

Couture C, Saveanu A, Barlier A et al (2012) Phenotypic homogeneity and genotypic variability in a large series of congenital isolated ACTH-deficiency patients with TPIT gene mutations. J Clin Endocrinol Metab 97:E486–E495. https://doi.org/10.1210/jc.2011-1659

Coya R, Vela A, Perez de Nanclares G, Rica I, Castano L, Busturia MA, Martul P (2007) Panhypopituitarism: genetic versus acquired etiological factors. J Pediatr Endocrinol Metab 20:27–36. https://doi.org/10.1515/JPEM.2007.20.1.27

Dasen JS, O'Connell SM, Flynn SE et al (1999) Reciprocal interactions of Pit1 and GATA2 mediate signaling gradient-induced determination of pituitary cell types. Cell 97:587–598. https://doi.org/10.1016/S0092-8674(00)80770-9

Dateki S, Fukami M, Sato N, Muroya K, Adachi M, Ogata T (2008) OTX2 mutation in a patient with anophthalmia, short stature, and partial growth hormone deficiency: functional studies

using the IRBP, HESX1, and POU1F1 promoters. J Clin Endocrinol Metab 93:3697–3702. https://doi.org/10.1210/jc.2008-0720
Dateki S, Fukami M, Uematsu A et al (2010a) Mutation and gene copy number analyses of six pituitary transcription factor genes in 71 patients with combined pituitary hormone deficiency: identification of a single patient with LHX4 deletion. J Clin Endocrinol Metab 95:4043–4047. https://doi.org/10.1210/jc.2010-0150
Dateki S, Kosaka K, Hasegawa K et al (2010b) Heterozygous orthodenticle homeobox 2 mutations are associated with variable pituitary phenotype. J Clin Endocrinol Metab 95:756–764. https://doi.org/10.1210/jc.2009-1334
Dattani MT (2005) Growth hormone deficiency and combined pituitary hormone deficiency: does the genotype matter? Clin Endocrinol 63:121–130. https://doi.org/10.1111/j.1365-2265.2005.02289.x
Dattani MT, Martinez-Barbera JP, Thomas PQ et al (1998) Mutations in the homeobox gene HESX1/Hesx1 associated with septo-optic dysplasia in human and mouse. Nat Genet 19:125–133. https://doi.org/10.1038/477
Davis SW, Camper SA (2007) Noggin regulates Bmp4 activity during pituitary induction. Dev Biol 305:145–160. https://doi.org/10.1016/j.ydbio.2007.02.001
Davis EE, Frangakis S, Katsanis N (2014) Interpreting human genetic variation with in vivo zebrafish assays. Biochim Biophys Acta 1842:1960–1970. https://doi.org/10.1016/j.bbadis.2014.05.024
Davis SW, Keisler JL, Perez-Millan MI, Schade V, Camper SA (2016) All hormone-producing cell types of the pituitary intermediate and anterior lobes derive from Prop1-expressing progenitors. Endocrinology 157:1385–1396. https://doi.org/10.1210/en.2015-1862
Day RN, Koike S, Sakai M, Muramatsu M, Maurer RA (1990) Both Pit-1 and the estrogen receptor are required for estrogen responsiveness of the rat prolactin gene. Mol Endocrinol 4:1964–1971. https://doi.org/10.1210/mend-4-12-1964
De Rienzo F, Mellone S, Bellone S et al (2015) Frequency of genetic defects in combined pituitary hormone deficiency: a systematic review and analysis of a multicentre Italian cohort. Clin Endocrinol 83:849–860. https://doi.org/10.1111/cen.12849
Delahaye A, Bitoun P, Drunat S et al (2012) Genomic imbalances detected by array-CGH in patients with syndromal ocular developmental anomalies. Eur J Hum Genet 20:527–533. https://doi.org/10.1038/ejhg.2011.233
Demurger F, Ichkou A, Mougou-Zerelli S et al (2015) New insights into genotype-phenotype correlation for GLI3 mutations. Eur J Hum Genet 23:92–102. https://doi.org/10.1038/ejhg.2014.62
Di Iorgi N, Morana G, Allegri AE et al (2016) Classical and non-classical causes of GH deficiency in the paediatric age. Best Pract Res Clin Endocrinol Metab 30:705–736. https://doi.org/10.1016/j.beem.2016.11.008
Diaczok D, Romero C, Zunich J, Marshall I, Radovick S (2008) A novel dominant negative mutation of OTX2 associated with combined pituitary hormone deficiency. J Clin Endocrinol Metab 93:4351–4359. https://doi.org/10.1210/jc.2008-1189
Drolet DW, Scully KM, Simmons DM, Wegner M, Chu KT, Swanson LW, Rosenfeld MG (1991) TEF, a transcription factor expressed specifically in the anterior pituitary during embryogenesis, defines a new class of leucine zipper proteins. Genes Dev 5:1739–1753. https://doi.org/10.1101/gad.5.10.1739
Dubourg C, Lazaro L, Pasquier L et al (2004) Molecular screening of SHH, ZIC2, SIX3, and TGIF genes in patients with features of holoprosencephaly spectrum: mutation review and genotype-phenotype correlations. Hum Mutat 24:43–51. https://doi.org/10.1002/humu.20056
Dusatkova P, Pfäffle R, Brown MR et al (2016) Genesis of two most prevalent PROP1 gene variants causing combined pituitary hormone deficiency in 21 populations. Eur J Hum Genet 24:415–420. https://doi.org/10.1038/ejhg.2015.126
El-Jaick KB, Powers SE, Bartholin L et al (2007) Functional analysis of mutations in TGIF associated with holoprosencephaly. Mol Genet Metab 90:97–111. https://doi.org/10.1016/j.ymgme.2006.07.011

Ergin AB, Kennedy AL, Gupta MK, Hamrahian AH (2015) The Cleveland Clinic manual of dynamic endocrine testing. Springer International, Cham. https://doi.org/10.1007/978-3-319-13048-4

Errichiello E, Gorgone C, Giuliano L et al (2018) SOX2: not always eye malformations. Severe genital but no major ocular anomalies in a female patient with the recurrent c.70del20 variant. Eur J Med Genet 61:335–340. https://doi.org/10.1016/j.ejmg.2018.01.011

Fang Q, Benedetti AF, Ma Q et al (2016a) HESX1 mutations in patients with congenital hypopituitarism: variable phenotypes with the same genotype. Clin Endocrinol 85:408–414. https://doi.org/10.1111/cen.13067

Fang Q, George AS, Brinkmeier ML et al (2016b) Genetics of combined pituitary hormone deficiency: roadmap into the genome era. Endocr Rev 37:636–675. https://doi.org/10.1210/er.2016-1101

Fauquier T, Rizzoti K, Dattani M, Lovell-Badge R, Robinson IC (2008) SOX2-expressing progenitor cells generate all of the major cell types in the adult mouse pituitary gland. Proc Natl Acad Sci USA 105:2907–2912. https://doi.org/10.1073/pnas.0707886105

Flemming GM, Klammt J, Ambler G et al (2013) Functional characterization of a heterozygous GLI2 missense mutation in patients with multiple pituitary hormone deficiency. J Clin Endocrinol Metab 98:E567–E575. https://doi.org/10.1210/jc.2012-3224

Franca MM, Jorge AA, Carvalho LR et al (2013) Relatively high frequency of non-synonymous GLI2 variants in patients with congenital hypopituitarism without holoprosencephaly. Clin Endocrinol 78:551–557. https://doi.org/10.1111/cen.12044

Franco D, Sedmera D, Lozano-Velasco E (2017) Multiple roles of Pitx2 in cardiac development and disease. J Cardiovasc Dev Dis 4. https://doi.org/10.3390/jcdd4040016

Fuxman Bass JI, Sahni N, Shrestha S et al (2015) Human gene-centered transcription factor networks for enhancers and disease variants. Cell 161:661–673. https://doi.org/10.1016/j.cell.2015.03.003

Gallardo ME, Lopez-Rios J, Fernaud-Espinosa I et al (1999) Genomic cloning and characterization of the human homeobox gene SIX6 reveals a cluster of SIX genes in chromosome 14 and associates SIX6 hemizygosity with bilateral anophthalmia and pituitary anomalies. Genomics 61:82–91. https://doi.org/10.1006/geno.1999.5916

Gangat M, Radovick S (2017) Pituitary hypoplasia. Endocrinol Metab Clin N Am 46:247–257. https://doi.org/10.1016/j.ecl.2017.01.003

Gaston-Massuet C, Andoniadou CL, Signore M, Sajedi E, Bird S, Turner JM, Martinez-Barbera JP (2008) Genetic interaction between the homeobox transcription factors HESX1 and SIX3 is required for normal pituitary development. Dev Biol 324:322–333. https://doi.org/10.1016/j.ydbio.2008.08.008

Gaston-Massuet C, McCabe MJ, Scagliotti V et al (2016) Transcription factor 7-like 1 is involved in hypothalamo-pituitary axis development in mice and humans. Proc Natl Acad Sci USA 113: E548–E557. https://doi.org/10.1073/pnas.1503346113

Gat-Yablonski G, Lazar L, Pertzelan A, Phillip M (2002) A novel mutation in PIT-1: phenotypic variability in familial combined pituitary hormone deficiencies. J Pediatr Endocrinol Metab 15:325–330. https://doi.org/10.1515/JPEM.2002.15.3.325

Gergics P, Brinkmeier ML, Camper SA (2015) Lhx4 deficiency: increased cyclin-dependent kinase inhibitor expression and pituitary hypoplasia. Mol Endocrinol 29:597–612. https://doi.org/10.1210/me.2014-1380

Gerth-Kahlert C, Williamson K, Ansari M et al (2013) Clinical and mutation analysis of 51 probands with anophthalmia and/or severe microphthalmia from a single center. Mol Genet Genomic Med 1:15–31. https://doi.org/10.1002/mgg3.2

Giri D, Vignola ML, Gualtieri A et al (2017) Novel FOXA2 mutation causes hyperinsulinism, hypopituitarism with craniofacial and endoderm-derived organ abnormalities. Hum Mol Genet 26:4315–4326. https://doi.org/10.1093/hmg/ddx318

Gorbenko Del Blanco D, Romero CJ, Diaczok D, de Graaff LC, Radovick S, Hokken-Koelega AC (2012) A novel OTX2 mutation in a patient with combined pituitary hormone deficiency, pituitary malformation, and an underdeveloped left optic nerve. Eur J Endocrinol 167:441–452. https://doi.org/10.1530/EJE-12-0333

Gordon DF, Haugen BR, Sarapura VD, Nelson AR, Wood WM, Ridgway EC (1993) Analysis of Pit-1 in regulating mouse TSH beta promoter activity in thyrotropes. Mol Cell Endocrinol 96:75–84. https://doi.org/10.1016/0303-7207(93)90097-4

Goto M, Hojo M, Ando M et al (2015) Hes1 and Hes5 are required for differentiation of pituicytes and formation of the neurohypophysis in pituitary development. Brain Res 1625:206–217. https://doi.org/10.1016/j.brainres.2015.08.045

Gregory LC, Gaston-Massuet C, Andoniadou CL et al (2015a) The role of the sonic hedgehog signalling pathway in patients with midline defects and congenital hypopituitarism. Clin Endocrinol 82:728–738. https://doi.org/10.1111/cen.12637

Gregory LC, Humayun KN, Turton JP, McCabe MJ, Rhodes SJ, Dattani MT (2015b) Novel lethal form of congenital hypopituitarism associated with the first recessive LHX4 mutation. J Clin Endocrinol Metab 100:2158–2164. https://doi.org/10.1210/jc.2014-4484

Grosse SD, Van Vliet G (2011) Prevention of intellectual disability through screening for congenital hypothyroidism: how much and at what level? Arch Dis Child 96:374–379. https://doi.org/10.1136/adc.2010.190280

Gucev Z, Tasic V, Plaseska-Karanfilska D et al (2016) LHX4 gene alterations: patient report and review of the literature. Pediatr Endocrinol Rev 13:749–755

Haddad-Tovolli R, Paul FA, Zhang Y et al (2015) Differential requirements for Gli2 and Gli3 in the regional specification of the mouse hypothalamus. Front Neuroanat 9:34. https://doi.org/10.3389/fnana.2015.00034

Halasz Z, Toke J, Patócs A et al (2006) High prevalence of PROP1 gene mutations in Hungarian patients with childhood-onset combined anterior pituitary hormone deficiency. Endocrine 30:255–260. https://doi.org/10.1007/s12020-006-0002-7

Hayashizaki Y, Hiraoka Y, Endo Y, Miyai K, Matsubara K (1989) Thyroid-stimulating hormone (TSH) deficiency caused by a single base substitution in the CAGYC region of the beta-subunit. EMBO J 8:2291–2296. https://doi.org/10.1002/j.1460-2075.1989.tb08355.x

Hayes FJ, Seminara SB, Crowley WF Jr (1998) Hypogonadotropic hypogonadism. Endocrinol Metab Clin North Am 27:739–763, vii. https://doi.org/10.1016/S0889-8529(05)70039-6

Heinen CA, Losekoot M, Sun Y et al (2016) Mutations in TBL1X are associated with central hypothyroidism. J Clin Endocrinol Metab 101:4564–4573. https://doi.org/10.1210/jc.2016-2531

Henderson RH, Williamson KA, Kennedy JS et al (2009) A rare de novo nonsense mutation in OTX2 causes early onset retinal dystrophy and pituitary dysfunction. Mol Vis 15:2442–2447

Hendriks-Stegeman BI, Augustijn KD, Bakker B, Holthuizen P, van der Vliet PC, Jansen M (2001) Combined pituitary hormone deficiency caused by compound heterozygosity for two novel mutations in the POU domain of the Pitl/POU1F1 gene. J Clin Endocrinol Metab 86:1545–1550. https://doi.org/10.1210/jcem.86.4.7371

Hergott-Faure L, Borot S, Kleinclauss C, Abitbol M, Penfornis A (2012) Pituitary function and glucose tolerance in a family with a PAX6 mutation. Ann Endocrinol (Paris) 73:510–514. https://doi.org/10.1016/j.ando.2012.10.001

Hide T, Hatakeyama J, Kimura-Yoshida C et al (2002) Genetic modifiers of otocephalic phenotypes in Otx2 heterozygous mutant mice. Development 129:4347–4357

Hu Y, Yu H, Shaw G, Renfree MB, Pask AJ (2011) Differential roles of TGIF family genes in mammalian reproduction. BMC Dev Biol 11:58. https://doi.org/10.1186/1471-213X-11-58

Hughes JN, Aubert M, Heatlie J et al (2016) Identification of an IGSF1-specific deletion in a five-generation pedigree with X-linked central hypothyroidism without macroorchidism. Clin Endocrinol 85:609–615. https://doi.org/10.1111/cen.13094

Idrees F, Bloch-Zupan A, Free SL et al (2006) A novel homeobox mutation in the PITX2 gene in a family with Axenfeld-Rieger syndrome associated with brain, ocular, and dental phenotypes. Am J Med Genet B Neuropsychiatr Genet 141B:184–191. https://doi.org/10.1002/ajmg.b.30237

Inoue H, Mukai T, Sakamoto Y et al (2012) Identification of a novel mutation in the exon 2 splice donor site of the POU1F1/PIT-1 gene in Japanese identical twins with mild combined pituitary hormone deficiency. Clin Endocrinol 76:78–87. https://doi.org/10.1111/j.1365-2265.2011.04165.x

Izumi Y, Suzuki E, Kanzaki S et al (2014) Genome-wide copy number analysis and systematic mutation screening in 58 patients with hypogonadotropic hypogonadism. Fertil Steril 102:1130–1136.e1133. https://doi.org/10.1016/j.fertnstert.2014.06.017
Johnston JJ, Olivos-Glander I, Killoran C et al (2005) Molecular and clinical analyses of Greig cephalopolysyndactyly and Pallister-Hall syndromes: robust phenotype prediction from the type and position of GLI3 mutations. Am J Hum Genet 76:609–622. https://doi.org/10.1086/429346
Joustra SD, Roelfsema F, Endert E et al (2016) Pituitary hormone secretion profiles in IGSF1 deficiency syndrome. Neuroendocrinology 103:408–416. https://doi.org/10.1159/000439433
Juanes M, Di Palma I, Ciaccio M et al (2016) Two novel heterozygous missense variations within the GLI2 gene in two unrelated Argentine patients. Medicina (B Aires) 76:213–218
Jullien N, Romanet P, Philippon M et al (2018) Heterozygous LHX3 mutations may lead to a mild phenotype of combined pituitary hormone deficiency. Eur J Hum Genet. https://doi.org/10.1038/s41431-018-0264-6
Kang S, Graham JM Jr, Olney AH, Biesecker LG (1997) GLI3 frameshift mutations cause autosomal dominant Pallister-Hall syndrome. Nat Genet 15:266–268. https://doi.org/10.1038/ng0397-266
Kantaputra PN, Limwongse C, Tochareontanaphol C, Mutirangura A, Mevatee U, Praphanphoj V (2006) Contiguous gene syndrome of holoprosencephaly and hypotrichosis simplex: association with an 18p11.3 deletion. American J Med Genet A 140:2598–2602. https://doi.org/10.1002/ajmg.a.31386
Kapali J, Kabat BE, Schmidt KL et al (2016) Foxo1 is required for normal somatotrope differentiation. Endocrinology 157:4351–4363. https://doi.org/10.1210/en.2016-1372
Kelberman D, Rizzoti K, Avilion A et al (2006) Mutations within Sox2/SOX2 are associated with abnormalities in the hypothalamo-pituitary-gonadal axis in mice and humans. J Clin Invest 116:2442–2455. https://doi.org/10.1172/JCI28658
Kelberman D, Turton JP, Woods KS et al (2009) Molecular analysis of novel PROP1 mutations associated with combined pituitary hormone deficiency (CPHD). Clin Endocrinol 70:96–103. https://doi.org/10.1111/j.1365-2265.2008.03326.x
Klee EW, Hoppman-Chaney NL, Ferber MJ (2011) Expanding DNA diagnostic panel testing: is more better? Expert Rev Mol Diagn 11:703–709. https://doi.org/10.1586/erm.11.58
Kristrom B, Zdunek AM, Rydh A, Jonsson H, Sehlin P, Escher SA (2009) A novel mutation in the LIM homeobox 3 gene is responsible for combined pituitary hormone deficiency, hearing impairment, and vertebral malformations. J Clin Endocrinol Metab 94:1154–1161. https://doi.org/10.1210/jc.2008-0325
Krude H, Biebermann H, Luck W, Horn R, Brabant G, Gruters A (1998) Severe early-onset obesity, adrenal insufficiency and red hair pigmentation caused by POMC mutations in humans. Nat Genet 19:155–157. https://doi.org/10.1038/509
Kulig E, Camper SA, Kuecker S, Jin L, Lloyd RV (1998) Remodeling of hyperplastic pituitaries in hypothyroid alpha-subunit knockout mice after thyroxine and 17beta-estradiol treatment: role of apoptosis. Endocr Pathol 9:261–274. https://doi.org/10.1007/BF02739967
Laumonnier F, Ronce N, Hamel BC et al (2002) Transcription factor SOX3 is involved in X-linked mental retardation with growth hormone deficiency. Am J Hum Genet 71:1450–1455. https://doi.org/10.1086/344661
Leger J, Olivieri A, Donaldson M et al (2014) European Society for Paediatric Endocrinology consensus guidelines on screening, diagnosis, and management of congenital hypothyroidism. J Clin Endocrinol Metab 99:363–384. https://doi.org/10.1210/jc.2013-1891
Lek M, Karczewski KJ, Minikel EV et al (2016) Analysis of protein-coding genetic variation in 60,706 humans. Nature 536:285. https://doi.org/10.1038/nature19057
Li S, Crenshaw EB 3rd, Rawson EJ, Simmons DM, Swanson LW, Rosenfeld MG (1990) Dwarf locus mutants lacking three pituitary cell types result from mutations in the POU-domain gene pit-1. Nature 347:528–533. https://doi.org/10.1038/347528a0
Li MH, Eberhard M, Mudd P et al (2015) Total colonic aganglionosis and imperforate anus in a severely affected infant with Pallister-Hall syndrome. Am J Med Genet A 167A:617–620. https://doi.org/10.1002/ajmg.a.36915

Lim HT, Kim DH, Kim H (2017) PAX6 aniridia syndrome: clinics, genetics, and therapeutics. Curr Opin Ophthalmol 28:436–447. https://doi.org/10.1097/ICU.0000000000000405

Lin SC, Li S, Drolet DW, Rosenfeld MG (1994) Pituitary ontogeny of the Snell dwarf mouse reveals Pit-1-independent and Pit-1-dependent origins of the thyrotrope. Development 120:515–522

Lonero A, Delvecchio M, Primignani P et al (2016) A novel OTX2 gene frameshift mutation in a child with microphthalmia, ectopic pituitary and growth hormone deficiency. J Pediatr Endocrinol Metab 29:603–605. https://doi.org/10.1515/jpem-2015-0425

Lougaris V, Tabellini G, Vitali M et al (2015) Defective natural killer-cell cytotoxic activity in NFKB2-mutated CVID-like disease. J Allergy Clin Immunol 135:1641–1643. https://doi.org/10.1016/j.jaci.2014.11.038

Lowry RB, Gould DB, Walter MA, Savage PR (2007) Absence of PITX2, BARX1, and FOXC1 mutations in De Hauwere syndrome (Axenfeld-Rieger anomaly, hydrocephaly, hearing loss): a 25-year follow up. Am J Med Genet A 143A:1227–1230. https://doi.org/10.1002/ajmg.a.31732

Ma Y, Qi X, Du J et al (2009) Identification of candidate genes for human pituitary development by EST analysis. BMC Genomics 10:109. https://doi.org/10.1186/1471-2164-10-109

Macchiaroli A, Kelberman D, Auriemma RS et al (2014) A novel heterozygous SOX2 mutation causing congenital bilateral anophthalmia, hypogonadotropic hypogonadism and growth hormone deficiency. Gene 534:282–285. https://doi.org/10.1016/j.gene.2013.10.043

Machinis K, Pantel J, Netchine I et al (2001) Syndromic short stature in patients with a germline mutation in the LIM homeobox LHX4. Am J Hum Genet 69:961–968. https://doi.org/10.1086/323764

Madeira JL, Nishi MY, Nakaguma M et al (2017) Molecular analysis of brazilian patients with combined pituitary hormone deficiency and orthotopic posterior pituitary lobe reveals eight different PROP1 alterations with three novel mutations. Clin Endocrinol 87:725–732. https://doi.org/10.1111/cen.13430

Maione L, Dwyer AA, Francou B, Guiochon-Mantel A, Binart N, Bouligand J, Young J (2018) GENETICS IN ENDOCRINOLOGY: genetic counseling for congenital hypogonadotropic hypogonadism and Kallmann syndrome: new challenges in the era of oligogenism and next-generation sequencing. Eur J Endocrinol 178:R55–R80. https://doi.org/10.1530/EJE-17-0749

Man PS, Wells T, Carter DA (2014) Cellular distribution of Egr1 transcription in the male rat pituitary gland. J Mol Endocrinol 53:271–280. https://doi.org/10.1530/JME-14-0158

Marcinkiewicz M, Day R, Seidah NG, Chretien M (1993) Ontogeny of the prohormone convertases PC1 and PC2 in the mouse hypophysis and their colocalization with corticotropin and alpha-melanotropin. Proc Natl Acad Sci USA 90:4922–4926. https://doi.org/10.1073/pnas.90.11.4922

Martinez-Frias ML, Ocejo-Vinyals JG, Arteaga R et al (2014) Interstitial deletion 14q22.3-q23.2: genotype-phenotype correlation. Am J Med Genet A 164A:639–647. https://doi.org/10.1002/ajmg.a.36330

Matzuk MM, Kornmeier CM, Whitfield GK, Kourides IA, Boime I (1988) The glycoprotein alpha-subunit is critical for secretion and stability of the human thyrotropin beta-subunit. Mol Endocrinol 2:95–100. https://doi.org/10.1210/mend-2-2-95

McCabe MJ, Dattani MT (2014) Genetic aspects of hypothalamic and pituitary gland development. Handb Clin Neurol 124:3–15. https://doi.org/10.1016/b978-0-444-59602-4.00001-0

McNay DE, Turton JP, Kelberman D et al (2007) HESX1 mutations are an uncommon cause of septooptic dysplasia and hypopituitarism. J Clin Endocrinol Metab 92:691–697. https://doi.org/10.1210/jc.2006-1609

Metherell LA, Savage MO, Dattani M, Walker J, Clayton PE, Farooqi IS, Clark AJ (2004) TPIT mutations are associated with early-onset, but not late-onset isolated ACTH deficiency. Eur J Endocrinol 151:463–465

Mishra R, Gorlov IP, Chao LY, Singh S, Saunders GF (2002) PAX6, paired domain influences sequence recognition by the homeodomain. J Biol Chem 277:49488–49494. https://doi.org/10.1074/jbc.M206478200

Molitch ME, Clemmons DR, Malozowski S, Merriam GR, Vance ML, Endocrine Society (2011) Evaluation and treatment of adult growth hormone deficiency: an Endocrine Society clinical practice guideline. J Clin Endocrinol Metab 96:1587–1609. https://doi.org/10.1210/jc.2011-0179

Mukhopadhyay S, Dermawan JK, Lanigan CP, Farver CF (2019) Insulinoma-associated protein 1 (INSM1) is a sensitive and highly specific marker of neuroendocrine differentiation in primary lung neoplasms: an immunohistochemical study of 345 cases, including 292 whole-tissue sections. Mod Pathol 32:100–109. https://doi.org/10.1038/s41379-018-0122-7

Nakamura A, Bak B, Silander TL et al (2013) Three novel IGSF1 mutations in four Japanese patients with X-linked congenital central hypothyroidism. J Clin Endocrinol Metab 98:E1682–E1691. https://doi.org/10.1210/jc.2013-1224

Narumi Y, Kosho T, Tsuruta G et al (2010) Genital abnormalities in Pallister-Hall syndrome: report of two patients and review of the literature. Am J Med Genet A 152A:3143–3147. https://doi.org/10.1002/ajmg.a.33720

Navardauskaite R, Dusatkova P, Obermannova B et al (2014) High prevalence of PROP1 defects in Lithuania: phenotypic findings in an ethnically homogenous cohort of patients with multiple pituitary hormone deficiency. J Clin Endocrinol Metab 99:299–306. https://doi.org/10.1210/jc.2013-3090

Nicholas AK, Jaleel S, Lyons G et al (2017) Molecular spectrum of TSHbeta subunit gene defects in central hypothyroidism in the UK and Ireland. Clin Endocrinol 86:410–418. https://doi.org/10.1111/cen.13149

Norppa AJ, Kauppala TM, Heikkinen HA, Verma B, Iwai H, Frilander MJ (2018) Mutations in the U11/U12-65K protein associated with isolated growth hormone deficiency lead to structural destabilization and impaired binding of U12 snRNA. RNA 24:396–409. https://doi.org/10.1261/rna.062844.117

Obermannova B, Pfaeffle R, Zygmunt-Gorska A et al (2011) Mutations and pituitary morphology in a series of 82 patients with PROP1 gene defects. Horm Res Paediatr 76:348–354. https://doi.org/10.1159/000332693

Osmundsen AM, Keisler JL, Taketo MM, Davis SW (2017) Canonical WNT signaling regulates the pituitary organizer and pituitary gland formation. Endocrinology 158:3339–3353. https://doi.org/10.1210/en.2017-00581

Patti G, Guzzeti C, Di Iorgi N, Maria Allegri AE, Napoli F, Loche S, Maghnie M (2018) Central adrenal insufficiency in children and adolescents. Best Pract Res Clin Endocrinol Metab 32:425–444. https://doi.org/10.1016/j.beem.2018.03.012

Pekic S, Doknic M, Miljic D et al (2011) Case seminar: a young female with acute hyponatremia and a sellar mass. Endocrine 40:325–331. https://doi.org/10.1007/s12020-011-9516-8

Pellegrini I, Roche C, Quentien MH et al (2006) Involvement of the pituitary-specific transcription factor pit-1 in somatolactotrope cell growth and death: an approach using dominant-negative pit-1 mutants. Mol Endocrinol 20:3212–3227. https://doi.org/10.1210/me.2006-0122

Perez Millan MI, Vishnopolska SA, Daly AZ et al (2018) Next generation sequencing panel based on single molecule molecular inversion probes for detecting genetic variants in children with hypopituitarism. Mol Genet Genomic Med. https://doi.org/10.1002/mgg3.395

Pfaeffle RW, Hunter CS, Savage JJ et al (2008) Three novel missense mutations within the LHX4 gene are associated with variable pituitary hormone deficiencies. J Clin Endocrinol Metab 93:1062–1071. https://doi.org/10.1210/jc.2007-1525

Pfäffle R (2006) Genetics of growth in the normal child. Eur J Endocrinol 155:S27–S33. https://doi.org/10.1530/eje.1.02234

Prasov L, Masud T, Khaliq S et al (2012) ATOH7 mutations cause autosomal recessive persistent hyperplasia of the primary vitreous. Hum Mol Genet 21:3681–3694. https://doi.org/10.1093/hmg/dds197

Pulichino AM, Vallette-Kasic S, Couture C et al (2003) Human and mouse TPIT gene mutations cause early onset pituitary ACTH deficiency. Genes Dev 17:711–716. https://doi.org/10.1101/gad.1065603

Quentien MH, Vieira V, Menasche M et al (2011) Truncation of PITX2 differentially affects its activity on physiological targets. J Mol Endocrinol 46:9–19. https://doi.org/10.1677/JME-10-0063

Raitila A, Lehtonen HJ, Arola J et al (2010) Mice with inactivation of aryl hydrocarbon receptor-interacting protein (Aip) display complete penetrance of pituitary adenomas with aberrant ARNT expression. Am J Pathol 177:1969–1976. https://doi.org/10.2353/ajpath.2010.100138

Rajab A, Kelberman D, de Castro SC et al (2008) Novel mutations in LHX3 are associated with hypopituitarism and sensorineural hearing loss. Hum Mol Genet 17:2150–2159. https://doi.org/10.1093/hmg/ddn114

Ramzan K, Bin-Abbas B, Al-Jomaa L, Allam R, Al-Owain M, Imtiaz F (2017) Two novel LHX3 mutations in patients with combined pituitary hormone deficiency including cervical rigidity and sensorineural hearing loss. BMC Endocr Disord 17:17. https://doi.org/10.1186/s12902-017-0164-8

Rauchman M, Hoffman WH, Hanna JD, Kulharya AS, Figueroa RE, Yang J, Tuck-Miller CM (2001) Exclusion of SIX6 hemizygosity in a child with anophthalmia, panhypopituitarism and renal failure. Am J Med Genet 104:31–36. https://doi.org/10.1002/ajmg.10016

Regal M, Paramo C, Sierra SM, Garcia-Mayor RV (2001) Prevalence and incidence of hypopituitarism in an adult Caucasian population in northwestern Spain. Clin Endocrinol 55:735–740. https://doi.org/10.1046/j.1365-2265.2001.01406.x

Rentzsch P, Witten D, Cooper GM, Shendure J, Kircher M (2019) CADD: predicting the deleteriousness of variants throughout the human genome. Nucleic Acids Res 47:D886–D894. https://doi.org/10.1093/nar/gky1016

Reynaud R, Albarel F, Saveanu A et al (2011) Pituitary stalk interruption syndrome in 83 patients: novel HESX1 mutation and severe hormonal prognosis in malformative forms. Eur J Endocrinol 164:457–465. https://doi.org/10.1530/eje-10-0892

Reynaud R, Jayakody SA, Monnier C et al (2012) PROKR2 variants in multiple hypopituitarism with pituitary stalk interruption. J Clin Endocrinol Metab 97:E1068–E1073. https://doi.org/10.1210/jc.2011-3056

Richards S, Aziz N, Bale S et al (2015) Standards and guidelines for the interpretation of sequence variants: a joint consensus recommendation of the American College of Medical Genetics and Genomics and the Association for Molecular Pathology. Genet Med 17:405–424. https://doi.org/10.1038/gim.2015.30

Richter T, Nestler-Parr S, Babela R et al (2015) Rare disease terminology and definitions-a systematic global review: report of the ISPOR rare disease special interest group. Value Health 18:906–914. https://doi.org/10.1016/j.jval.2015.05.008

Rizzoti K, Brunelli S, Carmignac D, Thomas PQ, Robinson IC, Lovell-Badge R (2004) SOX3 is required during the formation of the hypothalamo-pituitary axis. Nat Genet 36:247–255. https://doi.org/10.1038/ng1309

Rizzoti K, Akiyama H, Lovell-Badge R (2013) Mobilized adult pituitary stem cells contribute to endocrine regeneration in response to physiological demand. Cell Stem Cell 13:419–432. https://doi.org/10.1016/j.stem.2013.07.006

Rochette C, Jullien N, Saveanu A et al (2015) Identifying the deleterious effect of rare LHX4 allelic variants, a challenging issue. PLoS One 10:e0126648. https://doi.org/10.1371/journal.pone.0126648

Roessler E, Ermilov AN, Grange DK, Wang A, Grachtchouk M, Dlugosz AA, Muenke M (2005) A previously unidentified amino-terminal domain regulates transcriptional activity of wild-type and disease-associated human GLI2. Hum Mol Genet 14:2181–2188. https://doi.org/10.1093/hmg/ddi222

Rostomyan L, Potorac I, Beckers P, Daly AF, Beckers A (2017) AIP mutations and gigantism. Ann Endocrinol (Paris) 78:123–130. https://doi.org/10.1016/j.ando.2017.04.012

Sato N, Kamachi Y, Kondoh H, Shima Y, Morohashi K, Horikawa R, Ogata T (2007) Hypogonadotropic hypogonadism in an adult female with a heterozygous hypomorphic mutation of SOX2. Eur J Endocrinol 156:167–171. https://doi.org/10.1530/EJE-06-0606

Schaum N, Karkanias J, Neff NF et al (2018) Single-cell transcriptomics of 20 mouse organs creates a Tabula Muris. Nature 562:367–372. https://doi.org/10.1038/s41586-018-0590-4

Schilter KF, Schneider A, Bardakjian T, Soucy JF, Tyler RC, Reis LM, Semina EV (2011) OTX2 microphthalmia syndrome: four novel mutations and delineation of a phenotype. Clin Genet 79:158–168. https://doi.org/10.1111/j.1399-0004.2010.01450.x

Schilter KF, Reis LM, Schneider A et al (2013) Whole-genome copy number variation analysis in anophthalmia and microphthalmia. Clin Genet 84:473–481. https://doi.org/10.1111/cge.12202

Schneider A, Bardakjian T, Reis LM, Tyler RC, Semina EV (2009) Novel SOX2 mutations and genotype-phenotype correlation in anophthalmia and microphthalmia. Am J Med Genet A 149A:2706–2715. https://doi.org/10.1002/ajmg.a.33098

Seifi M, Walter MA (2018) Axenfeld-Rieger syndrome. Clin Genet 93:1123–1130. https://doi.org/10.1111/cge.13148

Semina EV, Reiter R, Leysens NJ et al (1996) Cloning and characterization of a novel bicoid-related homeobox transcription factor gene, RIEG, involved in Rieger syndrome. Nat Genet 14:392–399. https://doi.org/10.1038/ng1296-392

Seminara SB, Oliveira LM, Beranova M, Hayes FJ, Crowley WF Jr (2000) Genetics of hypogonadotropic hypogonadism. J Endocrinol Investig 23:560–565. https://doi.org/10.1007/BF03343776

Shimada A, Takagi M, Nagashima Y, Miyai K, Hasegawa Y (2016) A novel mutation in OTX2 causes combined pituitary hormone deficiency, bilateral microphthalmia, and agenesis of the left internal carotid artery. Horm Res Paediatr 86:62–69. https://doi.org/10.1159/000446280

Shimo N, Yasuda T, Kitamura T et al (2014) Aniridia with a heterozygous PAX6 mutation in which the pituitary function was partially impaired. Intern Med 53:39–42. https://doi.org/10.2169/internalmedicine.53.1184

Shirakawa T, Nakashima Y, Watanabe S et al (2018) A novel heterozygous GLI2 mutation in a patient with congenital urethral stricture and renal hypoplasia/dysplasia leading to end-stage renal failure. CEN Case Rep 7:94–97. https://doi.org/10.1007/s13730-018-0302-9

Simm F, Griesbeck A, Choukair D et al (2018) Identification of SLC20A1 and SLC15A4 among other genes as potential risk factors for combined pituitary hormone deficiency. Genet Med 20:728–736. https://doi.org/10.1038/gim.2017.165

Skowronska-Krawczyk D, Ma Q, Schwartz M et al (2014) Required enhancer-matrin-3 network interactions for a homeodomain transcription program. Nature 514:257–261. https://doi.org/10.1038/nature13573

Sobrier ML, Maghnie M, Vie-Luton MP, Secco A, di Iorgi N, Lorini R, Amselem S (2006) Novel HESX1 mutations associated with a life-threatening neonatal phenotype, pituitary aplasia, but normally located posterior pituitary and no optic nerve abnormalities. J Clin Endocrinol Metab 91:4528–4536. https://doi.org/10.1210/jc.2006-0426

Sobrier ML, Brachet C, Vié-Luton MP et al (2012) Symptomatic heterozygotes and prenatal diagnoses in a nonconsanguineous family with syndromic combined pituitary hormone deficiency resulting from two novel LHX3 mutations. J Clin Endocrinol Metab 97:E503–E509. https://doi.org/10.1210/jc.2011-2095

Sobrier ML, Tsai YC, Pérez C et al (2015) Functional characterization of a human POU1F1 mutation associated with isolated growth hormone deficiency (IGHD): a novel etiology for IGHD. Hum Mol Genet. https://doi.org/10.1093/hmg/ddv486

Sobrier ML, Tsai YC, Pérez C et al (2016) Functional characterization of a human POU1F1 mutation associated with isolated growth hormone deficiency: a novel etiology for IGHD. Hum Mol Genet 25:472–483. https://doi.org/10.1093/hmg/ddv486

Solomon BD et al (2009) Compound heterozygosity for mutations in PAX6 in a patient with complex brain anomaly, neonatal diabetes mellitus, and microophthalmia. Am J Med Genet A 149A:2543–2546. https://doi.org/10.1002/ajmg.a.33081

Sornson MW, Pineda-Alvarez DE, Balog JZ et al (1996) Pituitary lineage determination by the Prophet of Pit-1 homeodomain factor defective in Ames dwarfism. Nature 384:327–333. https://doi.org/10.1038/384327a0

Strande NT, Riggs ER, Buchanan AH et al (2017) Evaluating the clinical validity of gene-disease associations: an evidence-based framework developed by the clinical genome resource. Am J Hum Genet 100:895–906. https://doi.org/10.1016/j.ajhg.2017.04.015

Sun Y, Bak B, Schoenmakers N et al (2012) Loss-of-function mutations in IGSF1 cause an X-linked syndrome of central hypothyroidism and testicular enlargement. Nat Genet 44:1375–1381. https://doi.org/10.1038/ng.2453

Sutton E, Hughes J, White S et al (2011) Identification of SOX3 as an XX male sex reversal gene in mice and humans. J Clin Invest 121:328–341. https://doi.org/10.1172/JCI42580

Tajima T, Hattorri T, Nakajima T et al (2003) Sporadic heterozygous frameshift mutation of HESX1 causing pituitary and optic nerve hypoplasia and combined pituitary hormone deficiency in a Japanese patient. J Clin Endocrinol Metab 88:45–50. https://doi.org/10.1210/jc.2002-020818

Tajima T, Ohtake A, Hoshino M, Amemiya S, Sasaki N, Ishizu K, Fujieda K (2009) OTX2 loss of function mutation causes anophthalmia and combined pituitary hormone deficiency with a small anterior and ectopic posterior pituitary. J Clin Endocrinol Metab 94:314–319. https://doi.org/10.1210/jc.2008-1219

Tajima T, Nakamura A, Ishizu K (2013) A novel mutation of IGSF1 in a Japanese patient of congenital central hypothyroidism without macroorchidism. Endocr J 60:245–249. https://doi.org/10.1507/endocrj.EJ13-0009

Takagi M, Ishii T, Torii C, Kosaki K, Hasegawa T (2014a) A novel mutation in SOX3 polyalanine tract: a case of Kabuki syndrome with combined pituitary hormone deficiency harboring double mutations in MLL2 and SOX3. Pituitary 17:569–574. https://doi.org/10.1007/s11102-013-0546-5

Takagi M, Narumi S, Asakura Y, Muroya K, Hasegawa Y, Adachi M, Hasegawa T (2014b) A novel mutation in SOX2 causes hypogonadotropic hypogonadism with mild ocular malformation. Horm Res Paediatr 81:133–138. https://doi.org/10.1159/000355279

Takagi M, Nagasaki K, Fujiwara I et al (2015) Heterozygous defects in PAX6 gene and congenital hypopituitarism. Eur J Endocrinol 172:37–45. https://doi.org/10.1530/eje-14-0255

Takagi M, Takahashi M, Ohtsu Y, Sato T, Narumi S, Arakawa H, Hasegawa T (2016) A novel mutation in HESX1 causes combined pituitary hormone deficiency without septo optic dysplasia phenotypes. Endocr J 63:405–410. https://doi.org/10.1507/endocrj.EJ15-0409

Takagi M, Kamasaki H, Yagi H, Fukuzawa R, Narumi S, Hasegawa T (2017) A novel heterozygous intronic mutation in POU1F1 is associated with combined pituitary hormone deficiency. Endocr J 64:229–234. https://doi.org/10.1507/endocrj.EJ16-0361

Tasdemir S, Sahin I, Cayır A et al (2014) Holoprosencephaly: ZIC2 mutation in a case with panhypopituitarism. J Pediatr Endocrinol Metab 27:777–781. https://doi.org/10.1515/jpem-2013-0449

Tatsi C, Sertedaki A, Voutetakis A et al (2013) Pituitary stalk interruption syndrome and isolated pituitary hypoplasia may be caused by mutations in holoprosencephaly-related genes. J Clin Endocrinol Metab 98:E779–E784. https://doi.org/10.1210/jc.2012-3982

Tenenbaum-Rakover Y, Turgeon MO, London S, Hermanns P, Pohlenz J, Bernard DJ, Bercovich D (2016) Familial central hypothyroidism caused by a novel IGSF1 gene mutation. Thyroid 26:1693–1700. https://doi.org/10.1089/thy.2015.0672

Thomas PQ, Dattani MT, Brickman JM et al (2001) Heterozygous HESX1 mutations associated with isolated congenital pituitary hypoplasia and septo-optic dysplasia. Hum Mol Genet 10:39–45. https://doi.org/10.1093/hmg/10.1.39

Tommiska J, Känsäkoski J, Skibsbye L et al (2017) Two missense mutations in KCNQ1 cause pituitary hormone deficiency and maternally inherited gingival fibromatosis. Nat Commun 8:1289. https://doi.org/10.1038/s41467-017-01429-z

Treier M, O'Connell S, Gleiberman A et al (2001) Hedgehog signaling is required for pituitary gland development. Development 128:377–386

Trujillano D, Bertoli-Avella AM, Kumar Kandaswamy K et al (2017) Clinical exome sequencing: results from 2819 samples reflecting 1000 families. Eur J Hum Genet 25:176–182. https://doi.org/10.1038/ejhg.2016.146

Tsai EA, Grochowski CM, Falsey AM et al (2015) Heterozygous deletion of FOXA2 segregates with disease in a family with heterotaxy, panhypopituitarism, and biliary atresia. Hum Mutat 36:631–637. https://doi.org/10.1002/humu.22786

Turton JP, Mehta A, Raza J et al (2005a) Mutations within the transcription factor PROP1 are rare in a cohort of patients with sporadic combined pituitary hormone deficiency (CPHD). Clin Endocrinol 63:10–18. https://doi.org/10.1111/j.1365-2265.2005.02291.x

Turton JP, Reynaud R, Mehta A et al (2005b) Novel mutations within the POU1F1 gene associated with variable combined pituitary hormone deficiency. J Clin Endocrinol Metab 90:4762–4770. https://doi.org/10.1210/jc.2005-0570

Turton JP, Strom M, Langham S, Dattani MT, Le Tissier P (2012) Two novel mutations in the POU1F1 gene generate null alleles through different mechanisms leading to combined pituitary hormone deficiency. Clin Endocrinol 76:387–393. https://doi.org/10.1111/j.1365-2265.2011.04236.x

Vajravelu ME, Chai J, Krock B, Baker S, Langdon D, Alter C, De Leon DD (2018) Congenital hyperinsulinism and hypopituitarism attributable to a mutation in FOXA2. J Clin Endocrinol Metab 103:1042–1047. https://doi.org/10.1210/jc.2017-02157

Vallette-Kasic S, Pellegrini-Bouiller I, Sampieri F et al (2001) Combined pituitary hormone deficiency due to the F135C human Pit-1 (pituitary-specific factor 1) gene mutation: functional and structural correlates. Mol Endocrinol 15:411–420. https://doi.org/10.1210/mend.15.3.0601

Vallette-Kasic S, Brue T, Pulichino AM et al (2005) Congenital isolated adrenocorticotropin deficiency: an underestimated cause of neonatal death, explained by TPIT gene mutations. J Clin Endocrinol Metab 90:1323–1331. https://doi.org/10.1210/jc.2004-1300

van Tijn DA, de Vijlder JJ, Verbeeten B Jr, Verkerk PH, Vulsma T (2005) Neonatal detection of congenital hypothyroidism of central origin. J Clin Endocrinol Metab 90:3350–3359. https://doi.org/10.1210/jc.2004-2444

Vaquerizas JM, Kummerfeld SK, Teichmann SA, Luscombe NM (2009) A census of human transcription factors: function, expression and evolution. Nat Rev Genet 10:252–263. https://doi.org/10.1038/nrg2538

Vincent A, Forster N, Maynes JT et al (2014) OTX2 mutations cause autosomal dominant pattern dystrophy of the retinal pigment epithelium. J Med Genet 51:797–805. https://doi.org/10.1136/jmedgenet-2014-102620

Vivenza D, Godi M, Faienza MF et al (2011) A novel HESX1 splice mutation causes isolated GH deficiency by interfering with mRNA processing. Eur J Endocrinol 164:705–713. https://doi.org/10.1530/EJE-11-0047

Warr A, Robert C, Hume D, Archibald A, Deeb N, Watson M (2015) Exome sequencing: current and future perspectives. G3 (Bethesda) 5:1543–1550. https://doi.org/10.1534/g3.115.018564

Webb EA, AlMutair A, Kelberman D et al (2013) ARNT2 mutation causes hypopituitarism, post-natal microcephaly, visual and renal anomalies. Brain 136:3096–3105. https://doi.org/10.1093/brain/awt218

Welcker JE, Hernandez-Miranda LR, Paul FE, Jia S, Ivanov A, Selbach M, Birchmeier C (2013) Insm1 controls development of pituitary endocrine cells and requires a SNAG domain for function and for recruitment of histone-modifying factors. Development 140:4947–4958. https://doi.org/10.1242/dev.097642

Wingender E, Schoeps T, Haubrock M, Donitz J (2015) TFClass: a classification of human transcription factors and their rodent orthologs. Nucleic Acids Res 43:D97–102 https://doi.org/10.1093/nar/gku1064

Woods KS, Cundall M, Turton J et al (2005) Over- and underdosage of SOX3 is associated with infundibular hypoplasia and hypopituitarism. Am J Hum Genet 76:833–849. https://doi.org/10.1086/430134

Zhao L, Bakke M, Krimkevich Y, Cushman LJ, Parlow AF, Camper SA, Parker KL (2001) Steroidogenic factor 1 (SF1) is essential for pituitary gonadotrope function. Development 128:147–154

Zwaveling-Soonawala N, Alders M, Jongejan A et al (2018) Clues for polygenic inheritance of pituitary stalk interruption syndrome from exome sequencing in 20 patients. J Clin Endocrinol Metab 103:415–428. https://doi.org/10.1210/jc.2017-01660

Chapter 14
Hereditary Neurohypophyseal Diabetes Insipidus

Jonas Rutishauser, Nicole Beuret, Cristina Prescianotto-Baschong, and Martin Spiess

Abstract Neurohypophyseal diabetes insipidus (DI) is most often caused by trauma, including operations, and infiltrating processes in the hypothalamic-pituitary region. Irradiation, ischemia, infections, or autoimmunity can also underlie the disease. Since the middle of the nineteenth century, familial forms of neurohypophyseal DI have been described. Most commonly, the disease is transmitted in an autosomal dominant fashion; very rarely, autosomal recessive inheritance has been observed. Hereditary neurohypophyseal DI is caused by mutations in the gene encoding the antidiuretic hormone vasopressin (AVP) and its carrier protein neurophysin II (NPII). Symptoms result from the lack of hormone, or from the inability of mutant AVP to activate its renal receptor, and respond to treatment with desmopressin (DDAVP). Dominant mutations cause retention of the hormone precursor in the endoplasmic reticulum (ER) of vasopressinergic neurons in the hypothalamus, resulting in cellular dysfunction and eventually neuronal death. This so-called neurotoxicity hypothesis was initially established on the basis of autopsy studies in affected humans and has been supported by heterologous cell culture expression experiments and murine knock-in models. Current data show that retained mutants fail to be eliminated by the cell's quality control system and accumulate in fibrillar aggregations within the ER. Autosomal dominant neurohypophyseal DI may thus be viewed as a neurodegenerative disease confined to vasopressinergic neurons.

Keywords Diabetes insipidus · Neurohypophyseal · Vasopressin · Neurophysin · Hereditary · Endoplasmic reticulum · Aggregation · Wolfram syndrome

J. Rutishauser (✉) · N. Beuret · C. Prescianotto-Baschong · M. Spiess
Biozentrum, University of Basel, Basel, Switzerland
e-mail: j.rutishauser@unibas.ch

P. Igaz, A. Patócs (eds.), *Genetics of Endocrine Diseases and Syndromes*,
Experientia Supplementum 111, https://doi.org/10.1007/978-3-030-25905-1_14

List of Abbreviations

aa	Amino acid
AQP	Aquaporin
ATP	Adenosine triphosphate
AVP	Vasopressin; antidiuretic hormone
AVPR2	Vasopressin V2 receptor
cAMP	Cyclic adenosine monophosphate
CFTR	Cystic fibrosis transmembrane conductance regulator
DDAVP	Desmopressin
DI	Diabetes insipidus
DIDMOAD	Diabetes insipidus, diabetes mellitus, optic atrophy, sensorineural deafness
ER	Endoplasmic reticulum
ERAD	Endoplasmic reticulum-associated degradation
NPII	Neurophysin II
OMIM	Online Mendelian Inheritance in Man database
OT	Oxytocin
PKA	Protein kinase A
SP	Signal peptide
UPR	Unfolded protein response

14.1 Introduction

The term "diabetes insipidus" (DI) refers to the excretion of copious amounts of diluted urine (*diabetes*, flow; *insipidus*, tasteless), setting the disorder apart from diabetes mellitus (*mellitus*: sweet) and exemplifying the former practice of evaluating a differential diagnosis by tasting the patients' urine. Polydipsia (excessive thirst) ensues as a consequence of polyuria. Under physiological circumstances, the antidiuretic hormone arginine vasopressin, AVP, is synthesized in specialized hypothalamic neurons that extend to the posterior pituitary, from where it is secreted when plasma osmolality rises or circulating blood volume falls. AVP promotes free water reabsorption from the tubular lumen across renal collecting duct cells into the interstitial and intravasal spaces (Fig. 14.1). If this antidiuretic axis is disturbed, DI results.

Hereditary DI is a monogenetic disorder and usually follows a clear pattern of inheritance, reflecting either autosomal dominant, autosomal recessive, or X-linked transmission. Rarely, additional signs and symptoms are present. In these patients, DI thus constitutes a component of a syndromic disorder.

In this chapter, we will discuss the features of hereditary neurohypophyseal DI, focusing on both clinical and pathophysiological aspects.

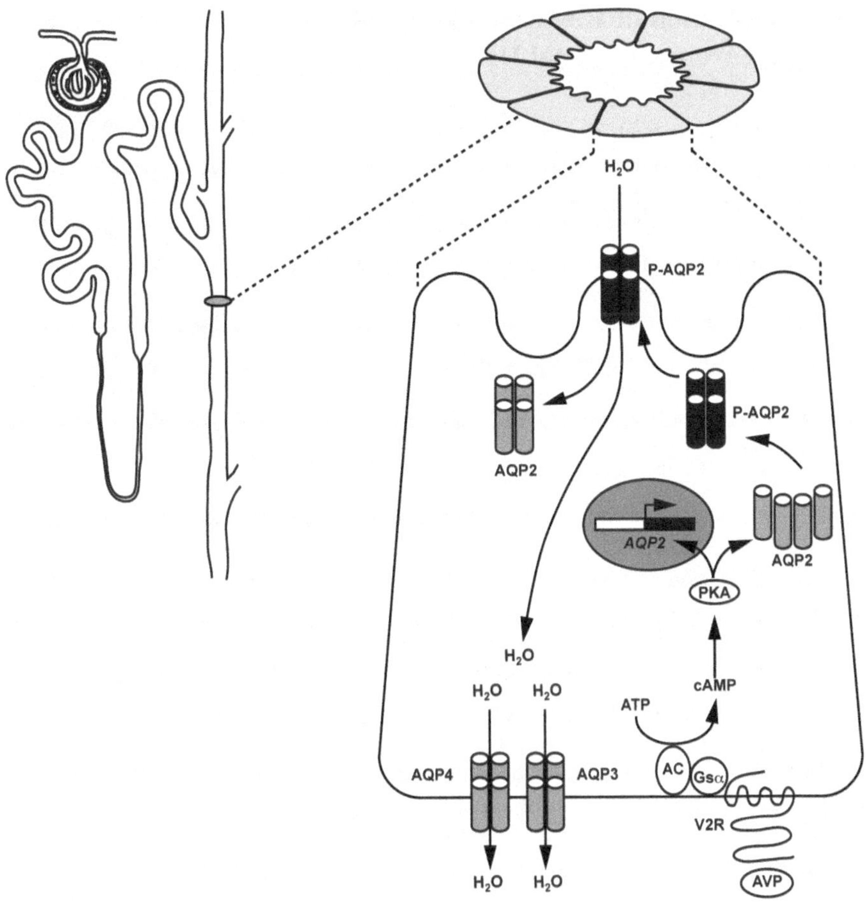

Fig. 14.1 Schematic of the AVP-mediated antidiuretic mechanism. A polarized principal cell of the renal collecting duct is shown on the right. Circulating AVP binds to its renal receptor (V2R), a G protein-coupled seven transmembrane domain receptor, which is located at the basolateral membrane. Coupling of the receptor to the stimulatory G protein (Gs) activates adenylyl cyclase (AC), which in turn converts adenosine triphosphate (ATP) to cyclic adenosine monophosphate (cAMP). cAMP then activates the protein kinase A (PKA) pathway, which exerts two effects. PKA activates nuclear factors, which increases the transcription of the aquaporin 2 (AQP2) water channel gene. PKA phosphorylates AQP2, which leads to the formation of homotetramers (P-AQP2), the functional water channel unit, which is inserted into the apical membrane and allows free water flow from the collecting duct lumen into the cell. Water molecules exit the cell into the interstitial space through aquaporin 3 and 4 water channels (AQP3, AQP4), located at the basolateral membrane. Dephosphorylation of the P-AQP2 homotetramers is followed by their internalization and dissociation. [Reproduced, with permission, from Rutishauser et al. (2016)]

14.2 Evolution of Research on Hereditary Neurohypophyseal DI

Hereditary DI has been described as early as 1841 (Lacombe 1841). In the late nineteenth and early twentieth century, large autosomal dominant pedigrees were reported in the German literature (Weil 1884, 1908; Gänsslen and Fritz 1924). While the molecular basis of the disorder was still unknown, important etiological insight came from post-mortem studies in patients with hereditary or "idiopathic" neurogenic DI (Gaupp 1941; Blotner 1958; Braverman et al. 1965; Green et al. 1967; Bergeron et al. 1991; Nagai et al. 1984). These investigations showed loss of vasopressinergic magnocellular neurons and mild gliosis in supraoptic and paraventricular hypothalamic nuclei, suggesting that neuronal damage had occurred specifically to AVP-producing cells and establishing the basis of the so-called neurotoxicity hypothesis. If a cell type-specific toxic effect, conferred e.g. by a mutant protein, could lead to cell death and eliminate AVP secretion, this would explain the autosomal dominant transmission observed in inherited neurogenic DI. In addition, a neurotoxic agent typically leads to progressive cell damage over a prolonged period of time, which would be in accordance with the clinical observation that the disease develops gradually after the initial manifestation several months to years after birth, albeit with high penetrance.

The gene encoding the precursor of AVP was an obvious candidate to cause hereditary neurogenic DI. The human genes for prepro-AVP and its homolog prepro-oxytocin (OT) were cloned over 30 years ago (Sausville et al. 1985). In 1991, the first paper reporting a heterozygous mutation in the AVP gene was published (Ito et al. 1991). Currently, 71 mutations are listed in the public domain of the Human Gene Mutation Database (HGMD, http://www.hgmd.cf.ac.uk).

Several animal models for neurohypophyseal DI have been described (Bernal et al. 2016). In the Brattleboro rat, studied since the 1960s (Valtin and Schroeder 1964), DI is transmitted in an autosomal recessive manner and results from a single base deletion in the *AVP* gene, which causes a frame shift and leads to inefficient translation of the mutant mRNA (Schmale et al. 1984). The first mouse model to reproduce many facets of human autosomal dominant neurohypophyseal DI was reported in 2003 (Russell et al. 2003). In these animals, a naturally occurring heterozygous human truncation mutation of the AVP precursor protein was introduced, resulting in a clear DI phenotype. Since then, additional rat (Si-Hoe et al. 2000; Davies and Murphy 2002; Castino et al. 2005) and mouse (Hayashi et al. 2009; Hagiwara et al. 2014) models have been published, with varying results regarding recapitulation of clinical polyuria/polydipsia and histological evidence of cytotoxicity in vasopressinergic neurons.

Since the 1990s, numerous expression studies have analysed intracellular trafficking of mutant vs. wild-type AVP hormone precursors (Olias et al. 1996; Beuret et al. 1999; Siggaard et al. 2005). In autosomal dominant neurogenic DI, retention of pathogenic AVP mutants in the endoplasmic reticulum (ER) has uniformly been found. Recent work has focused on aggregation of misfolded precursors in the ER and on

ER-associated degradation, suggesting that insoluble fibrillar aggregates may contribute to or even cause cell death in dominant neurogenic DI (Rutishauser et al. 2016).

14.3 Differential Diagnosis of Hereditary Diabetes Insipidus (OMIM 192340; 125700)

In adults with ad libitum access to fluids, polyuria is defined as a 24-h urinary output of >45–50 ml/kg body weight (Robertson 2001). Polyuria should be quantified, as estimations by patients tend to be imprecise. Uncontrolled diabetes mellitus resulting in glucosuria and thus solute diuresis must be excluded. The differential diagnosis between neurohypophyseal DI, nephrogenic DI, and primary polydipsia can be facilitated by measuring copeptin concentrations at baseline and after sufficient stimulation (i.e. serum [Na] $\geq$ 150 mM) by water deprivation and/or hypertonic saline infusion (Timper et al. 2015; Fenske et al. 2018).

Although de novo mutations in previously unaffected families can occur (Rutishauser et al. 2002; Bourdet et al. 2016; Joshi et al. 2017), a positive family history of polyuria and polydipsia is usually present in hereditary forms (Babey et al. 2011). The mode of transmission and consideration of clinical characteristics often allow to make a presumptive diagnosis, but confirmatory genetic analysis is advocated for both nephrogenic and neurogenic familial DI (Bichet and Bockenhauer 2016; Rutishauser et al. 2016; Joshi et al. 2018). The majority of patients with hereditary nephrogenic DI have mutations in the vasopressin V2 receptor (*AVPR2*) gene, which is encoded on the X chromosome. Autosomal recessive or, less common, dominant transmission is associated with mutations in the gene encoding aquaporin 2 water channels. Hereditary nephrogenic DI, particularly the X-linked and recessive types, is present at birth and characterized by potentially life-threatening dehydration. Conversely, symptoms of familial neurohypophyseal DI typically develop gradually, manifesting months or even years after birth.

In hereditary neurohypophyseal DI, both autosomal recessive and, much more commonly, dominant transmission occur. Since these disorders have distinct pathophysiologies, they will be considered separately.

14.4 The Vasopressin Gene and Its Product

The homologous genes encoding prepro-vasopressin (*AVP* gene) and prepro-oxytocin (*OT* gene) are located in a head-to-head orientation on chromosome 20p13, separated by a ~12 kilobase intervening sequence. The *AVP* gene (Fig. 14.2) consists of three exons, encoding the 19-amino acid (aa) N-terminal signal peptide (SP), the AVP nonapeptide hormone, a 93-aa neurophysin II (NPII) moiety, and a C-terminal 39-aa glycoprotein. The latter, called copeptin, represents

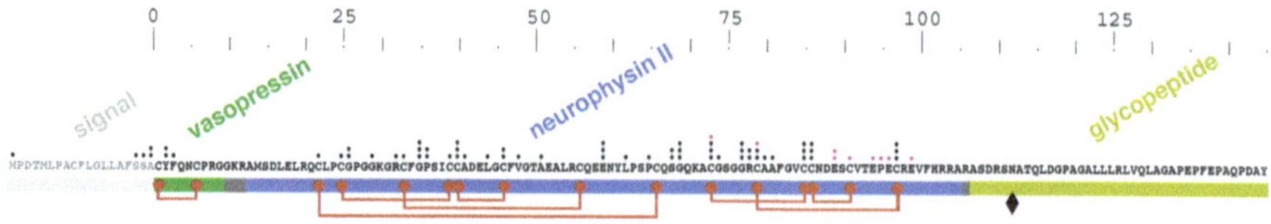

Fig. 14.2 Domain organization of prepro-vasopressin neurophysin II. The hormone precursor consists of the 19-amino acid (aa) signal peptide (grey), the vasopressin nonapeptide (green), the 93-aa carrier protein neurophysin II, and the C-terminal glycopeptide, copeptin (yellow). The glycosylation site is indicated by a black diamond. There are a total of eight disulfide bridges, seven in the neurophysin II and one in the vasopressin moieties, respectively, indicated by red lines. Dots indicate heterozygous mutations associated with autosomal dominant neurohypophyseal diabetes insipidus; missense or deletion in black and nonsense or frameshift in pink. [Reproduced, with permission, from Beuret et al. (2017)]

the main distinctive feature between the *AVP* and *OT* genes, as it is present only in the AVP precursor protein. After directing the nascent polypeptide chain to the ER, the SP is cleaved during cotranslational translocation. Prohormone folding in the ER implies AVP binding into a binding pocket of NPII (Wu et al. 2001; De Bree et al. 2003) and stabilization by eight disulfide bonds. After ER exit, the prohormone is transported through the Golgi apparatus to the trans-Golgi network, where it is sorted into neurosecretory granules and cleaved into AVP, NPII, and copeptin. In addition, AVP is C-terminally amidated. The three proteins are secreted into the circulation from nerve endings in the posterior pituitary by regulated exocytosis. Upon secretion, NPII and copeptin have no clinically appreciated function.

The majority of mutations in hereditary neurogenic DI are missense or nonsense point mutations, but deletions (Christensen et al. 2013; Luo et al. 2012) and indels have also been found (see http://www.hgmd.cf.ac.uk), as well as mutations altering splice sites (see below). No mutations have been described in the copeptin moiety.

14.5 Autosomal Recessive Neurohypophyseal DI

Compared to the much more common dominant type, this mode of inheritance in hereditary neurogenic DI is exceedingly rare. A recurrent recessive point mutation has been reported in two apparently unrelated Palestinian families originating from Texas (Willcutts et al. 1999) and Israel (Abu Libdeh et al. 2010). The mutation, passed on to the affected offspring by each of the heterozygous consanguineous parents, replaces proline at position 7 of the AVP moiety by leucin (P7L). Polyuria and polydipsia developed by the age of 15–24 months in affected children of one family and in the neonatal period in the other, but the reason for this discrepancy is unclear. Symptoms were successfully treated with desmopressin (DDAVP). At the cellular level, it was shown that the mutation caused a ~30-fold decrease in binding of AVP to its renal receptor. Conversely, when the P7L mutant was later expressed in cultured cells, its intracellular trafficking and secretion was normal (Birk et al. 2009).

Another child with very early-onset recessive neurogenic DI, born to consanguineous parents, was reported in 2013 (Christensen et al. 2013). Hypernatremia and urinary hypoosmolality were correctable by the administration of DDAVP, suggesting that the disorder was not caused by a defective AVPR2. Rather, a chromosomal deletion of ~10 kilobases in the *AVP* gene was identified on both alleles, assumedly abolishing gene transcription.

More recently, Canadian paediatricians reported on a child of Lebanese descent, born to asymptomatic parents and presenting with neurohypophyseal DI. Polyuria and polydipsia responded to DDAVP treatment, as did growth retardation. Sequence analysis of the *AVP* gene in the patient revealed a compound heterozygous state, with one allele carrying the known P7L mutation and the other a novel variant in the splice acceptor site of intron 1 (Bourdet et al. 2016). This case underscores the importance of genetic testing, even in the absence of a suggestive family history, in childhood-onset DI of uncertain origin.

14.6 Autosomal Dominant Neurohypophyseal DI

In the vast majority of published families with hereditary central DI, disease transmission follows a dominant pattern. Affected individuals gradually develop polyuria and polydipsia due to progressive AVP deficiency. Symptoms and signs typically start to manifest in infancy to early childhood. Disease penetrance is complete and symptoms are usually severe, although signal peptide mutations causing inefficient signal cleavage have been associated with later manifestation and a partial phenotype (McLeod et al. 1993; Siggaard et al. 2005; Toustrup et al. 2018). If children are deprived of adequate access to fluids, failure to thrive may occur, which is reversible by treatment with DDAVP (Brachet et al. 2011). Interestingly, the same mutation may result in variable disease severity, even among affected members of the same family (Repaske et al. 1997). Another peculiarity is partial recovery of polyuria in elderly males with familial neurohypophyseal DI (Rutishauser et al. 1996; Babey et al. 2011). The physiological basis of these observations is unclear.

14.6.1 ER Retention and Possible Links to Neuronal Cell Loss

Much insight has emerged from heterologous expression studies in cell culture experiments. The common denominator of all dominant neurogenic DI variants is that the mutant prohormone is retained in the ER by the ER quality control system, a machinery that ensures that only correctly folded proteins exit the ER (Araki and Nagata 2011). ER retention is common to the large group of "ER storage diseases", such as cystic fibrosis (retention of the mutant CFTR chloride channel), LDL receptor defect, or nephrogenic DI (retention of mutant AVPR2 or aquaporin 2) (Rutishauser and Spiess 2002). However, as opposed to the majority of these disorders, in autosomal dominant neurohypophyseal DI, the disease does not result from the mere lack of functional protein, which should be compensated by the wild-type allele, but from a dominant-negative effect of the mutant over the wild-type counterpart.

ER retention can be demonstrated by pulse-chase and immunoprecipitation experiments using cells expressing mutant or wild-type (control) provasopressin (Fig. 14.3). ER-retained proteins produce a typical reticular or more densely packed aggregate pattern when visualized by immunofluorescence, co-localizing with ER-resident marker proteins (Fig. 14.4).

Disruption of ER homeostasis, i.e. the mismatch between the load of proteins populating the ER and the ER folding and secretory capacity, activates a program of pathways signalling from the ER lumen to the cytoplasm and the nucleus (Chapman et al. 1998; Mori 2000). This program, termed ER stress response or unfolded protein response (UPR), is made up of several distinct components; e.g. upregulation of ER-resident chaperones and folding enzymes occurs, or programmed cell death pathways may become activated (Oyadomari and Mori 2004). In autosomal dominant neurohypophyseal DI, while the mechanism of neurotoxicity appears to be different from apoptosis (Ito and Jameson 1997), a heterozygous knock-in mouse model, carrying a human truncation provasopressin mutant, reproduced not only the clinical phenotype of AVP-deficient DI, but also demonstrated by immunostaining an apparent reduction in vasopressinergic neurons in the hypothalamus (Russell et al. 2003). This seemingly direct evidence for the neurotoxicity hypothesis has been questioned, however, in later experiments with mice carrying the same heterozygous truncation mutant. By in situ hybridization for AVP mRNA, vasopressinergic neurons were detectable despite the presence of polyuria in the mutant mice (Hayashi et al. 2009). The polyuria phenotype thus preceded neuronal loss. In the ER and nuclei of vasopressinergic cells, large aggregations were detected which contained markers of autophagy, a lysosomal clearance mechanism of intracellular protein waste (Hagiwara et al. 2014). Thus, in the pathophysiology of autosomal dominant neurogenic DI, the autophagy pathway may be involved, but the exact nature of the link between ER retention and toxic impact on neurons remains unclear.

14.6.2 Degradation and Fibrillar Aggregation of Pathogenic Provasopressin Mutants

ER-retained misfolded proteins are retrotranslocated from the ER lumen into the cytosol and targeted for ER-associated degradation (ERAD) by the proteasome (Ciechanover and Schwartz 1998; Hershko et al. 2000). This process has been demonstrated in the case of pathogenic provasopressin mutants in cell culture

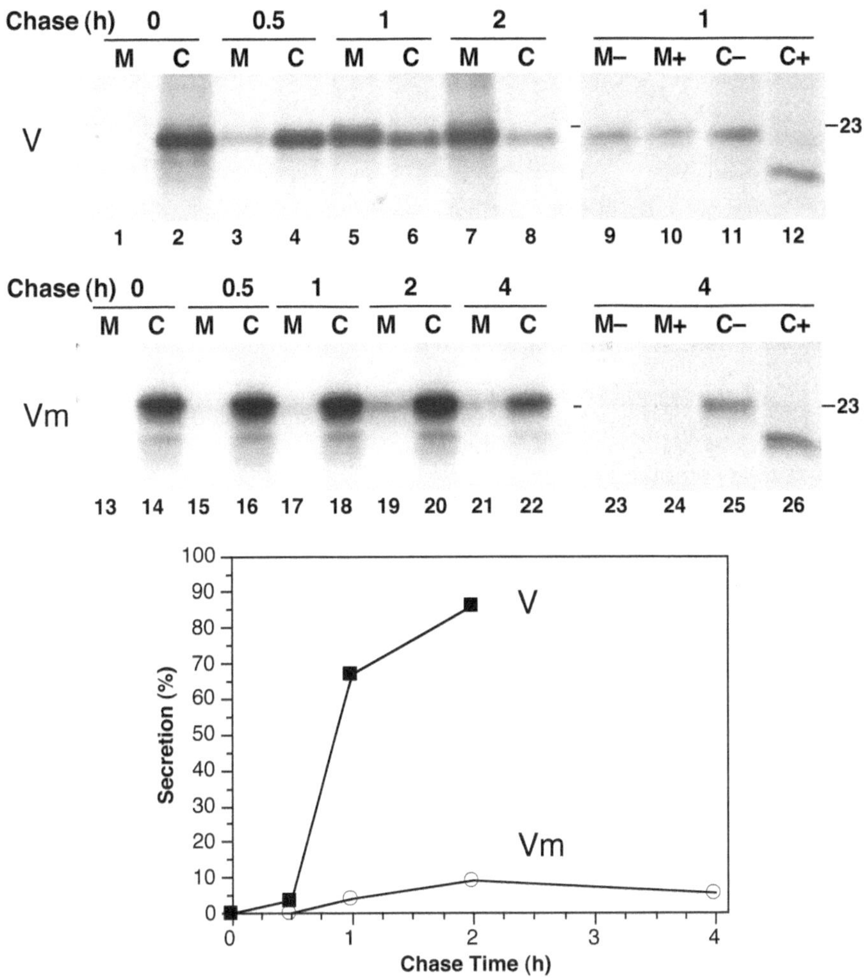

Fig. 14.3 ER retention of a dominant DI mutation. Wild-type vasopressin precursor (V) and the pathogenic mutant ΔG227 [Vm; see Rutishauser et al. (1996)] were expressed in transiently transfected COS-7 fibroblast cells. After pulse labelling for 30 min with [^{35}S]methionine, cells were chased for the indicated durations with excess unlabelled methionine. Media (M) and cell lysates (C) were immunoprecipitated and subjected to gel electrophoresis and autoradiography. The wild-type protein was rapidly secreted into the medium (lanes 1–8), while the mutant was retained quantitatively in the cells even after a chase of 4 h (lanes 13–22). Some samples were incubated with (+) or without (−) endoglycosidase H. Cell lysates (lanes 11, 12 and 25, 26) were sensitive to this treatment, indicating high-mannose glycosylation typical for the ER. In contrast, wild-type protein found in the media (lanes 9, 10) was endoglycosidase H-resistant, indicating that it had adopted complex glycosylation in the Golgi apparatus. (Reproduced with permission. This research was originally published in the Journal of Biological Chemistry. Beuret N., Rutishauser J., Bider M.D., Spiess M. Mechanism of endoplasmic reticulum retention of mutant vasopressin precursor caused by a signal peptide truncation associated with diabetes insipidus. J. Biol. Chem. 1999; 274(27): 18965–18972. © The American Society for Biochemistry and Molecular Biology)

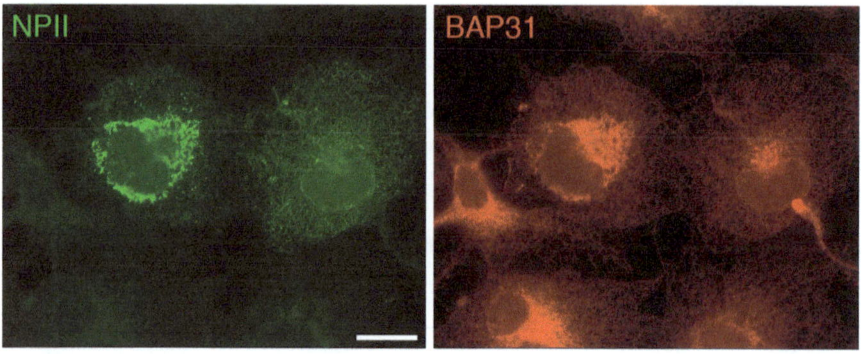

Fig. 14.4 ER localization of a dominant DI mutant by immunofluorescence. COS-1 fibroblast cells were transiently transfected with the dominant mutant C28Y. Cells were stained with antibodies against NP II (left panel) or the ER-resident protein BAP31 (right panel). The mutant protein produces a reticular staining pattern typical for the ER (NPII staining, right cell). Some cells show a more aggregate pattern (NPII staining, left cell). Anti-BAP31 staining shows co-localization with the C28Y mutant. Size bar: 20 μm [Adapted, with permission, from Rutishauser et al. (2016)]

experiments where proteasome inhibitors were used (Friberg et al. 2004) (Fig. 14.5). Interestingly, it was found that not only mutant but also a portion of wild-type precursors were degraded by the proteasome pathway. Indirect evidence for a "system overload" came from the early observation that a dominant AVP mutant associated with severe DI formed disulfide-linked oligomers (Beuret et al. 1999). It was later confirmed that these homo-oligomers accumulated in cells transfected with pathogenic AVP mutants (Birk et al. 2009). Further analysis of transfected cells by immunofluorescence staining and immunogold electron microscopy revealed that large aggregations with a fibrillar substructure gradually accumulated in the ER lumen (Birk et al. 2009; Beuret et al. 2017) (Fig. 14.6). These findings indicated that autosomal dominant neurohypophyseal DI shares essential characteristics with neurodegenerative disorders such as Huntington's, Alzheimer's, or Parkinson's disease associated with fibrillar (amyloid) aggregation.

Recent studies have shown that two sequences within the provasopressin prohormone independently confer the ability to form fibrils, namely, the AVP nonapeptide and the C-terminal copeptin (Beuret et al. 2017). Interestingly, the same two sequences also mediate physiological aggregation and sorting of the prohormone into neurosecretory granules (Beuret et al. 2017), lending support to the proposal that secretory granules are "functional amyloids" (Maji et al. 2009).

The current hypothesis thus states that the amount of mutant AVP precursor molecules exceeds the capacity of the degradation machinery, leading to accumulation and deposition of large fibrillar aggregations in the ER and, potentially, to neuronal damage by undefined mechanisms. Recent experimental work has addressed the role of the ER quality control and degradation system in the context of vasopressin physiology. Remarkably, mice with an intact *AVP* gene, but deficient in Sel1L protein, a component of the ERAD complex, develop AVP-deficient DI without showing

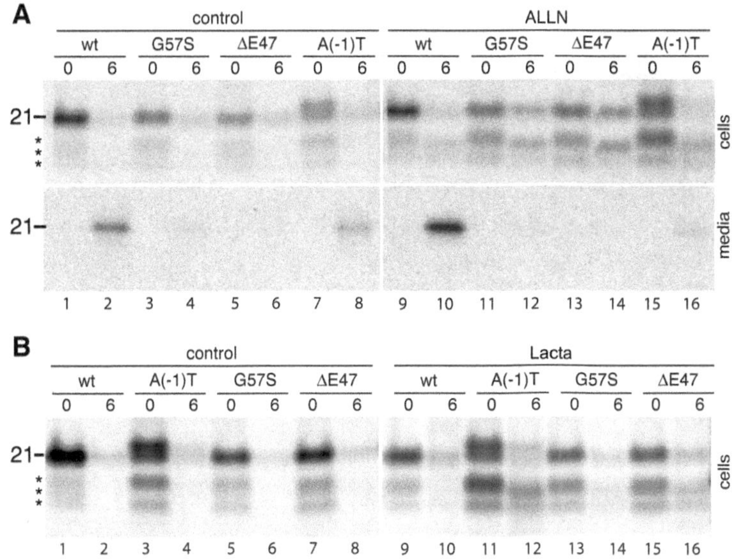

Fig. 14.5 Degradation of provasopressin by the proteasome. Wild-type (wt) and three different dominant DI mutants were expressed in transiently transfected COS-1 cells. G57S and ΔE47 are two mutations in the NPII moiety of the precursor. The signal peptide mutant A(−1)T causes partial signal cleavage deficiency. Cells were pulse-labelled with [^{35}S]methionine and chased for 0 or 6 h in the absence (control; lanes 1–8) or presence (lanes 9–16) of proteasomal inhibitors, 250 μM ALLN (panel **a**) or 25 μM lactacystin (panel **b**). Cell lysates (panel **a**, top) and media (panel **a**, bottom) were subjected to immunoprecipitation, gel electrophoresis, and autoradiography. After labelling, the precursor was detected as a major cytosolic ~21 kDa species, corresponding to glycosylated provasopressin. In the case of the A(−1)T mutant, a slightly larger band was also visible, representing uncleaved prepro-vasopressin. After 6 h of chase, wild-type and the signal-cleaved fraction of the A(−1)T mutant were detected in the media. Hardly any secretion-deficient mutants were detectable in the cells after 6 h, suggesting that they had been almost completely degraded. The addition of the proteasome inhibitors ALLN and lactacystin, but not the lysosomal inhibitors leupeptin and pepstatin (not shown), stabilized the cytosolic 21 kDa mutant and wild-type proteins. In addition to the full-length precursor, three cytosolic degradation intermediates of ~17–19 kDa [asterisks; panel **a** top and panel **b**] were also produced after labelling. These bands were equally stabilized by ALLN and lactacystin. These results indicate that retained dominant DI mutants—and to a smaller degree also wild-type provasopressin—is degraded by proteasomes. (Reproduced with permission. This research was originally published in the Journal of Biological Chemistry. Friberg M.A., Spiess M., Rutishauser J. Degradation of Wild-type Vasopressin Precursor and Pathogenic Mutants by the Proteasome. J. Biol. Chem. 2004; 279(29): 19441–19447. © The American Society for Biochemistry and Molecular Biology)

evidence of damage in magnocellular neurons (Shi et al. 2017). In a mouse neuroblastoma cell line deficient in Sel1L, wild-type and mutant vasopressin precursors accumulate in amyloid-like fibrillar aggregations (Shi et al. 2017). These data show that a functional ERAD is essential for maintaining the antidiuretic system in the wild-type context already and support the pathophysiological concepts outlined above which underlie autosomal dominant neurohypophyseal DI.

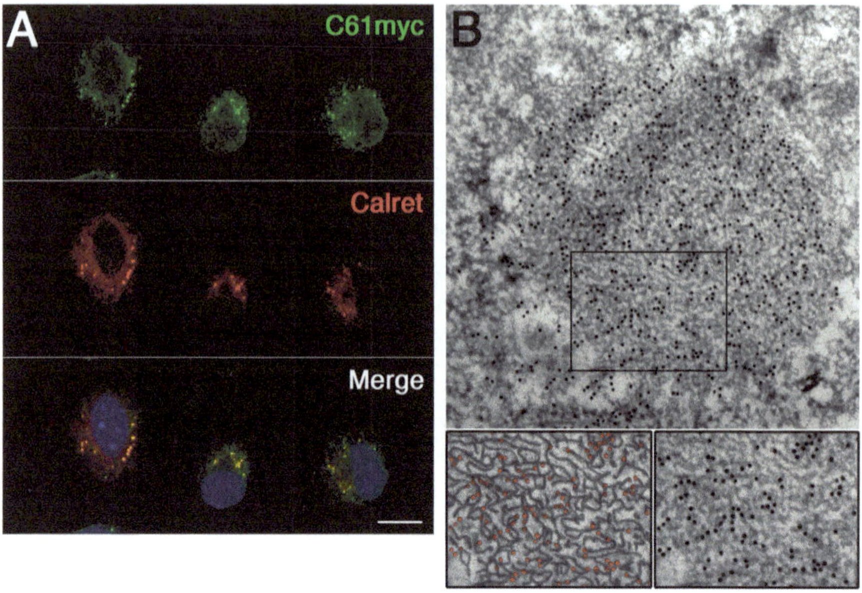

Fig. 14.6 ER aggregation of a C-terminally truncated DI mutant. In the shortest known naturally occurring dominant DI mutant, C61X, the codon for cysteine at position 61 is altered to a stop codon. This truncation mutant is not recognized by anti-provasopressin antibody raised against the C-terminal portion of NPII and copeptin and was myc-tagged for detection by anti-myc antibody. The C61myc mutant was expressed in transiently transfected mouse hippocampal HN10 neuroblastoma cells and analysed by immunofluorescence microscopy after co-staining for myc and the ER chaperone calreticulin (panel **a**, top and middle). Nuclei were stained with DAPI (blue). The two proteins co-localized in aggregations (panel **a**, bottom), indicating that the mutant was retained in the ER. Immunogold electron microscopy demonstrated that the provasopressin aggregates consisted of a network of fibrils, decorated by gold particles seen as black dots (panel **b**, top and bottom right). To enhance clarity, the fibrils were manually highlighted and the black dots coloured in red (panel **b**, bottom left). Size bar: 200 nm. [Reproduced, with permission, from Beuret et al. (2017)]

14.7 X-Linked Neurohypophyseal DI

Only one family tree with apparent X-linked transmission of neurogenic DI has been reported in abstract form (Habiby et al. 1996). Females are unaffected, and males show desmopressin-responsive DI of varying severity, manifesting months to years after birth (Babey et al. 2011). The phenotype has been linked to a region on chromosome Xq28. Importantly, both the *AVP* and *AVPR2* genes in affected males are normal. The gene causing this form of hereditary DI has not been identified so far.

14.8 Desmopressin-Responsive Diabetes Insipidus in the Context of the Wolfram Syndrome 1 (DIDMOAD Syndrome)

Patients affected with this rare autosomal recessive syndrome, first described in 1938 (Wolfram and Wagener 1938), carry homozygous or compound heterozygous mutations in the *WFS1* gene (Inoue et al. 1998; Strom et al. 1998) (OMIM 222300). Diabetes insipidus, diabetes mellitus, optic atrophy, and sensorineural deafness (DIDMOAD) are the components of the complex disorder, with DI manifesting in up to 70% of affected individuals (Barrett et al. 1995). Insulin-dependent diabetes mellitus and bilateral optic atrophy are the two features requested to make a diagnosis, but besides DI and deafness, psychiatric illness associated with a high risk of suicide (Swift et al. 1991, 1998) and brain stem and cerebellar disease (Chaussenot et al. 2011) have also been observed. Prognosis is poor when patients develop neurological dysfunction.

The *WFS1* gene, located in chromosome 4p16.1, encodes wolframin, an ER-resident transmembrane protein which is believed to control ER calcium levels and attenuate ER stress in pancreatic beta cells (Fonseca et al. 2005; Rigoli et al. 2018). Heterozygous mutations in *WFS1*, resulting in deficiency in wolframin, may trigger the ER stress response and eventually activation of pro-apoptotic pathways (Delprat et al. 2018).

14.9 Conclusions

The clinical presentation, along with a careful medical history, will often allow a correct differential diagnosis in hereditary DI, which is confirmed by functional tests and genetic analysis. The neurogenic form is most often transmitted in an autosomal dominant fashion, and symptoms develop gradually, rarely endangering affected individuals. In abrupt neonatal onset, much more often caused by nephrogenic than neurogenic DI, rapid hydration treatment is key. Mutational analysis is recommended in all patients with suspected hereditary DI; importantly, a genetic basis should be considered in idiopathic childhood DI even in the absence of a family history, because de novo mutations in the responsible gene may occur.

References

Abu Libdeh A, Levy-Khademi F, Abdulhadi-Atwan M, Bosin E, Korner M, White PC, Zangen DH (2010) Autosomal recessive familial neurohypophyseal diabetes insipidus: onset in early infancy. Eur J Endocrinol 162(2):221–226. https://doi.org/10.1530/EJE-09-0772

Araki K, Nagata K (2011) Protein folding and quality control in the ER. Cold Spring Harb Perspect Biol 3(11):a007526. https://doi.org/10.1101/cshperspect.a015438

Babey M, Kopp P, Robertson GL (2011) Familial forms of diabetes insipidus: clinical and molecular characteristics. Nat Rev Endocrinol 7(12):701–714. https://doi.org/10.1038/nrendo.2011.100

Barrett TG, Bundey SE, Macleod AF (1995) Neurodegeneration and diabetes: UK nationwide study of Wolfram (DIDMOAD) syndrome. Lancet 346(8988):1458–1463

Bergeron C, Kovacs K, Ezrin C, Mizzen C (1991) Hereditary diabetes insipidus: an immunohistochemical study of the hypothalamus and pituitary gland. Acta Neuropathol 81(3):345–348

Bernal A, Mahía J, Puerto A (2016) Animal models of central diabetes insipidus: human relevance of acquired beyond hereditary syndromes and the role of oxytocin. Neurosci Biobehav Rev 66:1–14. https://doi.org/10.1016/j.neubiorev.2016.02.023

Beuret N, Rutishauser J, Bider MD, Spiess M (1999) Mechanism of endoplasmic reticulum retention of mutant vasopressin precursor caused by a signal peptide truncation associated with diabetes insipidus. J Biol Chem 274(27):18965–18972

Beuret N, Hasler F, Prescianotto-Baschong C, Birk J, Rutishauser J, Spiess M (2017) Amyloid-like aggregation of provasopressin in diabetes insipidus and secretory granule sorting. BMC Biol 15 (1):5. https://doi.org/10.1186/s12915-017-0347-9

Bichet DG, Bockenhauer D (2016) Genetic forms of nephrogenic diabetes insipidus (NDI): vasopressin receptor defect (X-linked) and aquaporin defect (autosomal recessive and dominant). Best Pract Res Clin Endocrinol Metab 30(2):263–276. https://doi.org/10.1016/j.beem.2016.02.010

Birk J, Friberg MA, Prescianotto-Baschong C, Spiess M, Rutishauser J (2009) Dominant pro-vasopressin mutants that cause diabetes insipidus form disulfide-linked fibrillar aggregates in the endoplasmic reticulum. J Cell Sci 122(Pt 21):3994–4002. https://doi.org/10.1242/jcs.051136

Blotner H (1958) Primary or idiopathic diabetes insipidus: a system disease. Metabolism 7 (3):191–200

Bourdet K, Vallette S, Deladoëy J, Van Vliet G (2016) Early-onset central diabetes insipidus due to compound heterozygosity for AVP mutations. Horm Res Pediatr 85(4):283–287. https://doi.org/10.1159/000441844

Brachet C, Birk J, Christophe C, Tenoutasse S, Velkeniers B, Heinrichs C, Rutishauser J (2011) Growth retardation in untreated autosomal dominant familial neurohypophyseal diabetes insipidus caused by one recurring and two novel mutations in the vasopressin-neurophysin II gene. Eur J Endocrinol 164(2):179–187. https://doi.org/10.1530/EJE-10-0823

Braverman LE, Mancini JP, Mc Goldrick DM (1965) Hereditary idiopathic diabetes insipidus. A case report with autopsy findings. Ann Intern Med 63:503–508

Castino R, Davies J, Beaucourt S, Isidoro C, Murphy D (2005) Autophagy is a prosurvival mechanism in cells expressing an autosomal dominant familial neurohypophyseal diabetes insipidus mutant vasopressin transgene. FASEB J 19(8):1021–1023

Chapman R, Sidrauski C, Walter P (1998) Intracellular signaling from the endoplasmic reticulum to the nucleus. Annu Rev Cell Dev Biol 14:459–485

Chaussenot A, Bannwarth S, Rouzier C et al (2011) Neurologic features and genotype-phenotype correlation in Wolfram syndrome. Ann Neurol 69:501–508. https://doi.org/10.1002/ana.22160

Christensen JH, Kvistgaard H, Knudsen J et al (2013) A novel deletion partly removing the AVP gene causes autosomal recessive inheritance of early-onset neurohypophyseal diabetes insipidus. Clin Genet 83(1):44–52. https://doi.org/10.1111/j.1399-0004.2011.01833.x

Ciechanover A, Schwartz AL (1998) The ubiquitin-proteasome pathway: the complexity and myriad functions of proteins death. Proc Natl Acad Sci USA 95(6):2727–2730

Davies J, Murphy D (2002) Autophagy in hypothalamic neurones of rats expressing a familial neurohypophysial diabetes insipidus transgene. J Neuroendocrinol 14(8):629–637

De Bree FM, Van der Kleij AAM, Nijenhuis M, Zalm R, Murphy D, Burbach JPH (2003) The hormone domain of the vasopressin prohormone is required for the correct prohormone trafficking through the secretory pathway. Neuroendocrinology 15:1156–1163

Delprat B, Maurice T, Delettre C (2018) Wolfram syndrome: MAMs' connection? Cell Death Dis 9 (3):364. https://doi.org/10.1038/s41419-018-0406-3

Fenske W, Refardt J, Chifu I et al (2018) A copeptin-based approach in the diagnosis of diabetes insipidus. N Engl J Med 379(5):428–439. https://doi.org/10.1056/NEJMoa1803760
Fonseca SG, Fukuma M, Lipson KL, Nguyen LX, Allen JR, Oka Y, Urano F (2005) WFS1 is a novel component of the unfolded protein response and maintains homeostasis of the endoplasmic reticulum in pancreatic beta-cells. J Biol Chem 280(47):39609–39615
Friberg MA, Spiess M, Rutishauser J (2004) Degradation of wild-type vasopressin precursor and pathogenic mutants by the proteasome. J Biol Chem 279(19):19441–19447
Gänsslen F (1924) Über diabetes insipidus. Klin Wochenschr 3(1):22–23
Gaupp R (1941) Über den diabetes insipidus. Z Ges Neurol Psychiat 171:514–546
Green JR, Buchan GC, Alvorg EC, Swanson AG (1967) Hereditary and idiopathic types of diabetes insipidus. Brain 90:707–714
Habiby R, Robertson GL, Kaplowitz PB, Rittig S (1996) A novel X-linked form of familial neurohypophyseal diabetes insipidus [abstract]. J Investig Med 44:341A
Hagiwara D, Arima H, Morishita Y et al (2014) Arginine vasopressin neuronal loss results from autophagy-associated cell death in a mouse model for familial neurohypophysial diabetes insipidus. Cell Death Dis 5:e1148. https://doi.org/10.1038/cddis.2014.124
Hayashi M, Arima H, Ozaki N et al (2009) Progressive polyuria without vasopressin neuron loss in a mouse model for familial neurohypophysial diabetes insipidus. Am J Physiol Regul Integr Comp Physiol 296(5):R1641–R1649. https://doi.org/10.1152/ajpregu.00034.2009
Hershko A, Ciechanover A, Varshavsky A (2000) Basic medical research award. The ubiquitin system. Nat Med 6(10):1073–1081
Inoue H, Tanizawa Y, Wasson J et al (1998) A gene encoding a transmembrane protein is mutated in patients with diabetes mellitus and optic atrophy (Wolfram syndrome). Nat Genet 20 (2):143–148
Ito M, Jameson JL (1997) Molecular basis of autosomal dominant neurohypophyseal diabetes insipidus. Cellular toxicity caused by the accumulation of mutant vasopressin precursors within the endoplasmic reticulum. J Clin Invest 99(8):1897–1905
Ito M, Mori Y, Oiso Y, Saito H (1991) A single base substitution in the coding region for neurophysin II associated with familial central diabetes insipidus. J Clin Invest 87(2):725–728
Joshi S, Brandstrom P, Gregersen N, Rittig S, Christensen JH (2017) Novel de novo AVPR2 variant in a patient with congenital nephrogenic diabetes insipidus. Case Rep Nephrol Dial 7 (3):130–137. https://doi.org/10.1159/000480009
Joshi S, Kvistgaard H, Kamperis K et al (2018) Novel and recurrent variants in AVPR2 in 19 families with X-linked congenital nephrogenic diabetes insipidus. Eur J Pediatr 177 (9):1399–1405. https://doi.org/10.1007/s00431-018-3132-z
Lacombe LU (1841) De la polydipsie. L'Expérience 203–208:305–391
Luo Y, Wang B, Qiu Y et al (2012) Clinical and molecular analysis of a Chinese family with autosomal dominant neurohypophyseal diabetes insipidus associated with a novel missense mutation in the vasopressin–neurophysin II gene. Endocrine 42(1):208–213. https://doi.org/10.1007/s12020-012-9606-2
Maji SK, Perrin MH, Sawaya MR et al (2009) Functional amyloids as natural storage of peptide hormones in pituitary secretory granules. Science 325(5938):328–332. https://doi.org/10.1126/science.1173155
McLeod JF, Kovács L, Gaskill MB, Rittig S, Bradley GS, Robertson GL (1993) Familial neurohypophyseal diabetes insipidus associated with a signal peptide mutation. J Clin Endocrinol Metab 77(3):599A–599G
Mori K (2000) Tripartite management of unfolded proteins in the endoplasmic reticulum. Cell 101 (5):451–454
Nagai I, Li CH, Hsieh SM, Kizaki T, Urano Y (1984) Two cases of hereditary diabetes insipidus, with an autopsy finding in one. Acta Endocrinol 105:318–323
Olias G, Richter D, Schmale H (1996) Heterologous expression of human vasopressin-neurophysin precursors in a pituitary cell line: defective transport of a mutant protein from patients with familial diabetes insipidus. DNA Cell Biol 15(11):929–935

Oyadomari S, Mori M (2004) Roles of CHOP/GADD153 in endoplasmic reticulum stress. Cell Death Differ 11(4):381–389

Repaske DR, Medlej R, Gültekin EK, Krishnamani MR, Halaby G, Findling JW, Phillips JA (1997) Heterogeneity in clinical manifestation of autosomal dominant neurohypophyseal diabetes insipidus caused by a mutation encoding Ala-1→Val in the signal peptide of the arginine vasopressin/neurophysin II/copeptin precursor. J Clin Endocrinol Metab 82(1):51–56

Rigoli L, Bramanti P, Di Bella C, De Luca F (2018) Correction: genetic and clinical aspects of Wolfram syndrome 1, a severe neurodegenerative disease. Pediatr Res 84(5):787. https://doi.org/10.1038/s41390-018-0146-1

Robertson GL (2001) Antidiuretic hormone. Normal and disordered function. Endocrinol Metab Clin N Am 30(3):671–694

Russell TA, Ito M, Ito M, Yu RN, Martinson FA, Weiss J, Jameson JL (2003) A murine model of autosomal dominant neurohypophyseal diabetes insipidus reveals progressive loss of vasopressin-producing neurons. J Clin Invest 112(11):1697–1706

Rutishauser J, Spiess M (2002) Endoplasmic reticulum storage diseases. Swiss Med Wkly 132 (17–18):211–222

Rutishauser J, Böni-Schnetzler M, Böni J, Wichmann W, Huisman T, Vallotton MB, Froesch ER (1996) A novel point mutation in the translation initiation codon of the pre-pro-vasopressin-neurophysin II gene: cosegregation with morphological abnormalities and clinical symptoms in autosomal dominant neurohypophyseal diabetes insipidus. J Clin Endocrinol Metab 81 (1):192–198

Rutishauser J, Kopp P, Gaskill MB, Kotlar TJ, Robertson GL (2002) Clinical and molecular analysis of three families with autosomal dominant neurohypophyseal diabetes insipidus associated with a novel and recurrent mutations in the vasopressin-neurophysin II gene. Eur J Endocrinol 146(5):649–656

Rutishauser J, Spiess M, Kopp P (2016) Genetic forms of neurohypophyseal diabetes insipidus. Best Pract Res Clin Endocrinol Metab 30(2):249–262. https://doi.org/10.1016/j.beem.2016.02.008

Sausville E, Carney D, Battey J (1985) The human vasopressin gene is linked to the oxytocin gene and is selectively expressed in a cultured lung cancer cell line. J Biol Chem 260 (18):10236–10241

Schmale H, Ivell R, Breindl M, Darmer D, Richter D (1984) The mutant vasopressin gene from diabetes insipidus (Brattleboro) rats is transcribed but the message is not efficiently translated. EMBO J 3(13):3289–3293

Shi G, Somlo DRM, Kim GH et al (2017) ER-associated degradation is required for vasopressin prohormone processing and systemic water homeostasis. J Clin Invest 127(10):3897–3912. https://doi.org/10.1172/JCI94771

Siggaard C, Christensen JH, Corydon TJ et al (2005) Expression of three different mutations in the arginine vasopressin gene suggests genotype-phenotype correlation in familial neurohypophyseal diabetes insipidus kindreds. Clin Endocrinol 63(2):207–216

Si-Hoe SL, De Bree FM, Nijenhuis M et al (2000) Endoplasmic reticulum derangement in hypothalamic neurons of rats expressing a familial neurohypophyseal diabetes insipidus mutant vasopressin transgene. FASEB J 14(12):1680–1684

Strom TM, Hörtnagel K, Hofmann S et al (1998) Diabetes insipidus, diabetes mellitus, optic atrophy and deafness (DIDMOAD) caused by mutations in a novel gene (wolframin) coding for a predicted transmembrane protein. Hum Mol Genet 7(13):2021–2028

Swift RG, Perkins DO, Chase CL, Sadler DB, Swift M (1991) Psychiatric disorders in 36 families with Wolfram syndrome. Am J Psychiatry 148:775–779

Swift RG, Polymeropoulos MH, Torres R, Swift M (1998) Predisposition of Wolfram syndrome heterozygotes to psychiatric illness. Mol Psychiatry 3:86–91

Timper K, Fenske W, Kühn F et al (2015) Diagnostic accuracy of copeptin in the differential diagnosis of the polyuria-polydipsia syndrome: a prospective multicenter study. J Clin Endocrinol Metab 100(6):2268–2274. https://doi.org/10.1210/jc.2014-4507

Toustrup LB, Kvistgaard H, Palmfeldt J et al (2018) The novel Ser18del AVP variant causes inherited neurohypophyseal diabetes insipidus by mechanisms shared with other signal peptide variants. Neuroendocrinology 106(2):167–186. https://doi.org/10.1159/000477246
Valtin H, Schroeder H (1964) Familial hypothalamic diabetes insipidus in rats (Brattleboro strain). Am J Phys 206:425–430
Weil A (1884) Über die hereditäre Form des Diabetes insipidus. Virchows Arch 90:70–95
Weil A (1908) Über die hereditäre Form des Diabetes insipidus. Arch Klin Med 93:180–200
Willcutts MD, Felner E, White PC (1999) Autosomal recessive familial neurohypophyseal diabetes insipidus with continued secretion of mutant weakly active vasopressin. Hum Mol Genet 8 (7):1303–1307
Wolfram DJ, Wagener HP (1938) Diabetes mellitus and simple optic atrophy among siblings: report of four cases. Mayo Clin Proc 13:715–718
Wu CK, Hu B, Rose JP et al (2001) Structures of an unliganded neurophysin and its vasopressin complex: implications for binding and allosteric mechanisms. Protein Sci 10:1869–1880

Chapter 15
Nephrogenic Diabetes Insipidus

András Balla and László Hunyady

Abstract Body fluid homeostasis is essential for normal life. In the maintenance of water balance, the most important factor and regulated process is the excretory function of the kidneys. The kidneys are capable to compensate not only the daily fluctuations of water intake but also the consequences of fluid loss (respiration, perspiration, sweating, hemorrhage). The final volume and osmolality of the excreted urine is set in the collecting duct via hormonal regulation. The hormone of water conservation is the vasopressin (AVP), and a large volume of urine is produced and excreted in the absence of AVP secretion or if AVP is ineffective in the kidneys. The aquaporin-2 water channel (AQP2) is expressed in the principal cells, and it plays an essential role in the reabsorption of water in the collecting ducts via type 2 vasopressin receptor (V2R)-mediated mechanism. If neural or hormonal regulation fails to operate the normal function of AVP-V2R-AQP2 system, it can result in various diseases such as diabetes insipidus (DI) or nephrogenic syndrome of inappropriate diuresis (NSIAD). The DI is characterized by excessive production of hyposmotic urine ("insipidus" means tasteless) due to the inability of the kidneys to concentrate urine. In this chapter, we focus and discuss the pathophysiology of nephrogenic DI (NDI) and the potential therapeutic interventions in the light of the current experimental data.

Keywords *AQP2* gene · *AVPR2* gene · Diabetes insipidus · G protein-coupled receptor (GPCR) · Nephrogenic diabetes insipidus · NDI · Signal transduction · Type 2 vasopressin receptor (V2R)

A. Balla · L. Hunyady (✉)
Faculty of Medicine, Department of Physiology, Semmelweis University, Budapest, Hungary

MTA-SE Laboratory of Molecular Physiology, Hungarian Academy of Sciences, Semmelweis University, Budapest, Hungary
e-mail: hunyady.laszlo@med.semmelweis-univ.hu

P. Igaz, A. Patócs (eds.), *Genetics of Endocrine Diseases and Syndromes*, Experientia Supplementum 111, https://doi.org/10.1007/978-3-030-25905-1_15

List of Abbreviations

ADH	Antidiuretic hormone
ANP	Atrial natriuretic peptide
AQP	Aquaporin water channel
AVP	Vasopressin
cAMP	3′,5′-Cyclic adenosine monophosphate
cNDI	Congenital forms of NDI
CREB	cAMP response element-binding protein
ddAVP	Desmopressin (1-deamino-8-D-arginine vasopressin)
DI	Diabetes insipidus
ENaC	Epithelial sodium channel
GPCR	G protein-coupled receptor
NaPi-2	Type 2 sodium-phosphate cotransporter
NBC1	Sodium-bicarbonate cotransporter
NDI	Nephrogenic diabetes insipidus
NCC	Na-Cl cotransporter
NKCC	Na^+-K^+-$2Cl^-$ cotransporter
NSIAD	Nephrogenic syndrome of inappropriate diuresis
PGE2	Prostaglandin E2
PKA	Protein kinase A
ROMK	Renal outer medullary potassium channel
SIADH	Syndrome of inappropriate antidiuretic hormone
V1R, V2R	Type 1 and type 2 arginine-vasopressin receptor

15.1 Introduction

The maintenance of constant volume and composition of the body fluids requires that the daily water intake and water loss are matched and tightly regulated. The balance between the water input and output is mainly regulated through the kidneys, although water intake is also controlled by thirst. Urine formation by the kidneys is the key regulatory factor in the maintenance of water and electrolyte homeostasis of the human body. The kidneys respond rapidly and appropriately to body fluid osmolality and volume fluctuations; however, the kidneys are able to fulfill these homeostatic tasks only under hormonal and neural regulatory mechanisms. Under normal conditions, the glomerular filtration by the kidneys produces approximately 120 ml of fluid in a minute, and the tubular system allows great variations in the rate of final fluid excretion. The volume of urine production can be greatly varied in antidiuresis (water deprivation) and in water diuresis (after excessive fluid load). Normally, about 1% of the filtered water is finally excreted as urine; the average urine output is ~0.5–1.5 ml/min. Some segments of the tubular system have permanent high water permeability because certain types of aquaporin water channels (AQP) reside constitutively on their apical and basolateral membranes. On the contrary, other segments are virtually water impermeable due to the lack of aquaporin water channels in the plasma membrane compartments. In healthy humans, approximately 85% of the filtered fluid is reabsorbed in the proximal tubule and in the loop of Henle, independently on the water homeostatic status of the body. Approximately 8–14.5% of the glomerular filtered fluid is reabsorbed in the collecting ducts, and it is under tight hormonal control via vasopressin (arginine vasopressin in humans, AVP; also called as antidiuretic hormone, ADH) and atrial natriuretic peptide (ANP) actions (Robertson 2001; Saito 2010). The AVP is synthesized as prohormone which is later cleaved to nonapeptide AVP in the supraoptic and paraventricular nuclei of the hypothalamus (Fliers et al. 1985; Sklar and Schrier 1983). The produced AVP is transported by axonal transport via the supraopticohypophyseal into the neurohypophysis and secreted from here in response to stimulation. A very sensitive mechanism allows that even less than 1% increase in osmolality stimulates osmoreceptors in the hypothalamus, which in turn induces the release of AVP into the systemic circulation. The secreted AVP circulates in the blood and primarily acts in the kidneys via V2R (type 2 AVP receptor). In addition to the AVP production and secretion, higher increase in extracellular osmolality leads to thirst perception, which drives drinking behavior helping to restore the normal osmolality and volume of the fluid compartments in the body. The vascular effects (vasoconstriction and total peripheral resistance increase) of AVP due to type 1 vasopressin receptor (V1R) activation are manifested only at greatly elevated AVP levels. This huge increase in AVP production and secretion can be seen only in response to baroreceptor activation reflex when blood volume changes reach at least 5–10%.

The collecting tubules are divided into subsegments such as cortical, outer medullary, and inner medullary collecting ducts but in all subsegments the AVP regulates the reabsorption of water. (The water permeability of the tight junctions between the epithelial cells of the collecting tubule is negligible.) The overall action of the AVP is the water conservation and formation of hyperosmotic urine. During antidiuresis, the AVP makes the luminal membrane of the principal cells in the collecting ducts water-permeable, and water is passively reabsorbed via AQP channels due to the existing osmotic gradient between the tubular fluid and the hyperosmotic interstitium. The effect of AVP is induced by the binding to and activation of the basolaterally located V2R in the collecting ducts which is followed by consequent signaling transduction steps leading to the translocation of AQP2 from endomembranes to the apical plasma membrane (Moeller et al. 2013). Under normal circumstances, the AQP2 is inserted in the luminal membrane of the principal cells as homotetrameric water channel.

AVP also regulates the urea permeability of the principal cells since its effect is required for the normal expression and function of urea transporters in the inner medullary collecting duct, enhancing the urea recycling and via this mechanism contributes to the buildup of corticopapillary osmotic gradient. This osmotic gradient is an important drive for the water reabsorption in the collecting tubule. It is important to note that the AVP is on top of the abovementioned effects in the collecting ducts and it also increases the activity of the Na^+-K^+-$2Cl^-$ cotransporter (NKCC) in the thick ascending limb of the loop of Henle, hence augmenting the corticopapillary osmotic gradient (Fenton and Knepper 2007). Moreover, AVP increases sodium reabsorption in the collecting duct by increasing the activity of the amiloride-sensitive epithelial sodium channel (ENaC) (Bankir et al. 2005).

The constant physiological regulation greatly varies the rate of water reabsorption in the collecting ducts, and finally 0.5–10% of the filtered water can be excreted. The rate of urine production is mainly regulated by water reabsorption through the aquaporin-2 channel's (AQP2) presence and thus the water permeability in the collecting duct principal cells. The water permeability of the collecting ducts is AVP-dependent and is under constant regulation. The huge variation of the water reabsorption in the collecting duct is the consequence of a specific chain of events which modify the water permeability and the AQP2 presence in the luminal (apical) membrane of the collecting tubule principal cells. Under maximal AVP influence, only ~0.3 ml fluid per minute is excreted; however, in lack of AVP-induced concentrating function of the kidneys, it can raise as much as ~12 ml urine production per minute. The osmolality of urine changes reciprocally with the volume of urine output; the osmolality can be as high as ~1300 mosm/kg water in maximal antidiuretic condition and as low as ~30 mosm/kg water in maximal diuresis in humans. After restoration of water balance, due to the termination of AVP secretion from the neurohypophysis and the elimination of circulating AVP molecules by kidney and liver vasopressinases, the AVP level decreases in a short time (10–30 min) (Czaczkes et al. 1964). Consequently, the V2R-induced mechanisms in principal cells diminish resulting in the relocation of AQP2 water channels into endomembrane compartments, which in turn greatly reduce the water permeability and reabsorption capacity of the collecting duct. Under normal conditions, the presence of AQP2 water channels in the luminal surface of the principal cells is the permissive factor for the water reabsorption.

Impaired regulatory mechanisms in the AVP action or genetic defects in the participating proteins can lead to disturbed renal function, and diseases such as diabetes insipidus (DI) or nephrogenic syndrome of inappropriate diuresis (NSIAD) depending on that loss-of-function or gain-of-function mutations are behind the restricted or exaggerated transport functions. Investigations of such disorders have contributed enormously to our understanding of the mechanisms of urinary concentration and identified the important proteins and revealed potential therapeutic interventions to cure or unburden the symptoms.

DI is a rare disease, and the prevalence is approximately 1 per 30,000 and characterized by the inability to normally concentrate urine resulting in several symptoms, such as polyuria (40–150 ml/kg/day, depending on the age), hyposthenuria (low specific gravity of urine, <290 mOsm/L), and compensatory polydipsia (Robertson 1995). This disease burdens normal life due to production and micturition of large volumes of urine all day long. Moreover, in severe forms of the disorder, the individuals must micturate and drink fluid even at night several times. The DI is frequently associated with urological complications, such as impaired bladder function, hydronephrosis, chronic renal failure, and large dilations of the urinary tract (Shalev et al. 2004; Boyd et al. 1980). The patients can be held in water balance as long as the fluid intake compensates the excessive urine output. The thirst sensation and its regulation are essential safety backup mechanisms since the compensatory water intake reflexes can avoid the development of severe hyperosmolality in the blood plasma. Unfortunately, if the water intake is limited, the patient becomes dehydrated and hypovolemic by reason of excessive water loss.

This chapter gives an overview of the various DI types focusing on nephrogenic DI, including the pathophysiology and potential therapeutic interventions in such disorders.

15.2 Nephrogenic Diabetes Insipidus (NDI)

In the NDI disorder, albeit the AVP production and its secretion are normally regulated by the hyperosmotic stimuli, the principal cells in the collecting ducts do not respond normally to the hormone. The irresponsiveness can be caused by several factors, such as genetic defects (familial or congenital nephrogenic diabetes insipidus due to mutations either in the *AVPR2* or *AQP2* genes), or can be acquired, i.e., from drug therapies. In adults, the acquired forms are more common, whereas children mostly present congenital forms of NDI (cNDI). In this chapter, we summarize the causes and the pathophysiological consequences of NDI; furthermore, we discuss the new treatment possibilities that have been proposed by the current research data in the literature to medicate or disburden the symptoms of NDI. The cited OMIM entries can be found at www.omim.org (Amberger and Hamosh 2017).

15.2.1 Types of NDI

15.2.1.1 Congenital Forms of NDI (cNDI)

The hereditary NDI syndromes are most commonly due to the mutations either in the *AVPR2* or in the *AQP2* genes (primary NDIs). Approximately 90% of the NDI cases are related to the malfunction of the V2R and its signaling, and ~10% is due to the autosomal mutations in the *AQP2* gene. Interestingly, the dysfunctions of V2R or AQP2 cause indistinguishable clinical symptoms, which are manifested immediately after birth. On top of the mutations in the *AVPR2* or *AQP2* gene, other genetic renal diseases can be in the background of the symptoms (secondary NDIs) (Bockenhauer and Bichet 2013). Most patients suffering from cNDI are diagnosed within the 3 years of life, with excessive vomiting, reduced growth, underweight, constipation, fever, and dehydration.

Disease-Causing Mutations of V2 Vasopressin Receptor (OMIM 304800)

The V2R belongs to the G protein-coupled receptor (GPCR) superfamily, composed by 371 amino acids that form 7 transmembrane domains. In the principal cells, the V2R acts mostly via coupling to G_s proteins, thus regulating the intracellular

3′,5′-cyclic adenosine monophosphate (cAMP) level in target cells. Members of the GPCR superfamily are the largest group of cell membrane receptors, and their mutations are responsible for numerous human diseases given the fact that more than 600 loss-of-function mutations of GPCRs have been identified (Schoneberg et al. 2004), including the majority of congenital NDI cases (Bichet 2009). The mutations in the V2R can cause failure in urine concentration due to several mechanisms including the inability to establish the corticopapillary osmotic gradient and the impaired water transport through collecting duct principal cells, but the most palpable dysfunction that defective V2R function in the principal cells induces is hyposmotic polyuria production. Under normal circumstances in healthy individuals, the AVP stimulation-induced V2R activation triggers cAMP signaling cascades, most importantly the activation of protein kinase A (PKA), which in turn phosphorylates the AQP2 on several residues that triggers the vesicular transport of AQP2-containing endomembranes into the apical membrane allowing water reabsorption in the collecting ducts (Nielsen et al. 2002) (Fig. 15.1a). Once the AVP secretion is diminished in response to the restored water balance, AQP2 abundance is also reduced due to its internalization through ubiquitin-mediated endocytosis and transport to storage vesicles and degradation (Kamsteeg et al. 2006). This regulation of AQP2 water channel localization is crucial to increase urine osmolality and to reduce urine output in humans (Moeller et al. 2013). In addition to the classical PKA activation pathway, it is important to emphasize that the increased intracellular cAMP directly binds and activates other effector signaling proteins, such as Epac (exchange factor directly activated by cAMP), which functions as guanine-nucleotide exchange factor for the small GTPase. It was demonstrated that the AQP2 abundance on the luminal surface of the principal cells mainly depends on the Epac activation and was independent of the PKA activity (Kortenoeven et al. 2012). Interestingly, during the aforementioned signaling processes, the AVP-bound V2R active receptor conformation is phosphorylated by GRK molecules, which leads to recognition and association with β-arrestin molecules, and the receptor is desensitized (although the AVP is still bound to the receptor). The arrestin recruitment initiates several important regulatory mechanisms. First, the arrestin molecules act as scaffold proteins to organize the endocytosis of the V2R which results in the decreased cell surface receptor density and the degradation of the receptor in the lysosomes (the AVP is bound so tightly that it can be dissociated from the receptor only upon breakdown of the receptor molecule). β-Arrestin-mediated receptor downregulation prevents exaggerated reabsorption in the collecting ducts and allows the possibility to regulate smoothly and rapidly the rate of water reabsorption.

AVP-induced V2R activation is necessary not just for the normal AQP2 trafficking pattern but also required for the normal AQP2 expression levels. It was demonstrated that although the intracellular cAMP level decays shortly after AVP stimulation, the AQP2 expression remains increased for days (DiGiovanni et al. 1994; Kortenoeven et al. 2012). Interestingly, the upregulatory effect of AVP on AQP2 expression level was dependent on extracellular signal-regulated kinase (ERK), Epac activation, and cAMP response element-binding protein (CREB), but

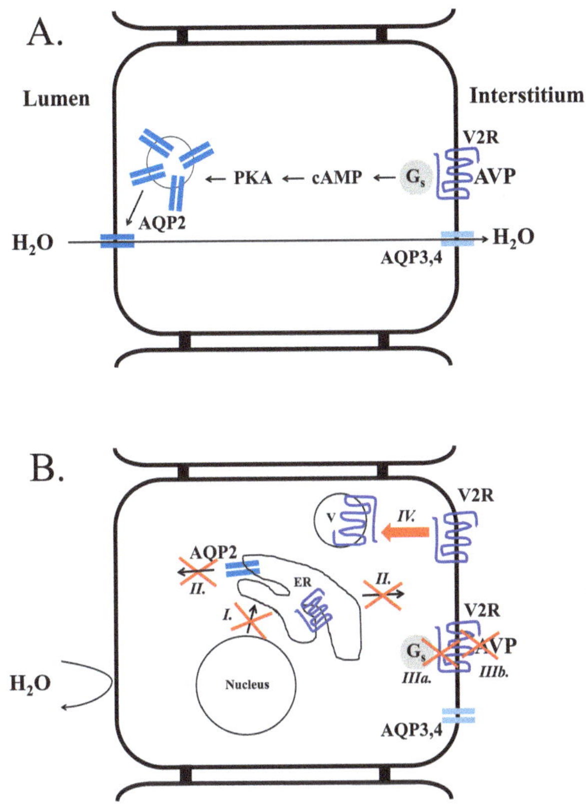

Fig. 15.1 Schematic illustration of AVP-induced AQP2 insertion into the apical surface of collecting duct principal cells (**a**) and the possible causes behind the development of NDI (**b**). Under normal circumstances (**a**), the AVP travels via the bloodstream to the kidneys where it binds to the basolaterally located V2R. This receptor is a G protein-coupled receptor and initiates cAMP signaling within the principal cells. The activation of PKA induces the vesicular trafficking of AQP2 containing endomembranes. Finally, the AQP2 is translocated into the apical surface making this water-permeable, and the water molecules are transported from the duct lumen to the kidney interstitium via the apically located AQP2 and the permanently located basolateral AQP3 and AQP4 water channels. (**b**) In cNDI, the impaired water transport is the consequence of mutations in the AVPR2 or AQP2 (labeled with roman numerals). Class ***I*** type of mutations can lead to impaired transcription, mRNA processing, or translation, class ***II*** mutations lead to endoplasmic reticulum (ER) retention, and class ***IIIa*** mutants display reduced G protein binding and/or G protein activation, whereas class ***IIIb*** mutations cause impaired ligand affinity, and class ***IV*** mutants display altered intracellular trafficking leading to receptor accumulation in intracellular vesicles

not on PKA activity (Umenishi et al. 2006; Kortenoeven et al. 2012). In addition to the abovementioned effects, the V2R normally contributes to the buildup of corticopapillary interstitial osmotic gradient as its function is required for the normal expression and function of urea transporters in the collecting duct and Na^+-K^+-$2Cl^-$ cotransporter in the thick ascending limb of the loop of Henle (Fenton and Knepper 2007). Moreover, the AVP increases sodium reabsorption in the collecting duct by increasing the activity of the amiloride-sensitive epithelial sodium channel (ENaC) (Bankir et al. 2005).

Several mutations have been identified causing congenital nephrogenic diabetes insipidus (cNDI) (Barak et al. 2001; Tao 2006; Wilbanks et al. 2002). cNDI is a rare disease and it is caused due to the mutations in either *AVPR2* or *AQP2* gene. Among the cNDI cases, approximately 90% of the patients are males with the X-linked recessive mutation in the *AVPR2* gene resulting in defective V2R in the kidney epithelial cells (Bichet 2009). The prevalence of this form (also called as type I cNDI or XNDI) is ~1 in 1,50,000 male births although mild forms of X-linked cNDI can be present in females as well. The *AVPR2* gene is located on chromosome region Xq28, which contains three exons and two introns, and shortly after its cloning, it was proposed that it could be responsible for congenital NDI (Seibold et al. 1993; Rosenthal et al. 1992; Birnbaumer et al. 1992). It was also demonstrated in early works that the patients with cNDI do not respond to desmopressin (dDAVP) treatment suggesting that the cAMP signaling is defective in these cases (Bichet et al. 1988, 1989).

As it was mentioned above, a few cNDI families were described in the literature, in which the female family members exhibit variable degrees, but usually mild symptoms of diabetes insipidus (Carroll et al. 2006; van Lieburg et al. 1999; Nomura et al. 1997). These heterozygous female individuals possess both normal and mutated *AVPR2* alleles. The studies on the skewed X-chromosome inactivation patterns of the female members suggested that the severity of symptoms were dependent on the rate of skewed methylation of X chromosome, and the NDI phenotype is caused by dominant methylation of the normal allele of *AVPR2* gene (Nomura et al. 1997; Arthus et al. 2000).

NDI caused by various mutations in V2R evolve their dysfunctions with different mechanisms (Arthus et al. 2000; Tao 2006). More than 260 mutations are described in the Human Gene Mutation Database (http://www.hgmd.cf.ac.uk/ac/gene.php?gene=AVPR2), and the majority of them are missense mutations (~61%), which act by different mechanisms (Spanakis et al. 2008). In addition, approximately 25% of the mutations are frameshift mutations due to nucleotide deletions or insertions, ~10% is nonsense mutations, and ~9% of the cases are large deletions, but infrequently complex rearrangements, splicing mutations, and in-frame deletions or insertions are also responsible for the X-linked NDI disorders (Bichet and Bockenhauer 2016). The V2R is composed by 371 amino acids that forms several domains, and mutations have been identified all over in the receptor, but most of the mutations are found in the transmembrane domains. The most frequent mutations are recurrent mutations, which have been identified in 35 ancestrally independent families, and mostly these occurred at potential mutational hot spots (a C-to-T or G-to-A nucleotide substitution occurred at a CpG dinucleotide) (Bichet and Bockenhauer 2016).

The mutations can also be classified by the nature of the impaired vasopressin receptor function. The classical classification of the mutations causing impaired V2R function is based on the pathophysiological and cellular consequences (Wesche et al. 2012). The AVP insensitivity can be the consequence of either decreased number of cell surface receptors or impaired receptor signal transduction (Fig. 15.1b). Class I mutations of the *AVPR2* gene can lead to impaired transcription, mRNA processing, or translation of the receptor resulting in truncated and usually rapidly degraded proteins. Taken together, the class I mutations prevent effective synthesis of the V2R. Class II mutations lead to the formation of misfolded full-length proteins, which are recognized by the quality control system of the endoplasmic reticulum (ER), resulting in defective intracellular trafficking of the V2R mutants, ER retention, and often degradation of the trapped receptors (Robben et al. 2006). In fact, the majority of *AVPR2* gene mutations are missense/nonsense mutations which result in class II mutant receptors. Class III mutants are another group of missense mutations, which reach the basolateral plasma membrane, but they display reduced G protein binding and/or G protein activation ability in response to AVP stimulation (class IIIa subtype), or their AVP binding is defective due to their impaired ligand affinity (class IIIb subtype), leading to inappropriate intracellular cAMP production and AQP2 trafficking. Class IV mutants have normal ligand binding, but their intracellular trafficking is altered causing impaired cAMP signal production mostly due to constitutive β-arrestin-dependent internalization even in the absence of ligands leading to decreased basolateral surface expression since the V2R accumulation in intracellular vesicles (Barak et al. 2001).

To complicate the picture further, the evaluation of the properties of a mutant V2R does not always lead to an unambiguous classification of the mutation. For example, the NDI causing R137H-V2R was classified as class IV mutation due to its constitutive β-arrestin-dependent internalization (Barak et al. 2001). Moreover, the R137H-V2R has also impaired G protein coupling (Rosenthal et al. 1993) and altered trafficking to the plasma membrane as well (Kocan et al. 2009). Interestingly, contrary to the symptoms of R137H, the R137C-V2R and R137L-V2R mutations lead to nephrogenic syndrome of inappropriate dieresis (NSIAD) due to the constitutive activity.

Gain-of-Function V2R Mutations Cause Nephrogenic Syndrome of Inappropriate Diuresis (NSIAD) (OMIM 300539)

Whereas the loss-of-function V2R mutations are responsible for the majority of the cNDI disorders, the gain-of-function mutations in the V2R lead to nephrogenic syndrome of inappropriate antidiuresis disease (NSIAD). This recently discovered syndrome may cause hyponatremia and especially in infants severe clinical symptoms such as convulsions. NSIAD is a very rare, X-linked disorder with monogenic inheritance, and to date, mutations of Phe229, Arg137, Ile130, and Leu312 have been identified as gain-of-function mutations in V2R (Carpentier et al. 2012; Erdelyi et al. 2015; Feldman et al. 2005; Tiulpakov et al. 2016). The clinical manifestation of NSIAD such as hyponatremia and reduced urinary dilution is undistinguishable from SIADH (syndrome of inappropriate ADH secretion), but very markedly the serum AVP level is low in NSIAD, whereas it is elevated in SIADH (Decaux et al. 2007). It was demonstrated that NSIAD causing gain-of-function mutation can lead to selective G protein activation and increased secondary messenger production in the cells.

The increased activity of V2R can be blocked by a V2R inverse agonist, such as tolvaptan, which could be a possible treatment option for patients with this type of V2R mutation (Erdelyi et al. 2015).

Congenital NDIs Due to Mutated AQP2 (OMIM 125800)

In the other main form of cNDI which corresponds approximately to ~10% of the inherited NDI cases, the patients suffer from autosomal mutation in the gene encoding the AQP2 water channel (Bichet 2009). The patients exhibit typical features of NDI similar to V2R loss-of-function mutation-caused symptoms, and the disorder is vasopressin resistant, but it is associated with nonfunctional water channels. This form of hereditary NDI is also called as type II form of cNDI, and the characteristic difference from the type I form is that the intracellular cAMP level increases in response to AVP stimulation (Zimmerman and Green 1975; Deen et al. 1994; Langley et al. 1991). The autosomal cNDI can be caused by heterozygous, homozygous, or compound heterozygous mutations in the *AQP2* gene, and both autosomal-recessive and autosomal-dominant modes of inheritance are described (Morello and Bichet 2001; van Lieburg et al. 1999; Deen et al. 1994). The chromosomal location of *AQP2* is 12q12-q13 and to date 61 mutations have been identified (http://www.hgmd.cf.ac.uk/ac/gene.php?gene=AQP2) (Bichet and Bockenhauer 2016). The majority of the mutations (48) are missense/nonsense mutations, but few splicing, small deletion, and insertion mutations are also presented in the databases. The consequences of *AQP2* gene mutations can be different depending on the nature of the mutation, but most commonly result in impaired vesicular transport of AQP2 water channels. Under such condition the AQP2 molecules are retained in the endosomes and not translocated into the apical (luminal) surface of the principal cells (Tamarappoo and Verkman 1998). As it was discussed in the case of the misfolded and misrouted V2R mutant proteins, theoretically, it is possible to intervene by the help of pharmacological chaperones which could facilitate the reverse of the intracellular retention of AQP2 mutant proteins. Most of the mutations are autosomal-recessive mutations leading to misfolding, ER retention, and degradation of the produced AQP2 mutants (Moeller et al. 2013; Wesche et al. 2012; Frick et al. 2014). Although the majority of the dominant mutations result in complete lack of functionality, some ER retention mutants, in which the misfolding is not severe, display reduced degradation and partial responsiveness to AVP stimulation (Canfield et al. 1997; Frick et al. 2014; Marr et al. 2001, 2002; Mulders et al. 1997). Interestingly, these dominant mutations cause less severe phenotype compared to patients with compound heterozygous or homozygous recessive mutations (Mulders et al. 1998; Bichet and Bockenhauer 2016). The dominant mutations affect the carboxyl terminus of AQP2, their folding is correct, and they are not retained in the ER, although due to the mutations, they are not able to cooperate fully with the wild type AQP2 molecules. It was demonstrated that such mutants form mixed tetramer complex with the wild type AQP2 but they are misrouted and retained in the Golgi compartment (Mulders et al. 1998; de Mattia et al. 2004; Kamsteeg et al. 1999).

"Complex" NDI

The *AVPR2* or *AQP2* gene mutation-caused symptoms are also called as "pure" NDI phenotypes since they display water loss but the electrolytes, including sodium, potassium, chloride, and calcium, are normally conserved (Bockenhauer and Bichet 2017). The "complex" NDI can be caused by mutant membrane proteins involved in sodium chloride reabsorption in the thick ascending limb of the loop of Henle leading to, not just loss of water, but also electrolyte loss. Such mutations can be found in the genes encoding the Na^{+}-K^{+}-$2Cl^{-}$ cotransporter, renal outer medullary potassium channel (ROMK), Barttin (Bartter syndrome, infantile, with sensorineural deafness), kidney-specific chloride channel ClC-Kb, and chloride channel Ka causing polyuria, polydipsia, and loss of sodium, chloride, calcium, magnesium, and potassium (Bockenhauer and Bichet 2017).

15.2.1.2 Acquired Forms of NDI

The majority of the NDI cases are acquired diseases caused by various factors, including complications of drug treatments, pathophysiological alterations such as electrolyte disturbances including hypokalemia and hypercalcemia, and diseases (sickle cell disease, sarcoidosis, amyloidosis, multiple myeloma, Sjogren's disease). Numerous data have been reported that NDI can be induced by various other drugs including lithium, demeclocycline, foscarnet, clozapine, cisplatin, or methoxyflurane (Bendz and Aurell 1999).

Consumption and uptake of trace amounts of lithium are essential for the normal brain, immune, and reproductive functions, and it is well known that lithium deficiency leads to serious health problems, including behavioral problems. Lithium treatment is still the most effective cure in bipolar disorders and has been used for decades despite the disadvantages such as renal side effects. Lithium-caused DI is a serious, well-studied side effect in the treatment of bipolar mood disorders leading to polyuria (and consequent dehydration, thirst, and polydipsia), elevated renal sodium excretion, and even chronic kidney disease (Nielsen et al. 2008). Lithium treatment induces vasopressin-resistant polyuria in 20–40% of the patients mostly due to the disruption of normal aquaporin function and increased sodium excretion as the result of epithelial sodium channel (ENaC) dysfunction in the kidney collecting ducts (Marples et al. 1995). The renal lithium handling is similar to that of sodium due to their similar size and charge. Lithium enters the distal tubule segments through the amiloride-sensitive ENaC in the distal tubule segments and leaves the cells via the Na^{+}/H^{+} exchanger (NHE1) to the interstitium. It is demonstrated that clinically relevant lithium concentrations reduced the mRNA transcription and protein expression of AQP2, which can be reversed by administration of amiloride; moreover, the lithium treatment disrupted the normal trafficking and distribution pattern of AQP2 (Kortenoeven et al. 2009; Li et al. 2006). In addition to the reduced AQP2 level in the apical surface, the transcellular water transport is greatly diminished due to the effect that lithium also decreases the expression of the basolaterally located AQP3 level in the collecting duct principal cells (Kwon et al. 2000). Chronic lithium treatment has been reported to inhibit the sodium transport through the amiloride-sensitive ENaC resulting in increased sodium excretion (Thomsen et al. 1999). Furthermore, it has been demonstrated that other sodium transport functions are also affected in response to lithium treatment. The thiazide-sensitive Na-Cl cotransporter (NCC) located in the distal convoluted tubule, the type 2 sodium-phosphate cotransporter (NaPi-2) located in the proximal tubule, and the electrogenic sodium bicarbonate cotransporter (NBC1) are downregulated during lithium treatment (Kwon et al. 2000). Lithium also reduces the water reabsorption ability by affecting the urea cycling that normally contributes to the buildup of corticopapillary interstitial osmotic gradient. It has been demonstrated that chronic lithium treatment induces decreased urea transporter abundance (Klein et al. 2002). Taken together, in addition to the dysfunctional AQP2, sodium wasting due to the impaired sodium cotransporter functions and the reduced urine concentrating ability due to the urea transporter deficiency also play important roles in the development of polyuria during chronic lithium treatment. The symptoms of the lithium-induced side effects can be alleviated by administration of thiazide and amiloride (Bedford et al. 2008a), angiotensin-converting enzyme inhibitors, AT1R angiotensin II receptor blockers, or spironolactone mineralocorticoid receptor blocker (Kwon et al. 2009).

Demeclocycline is a tetracycline derivative antibiotic. It has been demonstrated that chronic demeclocycline treatment has several side effects, including NDI (Singer and Rotenberg 1973). It was revealed that demeclocycline-induced NDI is the consequence of the decreased AQP2 expression and its cell surface abundance in response to the treatment (Kortenoeven et al. 2013). Interestingly, demeclocycline reduced the adenylate cyclase activity in kidney cells and its effect was independent on V2R signaling. Demeclocycline is not really used in the treatment of infections nowadays, but its renal side effects were utilized to alleviate the symptoms of syndrome of inappropriate antidiuretic hormone (SIADH). In SIADH, abnormally high levels of AVP are secreted by the pituitary tumors, which in turn results in excessive water reabsorption in the collecting ducts. The too high level of water retention causes volume expansion in the fluid compartments, whereas the osmolality of the extracellular and intracellular fluids becomes decreased compared with the normal levels. Moreover, the high level of AVP increases the Na^+ reabsorption through the NKCC cotransporter and epithelial sodium channel (ENaC) (Ecelbarger et al. 2001). The use of demeclocycline in SIADH is based on the fact that the drug reduces the AVP-evoked hyponatremia, although the development of V2 vasopressin receptor antagonists, the vaptans, supersedes its usage in the treatment of SIADH (Sherlock and Thompson 2010).

15.2.2 Treatment Possibilities for NDI

In contrary to central DI where desmopressin is widely and successfully used to cure the symptoms, the treatment of NDI patients is more difficult to achieve. In the past, several potential treatment possibilities of DI were described [reviewed recently by

Kalra et al. (2016)] such as the usage of carbamazepine (Rado 1976; Meinders et al. 1974), chlorpropamide (Wales and Fraser 1971), thiazide diuretics (Alon and Chan 1985; O'Doherty et al. 1962), amiloride (Bedford et al. 2008b; Kortenoeven et al. 2009), indapamide (Kocak et al. 1990), clofibrate (Moses et al. 1973), and indomethacin (Weinstock and Moses 1990). The treatment of cNDI was tuned during the years. The combination of amiloride and hydrochlorothiazide was found superior than the combination of hydrochlorothiazide and a prostaglandin synthase inhibitor (Alon and Chan 1985). The inhibitors of prostaglandin synthesis are also useful medicines to ameliorate the symptoms of cNDI, and among the tested inhibitors, indomethacin was much more effective than ibuprofen (Libber et al. 1986). In addition to these drugs, recent findings have suggested novel therapeutic possibilities.

The identification of the NDI-causing mutations and the determination of the altered properties and cellular consequences altered could help to define or suggest therapeutic strategies for the treatment of NDI patients. The potential therapeutic approaches deal with either bypassing the V2R signal transduction processes or improving AQP2 function. It is proposed and highly recommended to identify the potential genetic defect as soon as possible in case of the possibility of congenital NDI. Both *AVPR2* and *AQP2* genes can be sequenced with ease due to their relatively small size. The genetic testing of infants whose families may be associated with congenital NDI can be performed even in prenatal or perinatal periods from amniotic cells, chorionic villous samples, or cord blood (Bichet and Bockenhauer 2016). Since the inherited NDI is manifested immediately after birth, it is fundamental to correctly recognize the disorder, and especially in case of infants, it is essential to treat the affected individuals with abundant fluid intake in order to avoid the repeated episodes of dehydration since these episodes are probably responsible for the generation of mental and physical retardation.

Possible interventions include direct stimulation of cAMP signal generation in the principal cells, bypassing the necessity of vasopressin activation, and different strategies to rescue the impaired receptor function (Wesche et al. 2012). The most extensively investigated V2R mutants belong to the class II mutations, which cause ER retention. The ER has a quality control system that prevents misfolded proteins to reach their final subcellular destinations (Ellgaard and Helenius 2003). Pharmacological chaperons or pharmacochaperons are small, cell-permeable substances that improve the folding of misfolded mutated, otherwise functional proteins in the ER. As a result of pharmacochaperon action, the misfolded proteins can bypass the ER quality control system and become rescued from ER retention. This phenomenon proposed a therapeutic approach in which the chaperons can lead to increased plasma membrane expression of otherwise functional vasopressin receptor mutants. Numerous data have presented the usage of pharmacological chaperons to rescue dysfunctional V2R mutants. Pharmacological chaperones of the V2R can be antagonists (Bernier et al. 2004; Morello et al. 2000; Ranadive et al. 2009; Robben et al. 2007; Wuller et al. 2004) or agonists (Jean-Alphonse et al. 2009; Robben et al. 2009). The approach was also confirmed in clinical studies of X-linked NDI patients who suffer from ER retention V2R mutations. Administration of SR49059 V1a receptor nonpeptide antagonist significantly reduced the urine volume and water intake and increased the urine osmolarity suggesting that pharmacochaperons may offer a new therapeutic approach to the treatment of the NDI patients who suffer from ER retention V2R mutations (Bernier et al. 2006).

The altered mutant V2 receptor conformations can result in decreased potency of AVP and other ligands, such as dDAVP. Theoretically the potency of other agonists can be affected differently, and certain agonists may activate the mutant receptor despite the conformational change. Screening and testing drug libraries can yield ligands, which can work as personalized therapy in case of a certain mutation. In case of N321K-V2R mutation, which caused a conformation with altered agonist sensitivity, the mutant receptor can be stimulated and activated by dVDAVP proposing a therapeutic for patients with N321K mutation in the V2R (Erdelyi et al. 2014). Taken together, the promising experimental data suggest that personalized medicines can offer treatments for NDI patients with pathogenic mutations of V2R.

It is also promising that some interventions may bypass the V2R activation in order to generate cAMP signal for the PKA-mediated APQ2 translocation; thus, urinary concentration can be independent of V2R. In the collecting duct, locally produced autocrine and paracrine factors including bradykinin, ATP, adenosine, endothelin, nitric oxide, and prostaglandin E2 (PGE2) may also regulate the water permeability (Pearce et al. 2015; Sands and Layton 2014). It was demonstrated that PGE2 receptor EP4 activation promotes AQP2 translocation via cAMP signal and PKA activation; moreover, it also induces AQP2 expression in a cAMP response element-binding protein (CREB)-dependent manner (Gao et al. 2015). This finding suggests that EP4 receptor agonists are potential therapeutic drugs for the treatment of DI, irrespective of the type of the DI. It was also demonstrated that the agonist stimulation of (pro)renin receptor, which is also expressed in the collecting duct and is regulated by the PGE2 receptor EP4, induced AQP2 expression, whereas its inhibition partially prevented the decrease in urine volume and the increase in urine osmolality and AQP2 expression-induced water deprivation in in vivo animal studies (Wang et al. 2016). It was discovered recently that adenosine monophosphate kinase (AMPK) is capable to phosphorylate both AQP2 and urea transporter UT-A1 in rat inner medullary collecting ducts in response to metformin stimulation (Klein et al. 2016). The authors used metformin as AMPK activator, which is approved for the use in patients with type 2 diabetes mellitus and polycystic ovary syndrome. Metformin increased the apical membrane expression of AQP2, both osmotic water permeability and urea permeability in collecting ducts. Erlotinib, which is a receptor tyrosine kinase inhibitor selective for epidermal growth factor receptor (EGFR), is a medication in the treatment of some cancer including non-small cell lung cancer and pancreatic cancer. It was currently identified in a high-throughput chemical screening assay that erlotinib was effective to stimulate AQP2 translocation and reduced urine output by 45% in lithium-induced NDI model in a cAMP-independent manner (Cheung et al. 2016). Since animal studies suggest metformin and erlotinib as novel therapeutic options for NDI and given the fact that both are approved medications, it was suggested to initiate clinical trials to determine the benefits of these drugs in the treatment of various forms of diabetes insipidus (Bockenhauer and Bichet 2017; Bech et al. 2018). It was demonstrated that activation of cGMP-mediated signaling pathway could result in AQP2 translocation and administration of cGMP phosphodiesterase type 5 inhibitor sildenafil significantly increased the AQP2 insertion into the luminal membrane compartments. Sildenafil induced elevated intracellular cGMP levels and the plasma membrane accumulation of AQP2 was not dependent on V2R activation (Bouley et al. 2005). Another possibility to bypass the V2R-induced AQP2 translocation is the stimulation of β3 adrenergic receptor. The β3 adrenergic receptor is also expressed in the collecting duct, and it was demonstrated that its stimulation with the selective agonist BRL37344 induced cAMP signal and translocation of AQP2 in the principal cells and also increased the activity of Na^+-K^+-$2Cl^-$ cotransporter in the thick ascending limb of the loop of Henle. Taken together, administration of BRL37344 promoted a potent antidiuretic effect in AVPR2-deficient animals (Procino et al. 2016). Since the mirabegron, a β3 adrenergic receptor agonist, is already introduced in the clinical practice to treat overactive bladder, enticing the possibility to carry out clinical investigations to test the potential ameliorating effects of this drug in NDI patients (Cernecka et al. 2014; Chapple et al. 2014). Another possible therapeutic option can be the administration of simvastatin, a lipid-lowering medication, since it was recently demonstrated that it was able to reduce urine output and increase urine osmolality in hypercholesterolemic patients (Procino et al. 2016). A recent clinical study investigated the effects of sildenafil, metformin, and simvastatin on AVP-independent urine concentration in healthy volunteers, and only simvastatin had an effect on urine osmolality, although further studies are necessary to address the possible effects of these drugs in combination or in patients suffering from NDI (Bech et al. 2018).

15.3 Other Major Types of and Differential Diagnosis of Diabetes Insipidus

Early diagnosis and correct typing of the DI are critical, especially in infants and small children since the consecutive, repetitive dehydration episodes can lead to mental and physical retardation (Bichet 2009). The symptoms of untreated DI eventually may lead to death due to exsiccosis, electrolyte imbalances, hyperosmolality, and circulatory failure due to low blood volume. The clinical diagnosis of the DI is based on functional tests. The widely used tests are the water deprivation test and administration of the dDAVP (desmopressin) to distinguish between the various forms of DI (Di Iorgi et al. 2012).

DI can be inherited (less than 10% of the cases) or acquired (Fujiwara and Bichet 2005). The symptoms of DI can be the consequence of four fundamentally different reasons, which are used for the classification the various forms of DI (Fenske and Allolio 2012). In the clinical practice, it is essential to diagnose the type of syndrome for the proper treatment of the individual, especially in less severe forms of the symptoms (Robertson 1988).

The central (neurohypophyseal) DI (OMIM 125700) is due to the impaired AVP production or release from the central nervous system and can be acquired or congenital, and the syndromes are the consequence of deficient release of AVP from the neurohypophysis (Arima et al. 2016). Neurohypophyseal DI is discussed in detail in Chap. 14.

Gestational DI is a rare complication; the prevalence is approximately 1 per 30,000 pregnancies (Fenske and Allolio 2012). This form of DI is the consequence of the rapid elimination (metabolism) of the circulating AVP by the placental vasopressinase, also called placental cysteine aminopeptidase, secreted by the trophoblasts. In rare occasions, the disorder can be due to exaggeration of pre-existing mild forms of neurohypophyseal or nephrogenic DI. The symptoms usually manifest themselves in the third trimester of pregnancy, especially if carrying multiple fetuses (Ichaliotis and Lambrinopoulos 1965). The rapid elimination of the circulating AVP causes transient DI and usually can be treated by the administration of desmopressin, which is resistant to vasopressinase cleavage (Ananthakrishnan 2016). The transient GDI is usually resolved after delivery (within few weeks), although in subsequent pregnancies can cause even severe symptoms (Kalelioglu et al. 2007).

The most common dypsogenic or psychogenic DI can be caused by primary polydipsia, which is excessive water intake due to impaired thirst perception (dypsogenic DI) or psychological function (psychogenic DI). Primary polydipsia can be induced by either defective thirst sensation or perception and frequently is associated with schizophrenia, anxiety disorder, and depression, although an increasing number of cases demonstrate primary polydipsia in non-psychiatric patients sometimes induced by drugs causing sensation of dry mouth (Sailer et al. 2017).

15.4 Genetic Counseling

Early detection and providing abundant water supply or treatment for DI patients are essential to allow normal mental and physical development and normal lifespan (Bichet and Bockenhauer 2016). In case of infants and small children, it is highly recommended to sequence their DNAs to obtain correct genetic diagnosis, if hypernatremic dehydration episodes occur (Bockenhauer and Bichet 2017). Since both *AVPR2* and *AQP2* are small genes, their sequence can be easily sequenced, allowing not just perinatal and prenatal testing but the genetic testing of the carriers as well (Bichet and Bockenhauer 2016).

15.5 Conclusion

Diabetes insipidus is a rare disorder with diversity of backgrounds in which impairments affect either the V2 vasopressin receptor or the AQP2 water channel functions. It is essential to keep the patients in water balance either by the treatment of the disease or by providing a necessary amount of fluid intake. It is also pivotal to identify the nature of the disorder as early as possible to reveal the cause behind the disorder and to treat the patient appropriately. Although numerous potential new treatment possibilities have been proposed currently, more translational research is necessary to offer personalized medicine for the patients who suffer from distinct mutations leading to congenital forms of NDI.

Acknowledgments This work was supported by the Hungarian National Research, Development and Innovation Fund (NKFI K116954 and NVKP_16-1-2016-0039).

References

Alon U, Chan JC (1985) Hydrochlorothiazide-amiloride in the treatment of congenital nephrogenic diabetes insipidus. Am J Nephrol 5(1):9–13. https://doi.org/10.1159/000166896

Amberger JS, Hamosh A (2017) Searching online mendelian inheritance in man (OMIM): a knowledgebase of human genes and genetic phenotypes. Curr Protoc Bioinformatics 58:1 2 1–1 2 12. https://doi.org/10.1002/cpbi.27

Ananthakrishnan S (2016) Diabetes insipidus during pregnancy. Best Pract Res Clin Endocrinol Metab 30(2):305–315. https://doi.org/10.1016/j.beem.2016.02.005

Arima H, Azuma Y, Morishita Y, Hagiwara D (2016) Central diabetes insipidus. Nagoya J Med Sci 78(4):349–358. https://doi.org/10.18999/nagjms.78.4.349

Arthus MF, Lonergan M, Crumley MJ et al (2000) Report of 33 novel AVPR2 mutations and analysis of 117 families with X-linked nephrogenic diabetes insipidus. J Am Soc Nephrol 11(6):1044–1054

Bankir L, Fernandes S, Bardoux P, Bouby N, Bichet DG (2005) Vasopressin-V2 receptor stimulation reduces sodium excretion in healthy humans. J Am Soc Nephrol 16(7):1920–1928. https://doi.org/10.1681/ASN.2004121079

Barak LS, Oakley RH, Laporte SA, Caron MG (2001) Constitutive arrestin-mediated desensitization of a human vasopressin receptor mutant associated with nephrogenic diabetes insipidus. Proc Natl Acad Sci U S A 98(1):93–98. https://doi.org/10.1073/pnas.011303698

Bech AP, Wetzels JFM, Nijenhuis T (2018) Effects of sildenafil, metformin, and simvastatin on ADH-independent urine concentration in healthy volunteers. Physiol Rep 6(7):e13665. https://doi.org/10.14814/phy2.13665

Bedford JJ, Leader JP, Jing R, Walker LJ, Klein JD, Sands JM, Walker RJ (2008a) Amiloride restores renal medullary osmolytes in lithium-induced nephrogenic diabetes insipidus. Am J Physiol Renal Physiol 294(4):F812–F820. https://doi.org/10.1152/ajprenal.00554.2007

Bedford JJ, Weggery S, Ellis G, McDonald FJ, Joyce PR, Leader JP, Walker RJ (2008b) Lithium-induced nephrogenic diabetes insipidus: renal effects of amiloride. Clin J Am Soc Nephrol 3(5):1324–1331. https://doi.org/10.2215/CJN.01640408

Bendz H, Aurell M (1999) Drug-induced diabetes insipidus: incidence, prevention and management. Drug Saf 21(6):449–456. https://doi.org/10.2165/00002018-199921060-00002

Bernier V, Lagace M, Lonergan M, Arthus MF, Bichet DG, Bouvier M (2004) Functional rescue of the constitutively internalized V2 vasopressin receptor mutant R137H by the pharmacological chaperone action of SR49059. Mol Endocrinol 18(8):2074–2084. https://doi.org/10.1210/me.2004-0080

Bernier V, Morello JP, Zarruk A et al (2006) Pharmacologic chaperones as a potential treatment for X-linked nephrogenic diabetes insipidus. J Am Soc Nephrol 17(1):232–243. https://doi.org/10.1681/ASN.2005080854

Bichet DG (2009) V2R mutations and nephrogenic diabetes insipidus. Prog Mol Biol Transl Sci 89:15–29. https://doi.org/10.1016/S1877-1173(09)89002-9
Bichet DG, Bockenhauer D (2016) Genetic forms of nephrogenic diabetes insipidus (NDI): vasopressin receptor defect (X-linked) and aquaporin defect (autosomal recessive and dominant). Best Pract Res Clin Endocrinol Metab 30(2):263–276. https://doi.org/10.1016/j.beem.2016.02.010
Bichet DG, Razi M, Lonergan M, Arthus MF, Papukna V, Kortas C, Barjon JN (1988) Hemodynamic and coagulation responses to 1-desamino[8-D-arginine] vasopressin in patients with congenital nephrogenic diabetes insipidus. New Engl J Med 318(14):881–887. https://doi.org/10.1056/NEJM198804073181403
Bichet DG, Razi M, Arthus MF et al (1989) Epinephrine and dDAVP administration in patients with congenital nephrogenic diabetes insipidus. Evidence for a pre-cyclic AMP V2 receptor defective mechanism. Kidney Int 36(5):859–866
Birnbaumer M, Seibold A, Gilbert S et al (1992) Molecular cloning of the receptor for human antidiuretic hormone. Nature 357(6376):333–335. https://doi.org/10.1038/357333a0
Bockenhauer D, Bichet DG (2013) Inherited secondary nephrogenic diabetes insipidus: concentrating on humans. Am J Physiol Renal Physiol 304(8):F1037–F1042. https://doi.org/10.1152/ajprenal.00639.2012
Bockenhauer D, Bichet DG (2017) Nephrogenic diabetes insipidus. Curr Opin Pediatr 29(2):199–205. https://doi.org/10.1097/MOP.0000000000000473
Bouley R, Pastor-Soler N, Cohen O et al (2005) Stimulation of AQP2 membrane insertion in renal epithelial cells in vitro and in vivo by the cGMP phosphodiesterase inhibitor sildenafil citrate (Viagra). Am J Physiol Renal Physiol 288(6):F1103–F1112. https://doi.org/10.1152/ajprenal.00337.2004
Boyd SD, Raz S, Ehrlich RM (1980) Diabetes insipidus and nonobstructive dilation of urinary tract. Urology 16(3):266–269
Canfield MC, Tamarappoo BK, Moses AM, Verkman AS, Holtzman EJ (1997) Identification and characterization of aquaporin-2 water channel mutations causing nephrogenic diabetes insipidus with partial vasopressin response. Hum Mol Genet 6(11):1865–1871
Carpentier E, Greenbaum LA, Rochdi D et al (2012) Identification and characterization of an activating F229V substitution in the V2 vasopressin receptor in an infant with NSIAD. J Am Soc Nephrol 23(10):1635–1640. https://doi.org/10.1681/ASN.2012010077
Carroll P, Al-Mojalli H, Al-Abbad A et al (2006) Novel mutations underlying nephrogenic diabetes insipidus in Arab families. Genet Med 8(7):443–447
Cernecka H, Sand C, Michel MC (2014) The odd sibling: features of beta3-adrenoceptor pharmacology. Mol Pharmacol 86(5):479–484. https://doi.org/10.1124/mol.114.092817
Chapple CR, Cardozo L, Nitti VW, Siddiqui E, Michel MC (2014) Mirabegron in overactive bladder: a review of efficacy, safety, and tolerability. Neurourol Urodyn 33(1):17–30. https://doi.org/10.1002/nau.22505
Cheung PW, Nomura N, Nair AV et al (2016) EGF receptor inhibition by erlotinib increases aquaporin 2-mediated renal water reabsorption. J Am Soc Nephrol 27(10):3105–3116. https://doi.org/10.1681/ASN.2015080903
Czaczkes JW, Kleeman CR, Koenig M (1964) Physiologic studies of antidiuretic hormone by its direct measurement in human plasma. J Clin Invest 43:1625–1640. https://doi.org/10.1172/JCI105038
de Mattia F, Savelkoul PJ, Bichet DG et al (2004) A novel mechanism in recessive nephrogenic diabetes insipidus: wild-type aquaporin-2 rescues the apical membrane expression of intracellularly retained AQP2-P262L. Hum Mol Genet 13(24):3045–3056. https://doi.org/10.1093/hmg/ddh339
Decaux G, Vandergheynst F, Bouko Y, Parma J, Vassart G, Vilain C (2007) Nephrogenic syndrome of inappropriate antidiuresis in adults: high phenotypic variability in men and women from a large pedigree. J Am Soc Nephrol 18(2):606–612. https://doi.org/10.1681/ASN.2006090987
Deen PM, Verdijk MA, Knoers NV, Wieringa B, Monnens LA, van Os CH, van Oost BA (1994) Requirement of human renal water channel aquaporin-2 for vasopressin-dependent concentration of urine. Science 264(5155):92–95

Di Iorgi N, Napoli F, Allegri AE et al (2012) Diabetes insipidus–diagnosis and management. Horm Res Paediatr 77(2):69–84. https://doi.org/10.1159/000336333

DiGiovanni SR, Nielsen S, Christensen EI, Knepper MA (1994) Regulation of collecting duct water channel expression by vasopressin in Brattleboro rat. Proc Natl Acad Sci U S A 91 (19):8984–8988

Ecelbarger CA, Kim GH, Wade JB, Knepper MA (2001) Regulation of the abundance of renal sodium transporters and channels by vasopressin. Exp Neurol 171(2):227–234. https://doi.org/10.1006/exnr.2001.7775

Ellgaard L, Helenius A (2003) Quality control in the endoplasmic reticulum. Nat Rev Mol Cell Biol 4(3):181–191. https://doi.org/10.1038/nrm1052

Erdelyi LS, Balla A, Patocs A, Toth M, Varnai P, Hunyady L (2014) Altered agonist sensitivity of a mutant v2 receptor suggests a novel therapeutic strategy for nephrogenic diabetes insipidus. Mol Endocrinol 28(5):634–643. https://doi.org/10.1210/me.2013-1424

Erdelyi LS, Mann WA, Morris-Rosendahl DJ et al (2015) Mutation in the V2 vasopressin receptor gene, AVPR2, causes nephrogenic syndrome of inappropriate diuresis. Kidney Int 88(5):1070–1078. https://doi.org/10.1038/ki.2015.181

Feldman BJ, Rosenthal SM, Vargas GA et al (2005) Nephrogenic syndrome of inappropriate antidiuresis. New Engl J Med 352(18):1884–1890. https://doi.org/10.1056/NEJMoa042743

Fenske W, Allolio B (2012) Clinical review: current state and future perspectives in the diagnosis of diabetes insipidus: a clinical review. J Clin Endocrinol Metab 97(10):3426–3437. https://doi.org/10.1210/jc.2012-1981

Fenton RA, Knepper MA (2007) Mouse models and the urinary concentrating mechanism in the new millennium. Physiol Rev 87(4):1083–1112. https://doi.org/10.1152/physrev.00053.2006

Fliers E, Swaab DF, Pool CW, Verwer RW (1985) The vasopressin and oxytocin neurons in the human supraoptic and paraventricular nucleus; changes with aging and in senile dementia. Brain Res 342(1):45–53

Frick A, Eriksson UK, de Mattia F et al (2014) X-ray structure of human aquaporin 2 and its implications for nephrogenic diabetes insipidus and trafficking. Proc Natl Acad Sci U S A 111(17):6305–6310. https://doi.org/10.1073/pnas.1321406111

Fujiwara TM, Bichet DG (2005) Molecular biology of hereditary diabetes insipidus. J Am Soc Nephrol 16(10):2836–2846. https://doi.org/10.1681/ASN.2005040371

Gao M, Cao R, Du S et al (2015) Disruption of prostaglandin E2 receptor EP4 impairs urinary concentration via decreasing aquaporin 2 in renal collecting ducts. Proc Natl Acad Sci U S A 112(27):8397–8402. https://doi.org/10.1073/pnas.1509565112

Ichaliotis SD, Lambrinopoulos TC (1965) Serum oxytocinase in twin pregnancy. Obstet Gynecol 25:270–272

Jean-Alphonse F, Perkovska S, Frantz MC et al (2009) Biased agonist pharmacochaperones of the AVP V2 receptor may treat congenital nephrogenic diabetes insipidus. J Am Soc Nephrol 20 (10):2190–2203. https://doi.org/10.1681/ASN.2008121289

Kalelioglu I, Kubat Uzum A, Yildirim A, Ozkan T, Gungor F, Has R (2007) Transient gestational diabetes insipidus diagnosed in successive pregnancies: review of pathophysiology, diagnosis, treatment, and management of delivery. Pituitary 10(1):87–93. https://doi.org/10.1007/s11102-007-0006-1

Kalra S, Zargar AH, Jain SM et al (2016) Diabetes insipidus: the other diabetes. Indian J Endocrinol Metab 20(1):9–21. https://doi.org/10.4103/2230-8210.172273

Kamsteeg EJ, Wormhoudt TA, Rijss JP, van Os CH, Deen PM (1999) An impaired routing of wild-type aquaporin-2 after tetramerization with an aquaporin-2 mutant explains dominant nephrogenic diabetes insipidus. EMBO J 18(9):2394–2400. https://doi.org/10.1093/emboj/18.9.2394

Kamsteeg EJ, Hendriks G, Boone M, Konings IB, Oorschot V, van der Sluijs P, Klumperman J, Deen PM (2006) Short-chain ubiquitination mediates the regulated endocytosis of the aquaporin-2 water channel. Proc Natl Acad Sci U S A 103(48):18344–18349. https://doi.org/10.1073/pnas.0604073103

Klein JD, Gunn RB, Roberts BR, Sands JM (2002) Down-regulation of urea transporters in the renal inner medulla of lithium-fed rats. Kidney Int 61(3):995–1002. https://doi.org/10.1046/j.1523-1755.2002.00210.x

Klein JD, Wang Y, Blount MA, Molina PA, LaRocque LM, Ruiz JA, Sands JM (2016) Metformin, an AMPK activator, stimulates the phosphorylation of aquaporin 2 and urea transporter A1 in inner medullary collecting ducts. Am J Physiol Renal Physiol 310(10):F1008–F1012. https://doi.org/10.1152/ajprenal.00102.2016

Kocak M, Karademir BM, Tetiker T (1990) Antidiuretic effect of indapamide in central diabetes insipidus. Acta Endocrinol (Copenh) 123(6):657–660

Kocan M, See HB, Sampaio NG, Eidne KA, Feldman BJ, Pfleger KD (2009) Agonist-independent interactions between beta-arrestins and mutant vasopressin type II receptors associated with nephrogenic syndrome of inappropriate antidiuresis. Mol Endocrinol 23(4):559–571. https://doi.org/10.1210/me.2008-0321

Kortenoeven ML, Li Y, Shaw S, Gaeggeler HP, Rossier BC, Wetzels JF, Deen PM (2009) Amiloride blocks lithium entry through the sodium channel thereby attenuating the resultant nephrogenic diabetes insipidus. Kidney Int 76(1):44–53. https://doi.org/10.1038/ki.2009.91

Kortenoeven ML, Trimpert C, van den Brand M, Li Y, Wetzels JF, Deen PM (2012) In mpkCCD cells, long-term regulation of aquaporin-2 by vasopressin occurs independent of protein kinase A and CREB but may involve Epac. Am J Physiol Renal Physiol 302(11):F1395–F1401. https://doi.org/10.1152/ajprenal.00376.2011

Kortenoeven ML, Sinke AP, Hadrup N, Trimpert C, Wetzels JF, Fenton RA, Deen PM (2013) Demeclocycline attenuates hyponatremia by reducing aquaporin-2 expression in the renal inner medulla. Am J Physiol Renal Physiol 305(12):F1705–F1718. https://doi.org/10.1152/ajprenal.00723.2012

Kwon TH, Laursen UH, Marples D, Maunsbach AB, Knepper MA, Frokiaer J, Nielsen S (2000) Altered expression of renal AQPs and Na(+) transporters in rats with lithium-induced NDI. Am J Physiol Renal Physiol 279(3):F552–F564. https://doi.org/10.1152/ajprenal.2000.279.3.F552

Kwon TH, Nielsen J, Moller HB, Fenton RA, Nielsen S, Frokiaer J (2009) Aquaporins in the kidney. Handb Exp Pharmacol 190:95–132. https://doi.org/10.1007/978-3-540-79885-9_5

Langley JM, Balfe JW, Selander T, Ray PN, Clarke JT (1991) Autosomal recessive inheritance of vasopressin-resistant diabetes insipidus. Am J Med Genet 38(1):90–94. https://doi.org/10.1002/ajmg.1320380120

Li Y, Shaw S, Kamsteeg EJ, Vandewalle A, Deen PM (2006) Development of lithium-induced nephrogenic diabetes insipidus is dissociated from adenylyl cyclase activity. J Am Soc Nephrol 17(4):1063–1072. https://doi.org/10.1681/ASN.2005080884

Libber S, Harrison H, Spector D (1986) Treatment of nephrogenic diabetes insipidus with prostaglandin synthesis inhibitors. J Pediatr 108(2):305–311

Marples D, Christensen S, Christensen EI, Ottosen PD, Nielsen S (1995) Lithium-induced downregulation of aquaporin-2 water channel expression in rat kidney medulla. J Clin Invest 95(4):1838–1845. https://doi.org/10.1172/JCI117863

Marr N, Kamsteeg EJ, van Raak M, van Os CH, Deen PM (2001) Functionality of aquaporin-2 missense mutants in recessive nephrogenic diabetes insipidus. Pflugers Arch 442(1):73–77. https://doi.org/10.1007/s004240000498

Marr N, Bichet DG, Hoefs S et al (2002) Cell-biologic and functional analyses of five new Aquaporin-2 missense mutations that cause recessive nephrogenic diabetes insipidus. J Am Soc Nephrol 13(9):2267–2277

Meinders AE, Cejka V, Robertson GL (1974) The antidiuretic action of carbamazepine in man. Clin Sci Mol Med 47(4):289–299

Moeller HB, Rittig S, Fenton RA (2013) Nephrogenic diabetes insipidus: essential insights into the molecular background and potential therapies for treatment. Endocr Rev 34(2):278–301. https://doi.org/10.1210/er.2012-1044

Morello JP, Bichet DG (2001) Nephrogenic diabetes insipidus. Annu Rev Physiol 63:607–630. https://doi.org/10.1146/annurev.physiol.63.1.607

Morello JP, Salahpour A, Laperriere A et al (2000) Pharmacological chaperones rescue cell-surface expression and function of misfolded V2 vasopressin receptor mutants. J Clin Invest 105(7):887–895. https://doi.org/10.1172/JCI8688
Moses AM, Howanitz J, van Gemert M, Miller M (1973) Clofibrate-induced antidiuresis. J Clin Invest 52(3):535–542. https://doi.org/10.1172/JCI107213
Mulders SM, Knoers NV, Van Lieburg AF et al (1997) New mutations in the AQP2 gene in nephrogenic diabetes insipidus resulting in functional but misrouted water channels. J Am Soc Nephrol 8(2):242–248
Mulders SM, Bichet DG, Rijss JP et al (1998) An aquaporin-2 water channel mutant which causes autosomal dominant nephrogenic diabetes insipidus is retained in the Golgi complex. J Clin Invest 102(1):57–66. https://doi.org/10.1172/JCI2605
Nielsen S, Frokiaer J, Marples D, Kwon TH, Agre P, Knepper MA (2002) Aquaporins in the kidney: from molecules to medicine. Physiol Rev 82(1):205–244. https://doi.org/10.1152/physrev.00024.2001
Nielsen J, Kwon TH, Christensen BM, Frokiaer J, Nielsen S (2008) Dysregulation of renal aquaporins and epithelial sodium channel in lithium-induced nephrogenic diabetes insipidus. Semin Nephrol 28(3):227–244. https://doi.org/10.1016/j.semnephrol.2008.03.002
Nomura Y, Onigata K, Nagashima T, Yutani S, Mochizuki H, Nagashima K, Morikawa A (1997) Detection of skewed X-inactivation in two female carriers of vasopressin type 2 receptor gene mutation. J Clin Endocrinol Metab 82(10):3434–3437. https://doi.org/10.1210/jcem.82.10.4312
O'Doherty NJ, Rosser J, Slater RJ (1962) Diabetes insipidus: the influence of chlorothiazide therapy in affected children. Can Med Assoc J 86:559–567
Pearce D, Soundararajan R, Trimpert C, Kashlan OB, Deen PM, Kohan DE (2015) Collecting duct principal cell transport processes and their regulation. Clin J Am Soc Nephrol 10(1):135–146. https://doi.org/10.2215/CJN.05760513
Procino G, Carmosino M, Milano S et al (2016) beta3 adrenergic receptor in the kidney may be a new player in sympathetic regulation of renal function. Kidney Int 90(3):555–567. https://doi.org/10.1016/j.kint.2016.03.020
Rado JP (1976) Decreased antidiuretic response in diabetes insipidus during prolonged treatment with carbamazepine presumably due to enzym-induction. Endokrinologie 67(3):322–330
Ranadive SA, Ersoy B, Favre H, Cheung CC, Rosenthal SM, Miller WL, Vaisse C (2009) Identification, characterization and rescue of a novel vasopressin-2 receptor mutation causing nephrogenic diabetes insipidus. Clin Endocrinol 71(3):388–393. https://doi.org/10.1111/j.1365-2265.2008.03513.x
Robben JH, Knoers NV, Deen PM (2006) Cell biological aspects of the vasopressin type-2 receptor and aquaporin 2 water channel in nephrogenic diabetes insipidus. Am J Physiol Renal Physiol 291(2):F257–F270. https://doi.org/10.1152/ajprenal.00491.2005
Robben JH, Sze M, Knoers NV, Deen PM (2007) Functional rescue of vasopressin V2 receptor mutants in MDCK cells by pharmacochaperones: relevance to therapy of nephrogenic diabetes insipidus. Am J Physiol Renal Physiol 292(1):F253–F260. https://doi.org/10.1152/ajprenal.00247.2006
Robben JH, Kortenoeven ML, Sze M et al (2009) Intracellular activation of vasopressin V2 receptor mutants in nephrogenic diabetes insipidus by nonpeptide agonists. Proc Natl Acad Sci U S A 106(29):12195–12200. https://doi.org/10.1073/pnas.0900130106
Robertson GL (1988) Differential diagnosis of polyuria. Annu Rev Med 39:425–442. https://doi.org/10.1146/annurev.me.39.020188.002233
Robertson GL (1995) Diabetes insipidus. Endocrinol Metab Clin N Am 24(3):549–572
Robertson GL (2001) Antidiuretic hormone. Normal and disordered function. Endocrinol Metab Clin N Am 30(3):671–694, vii
Rosenthal W, Seibold A, Antaramian A et al (1992) Molecular identification of the gene responsible for congenital nephrogenic diabetes insipidus. Nature 359(6392):233–235. https://doi.org/10.1038/359233a0
Rosenthal W, Antaramian A, Gilbert S, Birnbaumer M (1993) Nephrogenic diabetes insipidus. A V2 vasopressin receptor unable to stimulate adenylyl cyclase. J Biol Chem 268(18):13030–13033

Sailer C, Winzeler B, Christ-Crain M (2017) Primary polydipsia in the medical and psychiatric patient: characteristics, complications and therapy. Swiss Med Wkly 147:w14514. https://doi.org/10.4414/smw.2017.14514
Saito Y (2010) Roles of atrial natriuretic peptide and its therapeutic use. J Cardiol 56(3):262–270. https://doi.org/10.1016/j.jjcc.2010.08.001
Sands JM, Layton HE (2014) Advances in understanding the urine-concentrating mechanism. Annu Rev Physiol 76:387–409. https://doi.org/10.1146/annurev-physiol-021113-170350
Schoneberg T, Schulz A, Biebermann H, Hermsdorf T, Rompler H, Sangkuhl K (2004) Mutant G-protein-coupled receptors as a cause of human diseases. Pharmacol Ther 104(3):173–206. https://doi.org/10.1016/j.pharmthera.2004.08.008
Seibold A, Rosenthal W, Bichet DG, Birnbaumer M (1993) The vasopressin type 2 receptor gene. Chromosomal localization and its role in nephrogenic diabetes insipidus. Regul Pept 45(1–2):67–71
Shalev H, Romanovsky I, Knoers NV, Lupa S, Landau D (2004) Bladder function impairment in aquaporin-2 defective nephrogenic diabetes insipidus. Nephrol Dial Transplant 19(3):608–613
Sherlock M, Thompson CJ (2010) The syndrome of inappropriate antidiuretic hormone: current and future management options. Eur J Endocrinol 162(Suppl 1):S13–S18. https://doi.org/10.1530/EJE-09-1057
Singer I, Rotenberg D (1973) Demeclocycline-induced nephrogenic diabetes insipidus. In-vivo and in-vitro studies. Ann Intern Med 79(5):679–683
Sklar AH, Schrier RW (1983) Central nervous system mediators of vasopressin release. Physiol Rev 63(4):1243–1280. https://doi.org/10.1152/physrev.1983.63.4.1243
Spanakis E, Milord E, Gragnoli C (2008) AVPR2 variants and mutations in nephrogenic diabetes insipidus: review and missense mutation significance. J Cell Physiol 217(3):605–617. https://doi.org/10.1002/jcp.21552
Tamarappoo BK, Verkman AS (1998) Defective aquaporin-2 trafficking in nephrogenic diabetes insipidus and correction by chemical chaperones. J Clin Invest 101(10):2257–2267. https://doi.org/10.1172/JCI2303
Tao YX (2006) Inactivating mutations of G protein-coupled receptors and diseases: structure-function insights and therapeutic implications. Pharm Ther 111(3):949–973. https://doi.org/10.1016/j.pharmthera.2006.02.008
Thomsen K, Bak M, Shirley DG (1999) Chronic lithium treatment inhibits amiloride-sensitive sodium transport in the rat distal nephron. J Pharmacol Exp Ther 289(1):443–447
Tiulpakov A, White CW, Abhayawardana RS et al (2016) Mutations of vasopressin receptor 2 including novel L312S have differential effects on trafficking. Mol Endocrinol 30(8):889–904. https://doi.org/10.1210/me.2016-1002
Umenishi F, Narikiyo T, Vandewalle A, Schrier RW (2006) cAMP regulates vasopressin-induced AQP2 expression via protein kinase A-independent pathway. Biochim Biophys Acta 1758(8):1100–1105. https://doi.org/10.1016/j.bbamem.2006.06.001
van Lieburg AF, Knoers NV, Monnens LA (1999) Clinical presentation and follow-up of 30 patients with congenital nephrogenic diabetes insipidus. J Am Soc Nephrol 10(9):1958–1964
Wales JK, Fraser TR (1971) The clinical use of chlorpropamide in diabetes insipidus. Acta Endocrinol (Copeng) 68(4):725–736
Wang F, Lu X, Peng K et al (2016) Antidiuretic action of collecting duct (pro)renin receptor downstream of vasopressin and PGE2 receptor EP4. J Am Soc Nephrol 27(10):3022–3034. https://doi.org/10.1681/ASN.2015050592
Weinstock RS, Moses AM (1990) Desmopressin and indomethacin therapy for nephrogenic diabetes insipidus in patients receiving lithium carbonate. South Med J 83(12):1475–1477
Wesche D, Deen PM, Knoers NV (2012) Congenital nephrogenic diabetes insipidus: the current state of affairs. Pediatr Nephrol 27(12):2183–2204. https://doi.org/10.1007/s00467-012-2118-8
Wilbanks AM, Laporte SA, Bohn LM, Barak LS, Caron MG (2002) Apparent loss-of-function mutant GPCRs revealed as constitutively desensitized receptors. Biochemistry 41(40):11981–11989

Wuller S, Wiesner B, Loffler A et al (2004) Pharmacochaperones post-translationally enhance cell surface expression by increasing conformational stability of wild-type and mutant vasopressin V2 receptors. J Biol Chem 279(45):47254–47263. https://doi.org/10.1074/jbc.M408154200

Zimmerman D, Green OC (1975) Nephrogenic diabetes-insipidus - type-II- defect distal to adenylate cyclase step. Pediatr Res 9(4):381–381

Chapter 16
Monogenic Forms of Male Infertility

Csilla Krausz and Antoni Riera-Escamilla

Abstract Male infertility is a multifactorial and heterogeneous pathological condition affecting 7% of the general male population. The genetic landscape of male infertility is highly complex as semen and testis histological phenotypes are extremely heterogeneous, and at least 2000 genes are predicted to be involved in spermatogenesis. Genetic factors have been described in each etiological category of male reproductive impairment: (1) hypothalamic–pituitary axis dysfunction; (2) quantitative and qualitative alterations of spermatogenesis; (3) ductal obstruction/dysfunction. In 25% of azoospermic and in 10% of oligozoospermic men, a genetic anomaly can be diagnosed with the current genetic testing. However, up to now, only a relatively low number of monogenic factors have a clear-cut cause–effect relationship with impaired reproductive function. Thanks to the widespread diffusion of Next-Generation Sequencing, a continuously increasing number of monogenic causes of male infertility are being discovered and their validation is currently ongoing. The identification of genetic factors is of outmost clinical importance since there is a risk of transmission of genetic defects through natural or assisted reproductive techniques. The benefit of the genetic diagnosis of infertility has an obvious clinical significance for the patient itself with implications not only for his reproductive health but in many instances also for his general health.

Keywords Male infertility · Spermatogenesis · Genetics · Gene · Hypogonadism · Azoospermia · Oligozoospermia · Teratozoospermia · NGS · Exome

---

C. Krausz (✉)
Department of Experimental and Clinical Biomedical Sciences "Mario Serio", University of Florence, Florence, Italy
e-mail: csilla.krausz@unifi.it

A. Riera-Escamilla
Andrology Department, Fundació Puigvert, Instituto de Investigaciones Biomédicas Sant Pau (IIB-Sant Pau), Universitat Autònoma de Barcelona, Barcelona, Catalonia, Spain

P. Igaz, A. Patócs (eds.), *Genetics of Endocrine Diseases and Syndromes*,
Experientia Supplementum 111, https://doi.org/10.1007/978-3-030-25905-1_16

List of Abbreviations

AIS	Androgen Insensitivity Syndrome
AOA	Artificial oocyte activation
ART	Assisted reproductive techniques
AZF	Azoospermia factor
CAIS	Complete Androgen Insensitivity
CAVD	Congentinal Absence of Vas Deferens
CBAVD	Congentinal Bilateral Absence of Vas Deferens
CFAP	Cilia and Flagella Associated Protein family
CHARGE	Coloboma, Heart defects, Atresia of choanae, Retardation of growth and/or development, Genital and/or urinary defects, Ear anomalies or deafness
CHH	Congenital hypogonadotropic hypogonadism
CPC	Chromosomal passenger complex
CPHD	Combined pituitary hormone deficiency
CUAVD	Congenital unilateral absence of vas deferens
DBD	DNA-binding domain
DFS	Dysplasia of fibrous sheath
DNA-DSB	DNA-Double Strand Breaks
DSD	Disorders of sexual development
D-WS	Dandy-Walker syndrome
FA	Fanconi anemia
FISH	Fluorescence in situ hybridization
GHS	Gordon Holmes syndrome
HS	Hartsfield syndrome
HTCA	Head-tail coupling apparatus
ICSI	Intracytoplasmic sperm injection
KS	Kallmann syndrome
LBD	Ligand-binding domain
MAIS	Mild androgen insensitivity
MGS	Morning glory syndrome
MMAF	Multiple Morphological Abnormalities of the sperm Flagella
NAHR	Nonallelic homologous recombination
NGS	Next-generation sequencing
NOA	Nonobstructive azoospermia
NTD	N-terminal domain
OA	Obstructive azoospermia
PAIS	Partial androgen insensitivity
PAR	Pseudoautosomal region
PCD	Primary ciliary dyskinesia
PCR	Polymerase chain reaction

PEPNS	Polyendocrine deficiencies and Polyneuropathies
PGD	Preimplantation genetic diagnosis
POI	Premature ovarian insufficiency
SHFM	Split-hand/foot malformation
SOD	Septo-optic dysplasia
TEM	Transmission electron microscopy
TESE	Testicular sperm extraction
WES	Whole-exome sequencing
WS	Waardenburg syndrome

16.1 Introduction

Infertility affects about 14% of the couples in the general population and globally male factor is contributing to it for about 50% of cases. In about 95% of cases, male factor implies quantitative or qualitative alterations of sperm parameters while in about 5% of cases it is related to semen deposition in vagina (aspermia, erectile dysfunction, retrograde ejaculation, etc.). Male infertility is a multifactorial complex pathological condition with highly heterogeneous phenotypic representations. Recently, male reproductive dysfunction has been classified into four etiologic categories: (1) hypothalamic–pituitary axis dysfunction; (2) quantitative alterations of spermatogenesis; (3) qualitative alterations of spermatogenesis; and (4) ductal obstruction/dysfunction (Tournaye et al. 2016). Genetic factors play an important role in each of these categories, with the highest prevalence in the severest form of quantitative alterations, i.e., azoospermia. In fact, karyotype (numerical and structural chromosomal anomalies) and Y chromosome microdeletions are found in about 15% of men affected by severe male factor infertility. In sharp contrast with the incidence of chromosomal anomalies, known monogenic alterations are relatively rare and their screening is restricted to congenital hypogonadotropic hypogonadism (CHH), absence of vas deferens, mild androgen insensitivity, and monomorphic terato/asthenozoospermia. In about 40% of quantitative disturbances of spermatogenesis, the etiology remains unknown and we refer to them as idiopathic infertility. Genetic factors are likely to play an important role in idiopathic testicular impairment/failure. A growing number of genes have been reported in idiopathic azoospermia/oligozoospermia but at the moment only a few of them have been validated by more than one study (Fig. 16.1). In this chapter, we are going to provide a detailed description of those genetic factors that are already included in the diagnostic workup of infertile men. In addition, a brief overview is given on genes with potential clinical interest.

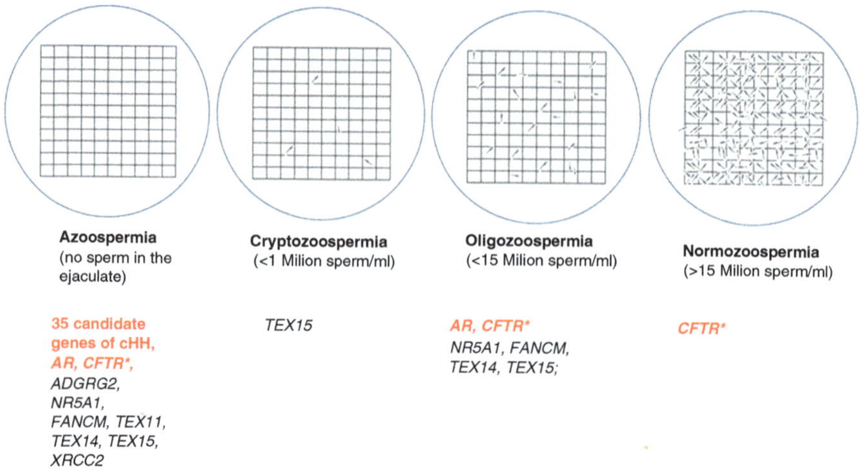

Fig. 16.1 Genotype–phenotype correlations, gene mutations versus semen phenotype. Genes in red with diagnostic value; genes in black with potential clinical value; *cHH* congenital Hypogonadotropic Hypogonadism, the complete list of genes is presented in Table 16.1. Asterisk mutations associated with unilateral congenital absence of vas deferens

16.2 Monogenic Causes with Diagnostic Value in the Four Etiologic Categories of Male Infertility

16.2.1 Genetic Causes of Hypothalamic–Pituitary Axis Dysfunction

A total of 35 candidate genes have been described in the literature to date (Boehm et al. 2015; Tournaye et al. 2016) with congenital hypogonadotropic hypogonadism (CHH) (Table 16.1). CHH is a rare, complex genetic disease (incidence of 1 in 8000 men) with variable expressivity, penetrance, and inheritance (Boehm et al. 2015). The classical phenotype of CHH is absent or delayed puberty, eunuchoid habitus, sparse or absent body hair, gynecomastia, cryptorchidism, micropenis, and very low testicular volume (<5 ml). However, in some cases, reduced spermatogenesis and mild hypoandrogenism are the only symptoms, resulting in a delayed CHH diagnosis after puberty. CHH can manifest itself with anosmia or hyposmia (Kallmann syndrome; KS) or as normosmic, isolated hypogonadotropic hypogonadism (Boehm et al. 2015). To note, KS can be associated with other developmental anomalies such as cleft lip or palate, dental agenesis, ear anomalies, congenital hearing impairment, renal agenesis, bimanual synkinesis, or skeletal anomalies (Boehm et al. 2015), whereas in normosmic CHH nonreproductive defects are absent. Some of the genes associated with CHH are also involved in different syndromic diseases (such as Gordon Holmes syndrome, CHARGE syndrome, and Waardenburg syndrome) (Boehm et al. 2015). Interestingly enough, "reversibility" of the gonadotropin deficiency after testosterone therapy has been described in about 10–15% of

Table 16.1 Monogenic causes with diagnostic value in the four major etiologic categories of male infertility

Etiology of reproductive impairment	Gene (OMIM)	Cytogenetic band	Other syndrome/ diseases	Protein function
Hypothalamic–pituitary axis dysfunction	*CHD7*[a] *(608892)*	8q12.2	CHARGE	Embryonic differentiation of GnRH neuron
	DUSP6[a] *(602748)*	12q21.33	–	
	FGF17[a] *(603725)*	8p21.3	D-WAS	
	FGF8[a] *(600483)*	10q24.32	CPHD	
	FGFR1[a] *(136350)*	8p11.23	CPHD, SOD, HS, SHFM	
	FLRT3 *(604808)*	20p12.1	–	
	HESX1 *(601802)*	3p14.3	CPHD, SOD	
	HS6ST1[a] *(604846)*	2q14.3	–	
	IL17RD *(606807)*	3p14.3	–	
	SOX10 *(602229)*	22q13.1	WS	
	SPRY4[a] *(607984)*	5q31.3		
	AXL *(109135)*	19q13.2	–	Migration of GnRH neurons
	CHD7[a] *(608892)*	8q12.2	CHARGE	
	FEZF1 *(613301)*	7q31.32		
	ANOS1 *(300836)*	Xp22.31		
	NSMF[a] *(608137)*	9q34.3		
	PROK2[a] *(607002)*	3p13		
	PROKR2[a] *(607123)*	20p12.3	CPHD; MGS	
	SEMA3A *(603961)*	7q21.11		
	SEMA3E *(608166)*	7q21.11		
	SEMA7A[a] *(607961)*	15q24.1		

(continued)

Table 16.1 (continued)

Etiology of reproductive impairment	Gene (OMIM)	Cytogenetic band	Other syndrome/ diseases	Protein function
	WDR11[a] *(606417)*	10q26.12	CPHD	
	TAC3 (162330)	12q13.3		Upstream and metabolic regulation of GnRH neuron function
	DMXL2 (612186)	15q21.2	PEPNS	
	KISS1 (603286)	1q32.1		
	KISS1R (604161)	19p13.3		
	LEP (164160)	7q32.1		
	LEPR (601007)	1p31.3		
	NR0B1 (300473)	Xp21.2		
	OTUD4 (611744)	4q31.21	GHS	
	PCSK1 (162150)	5q15		
	RNF216 (609948)	7p22.1	GHS	
	PNPLA6 (603197)	19p13.2	GHS	
	TAC3R (162332)	4q24		
	GnRH1 (152760)	8p21.2	–	GnRH synthesis
	GnRHR (138850)	4q13.2	–	GnRH receptor activation
Quantitative alterations of spermatogenesis	*AR (313700)*	Xq12	AIS	Steroid-hormone activated transcription factor
Qualitative alterations of spermatogenesis	*AURKC (603495)*	19q13.43		Chromosome alignment and segregation
	DNAH1 (603332)	3p21.1	PCD	Biogenesis of the axoneme
	DPY19L2 (613893)	12q14.2		Acrosome formation
	SUN5 (613942)	20q11.21		Anchoring sperm head to the tail

(continued)

Table 16.1 (continued)

Etiology of reproductive impairment	Gene (OMIM)	Cytogenetic band	Other syndrome/ diseases	Protein function
Ductal obstruction/ dysfunction	*CFTR (602421)*	7q31.2	Cystic fibrosis	Chloride transport

AIS Androgen Insensitivity Syndrome, *CHARGE* coloboma, heart defects, atresia of choanae, retardation of growth and/or development, genital and/or urinary defects, ear anomalies or deafness, *CPHD* combined pituitary hormone deficiency, *CTO* contributes to oligogenicity, *D-WS* Dandy-Walker syndrome; *GHS* Gordon Holmes syndrome, *HS* Hartsfield syndrome, *MGS* Morning Glory syndrome, *PCD* Primary Ciliary Dyskinesia, *PEPNS* polyendocrine deficiencies and polyneuropathies, *SHFM* split-hand/foot malformation, *SOD* septo-optic dysplasia, *WS* Waardenburg syndrome
[a]Gene responsible for both normosmic CHH and Kallmann syndrome

patients affected by KS or normosmic CHH (Quinton et al. 1999; Ribeiro et al. 2007; Raivio et al. 2007; Dwyer et al. 2016).

The 35 CHH genes are implicated either in the development/migration of the GnRH neurons or in the neuroendocrine regulation of GnRH secretion or action (Boehm et al. 2015). CHH presents a number of peculiar features from a genetic point of view: (1) in some cases the same gene (i.e., *FGFR1*, *PROKR2*) may cause both KS and normosmic CHH, implying that from a genetic point of view a clear distinction between the two clinical entities cannot be established; (2) it does not follow the rules of Mendelian inheritance since in about 20% of cases there is a digenic/oligogenic inheritance, i.e., two heterozygous mutations in two or more candidate genes.

16.2.1.1 Testing and Genetic Counseling

The indication for testing is restricted to patients with confirmed CHH after the exclusion of all secondary forms (pituitary tumors, empty sella, etc.). Currently, genetic testing is based on Next-Generation Sequencing (NGS) gene panel, which is able to provide the diagnosis in about 40% of cases (Boehm et al. 2015; Tournaye et al. 2016). Novel genes associated with CHH are expected to be discovered by whole-exome sequencing (WES) analysis in the near future.

Since in about 80% of CHH patients spermatogenesis can be induced by the administration of gonadotropins (Dwyer et al. 2015), gene mutations can be transmitted either spontaneously or by assisted reproductive techniques. Overall, the complexity of this disease (variable expressivity, penetrance, and inheritance pattern) makes predicting the exact health consequences for the offspring difficult. For this reason, the Preimplantation Genetic Diagnosis (PGD) or prenatal diagnosis should be offered to couples mainly for syndromic cases and for those cases where the gene mutation shows a clear-cut cause–effect relationship. A periodic suspension of the hormonal replacement therapy is recommended to all CHH patients in order to assess a potential recovery of the hypothalamic–pituitary axis. To note, genetic testing does not help in identifying patients with higher probability of "reversal," since this condition has been described in association with mutations in different CHH candidates (Dwyer et al. 2016).

16.2.2 *Genetic Causes of Quantitative Alterations of Spermatogenesis*

16.2.2.1 *AR* (Androgen Receptor Gene)

AR (OMIM: 313700) is the only gene that is included in the diagnostic testing of specific cases of male infertility. Mutations in *AR* gene are associated with Androgen Insensitivity Syndrome (AIS) characterized by resistance to circulating testosterone. AIS is the most frequent cause of Disorders of Sexual Development (DSD) and based on the residual degree of functional capacity of the mutated AR the clinical phenotype can be divided into three categories: (1) Complete Androgen Insensitivity (CAIS; Morris syndrome) leading to a female phenotype in 46,XY individuals; (2) Partial Androgen Insensitivity (PAIS; Reifenstein syndrome) characterized by undervirilized male phenotype with ambiguous genitalia; (3) Mild Androgen Insensitivity (MAIS) associated with impaired sperm production in the presence of normal male genitalia (Krausz and Chianese 2014). Using conventional and Cre/Lox conditional *Ar*-null male mice recreated human disorders (Yeh et al. 2002). They showed female external sex development and testis atrophy with spermatocyte-stage arrest, resembling AIS human pathology. Sertoli cell-selective KO of the AR causes spermatocytic arrest, indicating an important role for intratesticular testosterone in meiosis (De Gendt et al. 2004).

The AR gene is situated on the X chromosome (Xq11–12) and contains eight exons that encode a protein of 920 amino acid residues. The protein functions as a steroid hormone-activated transcription factor and contains three major functional domains: the N-terminal domain (NTD, transcriptional activation region encoded by exon 1), the DNA-binding domain (DBD, encoded by exons 2 and 3), and the ligand-binding domain (LBD, encoded by exon 4–8). More than 1000 *AR* mutations have been described so far (Gottlieb et al. 2012) and the large majority of them are missense mutations located in the AR-DBD or AR-LBD leading to impairment in DNA or AR binding, respectively.

The *AR* gene also contains two polymorphic sites in the N-terminal transactivation domain (exon1) of the receptor: a polyglutamine tract -(CAG)*n*- and a polyglycine tract (GGC)*n*, which were the subject of many publications related to male infertility (Davis-Dao et al. 2007). The most extensively studied polymorphism concerns the trinucleotide CAG. Based on in vitro studies, it has been hypothesized that carriers of longer CAG repeat have a higher risk for infertility and cryptorchidism due to impaired androgen effect (Gao et al. 1996; Davis-Dao et al. 2007). This hypothesis has been challenged by novel functional and observational studies reporting that both a longer CAG tract and a shorter CAG tract might have a negative effect on the receptor function; hence, an optimal number of CAG repeats are necessary for the highest transcription (Nenonen et al. 2011; Davis-Dao et al. 2012). We can speculate that the optimum range may vary between the genomic and non-genomic actions, and also in different tissues, because the effect of polyQ repeat on transactivation is cell-specific, presumably due to distinct profiles of co-regulator proteins (Krausz 2012).

Testing and Genetic Counseling

Given the variable clinical phenotypes, indications are different for each type of AIS. CAIS is suspected in case of a 46,XY woman with primary amenorrhea, normal breast development and pubertal growth, reduced or absent sexual hair, and absent female internal genitalia. Clinical management is complex and involves a multidisciplinary approach including psychologists, endocrinologists, urologists, and gynecologists. Because of malignancy risk, gonads, usually located in the abdomen or inguinal canal, are commonly removed, requiring subsequent estrogen replacement to maintain feminization. In case of PAIS, the phenotype is highly dependent on the degree of residual AR function, ranging from male-appearing genitalia to severe undermasculinization resembling female genitalia (Mongan et al. 2015). Management of severe forms of PAIS, including gender assignment, is rather complex. The hormone profile of AIS is typically represented by high Androgen Sensitivity Index (ASI), calculated as the product of serum testosterone x serum luteinizing hormone, i.e., high LH with relatively high testosterone levels. In hypoandrogenized infertile men with high ASI, *AR* testing is indicted. However, a routine screening to all infertile men is not advised, since the frequency of *AR* mutations in unselected infertile men varies from 0–1.7% (Ferlin et al. 2006; Rajender et al. 2007). The frequency of *AR* mutations in PAIS is 41%, whereas no official estimate is given in the available mutation databases for the MAIS phenotype (Gottlieb et al. 2012). The role of CAG repeats in male infertility is probably more complex than it has been previously proposed; there are still important unanswered questions such as: what range of *AR* CAG repeat lengths predisposes to impaired sperm production and what risk of infertility is associated with each length (Davis-Dao et al. 2007). These open questions limit the clinical use of (CAG)n testing.

16.2.2.2 Y Chromosome Linked Male Infertility

The Y chromosome contains genes essential for testis development and function, such as the genes residing in the azoospermia factor (AZF) regions and the master gene for testis determination (SRY; OMIM:480000). Y chromosome microdeletions, removing the entire AZF regions (complete deletions), are one of the leading causes of spermatogenic failure and the screening for AZF deletions became part of the routine diagnostic workup of men with severe oligozoospermia/azoospermia (Krausz et al. 2014). A peculiar feature of the boundary of the AZF regions is the presence of repeated homologous sequences that are predisposed to deletion or duplication through a mechanism called nonallelic homologous recombination (NAHR). These deletions remove more than one gene in block; hence, they will not be further discussed in this chapter (for review see Krausz and Casamonti 2017). The only monogenic Y-chromosome-linked cause of male infertility concerns the *SRY* gene. *SRY* encodes the critical testis-determining transcription factor that activates a number of downstream transcription factors involved in testes formation. The gene is located below the pseudoautosomal region (PAR) of the short arm of the Y chromosome, and the erroneous translocation can occur during meiosis when the two sex chromosomes recombine between their PAR regions (Wu et al. 2014). This translocation leads to the 46,XX male syndrome (also known as de la Chapelle syndrome). This syndrome has a frequency of 1 in 20,000 children according to Genetics Home Reference (https://ghr.nlm.nih.gov/). Men with 46,XX male syndrome have smaller stature and a higher incidence of maldescended testes and gynecomastia, and are azoospermic with no exceptions (Vorona et al. 2007).

Testing and Genetic Counseling

Testicular sperm extraction (TESE) is not advised in XX male patients owing to the lack of Y chromosome-linked azoospermia factor (AZF) genes, meaning focal sperm production in the testis is not possible (Skaletsky et al. 2003). These patients can have hypoandrogenism, so a careful endocrine assessment (including analysis of FSH, LH, and testosterone levels) and follow-up monitoring of testosterone level are advised.

16.2.3 *Genetic Causes of Qualitative Alterations of Spermatogenesis*

16.2.3.1 *DPY19L2* (Dpy-19 Like 2 Gene)

DPY19L2 (OMIM: 613893) is the only gene included in the routine genetic diagnostic workup of globozoospermia. Globozoospermia is very rare, affecting 0.1% of infertile men, and is characterized by the production of round-headed, acrosome-less spermatozoa that are unable to fertilize the oocyte, as no acrosome reaction can occur (Fig. 16.2a). In mouse models, globozoospermia has been observed as a consequence of >50 different gene mutations (Coutton et al. 2015), but in humans, only mutations in the *DPY19L2* gene have been validated to be associated with this disorder. In fact, mutations in *DPY19L2* have been found in 60–80% of globozoospermic patients. *DPY19L2* is located on chromosome 12 and encodes a protein required during spermatogenesis for sperm head elongation and acrosome formation. The most frequent mutation is the complete deletion of the gene, caused by a similar mechanism to that observed for AZF deletions. *DPY19L2* is located in a region flanked by

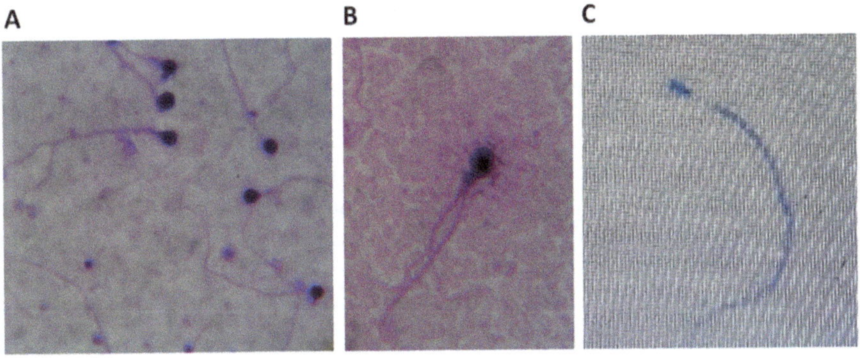

Fig. 16.2 Representative view of sperm morphology. (**a**) Roundheaded and acrosomeless spermatozoa. (**b**) Macrocephalic and multi-flagellated spermatozoa. (**c**) Acephalic spermatozoa

two 28 kb segmental duplications, which predisposes it to NAHR. The complete deletion of *DPY19L2* accounts for 80.4% of instances of *DPY19L2*-related globozoospermia, whereas the remaining instances are caused by intragenic deletions and point mutations (homozygous and compound heterozygous) (Ray et al. 2017).

Testing and Genetic Counseling

Mutations are mainly identified in patients with 100% globozoospermia; thus, genetic analysis should be restricted to this circumstance only. Given the high frequency of complete gene deletion, genetic testing can be easily performed using real-time quantitative PCR (Chianese et al. 2015) followed by breakpoint definition and mutation screening. Since *DPY19L2* deletions are not exceptionally rare in the general population (heterozygous carriers 1:85), screening in the female partners of male carriers prior intracytoplasmic sperm injection (ICSI) should be performed. The lack of phospholipase C-ζ, an acrosome phospholipase, is responsible for the absence of oocyte activation. Consequently, artificial oocyte activation (AOA) has been proposed as an option for patients with complete globozoospermia undergoing ICSI. However, the safety of AOA has been questioned as continued increases in intracellular calcium concentration can affect downstream molecular events, and it should be restricted to selected cases of 100% globozoospermia in which finding spermatozoa with residual acrosome is impossible (Kuentz et al. 2013).

16.2.3.2 *AURKC* (Aurora Kinase C)

To date, *AURKC* (OMIM: 603495) gene mutations are the only validated genetic causes macrozoospermia. Macrozoospermia, also known as sperm macrocephaly, affects <1% of the male population and it was reported for the first time in 1977 by Nistal and colleagues (1977). This qualitative disturbance is characterized by a high percentage of spermatozoa with large, irregular heads and multiple flagella (Fig. 16.2b). *AURKC* gene is located in chromosome 19 and encodes for a component of the chromosomal passenger complex (CPC) in meiotic cells and is essential for correct meiotic chromosomal segregation and cytokinesis (Dieterich et al. 2007). The *AURKC* mutations are associated with alterations of meiotic divisions leading to tetraploid spermatozoa. The most common mutation is the deletion of a cytosine in the exon 3 (c.144delC), observed in more than 85% of patients affected by macrozoospermia (Ray et al. 2017). Interestingly enough, the mutation is relatively common in heterozygosis in the Maghrebian population (1/50 men) and it has been proposed that heterozygote carriers may have a selective advantage due to a more relaxed meiotic checkpoint (Ben Khelifa et al. 2012). In Europeans, a recurrent stop gain mutation in exon 6 (p.Y248*) has been described (Ben Khelifa et al. 2012).

Testing and Genetic Counseling

All men with macrozoospermia should be tested for *AURKC* mutations before undergoing Assisted Reproductive Techniques (ART). After genetic testing, two different scenarios can occur: identification of homozygous or compound heterozygous mutations or an absence of mutations in this gene. In the first scenario, ICSI is not advised even after motile sperm organelle morphology examination, as all spermatozoa are polyploid (and are mostly tetraploid) and, therefore, normal embryonic development is not possible. By contrast, ART is not contraindicated in patients without mutations, but sperm FISH should be performed to evaluate the proportion of euploid sperm; hence, the likelihood of success. PGD can be proposed to those with intermediate rate of aneuploid spermatozoa.

16.2.3.3 *DNAH1* (Dynein Axonemal Heavy Chain 1)

DNAH1 gene (OMIM: 603332) mutations seems to be the major cause of Multiple Morphological Abnormalities of the sperm flagella (MMAF) (Ben Khelifa et al. 2014; Amiri-Yekta et al. 2016; Wang et al. 2017; Sha et al. 2017a; Tang et al. 2017; Coutton et al. 2018). MMAF, previously reported as dysplasia of fibrous sheath (DFS), is a rare disease defined as an asthenoteratozoospermia resulting from a mosaic of morphological abnormalities concerning the sperm flagella, including absent, coiled, bent, angulated, irregular, or short flagella (Ben Khelifa et al. 2014). In addition, lack of central microtubules and/or dynein arms may also be observed by transmission electron microscopy (TEM) in the sperm flagella of the affected subjects (Ben Khelifa et al. 2014). The incidence of MMAF has not already been investigated precisely. *DNAH1* is located on chromosome 3 and encodes an axonemal inner dynein arm heavy chain and when it is absent, the axoneme is grossly disorganized, often lacking the central pair (9 + 0 structure). Biallelic *DNAH1* mutations seem to be responsible for 30% of MMAF patients (Coutton et al. 2018).

Testing and Genetic Counseling

The screening for *DNAH1* mutations is recommended in patients affected by severe to complete asthenozoospermia due to sperm flagellar alterations. Flagellar abnormalities have been reported to be associated with an elevated frequency of aneuploidies and a poor ICSI outcome (Lewis-Jones et al. 2003; Baccetti et al. 2005; Collodel and Moretti 2006; Ghedir et al. 2014). However, patients with MMAF with mutated *DNHA1* showed low aneuploidy rate and normal sperm DNA integrity, indicating that not all patients with MMAF are at risk of chromosomal anomalies (Wambergue et al. 2016).

In 2015, a homozygous mutation in *DNAH1* was observed in two sisters affected by Primary ciliary dyskinesia (PCD) (Imtiaz et al. 2015), which is a disorder characterized by chronic respiratory tract infections, abnormally positioned internal organs, and infertility. This observation has prompted the novel hypothesis of a 'phenotypic continuum' ranging from infertile patients with PCD to patients with MMAF with no or mild PCD manifestations (Ray et al. 2017). Given the multitude of genes involved in ciliagenesis and function, MMAF could be a phenotypic variant of the classical form of PCD, and mutations affecting sperm flagella could be compensated for by other genes involved in other ciliated tissues. Therefore, it is still unclear the exact health consequences for the offspring and whether the female partner should be screened for *DNAH1* mutations.

16.2.3.4 *SUN5* (*Sad1* and *UNC84* Domain Containing 5 Gene)

The phenotype of the *SUN5*-mutated patients is characterized by acephalic spermatozoa with a variable but low proportion of abnormal head–tail junctions and tailless heads (Shang et al. 2017) (Fig. 16.2c). This sperm defect is due to the failure of centriole-tail attachment to the spermatid nucleus during the last phase of spermatogenesis. *SUN5* (OMIM: 613942) encodes a testis-specific protein localized in the neck region of spermatids. The disease is extremely rare and it is transmitted through recessive inheritance. Homozygous and compound heterozygous mutations were reported by four different authors (Zhu et al. 2016; Elkhatib et al. 2017; Shang et al. 2017; Sha et al. 2018b).

Testing and Genetic Counseling

Patients affected by acephalic spermatozoa should be screened for *SUN5* mutations. The only option for a biological paternity is ICSI through the selection of tailless sperm heads. The majority of papers report no pregnancy despite the presence of fertilized eggs. In five articles, nine couples obtained pregnancy after repeated ICSI attempts (Kamal et al. 1999; Porcu et al. 2003; Emery et al. 2004; Gambera et al. 2010; Shang et al. 2017).

16.2.4 Genetic Causes of Ductal Obstruction

16.2.4.1 *CFTR* (Cystic Fibrosis Transmembrane Conductance Regulator Gene)

Mutations in *CFTR* (OMIM: 602421) have been largely described in patients affected by Congenital Absence of Vas Deferens (CAVD). The CAVD may occur either as an isolated reproductive disorder or as an atypical symptom of Cystic Fibrosis, and accounts for up to 25% of patients with Obstructive Azoospermia (OA) (Oates and Amos 1994). It may affect one (CUAVD) or both vas deferens (CBAVD). The CUAVD is a rare condition associated with either oligo/or normozoospermia. In contrast, CBAVD associated with agenesis of seminal vesicles is characterized by typical semen alterations, such as low semen volume (<1 ml) with an acid pH (<7) and absence of spermatozoa. The *CFTR* gene is located on chromosome 7q31.2, contains 27 exons (Kerem et al. 1989; Riordan et al. 1989), and encodes a protein involved in chloride conduction across epithelial cell membranes. To date, more than 2000 variants have been identified in *CFTR* gene (http://www.genet.sickkids.on.ca/Home.html) and they are categorized in severe and mild mutations depending on their functional consequences. Although geographical and ethnic differences have been demonstrated in *CFTR* mutations, the most common mutations in CBAVD patients are F508del, 5T, and R117H (Yu et al. 2012). 5T is the shortest allele of IVS8-(T)*n*, which is a length variant of a polypyrimidine tract at the splice acceptor site of intron 8 of the *CFTR* gene. The length of the T tract (IVS8-5T, IVS8-7T, IVS8-9T) affects the splicing efficiency of exon 9 and thus the amount of normal *CFTR* mRNA. The phenotypic penetrance of 5 T allele depends on the length of adjacent TG repeats (12 or 13) and the M470 V missense mutation in exon 10, i.e., the 12TG-5T-V470 haplotype increases the risk of having CBAVD (de Meeus et al. 1998; Du et al. 2014).

Testing and Genetic Counseling

The screening for CFTR gene mutation is recommended in subjects with CAVD without renal agenesis (Jungwirth et al. 2012). In fact, subjects with CAVD and renal agenesis (in the majority of cases of unilateral agenesis of vas deferens) are considered to have different genetic basis, which may be attributed to defect of mesonephric duct development in the embryo (McCallum et al. 2001). This fact implies that all patients affected by CAVD should undergo an ultrasound scan of the pelvic region prior to genetic testing. Routine screening for *CTFR* variants is based on a panel of mutations (30–50 mutations) that are the most common for a given ethnic population (de Souza et al. 2017). In instances in which the two mutations are not identified using this panel (as CAVD is a recessive disease), the whole *CFTR* gene is subjected to sequencing in order to search for the second mutation. In those patients in whom pathogenic variants have been identified, genetic counseling is mandatory since patients with CBAVD are assumed to have normal testicular function, and they can undergo TESE–ICSI (as azoospermia is caused by obstruction) and generate their own biological children. Given that the carrier frequency of *CFTR* mutations in people of European descent is high (1 in 25), screening of the partner is mandatory in order to evaluate the risk of giving birth to a child affected by cystic fibrosis. If both parents are carriers, prenatal or PGD should be undertaken.

16.3 Additional Monogenic Causes of Male Infertility with Potential Clinical Interest

The diffusion of NGS platforms is allowing the identification of a number of genes involved in various semen phenotypes. However, only few of them have been validated by more than one independent study on a relatively high number of subjects (Table 16.2). In the following paragraphs we briefly describe those genes that were validated by more than one study and are potential candidates for diagnostic testing in the future.

16.3.1 Validated Candidate Genes Involved in Quantitative Alterations of Spermatogenesis

A total of six genes leading quantitative impairment of spermatogenesis have been validated by more than one independent study: *NR5A1* (OMIM: 184757), *TEX11* (OMIM: 300311), *TEX14* (OMIM: 605792), *TEX15* (OMIM: 605795), *FANCM* (OMIM: 609644), and *XRCC2* (OMIM: 600375). With the exception of *TEX11*, which is X-linked, the remaining genes are mapping to autosomes. Apart from *NR5A1*, which follows the Autosomal Dominant inheritance pattern, only recessive mutations lead to quantitative alterations of spermatogenesis.

NR5A1 encodes steroidogenic factor 1 (SF1), crucial in male and female gonadal development and steroidogenesis. Heterozygosis mutations in *NR5A1* have been associated with a variety of phenotypes ranging from primary adrenal insufficiency (AI) and complete 46,XY gonadal dysgenesis (Schimmer and White 2010; Ferraz-de-Souza et al. 2011) to 46,XY DSD including bilateral anorchia (Philibert et al. 2007; Brauner et al. 2011), hypospadias (Allali et al. 2011; Brandt et al. 2013), and hypogonadotropic hypogonadism (Hu et al. 2012).

Heterozygous mutations have also been reported in patients affected by severe oligozoospermia or azoospermia (Bashamboo et al. 2010; Ropke et al. 2013; Zare-Abdollahi et al. 2015; Ferlin et al. 2015; Tuttelmann et al. 2018) with a frequency ranging from 0.6% (Ropke et al. 2013) to 2.5% (Tuttelmann et al. 2018).

Concerning *TEX11*, *TEX14*, and *TEX15*, they belong to the family of Testis Expressed genes and, as their name indicates, they are over- or specifically expressed

Table 16.2 Monogenic causes of male infertility with potential clinical interest, validated in more than one study population

Etiology of reproductive impairment	Gene (OMIM)	Cytogenetic band	Cohort type	Associated semen/testis phenotype(s)	Genotype in affected individuals	References
Quantitative alterations of spermatogenesis	*FANCM (609644)*	14q21.2	Consanguineous family	NOA + Oligoasthenozoospermia	Homozygosis	Yin et al. (2019)
			Non-consanguineous family + sporadic cases	NOA	Homozygosis/ compound heterozygosis	Kasak et al. (2018)
	NR5A1 (184757)	9q33.3	Sporadic cases	NOA + Oligozoospermia	Heterozygosis	Bashamboo et al. (2010)
			Sporadic cases	NOA + Oligozoospermia	Heterozygosis	Ropke et al. (2013)
			Sporadic cases	NOA	Heterozygosis	Zare-Abdollahi et al. (2015)
			Sporadic cases	NOA + Oligozoospermia	Heterozygosis	Ferlin et al. (2015)
			Sporadic cases	NOA	Heterozygosis	Tuttelmann et al. (2018)
	TEX11 (300311)	Xp11	Sporadic cases	NOA	Hemizygosis	Yatsenko et al. (2015)
			Non-consanguineous family + sporadic cases	NOA	Hemizygosis	Yang et al. (2015)
			Non-consanguineous family	NOA	Hemizygosis	Sha et al. (2018a)
			Sporadic cases	NOA	Hemizygosis	Tuttelmann et al. (2018)
	TEX14 (605792)	17q22	Consanguineous family	NOA	Homozygosis	Gershoni et al. (2017)
			Consanguineous family + sporadic cases	NOA	Homozygosis	Fakhro et al. (2018)

	TEX15 (605795)	8p12	Consanguineous family	NOA+ Severe oligozoospermia	Homozygosis	Okutman et al. (2015)
			Non-consanguineous family	NOA	Compound heterozygosis	Colombo et al. (2017)
			Consanguineous family	Cryptozoospermia	Homozygosis	Wang et al. (2018)
	XRCC2 (600375)	7q36.1	Consanguineous family + sporadic cases	NOA	Homozygosis	Yang et al. (2018)
			Consanguineous family	NOA	Homozygosis	Zhang et al. (2019)
Qualitative alterations of spermatogenesis	*CFAP43 (617558)*	10q25.1	Consanguienous families + sporadic cases	MMAF	Compound heterozygosis	Tang et al. (2017)
			Consanguineous family + non consanguineous family + sporadic cases	MMAF	Homozygosis	Sha et al. (2017b)
			No data[a]	MMAF	Homozygosis/ compound heterozygosis	Coutton et al. (2018)
	CFAP44 (617559)	3q132	Consanguienous families + sporadic cases	MMAF	Homozygosis	Tang et al. (2017)
			Consanguineous family + non-consamnguineous family + sporadic cases	MMAF	Homozygosis and compound heterozygosis	Sha et al. (2017b)
			No data[a]	MMAF	Homozygosis	Coutton et al. (2018)
	CFAP69 (617949)	7q21.13	No data[a]	MMAF	Homozygosis/ compound heterozygosis	Dong et al. (2018)
			Consanguineous family + sporadic cases	MMAF	Homozygosis	He et al. (2019)

(continued)

Table 16.2 (continued)

Etiology of reproductive impairment	Gene (OMIM)	Cytogenetic band	Cohort type	Associated semen/testis phenotype(s)	Genotype in affected individuals	References
	WDR66 (618146)	12q21.31	No data[a]	MMAF	Homozygosis	kherraf et al. (2018)
			Consanguienous families + sporadic cases	MMAF	Homozygosis and compound heterozygosis	Li et al. (2019)
			Consanguineous family + sporadic cases	MMAF	Homozygosis and compound heterozygosis	Auguste et al. (2018)
	PMFBP1 (618085)	16q22.2	Consanguineous families + sporadic cases	Acephalic spermatozoa	Homozygosis/ compound heterozygosis	Zhu et al. (2018)
			Consanguineous family + sporadic case	Acephalic spermatozoa	Homozygosis/ compound heterozygosis	Sha et al. (2019)
	SPATA16 (609856)	3q23.31	Consanguineous family	Globozoospermia	Homozygosis	Dam et al. (2007)
			Sporadic cases	Globozoospermia	Homozygosis	Ellnati et al. (2016)
Ductal obstruction/ dysfunction	*ADGRG2 (300572)*	Xp22.13	Sporadic cases	CBAVD	Hemizygosis	Patat et al. (2016)
			Sporadic cases	CBAVD	Hemizygosis	Yang et al. (2017)
			Non-consanguienous family	CBAVD	Hemizygosis	Khan et al. (2018)

NOA nonobstructive azoospermia, *MMAF* Multiple Morphological Abnormalities of the sperm Flagella, *CBAVD* congenital bilateral absence of vas deferens
[a]Not precise data about but the type of cohort analyzed; however, they note that the majority of patients come from consanguineous families

in the testis. While *TEX15* is not associated with a clear-cut semen phenotype, since it has been found mutated both in patients with NOA and crypto/oligozoospermia (Okutman et al. 2015; Colombo et al. 2017; Wang et al. 2018), mutations in *TEX11* and *TEX14* are restricted to NOA (Yatsenko et al. 2015; Yang et al. 2015; Gershoni et al. 2017; Tuttelmann et al. 2018; Sha et al. 2018a; Fakhro et al. 2018). More precisely, *TEX11* mutations seem to be more frequent in NOA men with testis histology of meiotic arrest (Yatsenko et al. 2015) and should be tested in cases of suspected meiotic arrest.

FANCA (OMIM:607139), *FANCM*, and *XRCC2* are part of the Fanconi Anemia (FA) gene family. Proteins encoded by the FA gene family are involved in (DNA double strand breaks) DSB repair and are essential for mitosis and meiosis. By performing exome analysis, recessive *FANCA* mutations have been described in men affected by NOA (Sertoli Cell Only syndrome) and mild/borderline hematological alterations (Krausz et al. 2019). This finding underlies the importance of considering not only hormone dosage but also hematological parameters in the diagnostic workup of SCOS patients. Diagnosing occult FA is highly relevant since it is a medical condition that predisposes to specific FA-related cancers.

Mutations in *FANCM* are not associated with bone marrow failure and have been identified in both NOA and oligoasthenozoospermia (Kasak et al. 2018; Yin et al. 2019). Meiosis-specific mutations in the *XRCC2* gene were reported in NOA patient with spermatocytic arrest (Yang et al. 2018; Zhang et al. 2019). Interestingly enough, mutations in this gene also cause Premature Ovarian Insufficiency (POI) in females (Zhang et al. 2019). Hence, the genetic counseling should involve not only male but also female relatives in case of *XRCC2* mutations.

16.3.2 Validated Candidate Genes Involved in Qualitative Alterations of Spermatogenesis

Monomorhpic teratozoospermia defines a group of rare morphological anomalies, mainly globozoospermia, MMAF and sperm acephalia. The large majority of cases occur in consanguineous families since these are recessive diseases. In globozoospermia, besides the *DPY19L2* gene (see paragragh on routine screening), mutations in *SPATA16* (OMIM: 609856) have been reported in two independent studies (Elinati et al. 2016; Dam et al. 2007). This gene is located on chromosome 3 and encodes a testis-specific protein belonging to the tetratricopeptide repeat-like superfamily. The encoded protein localizes to the Golgi apparatus and is involved in the formation of sperm acrosome. Concerning the MMAF phenotype, besides *DNAH1* mutations, homozygous, and compound heterozygous mutations in *CFAP43* (OMIM: 617558), *CFAP44* (OMIM: 617559), *CFAP69* (OMIM: 617949), and *WDR66* (OMIM: 618146) have been reported in more than one study (Sha et al. 2017b; Tang et al. 2017; Coutton et al. 2018; Dong et al. 2018; Auguste et al. 2018; Kherraf et al. 2018; He et al. 2019). These genes encode a family of proteins belonging to the cilia and flagella associated protein family (CFAP) and are necessary to produce functional flagella. Interestingly enough, *CFAP43* and *CFAP44*, *WDR66* encode WD-repeat proteins, which confirm the importance of these type of proteins in human diseases and especially in male infertility. Overall, mutations in these genes may explain up to 50% of cases of MMAF (Li et al. 2019). Finally, in relationship with acephalic spermatozoa two independent studies reported homozygous and compound heterozygous mutations in *PMFBP1* (OMIM: 618085) (Zhu et al. 2018; Sha et al. 2019). PMFBP1 is localized at the head–tail coupling apparatus (HTCA) and cooperates with SUN5 and SPATA6 to connect sperm head to tail (Zhu et al. 2018). It has been postulated that mutations in *SUN5* and *PMFBP1* may explain 70% of cases of acephalic spermatozoa syndrome (Zhu et al. 2018); however, since mutations in *PMFBP1* have been only found in patients from Asia, further validation in other ethnic populations is needed.

16.3.3 Validated Candidate Genes Involved in Ductal Obstruction

After a comprehensive analysis of the *CFTR* gene, in about 20% of cases the origin of CAVD remains unknown. Recently, the *ADGRG2* gene (OMIM: 300572) has been identified as a new candidate gene in CBAVD in three independent studies (Patat et al. 2016; Yang et al. 2017; Khan et al. 2018). *ADGRG2* is an X-linked gene encoding an adhesion-class G protein-coupled receptor and is highly expressed in the efferent ducts (Obermann et al. 2003). Adgrg2-mutant mice develop fluid accumulation in the testes ducts, leading to an obstructive infertility phenotype, which resembles that described in men with *ADGRG2* mutation (Davies et al. 2004). Pathogenic *ADGRG2* variants were reported, accounting for 11%–15% of the CBAVD patients who are *CFTR*-negative (Patat et al. 2016; Yang et al. 2017).

16.4 Conclusions

Although more than 2000 genes have been predicted to be involved in human spermatogenesis, there are relatively few monogenic mutations that have been conclusively demonstrated and validated to cause male infertility in humans. Consequently, the current diagnostic genetic testing is restricted to a relatively small set of genes. Genetic counseling of the couple is an absolute requirement prior to assisted reproduction and in some instances includes testing of the female partner and recommendation for PGD. The major breakthrough in the discovery of genetic factors involved in male infertility occurred more than 30 years ago with the identification of the Y-chromosome-linked AZF region deletions (Vogt et al.

1996), which implied the deletion in block of more than one gene. While candidate gene re-sequencing studies were relatively successful in uncovering the genetic basis of CHH, this approach did not lead to novel diagnostic tests in idiopathic oligo/ azoospermia (Krausz and Riera-Escamilla 2018). Next-generation sequencing allowing the simultaneous analysis of several thousands of genes or the entire exome has contributed to major advances in the genetic diagnosis of monomorphic teratozoospermia, cHH, and in familial cases of idiopathic azoospermia. Exome studies are currently ongoing in quantitative impairment of spermatogenesis in large cohorts of sporadic patients. These studies have the potential to provide novel genetic diagnostic tests also in this category of patients. The clinical impact of discovering such factors became even more important in the era of in vitro fertilization, since these patients can now generate their own biological child through these techniques and the identification of transmissible genetic causes has relevance for their future children. Besides the consequences on reproductive health, an emerging issue is the possible genetic link between idiopathic impaired spermatogenesis and higher morbidity and mortality rates. This important topic is currently addressed by androgeneticists and will allow a more holistic clinical evaluation of our infertile patients.

References

Allali S, Muller J-B, Brauner R et al (2011) Mutation analysis of NR5A1 encoding steroidogenic factor 1 in 77 patients with 46, XY disorders of sex development (DSD) including hypospadias. PLoS One 6:e24117. https://doi.org/10.1371/journal.pone.0024117

Amiri-Yekta A, Coutton C, Kherraf Z-E et al (2016) Whole-exome sequencing of familial cases of multiple morphological abnormalities of the sperm flagella (MMAF) reveals new DNAH1 mutations. Hum Reprod 31:2872–2880. https://doi.org/10.1093/humrep/dew262

Auguste Y, Delague V, Desvignes J-P et al (2018) Loss of calmodulin- and radial-spoke-associated complex protein CFAP251 leads to immotile spermatozoa lacking mitochondria and infertility in men. Am J Hum Genet 103:413–420. https://doi.org/10.1016/j.ajhg.2018.07.013

Baccetti B, Collodel G, Estenoz M et al (2005) Gene deletions in an infertile man with sperm fibrous sheath dysplasia. Hum Reprod 20:2790–2794. https://doi.org/10.1093/humrep/dei126

Bashamboo A, Ferraz-de-Souza B, Lourenco D et al (2010) Human male infertility associated with mutations in NR5A1 encoding steroidogenic factor 1. Am J Hum Genet 87:505–512. https://doi.org/10.1016/j.ajhg.2010.09.009

Ben Khelifa M, Coutton C, Blum MGB et al (2012) Identification of a new recurrent aurora kinase C mutation in both European and African men with macrozoospermia. Hum Reprod 27:3337–3346. https://doi.org/10.1093/humrep/des296

Ben Khelifa M, Coutton C, Zouari R et al (2014) Mutations in DNAH1, which encodes an inner arm heavy chain dynein, lead to male infertility from multiple morphological abnormalities of the sperm flagella. Am J Hum Genet 94:95–104. https://doi.org/10.1016/j.ajhg.2013.11.017

Boehm U, Bouloux P-M, Dattani MT et al (2015) Expert consensus document: European Consensus Statement on congenital hypogonadotropic hypogonadism–pathogenesis, diagnosis and treatment. Nat Rev Endocrinol 11:547–564. https://doi.org/10.1038/nrendo.2015.112

Brandt T, Blanchard L, Desai K et al (2013) 46,XY disorder of sex development and developmental delay associated with a novel 9q33.3 microdeletion encompassing NR5A1. Eur J Med Genet 56:619–623. https://doi.org/10.1016/j.ejmg.2013.09.006

Brauner R, Neve M, Allali S et al (2011) Clinical, biological and genetic analysis of anorchia in 26 boys. PLoS One 6:e23292. https://doi.org/10.1371/journal.pone.0023292

Chianese C, Fino MG, Riera Escamilla A et al (2015) Comprehensive investigation in patients affected by sperm macrocephaly and globozoospermia. Andrology 3:203–212. https://doi.org/10.1111/andr.12016

Collodel G, Moretti E (2006) Sperm morphology and aneuploidies: defects of supposed genetic origin. Andrologia 38:208–215. https://doi.org/10.1111/j.1439-0272.2006.00742.x

Colombo R, Pontoglio A, Bini M (2017) Two novel TEX15 mutations in a family with nonobstructive azoospermia. Gynecol Obstet Investig 82:283–286. https://doi.org/10.1159/000468934

Coutton C, Escoffier J, Martinez G et al (2015) Teratozoospermia: spotlight on the main genetic actors in the human. Hum Reprod Update 21:455–485. https://doi.org/10.1093/humupd/dmv020

Coutton C, Vargas AS, Amiri-Yekta A et al (2018) Mutations in CFAP43 and CFAP44 cause male infertility and flagellum defects in Trypanosoma and human. Nat Commun 9:686. https://doi.org/10.1038/s41467-017-02792-7

Dam AHDM, Koscinski I, Kremer JAM et al (2007) Homozygous mutation in SPATA16 is associated with male infertility in human globozoospermia. Am J Hum Genet 81:813–820. https://doi.org/10.1086/521314

Davies B, Baumann C, Kirchhoff C et al (2004) Targeted deletion of the epididymal receptor HE6 results in fluid dysregulation and male infertility. Mol Cell Biol 24:8642–8648. https://doi.org/10.1128/MCB.24.19.8642-8648.2004

Davis-Dao CA, Tuazon ED, Sokol RZ, Cortessis VK (2007) Male infertility and variation in CAG repeat length in the androgen receptor gene: a meta-analysis. J Clin Endocrinol Metab 92:4319–4326. https://doi.org/10.1210/jc.2007-1110

Davis-Dao C, Koh CJ, Hardy BE et al (2012) Shorter androgen receptor CAG repeat lengths associated with cryptorchidism risk among Hispanic white boys. J Clin Endocrinol Metab 97: E393–E399. https://doi.org/10.1210/jc.2011-2439

De Gendt K, Swinnen JV, Saunders PTK et al (2004) A Sertoli cell-selective knockout of the androgen receptor causes spermatogenic arrest in meiosis. Proc Natl Acad Sci U S A 101:1327–1332. https://doi.org/10.1073/pnas.0308114100

de Meeus A, Guittard C, Desgeorges M et al (1998) Linkage disequilibrium between the M470V variant and the IVS8 polyT alleles of the CFTR gene in CBAVD. J Med Genet 35:594–596

de Souza DAS, Faucz FR, Pereira-Ferrari L et al (2017) Congenital bilateral absence of the vas deferens as an atypical form of cystic fibrosis: reproductive implications and genetic counseling. Andrology. https://doi.org/10.1111/andr.12450

Dieterich K, Soto Rifo R, Faure AK et al (2007) Homozygous mutation of AURKC yields large-headed polyploid spermatozoa and causes male infertility. Nat Genet 39:661–665. https://doi.org/10.1038/ng2027

Dong FN, Amiri-Yekta A, Martinez G et al (2018) Absence of CFAP69 causes male infertility due to multiple morphological abnormalities of the flagella in human and mouse. Am J Hum Genet 102:636–648. https://doi.org/10.1016/j.ajhg.2018.03.007

Du Q, Li Z, Pan Y et al (2014) The CFTR M470V, intron 8 poly-T, and 8 TG-repeats detection in Chinese males with congenital bilateral absence of the vas deferens. Biomed Res Int 2014:689185. https://doi.org/10.1155/2014/689185

Dwyer AA, Raivio T, Pitteloud N (2015) Gonadotrophin replacement for induction of fertility in hypogonadal men. Best Pract Res Clin Endocrinol Metab 29:91–103. https://doi.org/10.1016/j.beem.2014.10.005

Dwyer AA, Raivio T, Pitteloud N (2016) Management of endocrine disease: reversible hypogonadotropic hypogonadism. Eur J Endocrinol 174:R267–R274. https://doi.org/10.1530/EJE-15-1033

Ellnati E, Fossard C, Okutman O et al (2016) A new mutation identified in SPATA16 in two globozoospermic patients. J Assist Reprod Genet 33:815–820. https://doi.org/10.1007/s10815-016-0715-3

Elkhatib RA, Paci M, Longepied G et al (2017) Homozygous deletion of SUN5 in three men with decapitated spermatozoa. Hum Mol Genet 26:3167–3171. https://doi.org/10.1093/hmg/ddx200

Emery BR, Thorp C, Malo JW, Carrell DT (2004) Pregnancy from intracytoplasmic sperm injection of a sperm head and detached tail. Fertil Steril 81:686–688. https://doi.org/10.1016/j.fertnstert.2003.07.025

Fakhro KA, Elbardisi H, Arafa M et al (2018) Point-of-care whole-exome sequencing of idiopathic male infertility. Genet Med 20:1365–1373. https://doi.org/10.1038/gim.2018.10

Ferlin A, Vinanzi C, Garolla A et al (2006) Male infertility and androgen receptor gene mutations: clinical features and identification of seven novel mutations. Clin Endocrinol 65:606–610. https://doi.org/10.1111/j.1365-2265.2006.02635.x

Ferlin A, Rocca MS, Vinanzi C et al (2015) Mutational screening of NR5A1 gene encoding steroidogenic factor 1 in cryptorchidism and male factor infertility and functional analysis of seven undescribed mutations. Fertil Steril 104:163–9.e1. https://doi.org/10.1016/j.fertnstert.2015.04.017

Ferraz-de-Souza B, Lin L, Achermann JC (2011) Steroidogenic factor-1 (SF-1, NR5A1) and human disease. Mol Cell Endocrinol 336:198–205. https://doi.org/10.1016/j.mce.2010.11.006

Gambera L, Falcone P, Mencaglia L et al (2010) Intracytoplasmic sperm injection and pregnancy with decapitated sperm. Fertil Steril 93:1347.e7–1347.12. https://doi.org/10.1016/j.fertnstert.2008.12.087

Gao T, Marcelli M, McPhaul MJ (1996) Transcriptional activation and transient expression of the human androgen receptor. J Steroid Biochem Mol Biol 59:9–20

Gershoni M, Hauser R, Yogev L et al (2017) A familial study of azoospermic men identifies three novel causative mutations in three new human azoospermia genes. Genet Med. https://doi.org/10.1038/gim.2016.225

Ghedir H, Mehri A, Mehdi M et al (2014) Meiotic segregation and sperm DNA fragmentation in Tunisian men with dysplasia of the fibrous sheath (DFS) associated with head abnormalities. J Assist Reprod Genet 31:1167–1174. https://doi.org/10.1007/s10815-014-0290-4

Gottlieb B, Beitel LK, Nadarajah A et al (2012) The androgen receptor gene mutations database: 2012 update. Hum Mutat 33:887–894. https://doi.org/10.1002/humu.22046

He X, Li W, Wu H et al (2019) Novel homozygous CFAP69 mutations in humans and mice cause severe asthenoteratospermia with multiple morphological abnormalities of the sperm flagella. J Med Genet 56:96–103. https://doi.org/10.1136/jmedgenet-2018-105486

Hu SC, Ye J, Fathi AK et al (2012) Mutations in NR5A1 and PIN1 associated with idiopathic hypogonadotropic hypogonadism. Genet Mol Res 11:4575–4584. https://doi.org/10.4238/2012.October.9.6

Imtiaz F, Allam R, Ramzan K, Al-Sayed M (2015) Variation in DNAH1 may contribute to primary ciliary dyskinesia. BMC Med Genet 16:14. https://doi.org/10.1186/s12881-015-0162-5

Jungwirth A, Giwercman A, Tournaye H et al (2012) European Association of Urology guidelines on Male Infertility: the 2012 update. Eur Urol 62:324–332. https://doi.org/10.1016/j.eururo.2012.04.048

Kamal A, Mansour R, Fahmy I et al (1999) Easily decapitated spermatozoa defect: a possible cause of unexplained infertility. Hum Reprod 14:2791–2795

Kasak L, Punab M, Nagirnaja L et al (2018) Bi-allelic recessive loss-of-function variants in FANCM cause non-obstructive azoospermia. Am J Hum Genet 103:200–212. https://doi.org/10.1016/j.ajhg.2018.07.005

Kerem B, Rommens JM, Buchanan JA et al (1989) Identification of the cystic fibrosis gene: genetic analysis. Science 245:1073–1080

Khan MJ, Pollock N, Jiang H et al (2018) X-linked ADGRG2 mutation and obstructive azoospermia in a large Pakistani family. Sci Rep 8:16280. https://doi.org/10.1038/s41598-018-34262-5

Kherraf Z-E, Amiri-Yekta A, Dacheux D et al (2018) A homozygous ancestral SVA-insertion-mediated deletion in WDR66 induces multiple morphological abnormalities of the sperm flagellum and male infertility. Am J Hum Genet 103:400–412. https://doi.org/10.1016/j.ajhg.2018.07.014

Krausz C (2012) An encore for the repeats: new insights into an old genetic variant. J Clin Endocrinol Metab 97:764–767
Krausz C, Casamonti E (2017) Spermatogenic failure and the Y chromosome. Hum Genet 136 (5):637–655. https://doi.org/10.1007/s00439-017-1793-8
Krausz C, Chianese C (2014) Genetic testing and counselling for male infertility. Curr Opin Endocrinol Diabetes Obes 21:244–250. https://doi.org/10.1097/MED.0000000000000058
Krausz C, Riera-Escamilla A (2018) Genetics of male infertility. Nat Rev Urol 15(6):369–384. https://doi.org/10.1038/s41585-018-0003-3
Krausz C, Hoefsloot L, Simoni M, Tuttelmann F (2014) EAA/EMQN best practice guidelines for molecular diagnosis of Y-chromosomal microdeletions: state-of-the-art 2013. Andrology 2:5–19. https://doi.org/10.1111/j.2047-2927.2013.00173.x
Krausz C, Riera-Escamilla A, Chianese C et al (2019) From exome analysis in idiopathic azoospermia to the identification of a high-risk subgroup for occult Fanconi anemia. Genet Med Genet Med 21(1):189–194. https://doi.org/10.1038/s41436-018-0037-1
Kuentz P, Van den Meerschaut F, Elinati E et al (2013) Assisted oocyte activation overcomes fertilization failure in globozoospermic patients regardless of the DPY19L2 status. Hum Reprod 28:1054–1061. https://doi.org/10.1093/humrep/det005
Lewis-Jones I, Aziz N, Seshadri S et al (2003) Sperm chromosomal abnormalities are linked to sperm morphologic deformities. Fertil Steril 79:212–215
Li W, He X, Yang S et al (2019) Biallelic mutations of CFAP251 cause sperm flagellar defects and human male infertility. J Hum Genet 64:49–54. https://doi.org/10.1038/s10038-018-0520-1
McCallum T, Milunsky J, Munarriz R et al (2001) Unilateral renal agenesis associated with congenital bilateral absence of the vas deferens: phenotypic findings and genetic considerations. Hum Reprod 16:282–288
Mongan NP, Tadokoro-Cuccaro R, Bunch T, Hughes IA (2015) Androgen insensitivity syndrome. Best Pract Res Clin Endocrinol Metab 29:569–580. https://doi.org/10.1016/j.beem.2015.04.005
Nenonen HA, Giwercman A, Hallengren E, Giwercman YL (2011) Non-linear association between androgen receptor CAG repeat length and risk of male subfertility–a meta-analysis. Int J Androl 34:327–332. https://doi.org/10.1111/j.1365-2605.2010.01084.x
Nistal M, Paniagua R, Herruzo A (1977) Multi-tailed spermatozoa in a case with asthenospermia and teratospermia. Virchows Arch B Cell Pathol 26:111–118
Oates RD, Amos JA (1994) The genetic basis of congenital bilateral absence of the vas deferens and cystic fibrosis. J Androl 15:1–8
Obermann H, Samalecos A, Osterhoff C et al (2003) HE6, a two-subunit heptahelical receptor associated with apical membranes of efferent and epididymal duct epithelia. Mol Reprod Dev 64:13–26. https://doi.org/10.1002/mrd.10220
Okutman O, Muller J, Baert Y et al (2015) Exome sequencing reveals a nonsense mutation in TEX15 causing spermatogenic failure in a Turkish family. Hum Mol Genet 24:5581–5588. https://doi.org/10.1093/hmg/ddv290
Patat O, Pagin A, Siegfried A et al (2016) Truncating mutations in the adhesion G protein-coupled receptor G2 gene ADGRG2 cause an X-linked congenital bilateral absence of vas deferens. Am J Hum Genet 99:437–442. https://doi.org/10.1016/j.ajhg.2016.06.012
Philibert P, Zenaty D, Lin L et al (2007) Mutational analysis of steroidogenic factor 1 (NR5a1) in 24 boys with bilateral anorchia: a French collaborative study. Hum Reprod 22:3255–3261. https://doi.org/10.1093/humrep/dem278
Porcu G, Mercier G, Boyer P et al (2003) Pregnancies after ICSI using sperm with abnormal head-tail junction from two brothers: case report. Hum Reprod 18:562–567
Quinton R, Cheow HK, Tymms DJ et al (1999) Kallmann's syndrome: is it always for life? Clin Endocrinol 50:481–485
Raivio T, Falardeau J, Dwyer A et al (2007) Reversal of idiopathic hypogonadotropic hypogonadism. N Engl J Med 357:863–873. https://doi.org/10.1056/NEJMoa066494
Rajender S, Singh L, Thangaraj K (2007) Phenotypic heterogeneity of mutations in androgen receptor gene. Asian J Androl 9:147–179. https://doi.org/10.1111/j.1745-7262.2007.00250.x

Ray PF, Toure A, Metzler-Guillemain C et al (2017) Genetic abnormalities leading to qualitative defects of sperm morphology or function. Clin Genet 91:217–232. https://doi.org/10.1111/cge.12905

Ribeiro RS, Vieira TC, Abucham J (2007) Reversible Kallmann syndrome: report of the first case with a KAL1 mutation and literature review. Eur J Endocrinol 156:285–290. https://doi.org/10.1530/eje.1.02342

Riordan JR, Rommens JM, Kerem B et al (1989) Identification of the cystic fibrosis gene: cloning and characterization of complementary DNA. Science 245:1066–1073

Ropke A, Tewes A-C, Gromoll J et al (2013) Comprehensive sequence analysis of the NR5A1 gene encoding steroidogenic factor 1 in a large group of infertile males. Eur J Hum Genet 21:1012–1015. https://doi.org/10.1038/ejhg.2012.290

Schimmer BP, White PC (2010) Minireview: steroidogenic factor 1: its roles in differentiation, development, and disease. Mol Endocrinol 24:1322–1337. https://doi.org/10.1210/me.2009-0519

Sha Y, Yang X, Mei L et al (2017a) DNAH1 gene mutations and their potential association with dysplasia of the sperm fibrous sheath and infertility in the Han Chinese population. Fertil Steril 107:1312–1318.e2. https://doi.org/10.1016/j.fertnstert.2017.04.007

Sha Y-W, Wang X, Xu X et al (2017b) Novel mutations in CFAP44 and CFAP43 cause multiple morphological abnormalities of the sperm flagella (MMAF). Reprod Sci. https://doi.org/10.1177/1933719117749756

Sha Y, Zheng L, Ji Z et al (2018a) A novel TEX11 mutation induces azoospermia: a case report of infertile brothers and literature review. BMC Med Genet 19:63. https://doi.org/10.1186/s12881-018-0570-4

Sha Y-W, Xu X, Ji Z-Y et al (2018b) Genetic contribution of SUN5 mutations to acephalic spermatozoa in Fujian China. Gene 647:221–225. https://doi.org/10.1016/j.gene.2018.01.035

Sha Y-W, Wang X, Xu X et al (2019) Biallelic mutations in PMFBP1 cause acephalic spermatozoa. Clin Genet 95:277–286. https://doi.org/10.1111/cge.13461

Shang Y, Zhu F, Wang L et al (2017) Essential role for SUN5 in anchoring sperm head to the tail. Elife 6. https://doi.org/10.7554/eLife.28199

Skaletsky H, Kuroda-Kawaguchi T, Minx PJ et al (2003) The male-specific region of the human Y chromosome is a mosaic of discrete sequence classes. Nature 423:825–837. https://doi.org/10.1038/nature01722

Tang S, Wang X, Li W et al (2017) Biallelic mutations in CFAP43 and CFAP44 cause male infertility with multiple morphological abnormalities of the sperm flagella. Am J Hum Genet 100:854–864. https://doi.org/10.1016/j.ajhg.2017.04.012

Tournaye H, Krausz C, Oates RD (2016) Novel concepts in the aetiology of male reproductive impairment. Lancet Diabetes Endocrinol 5(7):544–553. https://doi.org/10.1016/S2213-8587(16)30040-7

Tuttelmann F, Ruckert C, Ropke A (2018) Disorders of spermatogenesis: perspectives for novel genetic diagnostics after 20 years of unchanged routine. Med Genet 30:12–20. https://doi.org/10.1007/s11825-018-0181-7

Vogt PH, Edelmann A, Kirsch S et al (1996) Human Y chromosome azoospermia factors (AZF) mapped to different subregions in Yq11. Hum Mol Genet 5:933–943

Vorona E, Zitzmann M, Gromoll J et al (2007) Clinical, endocrinological, and epigenetic features of the 46,XX male syndrome, compared with 47,XXY Klinefelter patients. J Clin Endocrinol Metab 92:3458–3465. https://doi.org/10.1210/jc.2007-0447

Wambergue C, Zouari R, Fourati Ben Mustapha S et al (2016) Patients with multiple morphological abnormalities of the sperm flagella due to DNAH1 mutations have a good prognosis following intracytoplasmic sperm injection. Hum Reprod 31:1164–1172. https://doi.org/10.1093/humrep/dew083

Wang X, Jin H, Han F et al (2017) Homozygous DNAH1 frameshift mutation causes multiple morphological anomalies of the sperm flagella in Chinese. Clin Genet 91:313–321. https://doi.org/10.1111/cge.12857

Wang X, Jin H-R, Cui Y-Q et al (2018) Case study of a patient with cryptozoospermia associated with a recessive TEX15 nonsense mutation. Asian J Androl 20:101–102
Wu Q-Y, Li N, Li W-W et al (2014) Clinical, molecular and cytogenetic analysis of 46, XX testicular disorder of sex development with SRY-positive. BMC Urol 14:70. https://doi.org/10.1186/1471-2490-14-70
Yang F, Silber S, Leu NA et al (2015) TEX11 is mutated in infertile men with azoospermia and regulates genome-wide recombination rates in mouse. EMBO Mol Med 7:1198–1210. https://doi.org/10.15252/emmm.201404967
Yang B, Wang J, Zhang W et al (2017) Pathogenic role of ADGRG2 in CBAVD patients replicated in Chinese population. Andrology 5:954–957. https://doi.org/10.1111/andr.12407
Yang Y, Guo J, Dai L et al (2018) XRCC2 mutation causes meiotic arrest, azoospermia and infertility. J Med Genet 55:628–636. https://doi.org/10.1136/jmedgenet-2017-105145
Yatsenko AN, Georgiadis AP, Ropke A et al (2015) X-linked TEX11 mutations, meiotic arrest, and azoospermia in infertile men. N Engl J Med 372:2097–2107. https://doi.org/10.1056/NEJMoa1406192
Yeh S, Tsai M-Y, Xu Q et al (2002) Generation and characterization of androgen receptor knockout (ARKO) mice: an in vivo model for the study of androgen functions in selective tissues. Proc Natl Acad Sci U S A 99:13498–13503. https://doi.org/10.1073/pnas.212474399
Yin H, Ma H, Hussain S et al (2019) A homozygous FANCM frameshift pathogenic variant causes male infertility. Genet Med 21:62–70. https://doi.org/10.1038/s41436-018-0015-7
Yu J, Chen Z, Ni Y, Li Z (2012) CFTR mutations in men with congenital bilateral absence of the vas deferens (CBAVD): a systemic review and meta-analysis. Hum Reprod 27:25–35. https://doi.org/10.1093/humrep/der377
Zare-Abdollahi D, Safari S, Mirfakhraie R et al (2015) Mutational screening of the NR5A1 in azoospermia. Andrologia 47:395–401. https://doi.org/10.1111/and.12274
Zhang Y-X, Li H-Y, He W-B et al (2019) XRCC2 mutation causes premature ovarian insufficiency as well as non-obstructive azoospermia in humans. Clin Genet 95(3):442–443
Zhu F, Wang F, Yang X et al (2016) Biallelic SUN5 mutations cause autosomal-recessive acephalic spermatozoa syndrome. Am J Hum Genet 99:942–949. https://doi.org/10.1016/j.ajhg.2016.08.004
Zhu F, Liu C, Wang F et al (2018) Mutations in PMFBP1 cause acephalic spermatozoa syndrome. Am J Hum Genet 103:188–199. https://doi.org/10.1016/j.ajhg.2018.06.010

Chapter 17
Genetic Causes of Female Infertility

Artur Beke

Abstract Nowadays, women's family planning intentions are postponed, and it is common that only later will the conditions be created for the woman to have children. Fortunately, in most cases, pregnancy is possible in this case, taking into account the increased genetic risk. However, this later childbirth may become impossible or significantly more difficult if we can detect sterility and infertility, and its genetic cause is revealed. Any procedure that can help to reduce the "aging" of society, the reproduction rate, must be treated as an important public health issue. It would be particularly important in cases where genetic causes can be detected in the background of female sterility and infertility. Endocrine causes, infections, immunological causes, psychic factors, stress, and weight problems may be among the causes of female infertility in addition to genetic causes and genetic developmental disorders. Infertility can also be caused by iatrogenic factors, previous interventions, and surgery. In this chapter we will discuss the diseases in which genetic factors play a role.

Keywords Female infertility · Sterility · Genetic causes · Monogenic forms

List of Abbreviations

AMH	Anti-Müllerian hormone
DSD	Disorder of sex development
FMR1	Fragile X mental retardation 1
GWAS	Genome-wide association study
HCG	Human chorionic gonadotropin
LH	Luteinizing hormone
PCOS	Polycystic ovary syndrome
POF	Premature ovarian failure

A. Beke (✉)
Department of Obstetrics and Gynecology, Semmelweis University, Budapest, Hungary
e-mail: beke.artur@med.semmelweis-univ.hu

P. Igaz, A. Patócs (eds.), *Genetics of Endocrine Diseases and Syndromes*,
Experientia Supplementum 111, https://doi.org/10.1007/978-3-030-25905-1_17

POI Premature ovarian insufficiency
SRY Sex-determining region Y

17.1 Introduction

The World Health Organization (WHO) defines infertility as "a disease of the reproductive system defined by the failure to achieve a clinical pregnancy after 12 months or more of regular unprotected sexual intercourse." In 85–90% of healthy couples, pregnancy occurs within 1 year with regular sex life.

According to the WHO, we are talking about primary infertility when a woman is not able to conceive (a woman is unable to ever bear a child), while secondary infertility is a condition when pregnancy has already occurred before (previous pregnancy or ability to carry a pregnancy to a live birth), but after which infertility develops (inability to become pregnant or to carry a pregnancy to a live birth) (WHO 1991).

Endocrine causes, infections, immunological causes, psychic factors, stress, and body weight problems can be the cause of female infertility in addition to genetic causes and genetic developmental disorders. Infertility can be caused by iatrogenic factors, previous interventions, and surgery (Shah et al. 2003). With age, the proportion of women with age-related infertility increases (ACOG 2014).

According to an earlier study by the World Health Organization (WHO), processing data from 8500 infertile couples in developed countries, female infertility can be found in 37% of the cases and male infertility in 8%, and in 35% male and female factors coexist in infertile couples. Twenty percent of the couples had no detectable cause of infertility, or pregnancy was established during the study.

In developed countries 24.8% of cases, ovulation disorders, in 5.7% endometriosis and in 12.4% pelvic adhesions, were found to be the cause of female infertility. In 22% of cases, infertility was due to fallopian tube pathologies (i.e., tubal obstruction in half of the cases). In 6.7% of cases, hyperprolactinemia was detected (WHO 1992).

In this chapter we will discuss the aspects in which genetic factors play a role.

17.2 Genes Involved in the Development of Female Genitals

Genes present in both sexes (*NR5A1*, *RSPO1*, *WNT4*, *NROB1*) play an important role in the development and formation of the genitals. In the presence of the Y chromosome, the *SOX9 gene*—activated by the *SRY* (sex-determining region Y) gene—plays a decisive role in blocking the function of *FOXL2* (forkhead box L2) and *WNT4* genes and promoting *FGF9* (fibroblast growth factor) and *AMH* (anti-Müllerian hormone) production. In the absence of SRY, the *NROB1* and *FOXL2* genes are relevant, and the function of the *SOX9* (SRY-related HMG-BOX gene 9) gene is blocked. Genes involved in development may affect female fertility.

The *SRY* gene is a testis determinant gene that triggers male development. Its mutation leads to Swyer syndrome, with gonadal dysgenesis and disorder of sex development (DSD). It results in insufficient initial follicle count (De Vos et al. 2010).

The *NR5A1* gene (formerly *SF-1* gene) plays a role in the production of *steroidogenic factor-1 (SF1)* transcription factor, which regulates many genes responsible for the activity of the adrenal and reproductive systems. It participates in the determination of sex as a transcriptional activator. Its mutation leads to Swyer syndrome and acute adrenal insufficiency, and 46,XX gonadal dysgenesis may occur (Bashamboo et al. 2009). Missense, frameshift, and in-frame mutations of the *NR5A1* gene can also lead to ovarian developmental and functional disorders. It causes 46,XY gonadal dysgenesis or sexual development disorder and 46,XX early ovarian depletion. Typically, it shows autosomal recessive inheritance, but in the study published by Lourenco of four families examined, three families were shown to have a dominant inheritance pattern and one family with recessive inheritance (Lourenço et al. 2009).

The SRY protein complexes with the *SF1* protein that acts as a transcription factor that enhances the production of other transcription factors, in particular the transcription of the *SOX9* gene. SOX9 induces the formation of the testis from the indifferent gonade during sex differentiation during the so-called *SOX9* autoregulation loop-induced process. SOX9 activates the *FGF9* (fibroblast growth factor 9) gene, which encodes the glia-activating factor protein, enhances the expression of SOX9 by positive feedback, and plays an important role in the development of Sertoli cells and blocks the WNT4 signaling pathway. The mutation of the gene causes a skeletal system disorder syndrome (camptomelic dysplasia), often associated with autosomal DSD and cleft palate (Dixon et al. 2011). Deletions and point mutations of SOX9 have been linked to the Pierre Robin sequences (Benko et al. 2009).

The *RSPO1* (R-spondin 1) gene as a ligand of the LGR4 receptor (leucine-rich repeat-containing G-protein coupled receptor 4) regulates and activates the *WNT4* signaling pathways. It plays an important role in ovarian development. By suppressing the *SOX9* gene, it contributes to the inhibition of male sex formation. As a result of its mutation, disorder of sex development (DSD) and palmoplantar hyperkeratosis can occur (Parma et al. 2006).

The *WNT4* (Wnt family member 4, formerly wingless-type MMTV integration site family, member 4) gene plays a role in the differentiation of cells and regulation of female development during embryogenesis. It affects the development of the uterus and the fallopian tubes. It is the determinant of the female sex. By suppressing the *SOX9* gene, it contributes to the inhibition of male sex formation. As an effect of this, the Müllerian ducts develop to form the uterus and uterine tubes. It is also involved in ovarian protection and follicular survival. The mutation of the *WNT4* gene may result in Mayer-Rokitansky-Küster-Hauser (MRKH) syndrome, which involves vaginal aplasia and abnormality of the Müllerian ducts (Chen et al. 2011a; Biason-Lauber et al. 2004).

The *FOXL2* gene is responsible for the female gonadogenesis as a transcription factor and has a postnatal role in the development of the ovaries; moreover, it is therefore a determining factor for female fertility. The inhibition of the *SOX9* gene prevents the male sex from developing. At its mutation, BPES (blepharophimosis-ptosis-epicanthus inversus syndrome) type I may develop, which is associated with premature ovarian insufficiency or BPES type II, where no POI is present. This disease shows autosomal dominant inheritance (Fraser et al. 1988; Mduri et al. 2010).

The cell type and promoter-dependent coactivator and corepressor of *NR5A1 (SF1)* gene is a regulatory molecule encoded by the *NR0B1* (nuclear receptor subfamily 1 group B member 1—formerly *DAX1*) gene. Its deletion was described in 46,XX DSD cases. Other functional loss-causing mutations were associated with congenital adrenal hypoplasia and hypogonadotropic hypogonadism.

17.3 Hypothalamic/Pituitary Infertility

One form of hypogonadotropic hypogonadism results from the inhibition of the pulsatile secretion of the gonadotropin-releasing hormone (GnRH). Reasons include excessive workout, eating disorders, weight loss, and stress. When women affected by hypothalamic amenorrhea were compared to controls, genetic variants were identified in many genes, suggesting genetic predisposition. In addition to the mutations of the *GNRHR gene* encoding the *GnRH receptor*, mutations of the various genes causing Kallmann syndrome have been identified. Hypothalamic hypogonadism is dealt with in more detail in Chap. 16 (Table 16.1). Six subtypes of Kallmann's syndrome are known. Here only mutations in the major genes responsible for the migration of GnRH-secreting neurons are mentioned. Mutations in the *KAL1* (Kallmann syndrome interval gene 1) gene encoding the anosmin 1 protein cause X-linked recessive hereditary disease (type 1). Mutations of the *FGFR1* (fibroblast growth factor receptor 1) gene, which encodes the fibroblast growth factor receptor 1, are associated with autosomal dominant inheritance (type 2). In the case of mutation of the *PROKR2* (prokineticin receptor 2) gene encoding the prokineticin receptor 2, an autosomal recessive (rarely dominant) inheritance can be observed (type 3). The prokineticin 2 protein is important for the development of the olfactory bulb, and for migration of GnRH neurons, an autosomal recessive (rarely dominant) inheritance pattern can be observed (type 4). In addition, type 5 can be distinguished, where mutations of the *CHD7* (encoding chromodomain helicase DNA-binding protein 7) gene have been detected and are responsible for the development of a complex developmental disorder (CHARGE syndrome—*c*oloboma, *h*eart defects, *a*tresia choanae, *r*etardation in growth, *g*enital anomalies, and *e*ar abnormality) showing an autosomal dominant inheritance pattern. In the case of mutations of fibroblast growth factor 8 *(FGF8* gene*)*, an autosomal dominant inheritance pattern can be observed (type 6).

17.4 Genes Involved in the Female Ovarian Cycle

The *TUBB8* (tubulin beta 8 class VIII) gene is required for proper follicular maturation. It encodes beta-tubulin unit of the microtubules. In the case of inherited or de novo mutations, follicular maturation processes cannot take place due to microtubule failure (Wang et al. 2018).

The expression of the *PADI6* (peptidylarginine deiminases type VI) gene is particularly high in the germinal vesicles of the oocytes in metaphase I and II and in the granulosa cells. Xu Y et al. explored the relationship between the mutation of the *PADI6* gene, inadequate early embryonic development, and female infertility. In one individual case, a homozygous nonsense mutation and in two cases heterozygous mutations were detected. In addition to the lower PAD16 expression in the affected follicles, seven other genes were involved, and the reduced amount of phosphorylated RNA polymerase II was observed (Xu et al. 2016).

The expression of the *HOXA7* (homeobox A7) gene in the primordial follicles is almost absent, but it is expressed in mature follicles. This gene regulates the proliferative activity and maturation of the ovarian follicles. There are two ways to modulate the growth of granulosa cells: through the epidermal growth factor receptor *(EGRF)* and the pre-B cell leukemia transcription factor *2 (PBX2)* forming dimers bound to a specific promoter region (Zhang et al. 2010).

Prostaglandins (PGs) have been shown to be involved in female reproduction, and they are particularly important in ovulation and implantation. *PGE2* induces many genes, including *Areg*, *Ereg*, *Has2*, and *Tnfaip6*, which are important in ovulation. PGE2 reduces the viscosity of the extracellular matrix by increasing cAMP levels and reduces the phagocytic activity of polymorphonuclear neutrophils (PMN). It is important for the proper function of the sperm and increases the ability to attach to the egg. It activates cytokines that promote decidua and trophoblast adhesion (CXCL12 and also stimulates CXCR4 expression), which promotes implantation (Niringiyumukiza et al. 2018).

17.5 Disorders and Genetics of Fertilization and Implantation

The *MTHFR* (methylenetetrahydrofolate reductase) gene is important for the metabolism of folic acid and the formation of methionine, which is necessary for methylation of DNA, RNA, proteins, and lipids. In a study of 120 patients diagnosed with recurrent implantation failure (RIF), in two cases mutation of the *MTHFR* gene was found (A1298C, C677T) (Choi et al. 2016). Thymidylate synthase (TS) encoded by the *TS* (thymidylate synthase) gene catalyzes the conversion of deoxyuridine monophosphate (dUMP) to deoxytimidine monophosphate (dTMP), an important enzyme in DNA synthesis. A correlation with the risk of early repetitive implantation failure (RIF) has been identified (Choi et al. 2016).

The *HOXA10* and the *HOXA11* (homeobox A10 and homeobox A11) genes are expressed in the endometrial glands and stroma during the menstrual cycle. These two homeobox genes are essential for embryo implantation. They act as important transcription modulators that either activate or suppress target genes. These genes include *β3 integrin* and *EMX2*, which themselves play an important role in embryo implantation. Although no mutations of the *HOXA10* or *HOXA11* genes have been described in humans, it has been shown that the expression of the *HOXA10* and *HOXA11* was also lower in those with observed implantation disorders. This means that the expression of these genes is necessary for proper implantation (Taylor 2000). The reduced implantation capability has been studied in a number of gynecological diseases leading to infertility. These include endometriosis, polycystic ovary syndrome (PCOS), leiomyoma, and hydrosalpinx. Compared to controls, the expression of the *HOXA10* and *HOXA11* was reduced in each of these diseases (Du and Taylor 2015).

In *Hoxa10*-deficient mice, during implantation of their own embryos or wild-type mice embryos, the implantation may take place and the embryos remain viable, but in the complete absence of Hoxa, the implantation is missed. In *Hoxa10*-deficient mice, the uterus appears to be anatomically physiological, but histological abnormalities have been detected. The front of the uterus is characterized by the transformation of an oviduct-like structure. *Hoxa11* homozygous mutation mice are also infertile due to implantation errors. In these mice, the number of endometrial glands and the secretion of leukemia inhibitory factor (LIF) were reduced (Du and Taylor 2015).

Estrogen receptors encoded by the *ESR1* (estrogen receptor 1) gene are essential for sexual development and reproductive function, but they also play a role in maintaining the balance of bone metabolism. Estrogen receptors are also involved in pathological processes, including breast cancer, endometrial cancer, and osteoporosis. The *ESR1* gene, together with the mutations of the *HK3* (hexokinase 3) and the *BRSK1* (BR serine/threonine kinase 1) genes, caused premature ovarian insufficiency in Chinese, Korean, and Dutch, but not in Serbian women (Qin et al. 2014). Swaminathan et al. studied two frequently tested single nucleotide polymorphisms (SNPs) of the *ESR1* gene (PvuII and XbaI) in India in a female infertile population of 114 members and a matched control group of 115 members, with at least one child or without a history of infertility or abortion. It was found that the XbaI heterozygosity was significantly higher in the control group, so this polymorphism could be a protective factor (Swaminathan et al. 2016).

17.6 Premature Ovarian Insufficiency (POI)

Premature ovarian insufficiency (POI) (previously called premature ovarian failure—POF) is an ovarian defect featured by premature depletion of ovarian follicles before the age of 40 years, and it has become a major cause of female infertility.

In human females, the processes of ovarian follicular maturation and folliculogenesis are a to a large extent regulated mechanisms. Females in the developing ovary have about seven million primordial follicles during their intrauterine life at the 20th gestation week. Only about one million primordial follicles are present at birth. Most of the follicles will be lost by atresia during fetal and postnatal life. Normally 400–500 follicles are maturated before physiological menopause, but in females with POF disease, the event of the menopause is premature. That's why it's important to filter out the genetic causes as soon as possible.

Many review publications deal with monogenic forms of premature ovarian failure. Some of the authors classify the genes based on their chromosomal position (genes on chromosome X or Y, genes on autosomal chromosomes), or on their function, or on whether the mutation of a given gene causes a syndrome (Persani et al. 2010; Fortuño and Labarta 2014; Chapman et al. 2015; Tucker et al. 2016; Thakur et al. 2018). The most important (major) genes whose mutations are associated with the POI disease are summarized in Table 17.1.

Several genes have been implicated in association with the POI disease (translocation of *DIAPH2* gene; *BMP15* gene variant; *PGRMC1* variant; complex diseases such as galactosemia, ataxia and teleangiectasia; and isolated diseases such as FSH/LH resistance, GDF9 variant) of which the premutation of the *FMR1* gene (increase in CGG repeat number) occurs most frequently (3–15%) (Persani et al. 2010).

17.6.1 FMR1 *Premutation*

The most common gene mutation associated with POI (4–10%) is the premutation of the *FMR1* (fragile X mental retardation 1) gene, which belongs to the trinucleotide repeat disorders, similar to Huntington's disease, Friedreich's ataxia, the majority of spinocerebellar ataxias, and myotonic dystrophy type 1 (DM1). (Myotonic dystrophy type 2 (DM2) is the consequence of a tetranucleotide expansion.)

The background of the disease is the expansion of (CGG)n repeats in the promoter region of the *FMR1* gene. The *FMR1* gene is located on the Xq27.3 locus in the so-called POF1 region (Beke et al. 2013). In addition to the normal repeat number, two additional allele types can be distinguished:

1. The premutation allele, where the number of CGG triplets is 55–200. The premutation allele causes the premature ovarian insufficiency (POI) and tremor/ataxia syndrome (FXTAS) associated with fragile X disease.
2. The full mutation allele, where the number of CGG triplets is >200. The full mutation is responsible for the formation of the fragile X syndrome (Martin-Bell syndrome), a dominant X-linked inheritance, which is a form of X-linked mental retardation.

We distinguish a so-called gray zone (CGG repeat number: 41–54). Recent observations suggest that patients with this allele are also associated with the symptoms associated with the premutation allele.

The *FMR1* gene encodes the FMRP protein, which is an RNA binding protein and plays a significant role in RNA transport processes, stabilization of RNA molecules, and mRNA translation. The FMRP protein is expressed in all tissues but has been

Table 17.1 Genes associated with premature ovarian insufficiency (POI)

Gene abbreviation	Gene name	Chromosomal localization
POI-associated X chromosome genes		
POF1 region (Xq26.2-q28)		
PGRMC1	Progesterone receptor membrane component 1	
UBE2A	Ubiquitin-conjugating enzyme E2A	
XPNPEP2	X-Prolyl aminopeptidase (aminopeptidase P) 2, membrane-bound	
TDPF3	Transcription factor DP family member 3	
HS6ST2	Heparan sulfate 6-O-sulfotransferase 2	
GPC3	Glypican 3	
RBMX	RNA binding motif protein X-linked	
FMR1	Fragile X mental retardation 1	
FMR2	Fragile X mental retardation 2	
POF 2 region (Xq13.3-q22)		
DIAPH2	Diaphanous-related formin (diaphanous homolog 2)	
DACH2	Dachshund family transcription factor 2	
POF1B	Premature ovarian failure, 1B	
Other X-region		
BMP15	Bone morphogenetic protein 15	Xp11.2
DBX	DEAD (Asp-Glu-Ala-Asp) box helicase 3, X-linked	Xp11.23-p11.3
USP9X	Ubiquitin-specific peptidase 9 X-linked	Xp11.4
POI-associated autosomal genes		
AARS2	Alanyl-TRNA synthetase 2, mitochondrial	6p21.1
AIRE	Autoimmune regulator	21q22.3
BMP4	Bone morphogenetic protein 4	14q22.2
BMP7	Bone morphogenetic protein 7	20q13.31
BMPR1B	Bone morphogenetic protein receptor, type IB	4q22
C10orf2	Chromosome 10 open reading frame 2 (mtDNS helicase)	10q24.31
CPEB1	Cytoplasmic polyadenylation element binding protein 1	15q25.2
DAZL	Deleted in azoospermia-like	3p24
eIF2B2	Eukaryotic translation initiation factor 2B subunit beta	14q24.3
eIF2B4	Eukaryotic translation initiation factor 2B subunit delta	2p23.3
eIF2B5	Eukaryotic translation initiation factor 2B subunit epsilon	3q27.1
EIF4EN1F1	Eukaryotic translation initiation factor 4E nuclear import factor 1	22q12.2
FIGLA	Folliculogenesis-specific BHLH transcription factor	2p13.3
FOXL2	Forkhead Box L2	3q23
FSHR	Follicle-stimulating hormone receptor	2p21.p16
GALT	Galactose-1-phosphate uridylyltransferase	9p13
GDF9	Growth differentiation factor 9	5q23.3
HSD17B4	Hydroxysteroid 17-beta dehydrogenase 4	5q23.1
INHA	Inhibin A	2q35
LHCGR	Luteinizing hormone/choriogonadotropin receptor	2p16.3

(continued)

Table 17.1 (continued)

Gene abbreviation	Gene name	Chromosomal localization
LHX8	LIM homeobox 8	1p31.1
LMNA	Lamin A/C	1q22
MRPS22	Mitochondrial small ribosomal subunit protein MS22	3q23
NANOS3	Nanos homolog 3 (*Drosophila*)	19p13.12
NBN	Nibrin	8q21.3
NOBOX	Murine newborn ovary box	7q35
NR5A1 (SF-1)	Nuclear receptor subfamily 5A1	9q33.3
PMM1	Phosphomannomutase 1	22q13.2
PMM2	Phosphomannomutase 2	16p13.2
POLG	DNA polymerase gamma, catalytic subunit (mtDNS polymeráz)	15q26.1
RCBTB1	Regulator of chromosome condensation (RCC1) and BTB (POZ) domain containing protein 1	13q14.2
SALL4	Spalt-like transcription factor 4	20q13.2
SGO2	Shugoshin 2	2q33.1
SOHLH1	Spermatogenesis and oogenesis-specific basic helix-loop-helix 1	9q34.3
STAR	Steroidogenic acute regulatory protein	8p11.23

expressed in specific amounts in the brain, ovaries, and testes. The disease develops, beyond the expansion of the CGG repeat number, due to hypermethylation (Lyons et al. 2015; Verkerk et al. 1991; O'Donnel and Warren 2002).

In later generations, premutation can be transformed into a full mutation. This process, in which the number of cytosine-guanine-guanine (CGG) repeats increases, is called expansion. CGG repeats may include adenine-guanine-guanine (AGG) interruptions. These interruptions stabilize the gene and reduce the risk of expansion. The larger the size of the premutation allele, and the less AGG interruptions in its sequence, the greater the chances of a full mutation allele.

The premutation CGG repeat number of the *FMR1* gene in the case of paternal inheritance is inherited in the next generation with nearly the same number of repeats. In the cases we investigated, CGG repeat number being increased to a full mutation state was not detected in the progeny generation in the case of paternal inheritance. In the examined samples, both the girl and the boy (female and male) progeny were found to have a premutation status (Beke et al. 2018)

In the case of maternal inheritance, the full mutation status is more likely to occur in the offspring, depending on the premutation CGG number and the number of AGG interruptions. The difference between paternal and maternal inheritance is due to the difference in maturation between male and female gametes (Beke et al. 2018) (Fig. 17.1).

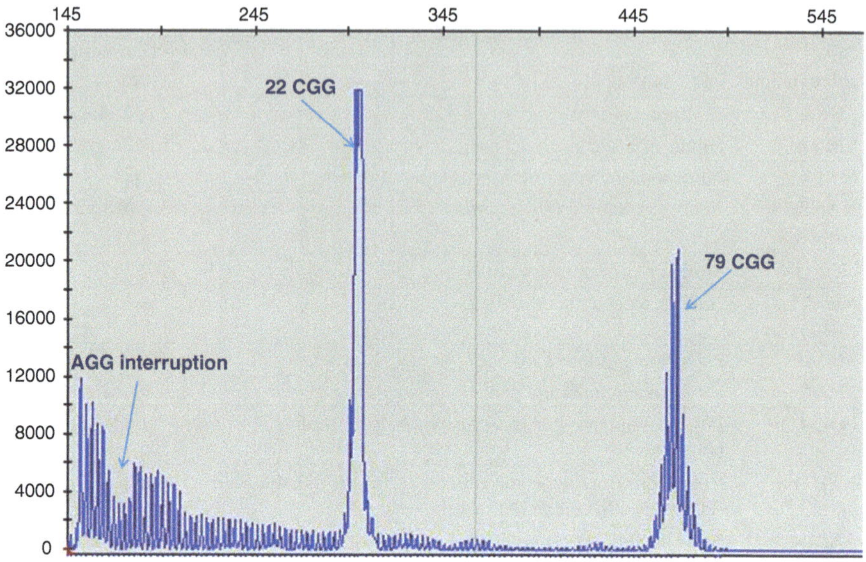

Fig. 17.1 Repeat-primed PCR (RP-PCR) result in a POI patient. The patient inherited the normal 22 CGG repeat number allele from the mother. The other allele was inherited from the father, where the paternal 75 CGG repeat number expanded to 79 was observed in the patient. There was no evidence of AGG interruptions in the father. The one AGG interruption is in accordance with the maternal allele. The patient's brother has full mutation (75→200 CGG repeat expansion) from paternal allele

Determining the number of AGG interruptions within the CGG repeats has a prominent role. If the number of AGG interruptions is 1 or 0, then the increase in CGG repeat number in the offspring should be taken into account, which, in any case with a gray zone carrier (41–54 CGG repetition number) mother, increases the risk of *FRAXA* premutation or full mutation (Beke et al. 2018)

If premutation of the *FMR1* gene is found in the background of premature ovarian insufficiency, the patient should be advised that genetic counseling is also recommended for the family members. It is also possible for a sister to have the disease, and the early detection of this will allow appropriate preventive treatments (e.g., egg freezing) before the symptoms occur. If a male relative (father, brother) carries the premutation of the *FMR1* gene, a neurological examination is recommended. In the case of pregnancy, prenatal diagnostic testing is important to exclude the possible full mutation fragile X mental retardation syndrome.

17.6.2 POI-Associated Syndromes

The following syndromes can be involved in the POI phenotype:

1. Turner syndrome which is an X chromosome aberration (see Chap. 20).
2. Fragile X syndrome (mentioned in Sect. 17.6.1).
3. Galactosemia which is an autosomal recessive disorder, and the prevalence of POI is 60–70% in female patients with galactosemia.
4. Blepharophimosis-ptosis-epicanthus inversus syndrome (BPES) which is an autosomal dominant disease.
5. Autoimmune polyendocrinopathy-candidiasis-ectodermal dystrophy (APECED)/autoimmune polyendocrine syndrome type 1 caused by mutation of the autoimmune regulator (*AIRE*) gene that can be associated with primary hypogonadism and ovarian insufficiency phenotype.
6. Steroidogenic enzyme defects that may involve several congenital enzyme defects and can disrupt estrogen synthesis resulting in a low estrogen level (Shelling 2010).

17.7 Polygenic Diseases Associated with Female Infertility

17.7.1 Polycystic Ovary Syndrome (PCOS)

Polycystic ovary syndrome (PCOS) is an extremely heterogeneous disease representing the most common cause of secondary amenorrhea in women, and the basis for its clinical diagnosis is hyperandrogenism, oligo-/anovulation, and ovarian polycystic morphology (Rotterdam criteria).

Several loci have been detected in PCOS that may be involved in the development of the disease. PCOS is a complex disease that also correlates with obesity, which is influenced by genetic factors as well (Chap. 19). In addition, environmental factors also play a role in the manifestation of the disease, such as diet and exercise.

Among the genetic alterations linked to PCOS, the following should be mentioned. Alterations of enzymes involved in steroid biosynthesis and metabolism, including the cholesterol side-chain cleavage enzyme catalyzing cholesterol-pregnenolone transformation, encoded by the *CYP11A* gene, and the 17α-hydroxylase/17,20-lyase enzyme encoded by the *CYP17* gene appear to be involved in the increased androgen production of the ovary. The increased steroid production in PCOS is also due to the increased activity of the 3β-hydroxysteroid dehydrogenase 2 enzyme encoded by the *HSD3B2* gene. Increased steroid production also extends to estrogen production. Androstenedione and testosterone produced in theca interna cells are converted to estrone and estradiol in granulosa cells by the aromatase enzyme encoded by the *CYP19*. The function of the theca interna cells is regulated by LH and the granulosa cells by FSH. Variants of the *CYP17* and *CYP19* genes have been associated with the development of PCOS (Park et al. 2008; Jin et al. 2009).

In addition to the ovaries, increased androgen production of the adrenal cortex is also involved in PCOS. Higher concentrations of peripheral dehydroepiandrosterone sulfate (DHEAS) could be detected in PCOS, presumably due to the increased function of the 17α-hydroxylase/17,20-lyase enzyme.

Disruption of cortisol metabolism may be also involved in the development of PCOS. The *steroid-5α-reductase 2* enzyme encoded by the *SRD5A2* gene converts cortisol to 5-α-dihydrocortisol in liver cells, thereby inactivating the biologically active hormone. Increased *5-α-reductase* activity was found in PCOS patients (Goodarzi et al. 2006). Another important enzyme in cortisol metabolism is the 11ß-hydroxysteroid dehydrogenase enzyme type 1 encoded by the *HSD11B1* gene. Its altered function has been linked to the adrenal androgenic hypersecretion that can be observed in PCOS (Grolmusz et al. 2014).

Hyperinsulinemia observed in PCOS stimulates ovarian androgen production. Insulin receptor (IR) encoded by the *INSR* gene and IRS-1 (insulin receptor substrate 1) signaling protein encoded by the *IRS-1* gene are serine-phosphorylated and inhibit insulin signaling, thereby causing insulin resistance and consequently hyperinsulinemia. Insulin and structurally very similar insulin-like growth factor-1 (IGF-1) stimulate LH-mediated androgen synthesis through their receptors. Insulin acts on follicular maturation, leading to early follicular atresia, contributing to the development of PCOS-specific anovulatory cycles (Dunaif 1997; Franks et al. 1992).

The function of the hypothalamus-pituitary-ovarian axis in PCOS is altered. One of the best-known neuroendocrine characteristic of the syndrome is the elevated LH/FSH ratio. High levels of LH contribute to the development of anovulatory cycles typical for PCOS and raise levels of ovarian androgen hormones. PCOS is characterized by an increased LH response to GnRH stimulation (increased sensitivity of LH production to GnRH), which may be associated with the presence of polymorphisms detected in the *LHCGR* (luteinizing hormone/choriogonadotropin receptor) gene encoding the LH receptor (Valkenburg et al. 2009).

Several GWAS (genome-wide association studies) have also been carried out which have contributed to our understanding of the genetic basis of PCOS. Chen et al. identified three loci: 2p16.3 (*LHCGR* gene), 2p21, and 9q33.3 (*DENND1A* gene) (Chen et al. 2011b). The *LHCGR* gene encodes the luteinizing hormone (LH) and human chorionic gonadotropin (HCG) receptors. The mutation of this gene is accompanied by increased LH, irregular menstruation, and lack of ovulation (anovulation), leading to infertility. The *DENND1A* (DENN domain containing 1A) gene is expressed in theca cells and is thought to play a role in steroidogenesis and contribute to hyperandrogenism in PCOS.

Shi et al. confirmed the role of these three loci in PCOS. In addition, eight other loci have been identified: 9q22.32, 11q22.1, 12q13.2, 12q14.3 (*HMGA2* gene), 16q12.1, 19p13.3 (*INSR* gene), 20q13.2, and 2p16.3.17 (*FSHR* gene) (Shi et al. 2012). Although the exact association of these with PCOS has not yet been proven, most of these genes play a role in reproductive hormone function, insulin signaling pathway, and type 2 diabetes. The *HMGA2* (high-mobility group AT-hook 2) gene encodes a protein that belongs to a non-histone chromosomal high-mobility group (HMG) and acts as a transcriptional regulatory factor, and its mutation plays a role in obesity.

In 2015, Lee et al. identified a new locus, 8q24.2, which is involved in *telomerase* activity and determines the length of the *telomer* (Lee et al. 2015). Shorter telomeres are also important in gluconeogenesis, mitochondrial metabolism, and pathogenesis of diabetes mellitus, all of which may play a role in PCOS. Hayes et al. identified two new loci: 11p14.1 which encodes the subunit of FSH-β and 8p23.1.28 where the *GATA4* (GATA binding protein 4) gene is involved as a *transcription factor* in gonadal function and steroidogenesis. The FDFT1 (farnesyl diphosphate farnesyl transferase) gene can also be found here, encoding the *farnesyl diphosphate farnesyl transferase*, which is necessary for the biosynthesis of cholesterol (Hayes et al. 2015).

Jones et al. showed the increased expression of the *STON1-GTF2A1L* gene and the *LHCGR* gene in non-obese patients and the decreased expression of the *INSR* gene in obese patients (Jones et al. 2015). This suggests that gene expression may differ between obese and non-obese patients and may contribute to the heterogeneity of PCOS.

17.7.2 Endometriosis

Endometriosis is known to play a role in the development of female infertility. The exact etiology of endometriosis is still unknown at present, with many factors contributing to its development. The first GWAS on endometriosis was conducted in Japan in 2010 including 1907 endometriosis patients and 5292 controls. It has been shown that the rs10965235 SNP of the *CDKN2B-AS* gene (locus 9p21) can be associated with the development of endometriosis. The gene is expressed in the uterus. The cyclin-dependent kinase inhibitor-2B-antisense RNA molecule, which is transcribed from this noncoding gene, was found to bind to messenger RNA transcribed from three tumor suppressor genes regulating cyclin kinases (*CDKN2*, cyclin-dependent kinase inhibitor 2A; *CDKN2B*, cyclin-dependent kinase inhibitor 2B; and *CDKN2A*, cyclin-dependent kinase inhibitor 2A). By regulating tumor suppressor protein function, the gene can also be associated with the development of several diseases, such as coronary diseases, diabetes mellitus, aortic aneurysm, cerebral aneurysm, and various tumors (melanoma, basal cell carcinoma, glioma). Hypermethylation of the promoter region of the gene and the described SNP may be associated with the development of endometriosis (Uno et al. 2010).

In addition, two SNPs within the *WNT4* gene (Wnt family member 1 or proto-oncogene Wnt-1 gene) have been associated with endometriosis; the gene was previously discussed in genes regulating female genital development (Uno et al. 2010). It is believed that the development of endometriosis can be explained by the abnormal development of female genital cells.

Among other genes associated with endometriosis, the *NFE2L3* (*nuclear factor, erythroid 2-like 3*) gene, expressed in the placenta of the *HOXA10* (homeobox A10) gene involved in uterine development, can also be mentioned (Painter et al. 2011). Based on their meta-analysis of eight GWAS studies, Rahmioglu et al. combined data of 11,506 cases and 32,678 controls (Rahmioglu et al. 2014). The *WNT4*,

GREB1 (growth-regulating estrogen receptor binding 1), *ID4* (inhibitor of DNA binding 4, HLH protein), *CDKN2BAS* (CDKN2B antisense RNA 1), and *VEZT* genes (vezatin, adherens junctions transmembrane protein) were considered to be of importance. The *GREB1* gene (growth-regulating estrogen receptor binding gene 1) is involved in the *estrogen* regulatory pathway.

The *ID4* gene (inhibitor of DNA binding 4, HLH protein) encodes the DNA-binding protein inhibitor ID4 protein involved in transcriptional control, which acts through the regulation of the *HOXA9* (homeobox A9) and the *CDKN1A* gene*s* (cyclin-dependent kinase inhibitor 1A). It plays a role in embryogenesis and has an enhanced expression in ovarian, endometrial, and breast cancers, in addition to other tumors. The *VEZT* gene (vezatin, adherens junctions transmembrane protein) encodes the component *of E-cadherin transmembrane protein*, which is essential for embryogenesis. The VEZT gene can also play a role in the regulation of cell migration and invasion, so it can contribute to the pathogenesis of endometriosis.

In the study conducted by De Conto et al., polymorphisms of the genes *GDF9* (growth differentiation factor 9), *AMHR2* (anti-Mullerian hormone receptor type 2), and *AMH* (anti-Mullerian hormone) were investigated, and neither the *GDF9* nor *AMHR2* gene polymorphism showed significant correlation with endometriosis; however, the *AMH* gene polymorphism was associated with endometriosis-related infertility (De Conto et al. 2017).

17.8 Genetic Counseling for Infertility Testing

In the case of infertility, genetic counseling should take into account other obstetric, endocrinological, and infectological examinations (tests) that have been carried out previously and other possible causes identified earlier. Genetic counseling should be conducted accordingly.

Female genital malformations and disorders of ovulation, fertilization, and implantation are reasons for genetic testing if they can influence personalized treatment. Most of the abnormalities detected can be treated so that proper treatment of polycystic ovarian syndrome can lead to pregnancy, and no further genetic testing is required.

The vast majority of genetic testing may be due to suspicion of premature ovarian insufficiency (POI). Genetic counseling should also be personalized in this case, as in such cases where the patient may be confronted with the depletion of her total ovarian reserve (follicular depletion), pregnancy can only occur with egg donation. In the case of premature ovarian failure, other factors such as psychological factors, osteoporosis, and cardiovascular risk factors should also be taken into account due to early menopause. By predicting premature ovarian failure, the patient and the medical staff will be able to prepare in time, and, if appropriate, other interventions can help to achieve the desired pregnancy before the ovarian function stops (egg freezing).

Nowadays, women's family planning intentions are postponed, and it is common that only later will the conditions be created for a woman to have a child. Some of the infertile couples have a more advanced age, so these genetic risks should also be taken into account during genetic counseling.

Special aspects of genetic counseling in infertility should be taken into account if pregnancy occurs after infertility treatment and the way the pregnancy was established. Traditional-assisted reproduction procedures do not increase the risk of fetal, genetic abnormalities, but intracytoplasmatic sperm injections (ICSI), performed partly due to male infertility, may increase the risk of fetal chromosome aberrations according to literature data, and therefore genetic counseling in such cases is recommended.

References

American College of Obstetricians and Gynecologists (ACOG) (2014) Committee on Gynecologic Practice and Practice Committee. Female age-related fertility decline. Committee Opinion No. 589. Fertil Steril 101:633–634. https://doi.org/10.1016/j.fertnstert.2013.12.032

Bashamboo A, Ravel C, Brauner R, McElreavey K (2009) NR5A1 and ovarian failure. Med Sci (Paris) 25:809–813. https://doi.org/10.1051/medsci/20092510809

Beke A, Piko H, Haltrich I et al (2013) Molecular cytogenetic analysis of Xq critical regions in premature ovarian failure. Mol Cytogenet 20(62):1–8. https://doi.org/10.1186/1755-8166-6-62

Beke A, Piko H, Haltrich I, Karcagi V, Rigo J Jr, Molnar MJ, Fekete G (2018) Study of patterns of inheritance of premature ovarian failure syndrome carrying maternal and paternal premutations. BMC Med Genet 19:113, 1–113, 9. doi: https://doi.org/10.1186/s12881-018-0634-5

Benko S, Fantes JA, Amiel J et al (2009) Highly conserved non-coding elements on either side of SOX9 associated with Pierre Robin sequence. Nat Genet 41:359–364. https://doi.org/10.1038/ng.329

Biason-Lauber A, Konrad D, Navratil F, Schoenle EJ (2004) A WNT4 mutation associated with Müllerian-duct regression and virilization in a 46,XX woman. N Engl J Med 351:792–798

Chapman C, Cree L, Shelling AN (2015) The genetics of premature ovarian failure: current perspectives. Int J Womens Health 7:799–810. https://doi.org/10.2147/IJWH.S64024

Chen B, Suo P, Wang B et al (2011a) Mutation analysis of the WNT4 gene in Han Chinese women with premature ovarian failure. Reprod Biol Endocrinol 9:75. https://doi.org/10.1186/1477-7827-9-75

Chen ZJ, Zhao H, He L et al (2011b) Genome-wide association study identifies susceptibility loci for polycystic ovary syndrome on chromosome 2p16.3, 2p21 and 9q33.3. Nat Genet 43:55–59. https://doi.org/10.1038/ng.732

Choi Y, Kim JO, Shim SH et al (2016) Genetic variation of methylenetetrahydrofolate reductase (MTHFR) and thymidylate synthase (TS) genes is associated with idiopathic recurrent implantation failure. PLoS One 11(8):e0160884. https://doi.org/10.1371/journal.pone.0160884

De Conto E, Matte Ú, Bilibio JP, Genro VK, Souza CA, Leão DP, Cunha-Filho JS (2017) Endometriosis-associated infertility: GDF-9, AMH, and AMHR2 genes polymorphisms. J Assist Reprod Genet 34:1667–1672. https://doi.org/10.1007/s10815-017-1026-z

De Vos M, Devroey P, Fauser BC (2010) Primary ovarian insufficiency. Lancet 376:911–921. https://doi.org/10.1016/S0140-6736(10)60355-8

Dixon MJ, Marazita ML, Beaty TH, Murray JC (2011) Cleft lip and palate: understanding genetic and environmental influences. Nat Rev Genet 12:167–178. https://doi.org/10.1038/nrg2933

Du H, Taylor HS (2015) The role of hox genes in female reproductive tract development, adult function, and fertility. Cold Spring Harb Perspect Med 6(1):a023002. https://doi.org/10.1101/cshperspect.a023002

Dunaif A (1997) Insulin resistance and the polycystic ovary syndrome: mechanism and implications for pathogenesis. Endocr Rev 18:774–800

Fortuño C, Labarta E (2014) Genetics of primary ovarian insufficiency: a review. J Assist Reprod Genet 31:1573–1585. https://doi.org/10.1007/s10815-014-0342-9

Franks S, Gilling-Smith C, Watson H, Willis D (1992) Insulin action in the normal and polycystic ovary. Endocrinol Metab Clin N Am 28:361–378

Fraser IS, Shearman RP, Smith A, Russell P (1988) An association among blepharophimosis, resistant ovary syndrome, and true premature menopause. Fertil Steril 50:747–751

Goodarzi MO, Shah NA, Antoine HJ et al (2006) Variants in the 5alpha-reductase type 1 and type 2 genes are associated with polycystic ovary syndrome and the severity of hirsutism in affected women. J Clin Endocrinol Metab 91:4085–4091

Grolmusz VK, Acs OD, Feldman-Kovács K et al (2014) Genetic variants of the HSD11B1 gene promoter may be protective against polycystic ovary syndrome. Mol Biol Rep 41:5961–5969. https://doi.org/10.1007/s11033-014-3473-2

Hayes MG, Urbanek M, Ehrmann DA et al (2015) Reproductive Medicine Network. Genome-wide association of polycystic ovary syndrome implicates alterations in gonadotropin secretion in European ancestry populations. Nat Commun 6:7502. https://doi.org/10.1038/ncomms8502

Jin JL, Sun J, Ge HJ et al (2009) Association between CYP19 gene SNP rs2414096 polymorphism and polycystic ovary syndrome in Chinese women. BMC Med Genet 10:139. https://doi.org/10.1186/1471-2350-10-139

Jones MR, Brower MA, Xu N et al (2015) Systems genetics reveals the functional context of PCOS loci and identifies genetic and molecular mechanisms of disease heterogeneity. PLoS Genet 11 (08):e1005455. https://doi.org/10.1371/journal.pgen.1005455

Lee H, Oh JY, Sung YA, Chung HW (2015) Genome-wide association study identified new susceptibility loci for polycystic ovary syndrome. Hum Reprod 30:723–731. https://doi.org/10.1093/humrep/deu352

Lourenço D, Brauner R, Lin L et al (2009) Mutations in NR5A1 associated with ovarian insufficiency. N Engl J Med 360:1200–1210. https://doi.org/10.1056/NEJMoa0806228

Lyons JI, Kerr GR, Mueller PW (2015) Fragile X syndrome. Scientific background and screening technologies. J Mol Diagn 17:463–471. https://doi.org/10.1016/j.jmoldx.2015.04.006

Mduri G, Bachelot A, Duflos C et al (2010) FOXL2 mutations lead to different ovarian phenotypes in BPES patients: case report. Hum Reprod 25:235–243. https://doi.org/10.1093/humrep/dep355

Niringiyumukiza JD, Cai H, Xiang W (2018) Prostaglandin E2 involvement in mammalian female fertility: ovulation, fertilization, embryo development and early implantation. Reprod Biol Endocrinol 16:43. https://doi.org/10.1186/s12958-018-0359-5

O'Donnel TW, Warren ST (2002) A decade of molecular studies of fragile X syndrome. Annu Rev Neurosci 25:315–338

Painter JN, Anderson CA, Nyholt DR et al (2011) Genome-wide association study identifies a locus at 7p15.2 associated with endometriosis. Nat Genet 43:51–54. https://doi.org/10.1038/ng.731

Park JM, Lee EJ, Ramakrishna S, Cha DH, Baek KH (2008) Association study for single nucleotide polymorphisms in the CYP17A1 gene and polycystic ovary syndrome. Int J Mol Med 22:249–254

Parma P, Radi O, Vidal V et al (2006) R-spondin1 is essential in sex determination, skin differentiation and malignancy. Nat Genet 38:1304–1309

Persani L, Rossetti R, Cacciatore C (2010) Genes involved in human premature ovarian failure. J Mol Endocrinol 45:257–279. https://doi.org/10.1677/JME-10-0070

Qin Y, Vujovic S, Li G et al (2014) Ethnic specificity of variants of the ESR1, HK3, BRSK1 genes and the 8q22.3 locus: no association with premature ovarian failure (POF) in Serbian women. Maturitas 77:64–67. https://doi.org/10.1016/j.maturitas.2013.09.006

Rahmioglu N, Nyholt DR, Morris AP et al (2014) Genetic variants underlying risk of endometriosis: insights from meta-analysis of eight genome-wide association and replication datasets. Hum Reprod Update 20:702–716

Shah K, Sivapalan G, Gibbons N et al (2003) The genetic basis of infertility. Reproduction 126:13–25
Shelling AN (2010) Premature ovarian failure. Reproduction 140:633–641. https://doi.org/10.1530/REP-09-0567
Shi Y, Zhao H, Shi Y et al (2012) Genome-wide association study identifies eight new risk loci for polycystic ovary syndrome. Nat Genet 44:1020–1025. https://doi.org/10.1038/ng.2384
Swaminathan M, Ganesh V, Koshy T, Venugopal P, Paul S, Venkatesan V (2016) A study on the role of estrogen receptor gene polymorphisms in female infertility. Genet Test Mol Biomarkers 20:692–695
Taylor HS (2000) The role of HOX genes in the development and function of the female reproductive tract. Semin Reprod Med 18:81–89
Thakur M, Feldman G, Puscheck EE (2018) Primary ovarian insufficiency in classic galactosemia: current understanding and future research opportunities. J Assist Reprod Genet 35:3–16. https://doi.org/10.1007/s10815-017-1039-7
Tucker EJ, Grover SR, Bachelot A, Touraine P, Sinclair AH (2016) Premature ovarian insufficiency: new perspectives on genetic cause and phenotypic spectrum. Endocr Rev 37:609–635
Uno S, Zembutsu H, Hirasawa A et al (2010) A genome-wide association study identifies genetic variants in the CDKN2BAS locus associated with endometriosis in Japanese. Nat Genet 42:707–710. https://doi.org/10.1038/ng.612
Valkenburg O, Uitterlinden AG, Piersma D et al (2009) Genetic polymorphisms of GnRH and gonadotrophic hormone receptors affect the phenotype of polycystic ovary syndrome. Hum Reprod 24:2014–2022. https://doi.org/10.1093/humrep/dep113
Verkerk AJ, Pieretti M, Sutcliffe JS et al (1991) Identification of a gene (FMR1) containing a CGG repeat coincident with a breakpoint cluster region exhibiting length variation in fragile X syndrome. Cell 65:905–914
Wang AC, Zhang YS, Wang BS et al (2018) Mutation analysis of the TUBB8 gene in primary infertile women with arrest in oocyte maturation. Gynecol Endocrinol 34:900–904. https://doi.org/10.1080/09513590.2018.1464138
WHO Technical Report Series. Recent Advances in Medically Assisted Conception Number 820 (1992) pp 1–111
WHO/MCH (1991) Infertility: a tabulation of available data on primary and secondary infertility. WHO, Geneva
Xu Y, Shi Y, Fu J et al (2016) Mutations in PADI6 cause female infertility characterized by early embryonic arrest. Am J Hum Genet 99:744–752. https://doi.org/10.1016/j.ajhg.2016.06.024
Zhang Y, Huang Q, Cheng JC, Nishi Y, Yanase T, Huang HF, Leung PC (2010) Homeobox A7 increases cell proliferation by up-regulation of epidermal growth factor receptor expression in human granulosa cells. Reprod Biol Endocrinol 8:61. https://doi.org/10.1186/1477-7827-8-61

Chapter 18
Monogenic Forms of Diabetes Mellitus

Zsolt Gaál and István Balogh

Abstract In addition to the common types of diabetes mellitus, two major monogenic diabetes forms exist. Maturity-onset diabetes of the young (MODY) represents a heterogenous group of monogenic, autosomal dominant diseases. MODY accounts for 1–2% of all diabetes cases, and it is not just underdiagnosed but often misdiagnosed to type 1 or type 2 diabetes. More than a dozen MODY genes have been identified to date, and their molecular classification is of great importance in the correct treatment decision and in the judgment of the prognosis. The most prevalent subtypes are *HNF1A*, *GCK*, and *HNF4A*. Genetic testing for MODY has changed recently due to the technological advancements, as contrary to the sequential testing performed in the past, nowadays all MODY genes can be tested simultaneously by next-generation sequencing. The other major group of monogenic diabetes is neonatal diabetes mellitus which can be transient or permanent, and often the diabetes is a part of a syndrome. It is a severe monogenic disease appearing in the first 6 months of life. The hyperglycemia usually requires insulin. There are two forms, permanent neonatal diabetes mellitus (PNDM) and transient neonatal diabetes mellitus (TNDM). In TNDM, the diabetes usually reverts within several months but might relapse later in life. The incidence of NDM is 1:100,000–1:400,000 live births, and PNDM accounts for half of the cases. Most commonly, neonatal diabetes is caused by mutations in *KCNJ11* and *ABCC8* genes encoding the ATP-dependent potassium channel of the β cell. Neonatal diabetes has experienced a quick and successful transition into the clinical practice since the discovery of the molecular background. In case of both genetic diabetes groups, recent guidelines recommend genetic testing.

Keywords Maturity-onset diabetes of the young · Neonatal diabetes mellitus · Autosomal dominant

Z. Gaál
4th Department of Medicine, Jósa András Teaching Hospital, Nyíregyháza, Hungary

I. Balogh (✉)
Division of Clinical Genetics, Department of Laboratory Medicine, Faculty of Medicine, University of Debrecen, Debrecen, Hungary
e-mail: balogh@med.unideb.hu

P. Igaz, A. Patócs (eds.), *Genetics of Endocrine Diseases and Syndromes*,
Experientia Supplementum 111, https://doi.org/10.1007/978-3-030-25905-1_18

List of Abbreviations

CEL	Carboxyl ester lipase
CRP	C-reactive protein
GCK	Glucokinase
GDM	Gestational diabetes mellitus
HNF1A	Hepatocyte nuclear factor 1A
HNF1B	Hepatocyte nuclear factor 1B
HNF4A	Hepatocyte nuclear factor 4A
MODY	Maturity-onset diabetes of the young
NDM	Neonatal diabetes mellitus
NGS	Next-generation sequencing
OMIM	Online Mendelian Inheritance in Man
PNDM	Permanent neonatal diabetes mellitus
TNDM	Transient neonatal diabetes mellitus

18.1 Introduction

Monogenic forms of diabetes mellitus are composed of two major group of disorders, maturity-onset diabetes of the young and neonatal diabetes. Each of these diseases has its own speciality, symptoms, age of onset, molecular background, and treatment options. Many of the monogenic diabetes genes are transcription factors. In the next sections, genetics of the maturity-onset diabetes of the young (MODY) and the genetics of neonatal diabetes are discussed in details.

Cammidge wrote in 1928 by analyzing diabetic pedigrees: "...it might well be that it behaved as a dominant, for with a dominant character (1) all the affected individuals have an affected parent; (2) in families where both affected and unaffected occur their numbers are, on the average, equal; (3) none of the unaffected, although springing from affected parents, have affected descendants," giving an accurate presentation of a dominantly transmitted diabetes (Cammidge 1928). Later, Fajans and Tattersall coined the term "maturity-onset diabetes of the young, MODY," and set the major criteria that are still in use:

1. Age of onset of diabetes in young adulthood, before 25 years.
2. Inheritance is autosomal dominant.
3. The lack of insulin deficiency during the early phase of the disease (Fajans and Conn 1960; Tattersall 1974).

1–2% of all diabetic cases are of monogenic causes (Edghill et al. 2008). Prevalence of the subtypes shows high degree of variability, which is at least partly due to the selection criteria used for patient recruitment. Approximately 80% of MODY patients are misdiagnosed as type 1 or type 2 diabetes (Shields et al. 2010). To reach the correct, molecular diagnosis, it might take as long as 10 years

(Thanabalasingham et al. 2012). In a high proportion of the patients, once the genetic diagnosis identifies the molecular background of the disease, the treatment is usually changed or even stopped, depending on the subtype (Shepherd et al. 2018). Major characteristics of the most common MODY subtypes in comparison with type 1 and type 2 diabetes mellitus are shown in Table 18.1.

18.2 The Role of MODY-Causing Transcription Factors in Pancreas Physiology

Both the embryonic development of the pancreas and its adaptation to the environmental challenges after birth are complex processes mediated by a concerted action of many transcription factors. The different cell types of the endocrine pancreas have well-defined roles in glucose homeostasis. The insulin-producing β cells and the glucagon-producing α cells are originated from a common early endocrine progenitor (van der Meulen and Huising 2015). Some of these transcription factors have a major role in the development of the organ, highlighted by the fact that their absence results in pancreas agenesis as exemplified by PDX1 (IPF1) (Jonsson et al. 1994; Stoffers et al. 1997b). Others are more involved in the lineage differentiation, as PAX4 and NEUROD1 (van der Meulen and Huising 2015). Their activity, however, is not restricted to the developmental processes. Fully differentiated β cells still require NEUROD1 and PDX1 (Ahlgren et al. 1998; Naya et al. 1997) for their proper functioning. PAX4-deficient mice lack β cells and die 3–5 days postpartum, i.e., due to hyperglycemia (Sosa-Pineda et al. 1997). During the development of the pancreas, PAX4 is expressed in every endocrine progenitor and later is required for the β cell development (Lorenzo et al. 2017). In adults, it is associated with increased β cell survival and implicated in β cell plasticity (Lorenzo et al. 2017). The available data about the role of PAX4 makes it a promising target for novel therapeutic approaches where regeneration of β cell mass would be the goal of the treatment (Lorenzo et al. 2017, 2018). PAX4 exerts its action by binding to promoters and enhancers in its target genes' sequences. Such sequences are present in glucagon, ghrelin, and insulin genes. Upon binding, inhibition occurs; thus, PAX4 is a repressor of these genes (Campbell et al. 1999; Petersen et al. 2000; Wang et al. 2008). The interaction of the pancreas-specific promoter of PAX4 with HNF1α, HNF4α, PDX1, and NEUROD1 sheds more light on the regulation of PAX4 expression (Smith et al. 2000) and adds valuable data to the pathogenesis of other MODY subtypes. HNF1B plays a significant role in the development of both endocrine and exocrine pancreas (Haumaitre et al. 2006), required for the differentiation of pancreatic progenitors from endodermal cells (Poll et al. 2006).

Table 18.1 Comparison of the most common MODY subtypes with type 1 and type 2 diabetes

	HNF1A-MODY HNF4A-MODY	HNF1B-MODY	GCK-MODY	T1DM	T2DM
Usual age at diagnosis	10–45 years	10–45 years	From birth	1–30 years	> 25 years
Ketoacidosis	Very rare	Very rare	–	Common	Rare
Positive family history	Present in majority (de novo mutations exist)	Present in majority (de novo mutations frequent)	Present in majority (often missed)	2–4%	~50%
Special phenomenon	Nonobese (both), macrosomia, transient hypoglycemia in the neonatal period (HNF4A), renal glucosuria (HNF1A)	Nonobese, renal abnormalities, hyperuricemia, abnormal liver function tests	Nonobese, often diagnosed during pregnancy	Nonobese, beta cell autoantibodies detected in majority, C-peptide low or absent	Obesity, insulin resistance
First-line treatment	Low-dose sulfonylurea	Metformin if possible	No pharmacological treatment except pregnancy	Insulin	Metformin

Some data are from Juszczak et al. (2016)

18.3 Maturity-Onset Diabetes of the Young (MODY)

It is difficult to estimate the frequency of the disease as the screening strategies are different in different countries and the cost associated with genetic testing in case of all diabetic patients is still too high.

18.3.1 HNF4A-*MODY*

HNF4α is a steroid hormone receptor protein. It is expressed in the liver, pancreas, kidney, and small intestine (Yamagata 2003). Similar to HNF1A-MODY, the causative mutations in *HNF4A* (OMIM 600281) gene (Yamagata et al. 1996a) are loss-of-function alterations resulting in haploinsufficiency (Ferrer 2002; Lausen et al. 2000). The gene has two promoters from which P2 is utilized in the pancreas (Thomas et al. 2001). The cross-regulation between HNF1α and HNF4α in the pancreatic β cells is proven by the fact that mutations in the binding sites of the other in any of these genes' promoter result in MODY (Gragnoli et al. 1997; Hansen et al. 2002). The clinical presentation of *HNF4A*-MODY is very similar to *HNF1A*-MODY with some difference. Macrosomia in mutation carriers compared to wild-type family members and a transient hypoglycemia in the neonatal period might be present due to a paradoxically caused fetal and neonatal hyperinsulinism (Pearson et al. 2007). In addition to its role in glucose metabolism, HNF4α regulates expression of various proteins involved in the lipid metabolism (Yamagata 2003). *HNF4A*-MODY represents approximately 5% of all MODY cases (Ellard et al. 2008). Mutations causing *HNF4A*-MODY are shown in Fig. 18.1.

18.3.2 GCK-*MODY*

Unusual among the MODY proteins, glucokinase (GCK) is not a transcription factor; it is an enzyme considered to be the glucose sensor of the pancreas as small changes in

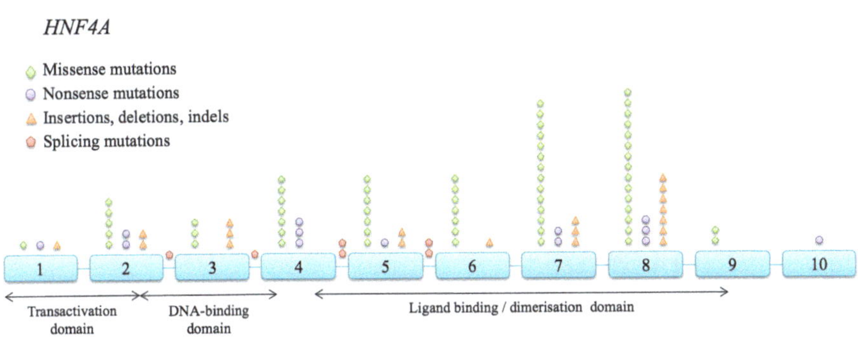

Fig. 18.1 Mutation distribution in *HNF4A* gene (Human Gene Mutation Database, assessed February 2019, small-scale mutations shown). Reference sequence: NM_175914.4

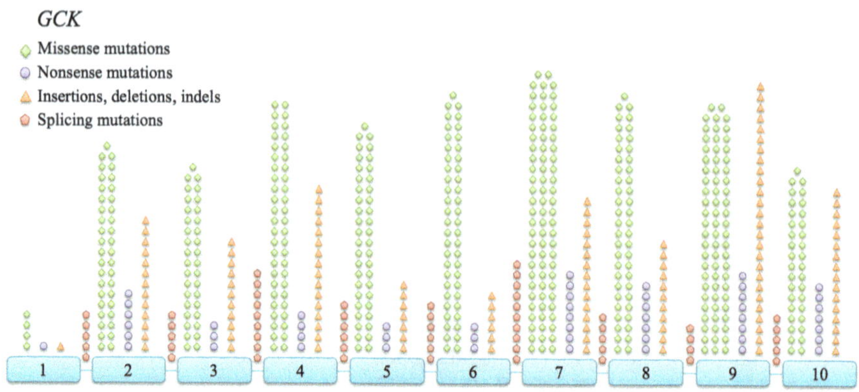

Fig. 18.2 Mutation distribution in *GCK* gene (Human Gene Mutation Database, assessed February 2019, small-scale mutations shown). Reference sequence: NM_000162.4

its activity alter the insulin secretion from the β cell (Matschinsky 1990). It was identified as a MODY-causing gene by analysis of large pedigrees (OMIM 138079) (Froguel et al. 1993; Hattersley et al. 1992). Heterozygous loss-of-function mutations causes a mildly elevated glucose level, which is present, contrary to other MODY subtypes from birth. This fasting hyperglycemia, however, is not associated with increased risk of micro- or macrovascular complications (Steele et al. 2014). One explanation for this interesting phenomenon is that even if the presence of the mutation sets the threshold of glucose levels to be higher where insulin is to be secreted, this secretion is still well regulated, and therefore the postprandial glucose excursions are limited (Ajjan and Owen 2014). There are no apparent mutational hotspots in the *GCK* gene. Most alterations are nucleotide substitutions resulting in amino acid change. Mutations causing *GCK*-MODY are shown in Fig. 18.2. The consequence of the mutation might affect the kinetic properties of the enzyme (Capuano et al. 2012; Valentinova et al. 2012) or predisposes to its misfolding and, consequently, aggregation (Negahdar et al. 2012; Negahdar et al. 2014). Large deletions in the *GCK* gene also occur (Ellard et al. 2007). *GCK*-MODY patients usually require no pharmacological treatment (Steele et al. 2014); however, they are frequently treated unnecessarily (Carmody et al. 2016). *GCK* mutations are frequently found in GDM (gestational diabetes mellitus) patients. In recent studies, 1–2% of GDM patients were shown to have GCK-MODY (Gjesing et al. 2017; Rudland et al. 2016). Prevalence of *GCK*-MODY among all MODY cases is similar to HNF1A, 20–50% (Ellard et al. 2008). A large pedigree of *GCK*-MODY is shown in Fig. 18.3.

18.3.3 HNF1A-*MODY*

HNF1α mainly acts as a regulator of differentiated cellular processes (Maestro et al. 2007) and controls β cell function and growth as well (Yamagata 2014). It is

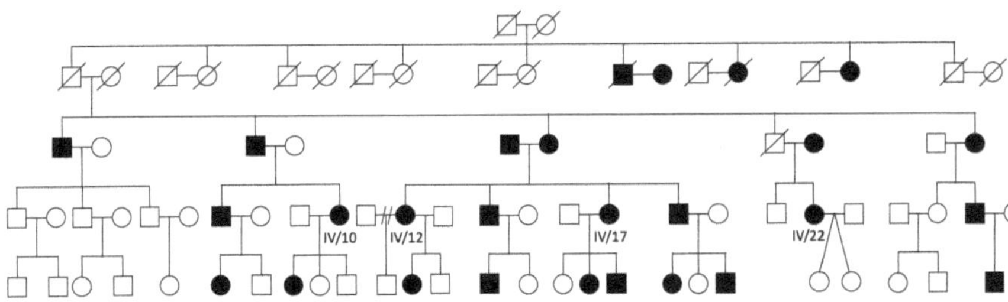

Fig. 18.3 Heterogeneity in a large Hungarian *GCK*-MODY pedigree. Index patient: IV/17. All descendants of the generation II were screened for MODY mutations. 44 patients were tested and *GCK*-MODY was present in 21 patients. Two patients who were negative for *GCK* mutations had type 2 diabetes. In patients IV/10, IV/12, IV/17, and IV/22 diabetes were diagnosed during pregnancy. Index patient has both *GCK*-MODY and type 1 diabetes. Diabetic patients are labeled with black fill

expressed in various organs, i.e., the liver, pancreas, stomach, kidney, and small intestine. HNF1α is an upstream regulator of HNF4α in the pancreas (Odom et al. 2004). In the case of the *HNF1A*-MODY (OMIM 142410) (Yamagata et al. 1996b), the mechanism is mainly haploinsufficiency due to loss-of-function mutations (Ferrer 2002; Thomas et al. 2002). In addition to the small-scale mutations, larger deletions can also be found (Ellard et al. 2007). *HNF1A*-MODY shows age-dependent high penetrance, 63% by the age of 25 years, 93.6% by the age of 50 years, and 98.7% by the age of 75 years (Shepherd et al. 2001). There is a correlation between the localization of the mutation and the age of diagnosis, as mutations that affect the C-terminal end of the transactivation domain of the transcription factor are usually diagnosed later (Bellanne-Chantelot et al. 2008; Harries et al. 2006) compared to those who harbor mutations in N-terminal part. *HNF1A*-MODY is the most prevalent subtype, depending on the population studied, and its proportion in all MODY cases can be as high as 60% (Ryffel 2001), but generally 20–50% is accepted (Ellard et al. 2008). Glycosuria is present in the disease (Menzel et al. 1998). *HNF1A*-MODY patients are sensitive to low-dose sulfonylureas (Pearson et al. 2003), and the switch to sulfonylureas might be possible for patients even after a long-term insulin treatment (Shepherd and Hattersley 2004). When compared to type 1 diabetes group, a long-term sulfonylurea treatment led to lower rate of diabetic complications, and 80% of the patients could remain on sulfonylurea only during the 7 years of follow-up (Bacon et al. 2016). The C-reactive protein (CRP) encoding *CRP* gene has HNF1α binding site in its promoter (Toniatti et al. 1990), and it was shown that CRP levels are significantly lower in *HNF1A*-MODY patients compared to other diabetic groups or healthy controls (Owen et al. 2010; Thanabalasingham et al. 2011). Mutations causing *HNF1A*-MODY are shown in Fig. 18.4.

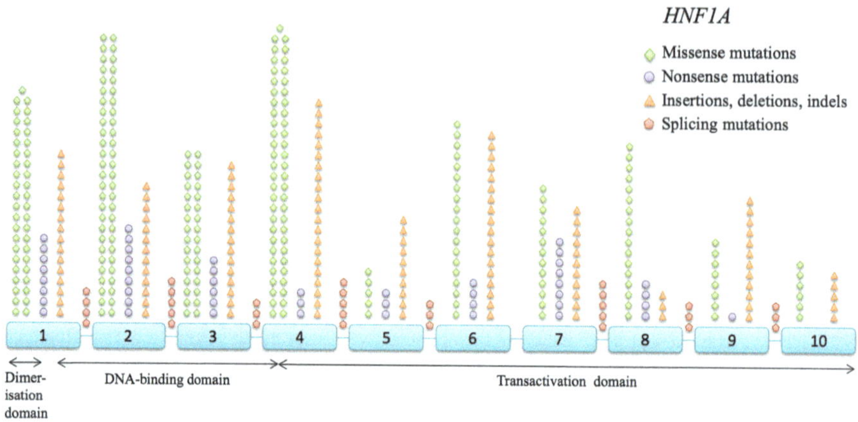

Fig. 18.4 Mutation distribution in HNF1A gene (Human Gene Mutation Database, assessed February 2019, small-scale mutations shown). Reference sequence: NM_000545.6

18.3.4 PDX1-*MODY*

Phylogenetically, PDX1 and PAX4 are closely related (Chakraborty et al. 2015). It is not surprising that *PDX1* heterozygous mutations result in MODY (Stoffers et al. 1997a). There are few reports where *PDX1* mutations (OMIM 600733) are described in MODY (Anik et al. 2015; Cockburn et al. 2004; Doddabelavangala Mruthyunjaya et al. 2017; Fajans et al. 2010; Mangrum et al. 2015). *PDX1*-MODY accounts for less than 1% of all MODY cases (Ellard et al. 2008). These are small deletions and small indel causing frameshift and premature stop codon as well as missense mutations. Used therapeutic approaches include dietary restriction and insulin and sitagliptin administrations. Average age of onset shows considerable interindividual variations.

18.3.5 HNF1B-*MODY*

HNF1B-MODY is caused by heterozygous mutations of the *HNF1B* gene (OMIM 189907) (Horikawa et al. 1997). Pancreas hypoplasia is present in *HNF1B*-MODY patients which results in β cell dysfunction and reduced insulin secretion. It is important to note that the pancreas is only one of the affected organs by the mutated gene as HNF1β is required for genes to be transcribed in the kidney, liver, and genitourinary tract (Ferre and Igarashi 2018). Although its mutation was discovered first in monogenic diabetic patients (Horikawa et al. 1997), it was soon realized that its haploinsufficiency is responsible for RCAD syndrome (renal cysts and diabetes) (Heidet et al. 2010; Ulinski et al. 2006). In line with the wide expression pattern, symptoms of patients with heterozygous *HNF1B* loss-of-function mutations might include abnormal liver enzyme levels, genital tract malformations, diabetes, and renal abnormalities. In fact, the diagnosis of the renal abnormalities often precedes the diabetes, which is partly due to the later age on onset of MODY which is 24 years of age on average (Chen et al. 2010). The age of onset of the diabetes varies to a great extent, from neonatal period (rare) through the most frequent early adulthood until the late middle age (Edghill et al. 2006a; Yorifuji et al. 2004). Hypomagnesemia and hypokalemia are present in approximately half of the patients (Adalat et al. 2009; Faguer et al. 2011). Exocrine pancreas dysfunction, albeit often subclinical, is seen (Bellanne-Chantelot et al. 2004). There is no apparent genotype-phenotype relationship; a large difference in symptoms and age of onset can be seen even in the same family (Heidet et al. 2010). Compared to the other MODY genes, *HNF1B* has two major peculiarities. First, half of the patients carry de novo mutations; therefore, neither the renal manifestations nor the diabetes can be recorded in the families of the affected patients (Edghill et al. 2006a; Heidet et al. 2010). Second, the same proportion of the patients carry a large heterozygous deletion (Bellanne-Chantelot et al. 2005). This mutational hotspot is due to a non-allelic homologous recombination event in chromosome 17q12 (Mefford et al. 2007) that includes more than a dozen genes in addition to *HNF1B* (Laffargue et al. 2015; Mefford et al. 2007). When this rearrangement is present, symptoms might include epilepsy, autism spectrum disorder, and developmental delay (Bockenhauer and Jaureguiberry 2016). Intellectual disability, however, was not restricted to deletion carriers but was present in patients with small-scale mutations too, altogether in 14% of the mutation-positive cases (Dubois-Laforgue et al. 2017).

Small-scale mutations are scattered in the entire gene which encodes a three-domain protein (Fig. 18.5) clustered mainly in exons 2 and 4. Phenotypically the large-scale and small-scale mutations do not differ, suggesting haploinsufficiency as a disease-causing mechanism (Clissold et al. 2015b).

The majority of the patients will need insulin eventually as the responsiveness to sulfonylureas is poor (Chen et al. 2010; Pearson et al. 2004). A *HNF1B*-MODY prevalence of 1–5% was reported (Beards et al. 1998; Ellard et al. 2008) among all MODY cases. To facilitate the clinical assessment for *HNF1B* genetic testing, a 17-parameter score system has been developed (Faguer et al. 2014). By using

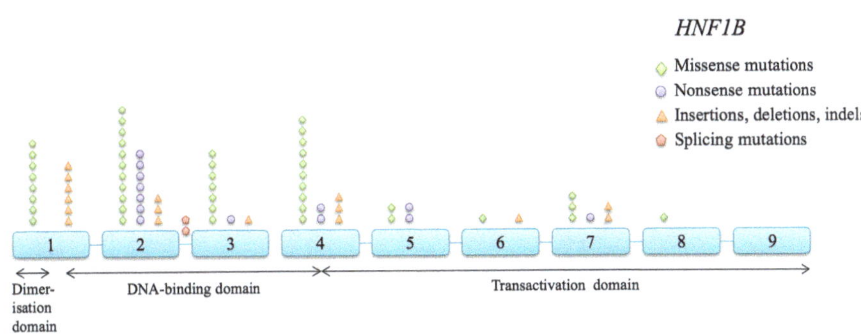

Fig. 18.5 Mutation distribution in *HNF1B* gene (Human Gene Mutation Database, assessed February 2019, small-scale mutations shown). Reference sequence: NM_000458.3. Note that a common large deletion is not shown

different characteristics (highest scores are given for hyperechogen kidney, renal cysts, MODY or hypoplasia of the tail and neck of the pancreas, or exocrine insufficiency and genital tract abnormality), a negative predictive value of 99% and a discrimination area under the curve of 0.78 could be reached. The score system was used on a retrospective dataset and found a negative predictive value of 85% and a discrimination area under the curve of 0.72 (Clissold et al. 2015a).

18.3.6 NEUROD1-*MODY*

Pancreas α and β cells are derived from a common progenitor. One of the transcription factors that are expressed during the differentiation of both cell types is NEUROD1 (van der Meulen and Huising 2015). In the process of β cell development, NEUROD1 is required for insulin expression (Naya et al. 1995). To date, less than 50 *NEUROD1*-MODY families have been described (Chapla et al. 2015; Gonsorcikova et al. 2008; Horikawa et al. 2018; Kristinsson et al. 2001; Liu et al. 2007; Malecki et al. 1999; Szopa et al. 2016), making *NEUROD1* mutations to be a very rare cause (OMIM 601724) [less than 1% (Ellard et al. 2008)] of MODY. There are variations both in the phenotype and the mutational spectrum. Missense, splicing mutations, and small insertions or deletions leading to frameshift have been described. Incomplete penetrance is likely, and in some cases episodes of diabetic ketosis (Horikawa et al. 2018) and retinopathy or nephropathy were observed (Horikawa et al. 2018; Szopa et al. 2016).

18.3.7 KLF11-*MODY*

KLF11 is a transcription factor involved in the fine-tuning of the insulin expression (Perakakis et al. 2012). Depending on the molecular context, KLF11 may act as stimulator or inhibitor, but it seems to be established that its activity on insulin gene promoter is dependent on p300 binding (Fernandez-Zapico et al. 2009; Perakakis et al. 2012), which protein is essential for *PDX1* function (Stanojevic et al. 2004). Missense mutations in the gene have been shown to be associated with MODY (Neve et al. 2005).

18.3.8 CEL-*MODY*

Carboxyl ester lipase (CEL) is a major constituent of the pancreatic juice. It is an enzyme involved in cholesterol ester hydrolysis in the duodenal lumen (Lombardo 2001). Unusual by its mechanism, *CEL*-MODY is not a primary endocrine disease as CEL is not expressed in β cells but expressed in the acinar tissue (Lombardo 2001). Frameshift mutations in the C-terminal of *CEL* have been shown to cause MODY (Raeder et al. 2006) with complete penetrance and with an age of onset in the

30s. Due to their localization, these mutations resist nonsense-mediated mRNA decay (Raeder et al. 2006); therefore, the mutant proteins are synthesized, and even their catalytic activity and secretion seem to be unaffected by the mutation (Johansson et al. 2011; Raeder et al. 2006). It has been suggested that *CEL*-MODY is a misfolding disease, where a dominant-negative effect is responsible for the pathology, which is a higher tendency to form aggregates both intra- and extracellularly (Johansson et al. 2011).

18.3.9 PAX4-*MODY*

PAX4-MODY was first described in 2007 (Plengvidhya et al. 2007). Later it was shown that the IVS7-1G>A mutation disrupts a splice acceptor site and results in a single amino acid deletion (p.Gln250del) with the consequence of an impaired repressor function of the mutant PAX4 (Sujjitjoon et al. 2016) as tested by functional analysis. Diabetic phenotype of the affected patients was rather severe. Similar decreased repressor effect was observed in the case of a missense mutation, p. Arg164Trp (Plengvidhya et al. 2007). Difference in expressitivity was observed in a *PAX4*-MODY family possessing a 39-basepair deletion (c.374-412del39) where one affected patient required insulin treatment, while his father was treated successfully with dietary restrictions only (Jo et al. 2011). In this case, functional analysis showed the skipping of exon 3, and the proposed mechanism was haploinsufficiency. In summary, although *PAX4* mutations have been proven to be causative in MODY, very few cases are described and mainly in Asian populations.

18.3.10 INS-*MODY*

Heterozygous mutations in the insulin (*INS*) gene (OMIM 176730) can cause MODY (Edghill et al. 2008). Age of onset and the required treatment show high degree of variations. The same mutation (p.Arg6Cys) results in diabetic phenotype at 15 and 65 years (Edghill et al. 2008), and the treatment could be diet only, oral agents, or insulin (Edghill et al. 2008). This position seems to be important as two other reports described causative alterations affecting Arg6 [p.Arg6His (Boesgaard et al. 2010; Meur et al. 2010)]. The molecular mechanism involves protein destabilization by disrupting a hydrogen bond (Molven et al. 2008), whose consequence can be endoplasmic reticulum stress as exemplified by p.Leu30Met (Meur et al. 2010) and p.Ala2Thr (Yan et al. 2017). Frameshift mutation has also been described [p. Gln78fs (Dusatkova et al. 2015)]. In some cases, insulin is required since diagnosis (Piccini et al. 2016).

18.3.11 BLK-*MODY*

BLK is a member of the Src family tyrosine kinases. Although it is mainly expressed in the B-cell lymphocyte lineage where it is involved in the signal transduction (Dymecki et al. 1990), BLK is expressed also in pancreatic β cells, hair follicles, salivary ducts, and thymus (Appel et al. 2002; Borowiec et al. 2009). The pathomechanism has not been clearly uncovered, but BLK upregulates PDX1 (Borowiec et al. 2009), and the described p.Ala71Thr missense mutation is associated with decreased insulin content of the β cells. This mutation has also been found in another patient (Mohan et al. 2018), and other possibly pathogenic missense alterations have also been described (Brahm et al. 2016; Doddabelavangala Mruthyunjaya et al. 2017).

18.3.12 ABCC8-*MODY*

By testing sulfonylurea-sensitive *HNF1A* and *HNF4A* mutation-negative MODY cases with no family history of neonatal diabetes, Bowman et al. identified *ABCC8* missense mutations as a cause of MODY (Bowman et al. 2012). In a similar approach (i.e., analysis of mutation-negative MODY cases), Johansson et al. identified a MODY-causing *ABCC8* mutation (Johansson et al. 2012) by exome sequencing. In addition, potential pathogenic alterations were also identified recently (Mohan et al. 2018) in *ABCC8*. Similar to *KCNJ11*-MODY, it seems that the same *ABCC8* mutation might cause NDM and MODY. The available data suggest that the K_{ATP} channel encoding genes (*ABCC8* and *KCNJ11*) are responsible for a small subset of MODY cases. Due to the sulfonylurea treatment option, identification of these cases is important as well as cascade testing among the members in the affected families.

18.3.13 KCNJ11-*MODY*

The fundamental role of *KCNJ11* in monogenic diabetes is well established, especially in neonatal diabetes mellitus (Gloyn et al. 2004; Hattersley and Ashcroft 2005; Massa et al. 2005; Sagen et al. 2004; Vaxillaire et al. 2004). Interestingly, the same mutation, p.Glu227Lys, can be responsible for neonatal diabetes (Girard et al. 2006) and MODY as well (Bonnefond et al. 2012). As this residue is not in a close proximity to the ATP-binding site of the channel, it exerts its effect indirectly. By functional analysis, it has been shown that the mutation reduces the sensitivity of the channel to inhibition by MgATP and increases its intrinsic open probability. In these cases, the recommended treatment is sulfonylurea (Bonnefond et al. 2012).

18.3.14 APPL1-*MODY*

APPL1, an adapter protein, regulates endocytic pathways (Zoncu et al. 2009). In addition to other tissues, its expression has been observed in the pancreas (Mitsuuchi et al. 1999) where it acts as a regulator of insulin secretion in the β cells (Cheng et al. 2012). Contrary to other MODY gene knockout (KO) mice models, *APPL1* KO mice show diabetes-related phenotype, like impaired glucose-stimulated insulin secretion (Wang et al. 2011). Data about the *APPL1*-MODY is very limited. Prudente et al. (2015) identified two mutations in two families with MODY be exome sequencing. Median age of onset of the disease was 38 years. It has been shown by in silico and functional analyses that both are loss-of-function mutations, as p.Leu552∗ truncates the mutant protein and is subjected to rapid proteolytic degradation and p.Asp94Asn, although the mutant protein stability is not affected, disrupts a salt bridge.

18.3.15 RFX6-*MODY*

Very recently a novel MODY gene was identified (Patel et al. 2017). *RFX6*, the gene which causes neonatal diabetes when recessive mutations are present (see below), causes MODY with reduced penetrance when protein truncation mutations are present in heterozygous form. The proposed mechanism is haploinsufficiency, and after 10 years of age on onset, 69% of the patients required insulin treatment (Patel et al. 2017). The RFX6 transcription factor has a significant role in the regulation of insulin secretion (Chandra et al. 2014).

18.3.16 Analysis of Large Cohorts for MODY Mutations

In a diet-treated GDM women cohort of 354 patients, 5.9% of them had possibly pathogenic mutations in MODY genes. This high prevalence data warrants testing for MODY in such a population (Gjesing et al. 2017). By sequencing 22 monogenic diabetes genes in 4016 type 2 diabetic patients, 40 patients were found to have known pathogenic alterations and 7 patients to have protein truncation variants (i.e., likely pathogenic or pathogenic) (Bansal et al. 2017). In a comprehensive UK study performed on pediatric diabetic population, where the testing pathway included urinary C-peptide creatinine ratio followed by DAD/IA2 islet autoantibody testing and subsequent genetic testing, 2.5% of the patients had monogenic diabetes (Shepherd et al. 2016). In a US study, 8.0% MODY cases were identified among autoantibody-negative youth diabetic population (other selection criterion was fasting C-peptide level of 0.8 ng/mL or greater) (Pihoker et al. 2013). An analysis using the Norwegian Childhood Diabetes Registry revealed that the minimum prevalence of monogenic diabetes among Norwegian children is 3.1/100.000 (Irgens et al. 2013), and a recent analysis of the same registry resulted in a 4.1% of likely pathogenic/pathogenic alterations in MODY genes in autoantibody-negative children (Johansson et al. 2017). In a retrospective Italian study involving 3781 pediatric diabetes cases, the prevalence of MODY was found to be 5.5% (Delvecchio et al. 2017). *GCK*-MODY was studied in 3345 Chinese subjects, in a cohort that included 545 diabetic patients (Ma et al. 2018). GCK-MODY prevalence of 0.21% in the whole population and 1.3% in the diabetic patients was found (Ma et al. 2018).

In order to help the clinician in the decision who to be tested, a MODY probability calculator was developed (Shields et al. 2012) which focuses on three major MODY genes (*HNF1A*, *HNF4A*, *GCK*). Among the studied ethnic groups, its performance seems to be the best in Europeans (Ang et al. 2016; Kwak et al. 2016). The MODY probability calculator can be used if the age of the patients at diagnosis is less than 35 years. The MODY criteria of multigeneration-affected members in the family need to be treated with caution as in many cases de novo mutations are responsible for the disease (Ang et al. 2016; Stanik et al. 2014).

18.3.17 Mutation Testing in MODY

With a few exceptions, there are no apparent mutational hotspots in the MODY genes. Therefore, mutational search of the coding regions of the genes has always been the most successful option. In the past, mutational screening methods, and as the gold standard, Sanger sequencing were used, frequently sequentially. In case of a classical MODY phenotype, usually *HNF1A* was sequenced as the most frequent cause and then *HNF4A* and *GCK* (Johansson et al. 2012). If a patient exhibited urogenital or pancreatic malformations and renal dysfunction, *HNF1B* was the most plausible candidate gene to test. Recently, in the era of next-generation sequencing (NGS), genetic testing of monogenic diabetes has been changed dramatically. Gene panel testing (Brahm et al. 2016; Doddabelavangala Mruthyunjaya et al. 2017; Johansson et al. 2017; Piccini et al. 2016) is widely used for molecular testing, with a subsequent confirmation of the detected variant(s) by Sanger sequencing. It is to be noted, however, that the analytical performance of each custom-made gene panel assay needs to be analyzed, and in some cases, NGS methods do not have the required analytical sensitivity (i.e., detection of the common deletion in *HNF1B*). Whole exome sequencing has been shown to be also an option (Bonnefond et al. 2012; Johansson et al. 2012; Johnson et al. 2018a, b; Kwak et al. 2016; Prudente et al. 2015; Yan et al. 2017). In the case of MODY, predictive/presymptomatic testing should be considered, especially in the advent of genomic medicine. More and more health insurance payers consider exome (genome) sequencing as a valuable and cost-effective tool for healthcare decision-making and even to prevent diseases with strong genetic background. MODY can easily be a good example as it is not an early-onset disease; therefore, preventive actions can be taken in order to delay the complications. In case of the clinical suspicion, the American Diabetes

Association recommends genetic testing for MODY (level of evidence "A") (American Diabetes 2019). In the case of similar later onset, albeit more severe genetic disorders, the ACMG (American College of Medical Genetics and Genomics) recommends to analyze exome/genome datasets for the detection of pathogenic mutations in the responsible genes in patient's sample irrespective of the original clinical question. In the case of transcription factor MODY subtypes, exome/genome sequencing performed in childhood due to any other reason might result in detection of a pathogenic mutation, which in turn in mutation-positive cases might result in presymptomatic diagnosis with a consequence of health benefit (early clinical diagnosis of hyperglycemia because of the increased awareness). In addition, these analyses might result in candidate testing which helps in decreasing the stress in unaffected family members. Moreover, it has been shown that MODY genetic testing in individuals with high expected pretest prevalence can be cost-effective with a benefit of improved quality of life and reduction of treatment costs (Brahm et al. 2016), especially when a patient is misdiagnosed with type 1 diabetes. An analysis within the frame of the SEARCH study resulted in 47 newly diagnosed MODY patients, 94% of them received insulin therapy preceding the diagnosis which could be stopped in most of the cases (Pihoker et al. 2013). Although next-generation sequencing strategies result in significantly higher mutation detection rate, their implementation to the routine genetic practice introduces new difficulties as many of the detected mutations are unique and yet to be functionally tested. Molecular genetic diagnostic rate for clinically suspected MODY patients varies but can reach to 40% (Brahm et al. 2016) in which the increase is mainly due to the use of the gene panel analysis by next-generation sequencing. The technological advancements in molecular testing methods make precision medicine possible in many situations. It has been shown that the outcome of pregnancy in both MODY and neonatal diabetes might depend on the fetal genotypes, as caused in *GCK*-MODY (Dickens and Naylor 2018) and in neonatal diabetes (Gaal et al. 2012). Fetal DNA analysis by noninvasive methods, such as circulating cell-free DNA sequencing (De Franco et al. 2017a), will allow personalized treatment decisions depending on the mutational status of the fetus and the mother.

18.4 Neonatal Diabetes

Neonatal diabetes mellitus is a severe monogenic disease appearing in the first 6 months of life. Hyperglycemia usually requires insulin. There are two forms: (1) permanent neonatal diabetes mellitus (PNDM) and (2) transient neonatal diabetes mellitus (TNDM). In TNDM the diabetes usually reverts within several months but might relapse later in life. Incidence of NDM is 1:100,000–1:400,000 live births (Iafusco et al. 2012; Shield 2000), and PNDM accounts for half of the cases.

18.4.1 Neonatal Diabetes Caused by KCNJ11 or ABCC8 Mutations

40–50% of the patients having neonatal diabetes possess mutations in the pancreas K_{ATP} channel genes (*ABCC8*, *KCNJ11*) (Hattersley and Patel 2017). The increased circulating glucose when entering the β cell is metabolized via the GCK enzyme. Under normal circumstances, the consequently increased ATP concentration leads to the closure of K_{ATP} channel that is composed of four Kir6.2 (encoded by *KCNJ11*) and four SUR1 (encoded by *ABCC8*) subunits. The channel closure results in membrane depolarization and in the elevation of intracellular Ca^{2+} level which will lead to the exocytosis of insulin-containing granules. The most common cause of PNDM is caused by activating mutations in *KCNJ11* (Gloyn et al. 2004) responsible for 30% of the cases. Mutations in *KCNJ11* might differ in consequence, as the phenotypic spectrum ranges from TNDM through PNDM without neurological involvement till DEND (developmental delay, epilepsy and neonatal diabetes, 20% of the cases) (Gloyn et al. 2006; Hattersley and Ashcroft 2005; Hattersley and Patel 2017). Later gain-of-function mutations in *ABCC8* leading to the same clinical phenotype (i.e., TNDM or PNDM) were also identified (Babenko et al. 2006; Proks et al. 2006). Such mutations in these two genes altogether are responsible for more than 40% of PNDM cases (De Franco et al. 2015; Edghill et al. 2008). In these patients, the recognition of the molecular background could be quickly translated into healthcare practice as the treatment is high-dose sulfonylureas (Pearson et al. 2006) which treatment results in the closure of the K_{ATP} channel by binding to SUR1 irrespectively to the intracellular ATP concentrations. The NDM-related K_{ATP} channel gene mutations have an impact on the management of pregnancy as the maternal genotype has a significant impact for the fetus (Shepherd et al. 2017). In case of an affected mother and unaffected fetus, sulfonylurea treatment leads to macrosomia and neonatal hyperinsulinemic hypoglycemia, while in the case of an affected fetus, normal birth weight was observed and even diabetes was not present after birth for 96 months (Gaal et al. 2012; Klupa et al. 2010; Myngheer et al. 2014; Unpublished observation of the authors). In such cases, the fetal DNA analysis during pregnancy by noninvasive methods will be of great benefit.

18.4.2 Neonatal Diabetes Caused by INS Mutations

In addition to *ABCC8* and *KCNJ11*, which cause PNDM more frequently than MODY, other MODY-causing genes might be in the background of NDM as well. One-fifth of PNDM are caused by *INS* mutations (Edghill et al. 2008; Stoy et al. 2007). These mutations might cause PNDM both in heterozygous and homozygous/compound heterozygous forms. In case of heterozygosity, the mechanism is dominant-negative effect (Park et al. 2010), while in recessive inheritance, insulin synthesis is impaired (Garin et al. 2010). In dominant mutations, which also can be de novo (Stoy et al. 2007), the mutant protein causes endoplasmic reticulum stress (Stoy et al. 2007) and probably results in defective β cell proliferation (Balboa et al. 2018). TNDM-causing mutations were also described (Stoy et al. 2010). Neurological symptoms are not present. *INS* mutation-caused NDM patients are treated with insulin.

18.4.3 Neonatal Diabetes Caused by GCK *Mutations*

Loss-of-function mutations that generate *GCK*-MODY in heterozygous form might be the cause of PNDM when they are homozygous, mainly in consanguineous families (Bennett et al. 2011; Njolstad et al. 2001). Missense, nonsense, and splice site mutations have been described (Bennett et al. 2011; Njolstad et al. 2003; Osbak et al. 2009; Rubio-Cabezas et al. 2008). Interestingly, homozygous *GCK* mutations have also been found in diabetic patients outside the neonatal period (Durmaz et al. 2012) and in infancy (Raimondo et al. 2014). The main pathomechanism is the instability of the mutant protein (Raimondo et al. 2014). Intrauterine growth retardation is observed. According to studies performed in mice model, *GCK* deficiency leads to impaired K_{ATP} signaling (Remedi et al. 2005). Sulfonylurea treatment was shown to improve glycemic control although insulin treatment could not be stopped (Turkkahraman et al. 2008), but the use of sulfonylurea does not always result in better glycemic control (Oriola et al. 2015).

18.4.4 Neonatal Diabetes Caused by PDX1 *Mutations*

Stoffers et al. described a clinical case of neonatal diabetes and pancreatic exocrine insufficiency due to a homozygous single base deletion in the *PDX1* gene. It was shown that the pancreas was absent (Stoffers et al. 1997b). Interestingly, permanent neonatal diabetes patients with biallelic *PDX1* mutations rarely show any sign of pancreatic agenesis (De Franco et al. 2013; Nicolino et al. 2010). This suggests hypomorphic effect of the mutations instead of loss of function, and to support this hypothesis, all patients with this phenotype had at least one missense mutation.

18.4.5 Neonatal Diabetes Caused by NEUROD1 *Mutations*

Since the first report of *NEUROD1*-MODY (Malecki et al. 1999), the role of the transcription factor in the development of monogenic diabetes is well established which is supported by the fact that homozygous loss-of-function mutations lead to permanent neonatal diabetes (Rubio-Cabezas et al. 2010) with severe neurological defects and visual impairment (Orosz et al. 2015; Rubio-Cabezas et al. 2010).

18.4.6 The Major Cause of TNDM: 6q24 Methylation Abnormalities

In addition to the insulin-requiring diabetes, intrauterine growth retardation and absence of ketoacidosis are typical in TNDM. The diabetes might relapse later; therefore, a follow-up is important (Docherty et al. 2013). In the majority of the cases, TDMN is caused by overexpression of the genes on chromosome 6q24 (Mackay et al. 2006) due to paternal uniparental disomy of chromosome 6, paternal duplication of 6q24, or maternal loss of methylation at the *PLAGL1* locus (Mackay and Temple 2010). This latter might be an isolated and epigenetic or might be a part of a multilocus imprinting disturbance (MLID) where facial dysmorphism, macroglossia, umbilical hernia, congenital heart defects, and neurological symptoms might associate with the diabetes (Touati et al. 2018). In a subset of MLID patients, recessive *ZFP57* mutations have been described (Boonen et al. 2013; Docherty et al. 2013; Touati et al. 2018). Clinical genetic counseling must be done knowing the cause because in epigenetic TNDM, there is no recurrence, while in inherited *ZFP57*, mutations represent a 25% recurrence risk when both parents are carriers (Touati et al. 2018). Paternal duplication might be de novo or inherited. Other rare causes of TNDM are discussed elsewhere in the chapter.

18.4.7 Other Rare Monogenic Forms of Neonatal Diabetes

Very rarely, mutation in *HNF1B* can also cause TNDM (De Franco et al. 2015; Edghill et al. 2006b; Yorifuji et al. 2004). In one of the reports, germline maternal mosaicism was found (Yorifuji et al. 2004), and another, de novo mutation was responsible for the disease (Edghill et al. 2006b). Interestingly, the same amino acid position (Ser148) was affected.

Recessive mutations in *GLIS3* cause PNDM, where polycystic kidney disease and congenital hypothyroidism are present as well (Senee et al. 2006). Recessive mutations in *NEUROG3* cause PNDM and enteric anendocrinosis (severe congenital malabsorptive diarrhea) (Rubio-Cabezas et al. 2011). Recessive mutations in *PAX6* are associated with NDM and severe ophthalmologic and neurologic anomalies (Solomon et al. 2009). Mutations in the *WFS1* gene are associated with a spectrum of phenotypes. In case of recessive mutations that cause Wolfram syndrome, no NDM is present. In contrast, possession of some dominant mutations results in early presentation of the symptoms, including neonatal or infancy-onset diabetes (De Franco et al. 2017b). Other symptoms are congenital cataracts, sensorineural deafness, and hypotonia. Pathomechanism of these dominant mutations might be induction of ER stress and consequently apoptosis (De Franco et al. 2017b). In some *SLC19A2* recessive mutations-caused TRMA (thiamine-responsive megaloblastic anemia) cases, NDM is present (Shaw-Smith et al. 2012; Sun et al. 2018). Thiamine supplementation has been shown to be beneficial in these patients (Sun et al. 2018).

The MNX1 transcription factor is involved in dorsal pancreas specification and β cell differentiation and proliferation (Pan et al. 2015). Recessive mutations found in consanguineous families result in NDM (Bonnefond et al. 2013; Flanagan et al. 2014a) as well as mutations in another pancreatic transcription factor, NKX2-2 (additional phenotypic features in this case are hypotonia, hearing impairment, cortical blindness, and impaired visual tracking) (Flanagan et al. 2014a). GATA4 transcription factor has a significant role in pancreas development, and mutation in *GATA4* results in NDM (D'Amato et al. 2010; Shaw-Smith et al. 2014). *GATA6* haploinsufficiency is a frequent cause of pancreas agenesis and neonatal diabetes (Allen et al. 2011). These patients also have congenital heart defects, but rarely no exocrine pancreas insufficiency is seen (Catli et al. 2013). Nonsense, splicing, and frameshift mutations have been described (Chao et al. 2015; Eifes et al. 2013; Suzuki et al. 2014; Tuhan et al. 2015). Homozygous or compound heterozygous mutations in *RFX6* usually result in a very severe phenotype with pancreas hypoplasia, neonatal diabetes, intestinal atresia, cholestatic disease, and gallbladder hypoplasia or aplasia (Chappell et al. 2008; Concepcion et al. 2014; Mitchell et al. 2004; Spiegel et al. 2011) which is not surprising as RFX6 is required for endocrine pancreas development and for insulin expression and secretion (Chandra et al. 2014). Interestingly, in some cases, the diabetic phenotype is childhood onset (Sansbury et al. 2015). Recessive mutations in *PTF1A* might be associated with syndromic pancreatic agenesis (with cerebellar agenesis) (Sellick et al. 2004) or with isolated pancreatic agenesis (Evliyaoglu et al. 2018; Gabbay et al. 2017; Weedon et al. 2014). Mutations might affect either the coding region of *PTF1A* or a distal enhancer sequence of the gene. Patients with immune dysregulation, polyendocrinopathy, enteropathy, and X-linked (IPEX) syndrome, which is due to hemizygous mutations in *FOXP3*, might also develop NDM (Rubio-Cabezas et al. 2009a). Rare recessive mutations in *SLC2A2* encoding GLUT2 glucose transporter result in Fanconi-Bickel syndrome, a carbohydrate metabolic disease. It is characterized by growth retardation, glycosuria, galactosuria, rickets, hepatomegaly, fasting hypoglycemia, and postprandial hyperglycemia (Khandelwal et al. 2018; Sansbury et al. 2012). In a small subset of the patients, TNDM or PNDM might occur (Sansbury et al. 2012). Activating mutations in *STAT3* are associated with PNDM and early-onset autoimmunity (Flanagan et al. 2014b). The mechanism that leads to the development of PNDM is not entirely known; an autoimmune attack on the endocrine pancreas, upregulated *NEUROG3* expression, and dysregulated insulin synthesis might all contribute (Flanagan et al. 2014b; Saarimaki-Vire et al. 2017; Velayos et al. 2017). PNDM is present in Wolcott-Rallison syndrome, an autosomal recessive disease characterized by spondyloepiphyseal dysplasia. The responsible gene, *EIF2AK3*, encodes a kinase located exclusively in the endoplasmic reticulum. Mutations are missense, splicing, frameshift, or nonsense (Brickwood et al. 2003; Rubio-Cabezas et al. 2009b). NDM caused by *EIF2AK3* mutations is very prevalent in consanguineous families (De Franco et al. 2015). Recessive mutations in *IER3IP1* gene result in a severe phenotype of microcephaly, epilepsy, and PND (Abdel-Salam et al. 2012; Shalev et al. 2014). Finally, recessive mutations in *LRBA* gene associated with NDM and autoimmune lymphoproliferative syndrome has been described (Johnson et al. 2017).

18.4.8 Mutation Testing in Neonatal Diabetes

According to the American Diabetes Association and the International Society for Pediatric and Adolescent Diabetes, every child with diabetes in the first 6 months of life should have immediate genetic testing for neonatal diabetes (evidence level "A") (American Diabetes 2019; Hattersley et al. 2018). Considering that NDM in these rare diseases in many cases precedes the appearance of the syndromic phenotype, and due to the considerable genetic heterogeneity in NDM, next-generation sequencing techniques, especially exome or genome sequencing, will soon be the ultimate choice of genetic testing.

References

Abdel-Salam GM, Schaffer AE, Zaki MS, Dixon-Salazar T, Mostafa IS, Afifi HH, Gleeson JG (2012) A homozygous IER3IP1 mutation causes microcephaly with simplified gyral pattern, epilepsy, and permanent neonatal diabetes syndrome (MEDS). Am J Med Genet A 158A:2788–2796. https://doi.org/10.1002/ajmg.a.35583

Adalat S, Woolf AS, Johnstone KA et al (2009) HNF1B mutations associate with hypomagnesemia and renal magnesium wasting. J Am Soc Nephrol 20:1123–1131. https://doi.org/10.1681/ASN.2008060633

Ahlgren U, Jonsson J, Jonsson L, Simu K, Edlund H (1998) Beta-cell-specific inactivation of the mouse Ipf1/Pdx1 gene results in loss of the beta-cell phenotype and maturity onset diabetes. Genes Dev 12:1763–1768

Ajjan RA, Owen KR (2014) Glucokinase MODY and implications for treatment goals of common forms of diabetes. Curr Diab Rep 14:559. https://doi.org/10.1007/s11892-014-0559-0

Allen HL, Flanagan SE, Shaw-Smith C et al (2011) GATA6 haploinsufficiency causes pancreatic agenesis in humans. Nat Genet 44:20–22. https://doi.org/10.1038/ng.1035

American Diabetes A (2019) 2. Classification and diagnosis of diabetes: standards of medical care in diabetes. Diabetes Care 42:S13–S28. https://doi.org/10.2337/dc19-S002

Ang SF, Lim SC, Tan CS et al (2016) A preliminary study to evaluate the strategy of combining clinical criteria and next generation sequencing (NGS) for the identification of monogenic diabetes among multi-ethnic Asians. Diabetes Res Clin Pract 119:13–22. https://doi.org/10.1016/j.diabres.2016.06.008

Anik A, Catli G, Abacı A et al (2015) Molecular diagnosis of maturity-onset diabetes of the young (MODY) in Turkish children by using targeted next-generation sequencing. J Pediatr Endocrinol Metab 28:1265–1271. https://doi.org/10.1515/jpem-2014-0430

Appel S, Filter M, Reis A et al (2002) Physical and transcriptional map of the critical region for keratolytic winter erythema (KWE) on chromosome 8p22-p23 between D8S550 and D8S1759. Eur J Hum Genet 10:17–25. https://doi.org/10.1038/sj.ejhg.5200750

Babenko AP, Polak M, Cavé H et al (2006) Activating mutations in the ABCC8 gene in neonatal diabetes mellitus. N Engl J Med 355:456–466. https://doi.org/10.1056/NEJMoa055068

Bacon S, Kyithar MP, Rizvi SR et al (2016) Successful maintenance on sulphonylurea therapy and low diabetes complication rates in a HNF1A-MODY cohort. Diabet Med 33:976–984. https://doi.org/10.1111/dme.12992

Balboa D, Saarimäki-Vire J, Borshagovski D et al (2018) Insulin mutations impair beta-cell development in a patient-derived iPSC model of neonatal diabetes. Elife 7. https://doi.org/10.7554/eLife.38519

Bansal V, Gassenhuber J, Phillips T et al (2017) Spectrum of mutations in monogenic diabetes genes identified from high-throughput DNA sequencing of 6888 individuals. BMC Med 15:213. https://doi.org/10.1186/s12916-017-0977-3

Beards F, Frayling T, Bulman M et al (1998) Mutations in hepatocyte nuclear factor 1beta are not a common cause of maturity-onset diabetes of the young in the UK. Diabetes 47:1152–1154

Bellanne-Chantelot C et al (2004) Clinical spectrum associated with hepatocyte nuclear factor-1beta mutations. Ann Intern Med 140:510–517

Bellanne-Chantelot C, Chauveau D, Gautier JF et al (2005) Large genomic rearrangements in the hepatocyte nuclear factor-1beta (TCF2) gene are the most frequent cause of maturity-onset diabetes of the young type 5. Diabetes 54:3126–3132

Bellanne-Chantelot C, Carette C, Riveline JP et al (2008) The type and the position of HNF1A mutation modulate age at diagnosis of diabetes in patients with maturity-onset diabetes of the young (MODY)-3. Diabetes 57:503–508. https://doi.org/10.2337/db07-0859

Bennett K, James C, Mutair A, Al-Shaikh H, Sinani A, Hussain K (2011) Four novel cases of permanent neonatal diabetes mellitus caused by homozygous mutations in the glucokinase gene. Pediatr Diabetes 12:192–196. https://doi.org/10.1111/j.1399-5448.2010.00683.x

Bockenhauer D, Jaureguiberry G (2016) HNF1B-associated clinical phenotypes: the kidney and beyond. Pediatr Nephrol 31:707–714. https://doi.org/10.1007/s00467-015-3142-2

Boesgaard TW, Pruhova S, Andersson EA et al (2010) Further evidence that mutations in INS can be a rare cause of Maturity-Onset Diabetes of the Young (MODY). BMC Med Genet 11:42. https://doi.org/10.1186/1471-2350-11-42

Bonnefond A, Philippe J, Durand E et al (2012) Whole-exome sequencing and high throughput genotyping identified KCNJ11 as the thirteenth MODY gene. PLoS One 7:e37423. https://doi.org/10.1371/journal.pone.0037423

Bonnefond A, Vaillant E, Philippe J et al (2013) Transcription factor gene MNX1 is a novel cause of permanent neonatal diabetes in a consanguineous family. Diabetes Metab 39:276–280. https://doi.org/10.1016/j.diabet.2013.02.007

Boonen SE, Mackay DJ, Hahnemann JM et al (2013) Transient neonatal diabetes, ZFP57, and hypomethylation of multiple imprinted loci: a detailed follow-up. Diabetes Care 36:505–512. https://doi.org/10.2337/dc12-0700

Borowiec M, Liew CW, Thompson R et al (2009) Mutations at the BLK locus linked to maturity onset diabetes of the young and beta-cell dysfunction. Proc Natl Acad Sci U S A 106:14460–14465. https://doi.org/10.1073/pnas.0906474106

Bowman P, Flanagan SE, Edghill EL et al (2012) Heterozygous ABCC8 mutations are a cause of MODY. Diabetologia 55:123–127. https://doi.org/10.1007/s00125-011-2319-x

Brahm AJ, Wang G, Wang J, McIntyre AD, Cao H, Ban MR, Hegele RA (2016) Genetic confirmation rate in clinically suspected maturity-onset diabetes of the young. Can J Diabetes 40:555–560. https://doi.org/10.1016/j.jcjd.2016.05.010

Brickwood S, Bonthron DT, Al-Gazali LI, Piper K, Hearn T, Wilson DI, Hanley NA (2003) Wolcott-Rallison syndrome: pathogenic insights into neonatal diabetes from new mutation and expression studies of EIF2AK3. J Med Genet 40:685–689

Cammidge PJ (1928) Diabetes mellitus and heredity. Br Med J 2:738–741

Campbell SC, Cragg H, Elrick LJ, Macfarlane WM, Shennan KI, Docherty K (1999) Inhibitory effect of pax4 on the human insulin and islet amyloid polypeptide (IAPP) promoters. FEBS Lett 463:53–57

Capuano M, Garcia-Herrero CM, Tinto N et al (2012) Glucokinase (GCK) mutations and their characterization in MODY2 children of southern Italy. PLoS One 7:e38906. https://doi.org/10.1371/journal.pone.0038906

Carmody D, Naylor RN, Bell CD et al (2016) GCK-MODY in the US National Monogenic Diabetes Registry: frequently misdiagnosed and unnecessarily treated. Acta Diabetol 53:703–708. https://doi.org/10.1007/s00592-016-0859-8

Catli G, Abaci A, Flanagan SE et al (2013) A novel GATA6 mutation leading to congenital heart defects and permanent neonatal diabetes: a case report. Diabetes Metab 39:370–374. https://doi.org/10.1016/j.diabet.2013.01.005

Chakraborty C, Bandyopadhyay S, Doss CG, Agoramoorthy G (2015) Exploring the genomic roadmap and molecular phylogenetics associated with MODY cascades using computational biology. Cell Biochem Biophys 71:1491–1502. https://doi.org/10.1007/s12013-014-0372-z

Chandra V, Albagli-Curiel O, Hastoy B et al (2014) RFX6 regulates insulin secretion by modulating Ca2+ homeostasis in human beta cells. Cell Rep 9:2206–2218. https://doi.org/10.1016/j.celrep.2014.11.010

Chao CS, McKnight KD, Cox KL, Chang AL, Kim SK, Feldman BJ (2015) Novel GATA6 mutations in patients with pancreatic agenesis and congenital heart malformations. PLoS One 10:e0118449. https://doi.org/10.1371/journal.pone.0118449

Chapla A, Mruthyunjaya MD, Asha HS et al (2015) Maturity onset diabetes of the young in India – a distinctive mutation pattern identified through targeted next-generation sequencing. Clin Endocrinol (Oxf) 82:533–542. https://doi.org/10.1111/cen.12541

Chappell L, Gorman S, Campbell F, Ellard S, Rice G, Dobbie A, Crow Y (2008) A further example of a distinctive autosomal recessive syndrome comprising neonatal diabetes mellitus, intestinal atresias and gall bladder agenesis. Am J Med Genet A 146A:1713–1717. https://doi.org/10.1002/ajmg.a.32304

Chen YZ, Gao Q, Zhao XZ et al (2010) Systematic review of TCF2 anomalies in renal cysts and diabetes syndrome/maturity onset diabetes of the young type 5. Chin Med J (Engl) 123:3326–3333

Cheng KK, Lam KS, Wu D et al (2012) APPL1 potentiates insulin secretion in pancreatic beta cells by enhancing protein kinase Akt-dependent expression of SNARE proteins in mice. Proc Natl Acad Sci U S A 109:8919–8924. https://doi.org/10.1073/pnas.1202435109

Clissold R, Shields B, Ellard S, Hattersley A, Bingham C (2015a) Assessment of the HNF1B score as a tool to select patients for HNF1B genetic testing. Nephron 130:134–140. https://doi.org/10.1159/000398819

Clissold RL, Hamilton AJ, Hattersley AT, Ellard S, Bingham C (2015b) HNF1B-associated renal and extra-renal disease-an expanding clinical spectrum. Nat Rev Nephrol 11:102–112. https://doi.org/10.1038/nrneph.2014.232

Cockburn BN, Bermano G, Boodram LL et al (2004) Insulin promoter factor-1 mutations and diabetes in Trinidad: identification of a novel diabetes-associated mutation (E224K) in an Indo-Trinidadian family. J Clin Endocrinol Metab 89:971–978. https://doi.org/10.1210/jc.2003-031282

Concepcion JP et al (2014) Neonatal diabetes, gallbladder agenesis, duodenal atresia, and intestinal malrotation caused by a novel homozygous mutation in RFX6. Pediatr Diabetes 15:67–72. https://doi.org/10.1111/pedi.12063

D'Amato E, Reh CS, Daniels M et al (2010) Genetic investigation in an Italian child with an unusual association of atrial septal defect, attributable to a new familial GATA4 gene mutation, and neonatal diabetes due to pancreatic agenesis. Diabet Med 27:1195–1200. https://doi.org/10.1111/j.1464-5491.2010.03046.x

De Franco E, Shaw-Smith C, Flanagan SE et al (2013) Biallelic PDX1 (insulin promoter factor 1) mutations causing neonatal diabetes without exocrine pancreatic insufficiency. Diabet Med 30: e197–e200. https://doi.org/10.1111/dme.12122

De Franco E, Flanagan SE, Houghton JA et al (2015) The effect of early, comprehensive genomic testing on clinical care in neonatal diabetes: an international cohort study. Lancet 386:957–963. https://doi.org/10.1016/S0140-6736(15)60098-8

De Franco E, Caswell R, Houghton JA, Iotova V, Hattersley AT, Ellard S (2017a) Analysis of cell-free fetal DNA for non-invasive prenatal diagnosis in a family with neonatal diabetes. Diabet Med 34:582–585. https://doi.org/10.1111/dme.13180

De Franco E, Flanagan SE, Yagi T et al (2017b) Dominant ER stress-inducing WFS1 mutations underlie a genetic syndrome of neonatal/infancy-onset diabetes, congenital sensorineural deafness, and congenital cataracts. Diabetes 66:2044–2053. https://doi.org/10.2337/db16-1296

Delvecchio M, Mozzillo E, Salzano G et al (2017) Monogenic diabetes accounts for 6.3% of cases referred to 15 Italian pediatric diabetes centers during 2007 to 2012. J Clin Endocrinol Metab 102:1826–1834. https://doi.org/10.1210/jc.2016-2490

Dickens LT, Naylor RN (2018) Clinical management of women with monogenic diabetes during pregnancy. Curr Diab Rep 18:12. https://doi.org/10.1007/s11892-018-0982-8

Docherty LE, Kabwama S, Lehmann A et al (2013) Clinical presentation of 6q24 transient neonatal diabetes mellitus (6q24 TNDM) and genotype-phenotype correlation in an international cohort of patients. Diabetologia 56:758–762. https://doi.org/10.1007/s00125-013-2832-1

Doddabelavangala Mruthyunjaya M, Chapla A, Hesarghatta Shyamasunder A et al (2017) Comprehensive maturity onset diabetes of the young (MODY) gene screening in pregnant women with diabetes in India. PLoS One 12:e0168656. https://doi.org/10.1371/journal.pone.0168656

Dubois-Laforgue D, Bellanné-Chantelot C, Charles P et al (2017) Intellectual disability in patients with MODY due to hepatocyte nuclear factor 1B (HNF1B) molecular defects. Diabetes Metab 43:89–92. https://doi.org/10.1016/j.diabet.2016.10.003

Durmaz E, Flanagan S, Berdeli A, Semiz S, Akcurin S, Ellard S, Bircan I (2012) Variability in the age at diagnosis of diabetes in two unrelated patients with a homozygous glucokinase gene mutation. J Pediatr Endocrinol Metab 25:805–808. https://doi.org/10.1515/jpem-2012-0077

Dusatkova L, Dusatkova P, Vosahlo J, Vesela K, Cinek O, Lebl J, Pruhova S (2015) Frameshift mutations in the insulin gene leading to prolonged molecule of insulin in two families with maturity-onset diabetes of the young. Eur J Med Genet 58:230–234. https://doi.org/10.1016/j.ejmg.2015.02.004

Dymecki SM, Niederhuber JE, Desiderio SV (1990) Specific expression of a tyrosine kinase gene, blk, in B lymphoid cells. Science 247:332–336

Edghill EL, Bingham C, Ellard S, Hattersley AT (2006a) Mutations in hepatocyte nuclear factor-1beta and their related phenotypes. J Med Genet 43:84–90. https://doi.org/10.1136/jmg.2005.032854

Edghill EL, Bingham C, Slingerland AS, Minton JA, Noordam C, Ellard S, Hattersley AT (2006b) Hepatocyte nuclear factor-1 beta mutations cause neonatal diabetes and intrauterine growth retardation: support for a critical role of HNF-1beta in human pancreatic development. Diabet Med 23:1301–1306. https://doi.org/10.1111/j.1464-5491.2006.01999.x

Edghill EL, Flanagan SE, Patch AM et al (2008) Insulin mutation screening in 1,044 patients with diabetes: mutations in the INS gene are a common cause of neonatal diabetes but a rare cause of diabetes diagnosed in childhood or adulthood. Diabetes 57:1034–1042. https://doi.org/10.2337/db07-1405

Eifes S, Chudasama KK, Molnes J et al (2013) A novel GATA6 mutation in a child with congenital heart malformation and neonatal diabetes. Clin Case Rep 1:86–90. https://doi.org/10.1002/ccr3.33

Ellard S, Thomas K, Edghill EL et al (2007) Partial and whole gene deletion mutations of the GCK and HNF1A genes in maturity-onset diabetes of the young. Diabetologia 50:2313–2317. https://doi.org/10.1007/s00125-007-0798-6

Ellard S, Bellanne-Chantelot C, Hattersley AT, European Molecular Genetics Quality Network Mg (2008) Best practice guidelines for the molecular genetic diagnosis of maturity-onset diabetes of the young. Diabetologia 51:546–553. https://doi.org/10.1007/s00125-008-0942-y

Evliyaoglu O, Ercan O, Ataoğlu E et al (2018) Neonatal diabetes: two cases with isolated pancreas agenesis due to homozygous PTF1A enhancer mutations and one with developmental delay, epilepsy, and neonatal diabetes syndrome due to KCNJ11 mutation. J Clin Res Pediatr Endocrinol 10:168–174. https://doi.org/10.4274/jcrpe.5162

Faguer S, Decramer S, Chassaing N et al (2011) Diagnosis, management, and prognosis of HNF1B nephropathy in adulthood. Kidney Int 80:768–776. https://doi.org/10.1038/ki.2011.225

Faguer S, Chassaing N, Bandin F et al (2014) The HNF1B score is a simple tool to select patients for HNF1B gene analysis. Kidney Int 86:1007–1015. https://doi.org/10.1038/ki.2014.202

Fajans SS, Conn JW (1960) Tolbutamide-induced improvement in carbohydrate tolerance of young people with mild diabetes mellitus. Diabetes 9:83–88

Fajans SS, Bell GI, Paz VP et al (2010) Obesity and hyperinsulinemia in a family with pancreatic agenesis and MODY caused by the IPF1 mutation Pro63fsX60. Transl Res 156:7–14. https://doi.org/10.1016/j.trsl.2010.03.003

Fernandez-Zapico ME, van Velkinburgh JC, Gutierrez-Aguilar R, Neve B, Froguel P, Urrutia R, Stein R (2009) MODY7 gene, KLF11, is a novel p300-dependent regulator of Pdx-1 (MODY4) transcription in pancreatic islet beta cells. J Biol Chem 284:36482–36490. https://doi.org/10.1074/jbc.M109.028852

Ferre S, Igarashi P (2018) New insights into the role of HNF-1beta in kidney (patho)physiology. Pediatr Nephrol. https://doi.org/10.1007/s00467-018-3990-7

Ferrer J (2002) A genetic switch in pancreatic beta-cells: implications for differentiation and haploinsufficiency. Diabetes 51:2355–2362

Flanagan SE, De Franco E, Lango Allen H et al (2014a) Analysis of transcription factors key for mouse pancreatic development establishes NKX2-2 and MNX1 mutations as causes of neonatal diabetes in man. Cell Metab 19:146–154. https://doi.org/10.1016/j.cmet.2013.11.021

Flanagan SE, Haapaniemi E, Russell MA et al (2014b) Activating germline mutations in STAT3 cause early-onset multi-organ autoimmune disease. Nat Genet 46:812–814. https://doi.org/10.1038/ng.3040

Froguel P, Zouali H, Vionnet N et al (1993) Familial hyperglycemia due to mutations in glucokinase. Definition of a subtype of diabetes mellitus. N Engl J Med 328:697–702. https://doi.org/10.1056/NEJM199303113281005

Gaal Z, Klupa T, Kantor I et al (2012) Sulfonylurea use during entire pregnancy in diabetes because of KCNJ11 mutation: a report of two cases. Diabetes Care 35:e40. https://doi.org/10.2337/dc12-0163

Gabbay M, Ellard S, De Franco E, Moises RS (2017) Pancreatic agenesis due to compound heterozygosity for a novel enhancer and truncating mutation in the PTF1A gene. J Clin Res Pediatr Endocrinol 9:274–277. https://doi.org/10.4274/jcrpe.4494

Garin I, Edghill EL, Akerman I et al (2010) Recessive mutations in the INS gene result in neonatal diabetes through reduced insulin biosynthesis. Proc Natl Acad Sci U S A 107:3105–3110. https://doi.org/10.1073/pnas.0910533107

Girard CA, Shimomura K, Proks P, Absalom N, Castano L, Perez de Nanclares G, Ashcroft FM (2006) Functional analysis of six Kir6.2 (KCNJ11) mutations causing neonatal diabetes. Pflugers Arch 453:323–332. https://doi.org/10.1007/s00424-006-0112-3

Gjesing AP, Rui G, Lauenborg J et al (2017) High prevalence of diabetes-predisposing variants in MODY genes among danish women with gestational diabetes mellitus. J Endocr Soc 1:681–690. https://doi.org/10.1210/js.2017-00040

Gloyn AL, Pearson ER, Antcliff JF et al (2004) Activating mutations in the gene encoding the ATP-sensitive potassium-channel subunit Kir6.2 and permanent neonatal diabetes. N Engl J Med 350:1838–1849. https://doi.org/10.1056/NEJMoa032922

Gloyn AL, Diatloff-Zito C, Edghill EL et al (2006) KCNJ11 activating mutations are associated with developmental delay, epilepsy and neonatal diabetes syndrome and other neurological features. Eur J Hum Genet 14:824–830. https://doi.org/10.1038/sj.ejhg.5201629

Gonsorcikova L, Pruhová S, Cinek O et al (2008) Autosomal inheritance of diabetes in two families characterized by obesity and a novel H241Q mutation in NEUROD1. Pediatr Diabetes 9:367–372. https://doi.org/10.1111/j.1399-5448.2008.00379.x

Gragnoli C, Lindner T, Cockburn BN, Kaisaki PJ, Gragnoli F, Marozzi G, Bell GI (1997) Maturity-onset diabetes of the young due to a mutation in the hepatocyte nuclear factor-4 alpha binding site in the promoter of the hepatocyte nuclear factor-1 alpha gene. Diabetes 46:1648–1651

Hansen SK, Parrizas M, Jensen ML et al (2002) Genetic evidence that HNF-1alpha-dependent transcriptional control of HNF-4alpha is essential for human pancreatic beta cell function. J Clin Invest 110:827–833. https://doi.org/10.1172/JCI15085

Harries LW, Ellard S, Stride A, Morgan NG, Hattersley AT (2006) Isomers of the TCF1 gene encoding hepatocyte nuclear factor-1 alpha show differential expression in the pancreas and define the relationship between mutation position and clinical phenotype in monogenic diabetes. Hum Mol Genet 15:2216–2224. https://doi.org/10.1093/hmg/ddl147

Hattersley AT, Ashcroft FM (2005) Activating mutations in Kir6.2 and neonatal diabetes: new clinical syndromes, new scientific insights, and new therapy. Diabetes 54:2503–2513

Hattersley AT, Patel KA (2017) Precision diabetes: learning from monogenic diabetes. Diabetologia 60:769–777. https://doi.org/10.1007/s00125-017-4226-2

Hattersley AT et al (1992) Linkage of type 2 diabetes to the glucokinase gene. Lancet 339:1307–1310

Hattersley AT, Greeley SAW, Polak M et al (2018) ISPAD Clinical Practice Consensus Guidelines 2018: the diagnosis and management of monogenic diabetes in children and adolescents. Pediatr Diabetes 19(Suppl 27):47–63. https://doi.org/10.1111/pedi.12772

Haumaitre C, Fabre M, Cormier S, Baumann C, Delezoide AL, Cereghini S (2006) Severe pancreas hypoplasia and multicystic renal dysplasia in two human fetuses carrying novel HNF1beta/ MODY5 mutations. Hum Mol Genet 15:2363–2375. https://doi.org/10.1093/hmg/ddl161

Heidet L, Decramer S, Pawtowski A et al (2010) Spectrum of HNF1B mutations in a large cohort of patients who harbor renal diseases. Clin J Am Soc Nephrol 5:1079–1090. https://doi.org/10.2215/CJN.06810909

Horikawa Y, Iwasaki N, Hara M et al (1997) Mutation in hepatocyte nuclear factor-1 beta gene (TCF2) associated with MODY. Nat Genet 17:384–385. https://doi.org/10.1038/ng1297-384

Horikawa Y, Enya M, Mabe H et al (2018) NEUROD1-deficient diabetes (MODY6): identification of the first cases in Japanese and the clinical features. Pediatr Diabetes 19:236–242. https://doi.org/10.1111/pedi.12553

Iafusco D, Massa O, Pasquino B et al (2012) Minimal incidence of neonatal/infancy onset diabetes in Italy is 1:90,000 live births. Acta Diabetol 49:405–408. https://doi.org/10.1007/s00592-011-0331-8

Irgens HU, Molnes J, Johansson BB et al (2013) Prevalence of monogenic diabetes in the population-based Norwegian Childhood Diabetes Registry. Diabetologia 56:1512–1519. https://doi.org/10.1007/s00125-013-2916-y

Jo W, Endo M, Ishizu K, Nakamura A, Tajima T (2011) A novel PAX4 mutation in a Japanese patient with maturity-onset diabetes of the young. Tohoku J Exp Med 223:113–118

Johansson BB, Torsvik J, Bjørkhaug L et al (2011) Diabetes and pancreatic exocrine dysfunction due to mutations in the carboxyl ester lipase gene-maturity onset diabetes of the young (CEL-MODY): a protein misfolding disease. J Biol Chem 286:34593–34605. https://doi.org/10.1074/jbc.M111.222679

Johansson S, Irgens H, Chudasama KK et al (2012) Exome sequencing and genetic testing for MODY. PLoS One 7:e38050. https://doi.org/10.1371/journal.pone.0038050

Johansson BB, Irgens HU, Molnes J et al (2017) Targeted next-generation sequencing reveals MODY in up to 6.5% of antibody-negative diabetes cases listed in the Norwegian Childhood Diabetes Registry. Diabetologia 60:625–635. https://doi.org/10.1007/s00125-016-4167-1

Johnson MB, De Franco E, Lango Allen H et al (2017) Recessively inherited LRBA mutations cause autoimmunity presenting as neonatal diabetes. Diabetes 66:2316–2322. https://doi.org/10.2337/db17-0040

Johnson SR, Leo P, Conwell LS, Harris M, Brown MA, Duncan EL (2018a) Clinical usefulness of comprehensive genetic screening in maturity onset diabetes of the young (MODY): a novel ABCC8 mutation in a previously screened family. J Diabetes 10:764–767. https://doi.org/10.1111/1753-0407.12778

Johnson SR, Leo PJ, McInerney-Leo AM et al (2018b) Whole-exome sequencing for mutation detection in pediatric disorders of insulin secretion: maturity onset diabetes of the young and congenital hyperinsulinism. Pediatr Diabetes 19:656–662. https://doi.org/10.1111/pedi.12638

Jonsson J, Carlsson L, Edlund T, Edlund H (1994) Insulin-promoter-factor 1 is required for pancreas development in mice. Nature 371:606–609. https://doi.org/10.1038/371606a0

Juszczak A, Pryse R, Schuman A, Owen KR (2016) When to consider a diagnosis of MODY at the presentation of diabetes: aetiology matters for correct management. Br J Gen Pract 66: e457–e459. https://doi.org/10.3399/bjgp16X685537

Khandelwal P, Sinha A, Jain V, Houghton J, Hari P, Bagga A (2018) Fanconi syndrome and neonatal diabetes: phenotypic heterogeneity in patients with GLUT2 defects. CEN Case Rep 7:1–4. https://doi.org/10.1007/s13730-017-0278-x

Klupa T, Kozek E, Nowak N et al (2010) The first case report of sulfonylurea use in a woman with permanent neonatal diabetes mellitus due to KCNJ11 mutation during a high-risk pregnancy. J Clin Endocrinol Metab 95:3599–3604. https://doi.org/10.1210/jc.2010-0096

Kristinsson SY, Thorolfsdottir ET, Talseth B et al (2001) MODY in Iceland is associated with mutations in HNF-1alpha and a novel mutation in NeuroD1. Diabetologia 44:2098–2103. https://doi.org/10.1007/s001250100016

Kwak SH, Jung CH, Ahn CH et al (2016) Clinical whole exome sequencing in early onset diabetes patients. Diabetes Res Clin Pract 122:71–77. https://doi.org/10.1016/j.diabres.2016.10.005

Laffargue F, Bourthoumieu S, Llanas B et al (2015) Towards a new point of view on the phenotype of patients with a 17q12 microdeletion syndrome. Arch Dis Child 100:259–264. https://doi.org/10.1136/archdischild-2014-306810

Lausen J, Thomas H, Lemm I et al (2000) Naturally occurring mutations in the human HNF4alpha gene impair the function of the transcription factor to a varying degree. Nucleic Acids Res 28:430–437

Liu L, Furuta H, Minami A, Zheng T, Jia W, Nanjo K, Xiang K (2007) A novel mutation, Ser159Pro in the NeuroD1/BETA2 gene contributes to the development of diabetes in a Chinese potential MODY family. Mol Cell Biochem 303:115–120. https://doi.org/10.1007/s11010-007-9463-0

Lombardo D (2001) Bile salt-dependent lipase: its pathophysiological implications. Biochim Biophys Acta 1533:1–28

Lorenzo PI, Juarez-Vicente F, Cobo-Vuilleumier N, Garcia-Dominguez M, Gauthier BR (2017) The diabetes-linked transcription factor PAX4: from gene to functional consequences. Genes (Basel) 8. https://doi.org/10.3390/genes8030101

Lorenzo PI, Cobo-Vuilleumier N, Gauthier BR (2018) Therapeutic potential of pancreatic PAX4-regulated pathways in treating diabetes mellitus. Curr Opin Pharmacol 43:1–10. https://doi.org/10.1016/j.coph.2018.07.004

Ma Y, Han X, Zhou X et al (2018) A new clinical screening strategy and prevalence estimation for glucokinase variant-induced diabetes in an adult Chinese population. Genet Med. https://doi.org/10.1038/s41436-018-0282-3

Mackay DJ, Temple IK (2010) Transient neonatal diabetes mellitus type 1. Am J Med Genet C Semin Med Genet 154C:335–342. https://doi.org/10.1002/ajmg.c.30272

Mackay DJ, Boonen SE, Clayton-Smith J et al (2006) A maternal hypomethylation syndrome presenting as transient neonatal diabetes mellitus. Hum Genet 120:262–269. https://doi.org/10.1007/s00439-006-0205-2

Maestro MA, Cardalda C, Boj SF, Luco RF, Servitja JM, Ferrer J (2007) Distinct roles of HNF1beta, HNF1alpha, and HNF4alpha in regulating pancreas development, beta-cell function and growth. Endocr Dev 12:33–45. https://doi.org/10.1159/000109603

Malecki MT, Jhala US, Antonellis A et al (1999) Mutations in NEUROD1 are associated with the development of type 2 diabetes mellitus. Nat Genet 23:323–328. https://doi.org/10.1038/15500

Mangrum C, Rush E, Shivaswamy V (2015) Genetically targeted dipeptidyl peptidase-4 inhibitor use in a patient with a novel mutation of MODY type 4. Clin Med Insights Endocrinol Diabetes 8:83–86. https://doi.org/10.4137/CMED.S31926

Massa O, Iafusco D, D'Amato E et al (2005) KCNJ11 activating mutations in Italian patients with permanent neonatal diabetes. Hum Mutat 25:22–27. https://doi.org/10.1002/humu.20124

Matschinsky FM (1990) Glucokinase as glucose sensor and metabolic signal generator in pancreatic beta-cells and hepatocytes. Diabetes 39:647–652

Mefford HC, Clauin S, Sharp AJ et al (2007) Recurrent reciprocal genomic rearrangements of 17q12 are associated with renal disease, diabetes, and epilepsy. Am J Hum Genet 81:1057–1069. https://doi.org/10.1086/522591

Menzel R, Kaisaki PJ, Rjasanowski I, Heinke P, Kerner W, Menzel S (1998) A low renal threshold for glucose in diabetic patients with a mutation in the hepatocyte nuclear factor-1alpha (HNF-1alpha) gene. Diabet Med 15:816–820. https://doi.org/10.1002/(SICI)1096-9136(199810)15:10<816::AID-DIA714>3.0.CO;2-P

Meur G, Simon A, Harun N et al (2010) Insulin gene mutations resulting in early-onset diabetes: marked differences in clinical presentation, metabolic status, and pathogenic effect through endoplasmic reticulum retention. Diabetes 59:653–661. https://doi.org/10.2337/db09-1091

Mitchell J, Punthakee Z, Lo B et al (2004) Neonatal diabetes, with hypoplastic pancreas, intestinal atresia and gall bladder hypoplasia: search for the aetiology of a new autosomal recessive syndrome. Diabetologia 47:2160–2167. https://doi.org/10.1007/s00125-004-1576-3

Mitsuuchi Y, Johnson SW, Sonoda G, Tanno S, Golemis EA, Testa JR (1999) Identification of a chromosome 3p14.3-21.1 gene, APPL, encoding an adaptor molecule that interacts with the oncoprotein-serine/threonine kinase AKT2. Oncogene 18:4891–4898. https://doi.org/10.1038/sj.onc.1203080

Mohan V, Radha V, Nguyen TT et al (2018) Comprehensive genomic analysis identifies pathogenic variants in maturity-onset diabetes of the young (MODY) patients in South India. BMC Med Genet 19:22. https://doi.org/10.1186/s12881-018-0528-6

Molven A, Ringdal M, Nordbø AM et al (2008) Mutations in the insulin gene can cause MODY and autoantibody-negative type 1 diabetes. Diabetes 57:1131–1135. https://doi.org/10.2337/db07-1467

Myngheer N, Allegaert K, Hattersley A et al (2014) Fetal macrosomia and neonatal hyperinsulinemic hypoglycemia associated with transplacental transfer of sulfonylurea in a mother with KCNJ11-related neonatal diabetes. Diabetes care 37:3333–3335. https://doi.org/10.2337/dc14-1247

Naya FJ, Stellrecht CM, Tsai MJ (1995) Tissue-specific regulation of the insulin gene by a novel basic helix-loop-helix transcription factor. Genes Dev 9:1009–1019

Naya FJ, Huang HP, Qiu Y, Mutoh H, DeMayo FJ, Leiter AB, Tsai MJ (1997) Diabetes, defective pancreatic morphogenesis, and abnormal enteroendocrine differentiation in BETA2/neuroD-deficient mice. Genes Dev 11:2323–2334

Negahdar M, Aukrust I, Johansson BB et al (2012) GCK-MODY diabetes associated with protein misfolding, cellular self-association and degradation. Biochim Biophys Acta 1822:1705–1715. https://doi.org/10.1016/j.bbadis.2012.07.005

Negahdar M, Aukrust I, Molnes J et al (2014) GCK-MODY diabetes as a protein misfolding disease: the mutation R275C promotes protein misfolding, self-association and cellular degradation. Mol Cell Endocrinol 382:55–65. https://doi.org/10.1016/j.mce.2013.08.020

Neve B, Fernandez-Zapico ME, Ashkenazi-Katalan V et al (2005) Role of transcription factor KLF11 and its diabetes-associated gene variants in pancreatic beta cell function. Proc Natl Acad Sci U S A 102:4807–4812. https://doi.org/10.1073/pnas.0409177102

Nicolino M, Claiborn KC, Senee V, Boland A, Stoffers DA, Julier C (2010) A novel hypomorphic PDX1 mutation responsible for permanent neonatal diabetes with subclinical exocrine deficiency. Diabetes 59:733–740. https://doi.org/10.2337/db09-1284

Njolstad PR, Søvik O, Cuesta-Muñoz A et al (2001) Neonatal diabetes mellitus due to complete glucokinase deficiency. N Engl J Med 344:1588–1592. https://doi.org/10.1056/NEJM200105243442104

Njolstad PR, Sagen JV, Bjørkhaug L et al (2003) Permanent neonatal diabetes caused by glucokinase deficiency: inborn error of the glucose-insulin signaling pathway. Diabetes 52:2854–2860

Odom DT, Zizlsperger N, Gordon DB et al (2004) Control of pancreas and liver gene expression by HNF transcription factors. Science 303:1378–1381. https://doi.org/10.1126/science.1089769

Oriola J, Moreno F, Gutierrez-Nogues A, Leon S, Garcia-Herrero CM, Vincent O, Navas MA (2015) Lack of glibenclamide response in a case of permanent neonatal diabetes caused by incomplete inactivation of glucokinase. JIMD Rep 20:21–26. https://doi.org/10.1007/8904_2014_383

Orosz O, Czeglédi M, Kántor I et al (2015) Ophthalmological phenotype associated with homozygous null mutation in the NEUROD1 gene. Mol Vis 21:124–130

Osbak KK, Colclough K, Saint-Martin C, Beer NL, Bellanne-Chantelot C, Ellard S, Gloyn AL (2009) Update on mutations in glucokinase (GCK), which cause maturity-onset diabetes of the young, permanent neonatal diabetes, and hyperinsulinemic hypoglycemia. Hum Mutat 30:1512–1526. https://doi.org/10.1002/humu.21110

Owen KR, Thanabalasingham G, James TJ, Karpe F, Farmer AJ, McCarthy MI, Gloyn AL (2010) Assessment of high-sensitivity C-reactive protein levels as diagnostic discriminator of maturity-onset diabetes of the young due to HNF1A mutations. Diabetes Care 33:1919–1924. https://doi.org/10.2337/dc10-0288

Pan FC, Brissova M, Powers AC, Pfaff S, Wright CV (2015) Inactivating the permanent neonatal diabetes gene Mnx1 switches insulin-producing beta-cells to a delta-like fate and reveals a facultative proliferative capacity in aged beta-cells. Development 142:3637–3648. https://doi.org/10.1242/dev.126011

Park SY, Ye H, Steiner DF, Bell GI (2010) Mutant proinsulin proteins associated with neonatal diabetes are retained in the endoplasmic reticulum and not efficiently secreted. Biochem Biophys Res Commun 391:1449–1454. https://doi.org/10.1016/j.bbrc.2009.12.090

Patel KA, Kettunen J, Laakso M et al (2017) Heterozygous RFX6 protein truncating variants are associated with MODY with reduced penetrance. Nat Commun 8:888. https://doi.org/10.1038/s41467-017-00895-9

Pearson ER, Starkey BJ, Powell RJ, Gribble FM, Clark PM, Hattersley AT (2003) Genetic cause of hyperglycaemia and response to treatment in diabetes. Lancet 362:1275–1281. https://doi.org/10.1016/S0140-6736(03)14571-0

Pearson ER, Badman MK, Lockwood CR, Clark PM, Ellard S, Bingham C, Hattersley AT (2004) Contrasting diabetes phenotypes associated with hepatocyte nuclear factor-1alpha and -1beta mutations. Diabetes Care 27:1102–1107

Pearson ER, Flechtner I, Njølstad PR et al (2006) Switching from insulin to oral sulfonylureas in patients with diabetes due to Kir6.2 mutations. N Engl J Med 355:467–477. https://doi.org/10.1056/NEJMoa061759

Pearson ER, Boj SF, Steele AM et al (2007) Macrosomia and hyperinsulinaemic hypoglycaemia in patients with heterozygous mutations in the HNF4A gene. PLoS Med 4:e118. https://doi.org/10.1371/journal.pmed.0040118

Perakakis N, Danassi D, Alt M et al (2012) Human Kruppel-like factor 11 differentially regulates human insulin promoter activity in beta-cells and non-beta-cells via p300 and PDX1 through the regulatory sites A3 and CACCC box. Mol Cell Endocrinol 363:20–26. https://doi.org/10.1016/j.mce.2012.07.003

Petersen HV, Jørgensen MC, Andersen FG et al (2000) Pax4 represses pancreatic glucagon gene expression. Mol Cell Biol Res Commun 3:249–254. https://doi.org/10.1006/mcbr.2000.0220

Piccini B, Artuso R, Lenzi L et al (2016) Clinical and molecular characterization of a novel INS mutation identified in patients with MODY phenotype. Eur J Med Genet 59:590–595. https://doi.org/10.1016/j.ejmg.2016.09.016

Pihoker C, Gilliam LK, Ellard S et al (2013) Prevalence, characteristics and clinical diagnosis of maturity onset diabetes of the young due to mutations in HNF1A, HNF4A, and glucokinase: results from the SEARCH for Diabetes in Youth. J Clin Endocrinol Metab 98:4055–4062. https://doi.org/10.1210/jc.2013-1279

Plengvidhya N, Kooptiwut S, Songtawee N et al (2007) PAX4 mutations in Thais with maturity onset diabetes of the young. J Clin Endocrinol Metab 92:2821–2826. https://doi.org/10.1210/jc.2006-1927

Poll AV, Pierreux CE, Lokmane L et al (2006) A vHNF1/TCF2-HNF6 cascade regulates the transcription factor network that controls generation of pancreatic precursor cells. Diabetes 55:61–69

Proks P, Arnold AL, Bruining J et al (2006) A heterozygous activating mutation in the sulphonylurea receptor SUR1 (ABCC8) causes neonatal diabetes. Hum Mol Genet 15:1793–1800. https://doi.org/10.1093/hmg/ddl101

Prudente S, Jungtrakoon P, Marucci A et al (2015) Loss-of-function mutations in APPL1 in familial diabetes mellitus. Am J Hum Genet 97:177–185. https://doi.org/10.1016/j.ajhg.2015.05.011

Raeder H, Johansson S, Holm PI et al (2006) Mutations in the CEL VNTR cause a syndrome of diabetes and pancreatic exocrine dysfunction. Nat Genet 38:54–62. https://doi.org/10.1038/ng1708

Raimondo A, Chakera AJ, Thomsen SK et al (2014) Phenotypic severity of homozygous GCK mutations causing neonatal or childhood-onset diabetes is primarily mediated through effects on protein stability. Hum Mol Genet 23:6432–6440. https://doi.org/10.1093/hmg/ddu360

Remedi MS, Koster JC, Patton BL, Nichols CG (2005) ATP-sensitive K+ channel signaling in glucokinase-deficient diabetes. Diabetes 54:2925–2931

Rubio-Cabezas O, Diaz Gonzalez F, Aragones A, Argente J, Campos-Barros A (2008) Permanent neonatal diabetes caused by a homozygous nonsense mutation in the glucokinase gene. Pediatr Diabetes 9:245–249. https://doi.org/10.1111/j.1399-5448.2007.00361.x

Rubio-Cabezas O, Minton JA, Caswell R et al (2009a) Clinical heterogeneity in patients with FOXP3 mutations presenting with permanent neonatal diabetes. Diabetes Care 32:111–116. https://doi.org/10.2337/dc08-1188

Rubio-Cabezas O, Patch AM, Minton JA et al (2009b) Wolcott-Rallison syndrome is the most common genetic cause of permanent neonatal diabetes in consanguineous families. J Clin Endocrinol Metab 94:4162–4170. https://doi.org/10.1210/jc.2009-1137

Rubio-Cabezas O, Minton JA, Kantor I, Williams D, Ellard S, Hattersley AT (2010) Homozygous mutations in NEUROD1 are responsible for a novel syndrome of permanent neonatal diabetes and neurological abnormalities. Diabetes 59:2326–2331. https://doi.org/10.2337/db10-0011

Rubio-Cabezas O, Jensen JN, Hodgson MI, Codner E, Ellard S, Serup P, Hattersley AT (2011) Permanent neonatal diabetes and enteric anendocrinosis associated with biallelic mutations in NEUROG3. Diabetes 60:1349–1353. https://doi.org/10.2337/db10-1008

Rudland VL, Hinchcliffe M, Pinner J et al (2016) Identifying glucokinase monogenic diabetes in a multiethnic gestational diabetes mellitus cohort: new pregnancy screening criteria and utility of HbA1c. Diabetes Care 39:50–52. https://doi.org/10.2337/dc15-1001

Ryffel GU (2001) Mutations in the human genes encoding the transcription factors of the hepatocyte nuclear factor (HNF)1 and HNF4 families: functional and pathological consequences. J Mol Endocrinol 27:11–29

Saarimaki-Vire J, Balboa D, Russell MA et al (2017) An activating STAT3 mutation causes neonatal diabetes through premature induction of pancreatic differentiation. Cell Rep 19:281–294. https://doi.org/10.1016/j.celrep.2017.03.055

Sagen JV, Raeder H, Hathout E et al (2004) Permanent neonatal diabetes due to mutations in KCNJ11 encoding Kir6.2: patient characteristics and initial response to sulfonylurea therapy. Diabetes 53:2713–2718

Sansbury FH, Flanagan SE, Houghton JA et al (2012) SLC2A2 mutations can cause neonatal diabetes, suggesting GLUT2 may have a role in human insulin secretion. Diabetologia 55:2381–2385. https://doi.org/10.1007/s00125-012-2595-0

Sansbury FH, Kirel B, Caswell R et al (2015) Biallelic RFX6 mutations can cause childhood as well as neonatal onset diabetes mellitus. Eur J Hum Genet 23:1744–1748. https://doi.org/10.1038/ejhg.2015.161

Sellick GS, Barker KT, Stolte-Dijkstra I et al (2004) Mutations in PTF1A cause pancreatic and cerebellar agenesis. Nat Genet 36:1301–1305. https://doi.org/10.1038/ng1475

Senee V, Chelala C, Duchatelet S et al (2006) Mutations in GLIS3 are responsible for a rare syndrome with neonatal diabetes mellitus and congenital hypothyroidism. Nat Genet 38:682–687. https://doi.org/10.1038/ng1802

Shalev SA, Tenenbaum-Rakover Y, Horovitz Y et al (2014) Microcephaly, epilepsy, and neonatal diabetes due to compound heterozygous mutations in IER3IP1: insights into the natural history of a rare disorder. Pediatr Diabetes 15:252–256. https://doi.org/10.1111/pedi.12086

Shaw-Smith C, Flanagan SE, Patch AM et al (2012) Recessive SLC19A2 mutations are a cause of neonatal diabetes mellitus in thiamine-responsive megaloblastic anaemia. Pediatr Diabetes 13:314–321. https://doi.org/10.1111/j.1399-5448.2012.00855.x

Shaw-Smith C, De Franco E, Lango Allen H et al (2014) GATA4 mutations are a cause of neonatal and childhood-onset diabetes. Diabetes 63:2888–2894. https://doi.org/10.2337/db14-0061

Shepherd M, Hattersley AT (2004) I don't feel like a diabetic any more': the impact of stopping insulin in patients with maturity onset diabetes of the young following genetic testing. Clin Med (Lond) 4:144–147

Shepherd M et al (2001) Predictive genetic testing in maturity-onset diabetes of the young (MODY). Diabet Med 18:417–421

Shepherd M, Shields B, Hammersley S et al (2016) Systematic population screening, using biomarkers and genetic testing, identifies 2.5% of the U.K. pediatric diabetes population with monogenic diabetes. Diabetes Care 39:1879–1888. https://doi.org/10.2337/dc16-0645

Shepherd M, Brook AJ, Chakera AJ, Hattersley AT (2017) Management of sulfonylurea-treated monogenic diabetes in pregnancy: implications of placental glibenclamide transfer. Diabet Med 34:1332–1339. https://doi.org/10.1111/dme.13388

Shepherd MH, Shields BM, Hudson M et al (2018) A UK nationwide prospective study of treatment change in MODY: genetic subtype and clinical characteristics predict optimal glycaemic control after discontinuing insulin and metformin. Diabetologia 61:2520–2527. https://doi.org/10.1007/s00125-018-4728-6

Shield JP (2000) Neonatal diabetes: new insights into aetiology and implications. Horm Res 53 (Suppl 1):7–11. https://doi.org/10.1159/000053198

Shields BM, Hicks S, Shepherd MH, Colclough K, Hattersley AT, Ellard S (2010) Maturity-onset diabetes of the young (MODY): how many cases are we missing? Diabetologia 53:2504–2508. https://doi.org/10.1007/s00125-010-1799-4

Shields BM, McDonald TJ, Ellard S, Campbell MJ, Hyde C, Hattersley AT (2012) The development and validation of a clinical prediction model to determine the probability of MODY in patients with young-onset diabetes. Diabetologia 55:1265–1272. https://doi.org/10.1007/s00125-011-2418-8

Smith SB, Watada H, Scheel DW, Mrejen C, German MS (2000) Autoregulation and maturity onset diabetes of the young transcription factors control the human PAX4 promoter. J Biol Chem 275:36910–36919. https://doi.org/10.1074/jbc.M005202200

Solomon BD, Pineda-Alvarez DE, Balog JZ et al (2009) Compound heterozygosity for mutations in PAX6 in a patient with complex brain anomaly, neonatal diabetes mellitus, and microophthalmia. Am J Med Genet A 149A:2543–2546. https://doi.org/10.1002/ajmg.a.33081

Sosa-Pineda B, Chowdhury K, Torres M, Oliver G, Gruss P (1997) The Pax4 gene is essential for differentiation of insulin-producing beta cells in the mammalian pancreas. Nature 386:399–402. https://doi.org/10.1038/386399a0

Spiegel R, Dobbie A, Hartman C, de Vries L, Ellard S, Shalev SA (2011) Clinical characterization of a newly described neonatal diabetes syndrome caused by RFX6 mutations. Am J Med Genet A 155A:2821–2825. https://doi.org/10.1002/ajmg.a.34251

Stanik J, Dusatkova P, Cinek O et al (2014) De novo mutations of GCK, HNF1A and HNF4A may be more frequent in MODY than previously assumed. Diabetologia 57:480–484. https://doi.org/10.1007/s00125-013-3119-2

Stanojevic V, Habener JF, Thomas MK (2004) Pancreas duodenum homeobox-1 transcriptional activation requires interactions with p300. Endocrinology 145:2918–2928. https://doi.org/10.1210/en.2003-1188

Steele AM, Shields BM, Wensley KJ, Colclough K, Ellard S, Hattersley AT (2014) Prevalence of vascular complications among patients with glucokinase mutations and prolonged, mild hyperglycemia. JAMA 311:279–286. https://doi.org/10.1001/jama.2013.283980

Stoffers DA, Ferrer J, Clarke WL, Habener JF (1997a) Early-onset type-II diabetes mellitus (MODY4) linked to IPF1. Nat Genet 17:138–139. https://doi.org/10.1038/ng1097-138

Stoffers DA, Zinkin NT, Stanojevic V, Clarke WL, Habener JF (1997b) Pancreatic agenesis attributable to a single nucleotide deletion in the human IPF1 gene coding sequence. Nat Genet 15:106–110. https://doi.org/10.1038/ng0197-106

Stoy J, Edghill EL, Flanagan SE et al (2007) Insulin gene mutations as a cause of permanent neonatal diabetes. Proc Natl Acad Sci U S A 104:15040–15044. https://doi.org/10.1073/pnas.0707291104

Stoy J, Steiner DF, Park SY, Ye H, Philipson LH, Bell GI (2010) Clinical and molecular genetics of neonatal diabetes due to mutations in the insulin gene. Rev Endocr Metab Disord 11:205–215. https://doi.org/10.1007/s11154-010-9151-3

Sujjitjoon J, Kooptiwut S, Chongjaroen N, Tangjittipokin W, Plengvidhya N, Yenchitsomanus PT (2016) Aberrant mRNA splicing of paired box 4 (PAX4) IVS7-1G>A mutation causing maturity-onset diabetes of the young, type 9. Acta Diabetol 53:205–216. https://doi.org/10.1007/s00592-015-0760-x

Sun C, Pei Z, Zhang M et al (2018) Recovered insulin production after thiamine administration in permanent neonatal diabetes mellitus with a novel solute carrier family 19 member 2 (SLC19A2) mutation. J Diabetes 10:50–58. https://doi.org/10.1111/1753-0407.12556

Suzuki S, Nakao A, Sarhat AR et al (2014) A case of pancreatic agenesis and congenital heart defects with a novel GATA6 nonsense mutation: evidence of haploinsufficiency due to nonsense-mediated mRNA decay. Am J Med Genet A. 164A:476–479. https://doi.org/10.1002/ajmg.a.36275

Szopa M, Ludwig-Galezowska AH, Radkowski P et al (2016) A family with the Arg103Pro mutation in the NEUROD1 gene detected by next-generation sequencing – clinical characteristics of mutation carriers. Eur J Med Genet 59:75–79. https://doi.org/10.1016/j.ejmg.2016.01.002

Tattersall RB (1974) Mild familial diabetes with dominant inheritance. Q J Med 43:339–357

Thanabalasingham G, Shah N, Vaxillaire M et al (2011) A large multi-centre European study validates high-sensitivity C-reactive protein (hsCRP) as a clinical biomarker for the diagnosis of diabetes subtypes. Diabetologia 54:2801–2810. https://doi.org/10.1007/s00125-011-2261-y

Thanabalasingham G, Pal A, Selwood MP et al (2012) Systematic assessment of etiology in adults with a clinical diagnosis of young-onset type 2 diabetes is a successful strategy for identifying maturity-onset diabetes of the young. Diabetes Care 35:1206–1212. https://doi.org/10.2337/dc11-1243

Thomas H, Jaschkowitz K, Bulman M et al (2001) A distant upstream promoter of the HNF-4alpha gene connects the transcription factors involved in maturity-onset diabetes of the young. Hum Mol Genet 10:2089–2097

Thomas H, Badenberg B, Bulman M et al (2002) Evidence for haploinsufficiency of the human HNF1alpha gene revealed by functional characterization of MODY3-associated mutations. Biol Chem 383:1691–1700. https://doi.org/10.1515/BC.2002.190

Toniatti C, Demartis A, Monaci P, Nicosia A, Ciliberto G (1990) Synergistic trans-activation of the human C-reactive protein promoter by transcription factor HNF-1 binding at two distinct sites. EMBO J 9:4467–4475

Touati A, Errea-Dorronsoro J, Nouri S et al (2018) Transient neonatal diabetes mellitus and hypomethylation at additional imprinted loci: novel ZFP57 mutation and review on the literature. Acta Diabetol. https://doi.org/10.1007/s00592-018-1239-3

Tuhan H, Catli G, Anik A, Ozmen D, Turkmen MA, Bober E, Abaci A (2015) Neonatal diabetes mellitus due to a novel mutation in the GATA6 gene accompanying renal dysfunction: a case report. Am J Med Genet A 167A:925–927. https://doi.org/10.1002/ajmg.a.36984

Turkkahraman D, Bircan I, Tribble ND, Akcurin S, Ellard S, Gloyn AL (2008) Permanent neonatal diabetes mellitus caused by a novel homozygous (T168A) glucokinase (GCK) mutation: initial response to oral sulphonylurea therapy. J Pediatr 153:122–126. https://doi.org/10.1016/j.jpeds.2007.12.037

Ulinski T, Lescure S, Beaufils S et al (2006) Renal phenotypes related to hepatocyte nuclear factor-1beta (TCF2) mutations in a pediatric cohort. J Am Soc Nephrol 17:497–503. https://doi.org/10.1681/ASN.2005101040

Valentinova L, Beer NL, Staník J et al (2012) Identification and functional characterisation of novel glucokinase mutations causing maturity-onset diabetes of the young in Slovakia. PLoS One 7: e34541. https://doi.org/10.1371/journal.pone.0034541

van der Meulen T, Huising MO (2015) Role of transcription factors in the transdifferentiation of pancreatic islet cells. J Mol Endocrinol 54:R103–R117. https://doi.org/10.1530/JME-14-0290

Vaxillaire M, Populaire C, Busiah K et al (2004) Kir6.2 mutations are a common cause of permanent neonatal diabetes in a large cohort of French patients. Diabetes 53:2719–2722

Velayos T, Martínez R, Alonso M et al (2017) An activating mutation in STAT3 results in neonatal diabetes through reduced insulin synthesis. Diabetes 66:1022–1029. https://doi.org/10.2337/db16-0867

Wang Q, Elghazi L, Martin S et al (2008) Ghrelin is a novel target of Pax4 in endocrine progenitors of the pancreas and duodenum. Dev Dyn 237:51–61. https://doi.org/10.1002/dvdy.21379

Wang Y, Cheng KK, Lam KS et al (2011) APPL1 counteracts obesity-induced vascular insulin resistance and endothelial dysfunction by modulating the endothelial production of nitric oxide and endothelin-1 in mice. Diabetes 60:3044–3054. https://doi.org/10.2337/db11-0666

Weedon MN, Cebola I, Patch AM et al (2014) Recessive mutations in a distal PTF1A enhancer cause isolated pancreatic agenesis. Nat Genet 46:61–64. https://doi.org/10.1038/ng.2826

Yamagata K (2003) Regulation of pancreatic beta-cell function by the HNF transcription network: lessons from maturity-onset diabetes of the young (MODY). Endocr J 50:491–499

Yamagata K (2014) Roles of HNF1alpha and HNF4alpha in pancreatic beta-cells: lessons from a monogenic form of diabetes (MODY). Vitam Horm 95:407–423. https://doi.org/10.1016/B978-0-12-800174-5.00016-8

Yamagata K, Furuta H, Oda N et al (1996a) Mutations in the hepatocyte nuclear factor-4alpha gene in maturity-onset diabetes of the young (MODY1). Nature 384:458–460. https://doi.org/10.1038/384458a0

Yamagata K, Oda N, Kaisaki PJ et al (1996b) Mutations in the hepatocyte nuclear factor-1alpha gene in maturity-onset diabetes of the young (MODY3). Nature 384:455–458. https://doi.org/10.1038/384455a0

Yan J, Jiang F, Zhang R et al (2017) Whole-exome sequencing identifies a novel INS mutation causative of maturity-onset diabetes of the young 10. J Mol Cell Biol 9:376–383. https://doi.org/10.1093/jmcb/mjx039

Yorifuji T, Kurokawa K, Mamada M et al (2004) Neonatal diabetes mellitus and neonatal polycystic, dysplastic kidneys: phenotypically discordant recurrence of a mutation in the hepatocyte nuclear factor-1beta gene due to germline mosaicism. J Clin Endocrinol Metab 89:2905–2908. https://doi.org/10.1210/jc.2003-031828

Zoncu R, Perera RM, Balkin DM, Pirruccello M, Toomre D, De Camilli P (2009) A phosphoinositide switch controls the maturation and signaling properties of APPL endosomes. Cell 136:1110–1121. https://doi.org/10.1016/j.cell.2009.01.032

Part V
Example of a Multifactorial Disease and Chromosomal Alterations in Endocrine Diseases

Chapter 19
Genetics of Obesity

Lotte Kleinendorst, Mieke M. van Haelst, and Erica L. T. van den Akker

Abstract Obesity is caused by an imbalance between energy intake and output, influenced by numerous environmental, biological, and genetic factors. Only a minority of people with obesity have a genetic defect that is the main cause of their obesity. A key symptom for most of these disorders is early-onset obesity and hyperphagia. For some genetic obesity disorders, the hyperphagia is the main characteristic, often caused by disruptions of the leptin-melanocortin pathway, the central pathway that regulates the body's satiety and energy balance. For other disorders, obesity is part of a distinct combination of other clinical features such as intellectual disability, dysmorphic facial features, or organ abnormalities. This chapter focuses on genetic obesity disorders and also summarizes the present knowledge on the genetics of the more common polygenic/multifactorial obesity.

Keywords Body weight regulation · Common obesity · Early-onset obesity · Hyperphagia · Leptin-melanocortin pathway · Genetic obesity · Non-syndromic obesity · Syndromic obesity

---

L. Kleinendorst
Obesity Center CGG, Erasmus MC, University Medical Center, Rotterdam, The Netherlands

Department of Clinical Genetics, Amsterdam UMC, Location AMC, Amsterdam, The Netherlands

Department of Clinical Genetics, Amsterdam UMC, Location VUmc, Amsterdam, The Netherlands

M. M. van Haelst
Department of Clinical Genetics, Amsterdam UMC, Location AMC, Amsterdam, The Netherlands

Department of Clinical Genetics, Amsterdam UMC, Location VUmc, Amsterdam, The Netherlands

E. L. T. van den Akker (✉)
Obesity Center CGG, Erasmus MC, University Medical Center, Rotterdam, The Netherlands

Division of Endocrinology, Department of Pediatrics, Erasmus MC-Sophia Children's Hospital, University Medical Center, Rotterdam, The Netherlands
e-mail: e.l.t.vandenakker@erasmusmc.nl

P. Igaz, A. Patócs (eds.), *Genetics of Endocrine Diseases and Syndromes*, Experientia Supplementum 111, https://doi.org/10.1007/978-3-030-25905-1_19

Abbreviations

ACTH	Adrenocorticotropic hormone
AgRP	Agouti-related protein
AHO	Albright hereditary osteodystrophy
BBS	Bardet-Biedl syndrome
BMI	Body mass index
CCK	Cholecystokinin
GLP-1	Glucagon-like peptide-1
ID	Intellectual disability
MC3R	Melanocortin 3 receptor
MC4R	Melanocortin 4 receptor
MSH	Melanocyte-stimulating hormone
NPY	Neuropeptide Y
PHP1a	Pseudohypoparathyroidism type 1a
POMC	Proopiomelanocortin
PWS	Prader-Willi syndrome
PYY	Peptide YY
UPD	Uniparental disomy

19.1 Introduction

Obesity is defined as fat accumulation that exceeds normal amounts, leading to an increased health risk. Obesity is one of the most common and serious health problems of our time (Williams et al. 2015), which can be seen in every health clinic in the world. Healthcare professionals determine an individual's weight status by using the body mass index (BMI), the calculation of body weight in relation to square height. Obesity starts at a BMI of 30 kg/m^2 (obesity and overweight 2018). In children, BMI standard deviation scores (SDS) are needed to assess overweight and obesity because BMI in children varies greatly while growing. They represent the deviation from the mean BMI in children of the same sex and same age.

Classification of Obesity for Adults

Below 18.5 kg/m^2 = underweight
- 18.5–24.9 = normal weight
- 25.0–29.9 = overweight
- 30.0–34.9 = obesity class I
- 35.0–39.9 = obesity class II
- 40 or higher = obesity class III

The health consequences of obesity extend to all organ systems. In the long term, this can result in cardio- and cerebrovascular diseases, cancer, and even premature death (Williams et al. 2015). Medical problems like osteoarthritis and polycystic ovary syndrome have a great impact on the well-being of people with obesity as well. Moreover, the impact of the stigma and its psychological effects are great threats to the quality of life of people with obesity. The consequences of obesity are even more alarming when considering the rising incidence and prevalence of obesity; according to recent estimations 20% of the world's population will be obese by 2025 (Collaboration 2016). Obesity and its related health consequences are therefore a large threat to our societal resources, not only because of high healthcare expenditure but also in productivity loss and reduced well-being.

The human body is an excellent energy battery. When little food is available, the body uses its energy storage; and when resources are superfluous, extra energy is stored in the form of fat. Day-to-day energy consumption and energy expenditure are regulated by a system of complex neurological and endocrine pathways, which will be discussed later in this chapter. This balance can be easily disrupted in our current environment, with numerous external factors that can lead to obesity. The causes of obesity are diverse, but the recent rise of its prevalence is mainly due to change in our environment (Hall 2018). Our society has become more obesogenic with easily accessible energy-dense food and a reduction in physical activity. Other factors such as sleep, stress, and medication can play a role in developing obesity as well. Somatic disorders such as Cushing's syndrome or hypothalamic damage are rare causes of obesity. These and other nongenetic causes of obesity are not further discussed in this chapter.

19.2 The Role of Genetics in Obesity

It is well known that environmental circumstances, such as sedentary lifestyle and fast-food consumption, are important players in the development of obesity, but variation in weight or BMI is also highly attributable to the genetic background. Multiple twin studies led to the conclusion that the heritability of weight can be as high as 70% (Polderman et al. 2015). In many people, obesity predisposition is probably polygenic and multifactorial, meaning that the combination of environmental factors and different genetic factors determine body weight. Currently, more than 100 genes are identified to be associated with obesity or BMI (Ignatieva et al. 2016). There are far less genes in which a single mutation leads to obesity regardless of environmental factors. However, there is growing evidence that there is a continuum between rare monogenic syndromic and common polygenic forms of obesity. Both the role of genetics in rare genetic obesity disorders and common polygenic obesity will be discussed in this chapter. Genetic obesity disorders are severe and disabling disorders with a variety of accompanying symptoms or features. These disorders are rare to extremely rare and can be difficult to diagnose. Genetic obesity disorders are more often diagnosed in children than in adult patient groups

(Kleinendorst et al. 2018). Syndromic obesity is the name used for genetic obesity disorders with intellectual disability/developmental delay, congenital anomalies, and/or organ dysfunction. There are however genetic disorders in which obesity is the main isolated symptom; they are often called non-syndromic obesity disorders. Hyperphagia (abnormally increased appetite with decreased satiety) is a key symptom in many patients with genetic obesity.

Hyperphagia

Hyperphagia, literally meaning excessive eating, is difficult to define in clinical features. Special hyperphagia questionnaires have been developed, for example, for Prader-Willi syndrome. Main topics of this questionnaire are the child's behavior regarding food (angry or sad when denied food), food-seeking behavior (nightly eating, going through trash to find something to eat), and the amount of time the child daily spends on food (talking about food, trying to acquire food) (Dykens et al. 2007). This questionnaire can also be used in other (suspected) hyperphagic obesity disorders. In many genetic obesity disorders hyperphagia plays an important role. However, there are genetic obesity disorders in which hyperphagia is less predominant and reduced energy expenditure can play a role.

19.3 Regulation of Body Weight

Maintaining adequate energy levels is crucial for every organism on earth. The body needs to be able to defend itself against starvation in times of scarcity and does this by building up fat mass. The arcuate nucleus of the hypothalamus plays the key role in the system of energy homeostasis through the leptin-melanocortin pathway (Fig. 19.1). For short-term regulation, it receives peripheral signals from gut hormones and pancreas hormones, giving information about food intake. For long-term regulation it receives signals from fat cell hormones, which give information about energy storage. Higher brain functions are also involved in the body's energy housekeeping. These mechanisms and the associated genes will be discussed in this paragraph.

19.3.1 Short-Term Regulation of Food Intake

Short-term regulation of appetite and satiety takes place through the senses and through gut hormones. When you see or smell food, or hear someone tell a story about a delicious meal, your brain's appetite regulating systems become active

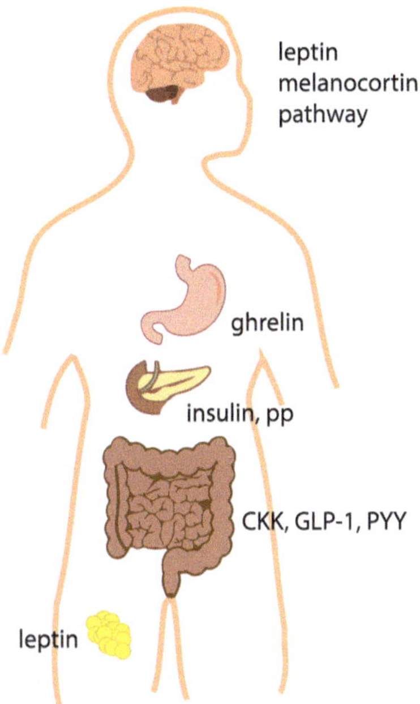

Hormone and receptor	Effect
Orexigenic	
AgRP - MC3R/MC4R	Antagonizes MC3R and MC4R in the hypothalamus leading to decreased satiety
NPY – NPYR	A reduction of Neuropeptide Y in the hypothalamus leads to an increase in satiety
Ghrelin – GHRH-R	The only known hormone that directly increases appetite, is produced in the stomach
Anorexigenic	
Alpha-MSH – MC4R	Activates MC4R in the hypothalamus, leading to satiety
CCK - CCK2R	Cholecystokinin decreases appetite in reaction to fatty food, is produced in the small intestine
GLP-1 – GLP-1R	Glucagon-like peptide-1 decreases appetite in reaction to protein and carbohydrate rich food, is produced in the small intestine
Insulin – Ins-R	Has effect on glucose uptake and on glycogen storage in the liver, is produced in the pancreas
Leptin – LepR	Stimulates alpha-MSH production, secreted by adipose tissue
PYY – NPY2R	Decreases appetite in reaction to fat and protein rich food, is produced in the small intestine and colon

Fig. 19.1 Schematic overview of the hormones and mechanisms involved in the regulation of satiety. Table: Orexigenic and anorexigenic hormones involved in the regulation of body weight

because the peripheral body signals are sent to the hypothalamus. And when the stomach is empty, it produces and secretes ghrelin. Ghrelin stimulates orexigenic neurons (agouti-related protein neurons) in the hypothalamus, leading to an increase in appetite and intestinal motility (which causes your stomach to growl when you are hungry). The gut hormones that are produced in the intestines following food intake have an opposite effect by inhibiting the agouti-related protein (AgRP) neurons in the hypothalamus and inducing satiety after a meal. Peptide YY (PYY) does this in response to protein intake, cholecystokinin in response to fat intake, and glucagon-like peptide 1 in response to carbohydrate intake (Fig. 19.1).

19.3.2 Long-Term Regulation of Food Intake

Adipose tissue secretes leptin. Leptin is a key player in the negative feedback regulation system of energy intake and expenditure. When leptin binds to its receptors, it sends a signal of the available energy storage. Leptin levels increase in the blood when a person gains fat mass. When the leptin receptor is active, it stimulates POMC expression. This precursor peptide is then cleaved into different hormones, of which adrenocorticotropic hormone (ACTH) and the melanocyte-stimulating hormones (MSH) are the most important with regard to genetic obesity disorders. MSH stimulates the different melanocortin receptors. Two subtypes of MSH, hormones α- and β-MSH, bind to the melanocortin 4 receptor (MC4R). Activation of MC4R leads to an anorexigenic signal, a decrease in food intake, and an increase in energy expenditure.

At the same time, elevated leptin levels suppress the neurons that lead to an orexigenic signal (AgRP). In this way, high amounts of leptin result in decreased food consumption and higher energy expenditure (Fig. 19.2). When this system is disturbed, people become hyperphagic.

19.3.3 Brain Reward System and Weight Regulation

Not only the leptin-melanocortin pathway is important in the regulation of our feeding behavior. It is evident that higher cortical functions, such as emotions, cognition, motivation, and tenacity, also play a role in the development and course of obesity. Our prefrontal cortex and mesolimbic dopamine system play a role in this. Two well-known neurotransmitters related to food are serotonin and dopamine. Dopamine is involved in the hedonic food circuit. Neurons release dopamine when a reward (in this case food) is anticipated and when the food is actually consumed. It is thought that dopamine release is lower in people with obesity (Wang et al. 2014), suggesting a lower feeling of reward while eating or after food consumption. To increase the feeling of reward, a person might eat more than normal.

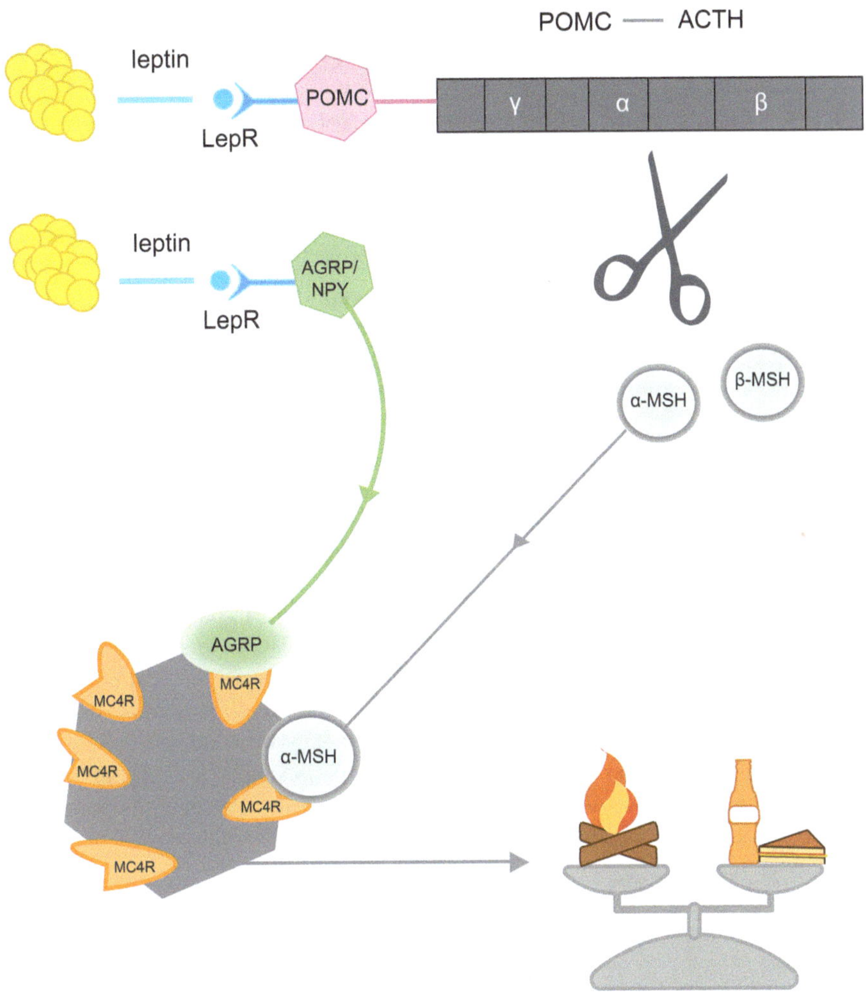

Fig. 19.2 Schematic overview of the leptin-melanocortin pathway

Serotonin is also involved in body weight regulation. It is sometimes viewed as the happiness hormone, but its functioning is far more complex, influencing functions as body temperature and sleep. Serotonin signaling appears to decrease food intake, and low serotonin signaling leads to increased appetite (Meguid et al. 2000). It influences the leptin-melanocortin pathway, since serotonin inhibits NPY and AgRP, whereas it activates alpha-MSH (la Fleur and Serlie 2014). In individuals with obesity, decreased serotonin signaling is seen in imaging studies (van Galen et al. 2018).

19.4 Genetic Obesity Disorders of the Leptin-Melanocortin Pathway (Non-syndromic Obesity)

19.4.1 Leptin and Leptin Receptor Deficiency

In 1997, Montague et al. reported the first patients with congenital leptin deficiency. These cousins from a consanguineous Pakistani family suffered from early-onset severe obesity and hyperphagia (Montague et al. 1997). The leptin gene was already discovered in obese mice 3 years before the identification of patients with leptin deficiency. The patients were screened for LEP mutations and indeed showed a homozygous frameshift mutation in *LEP*. Patients with congenital leptin deficiency have early-onset extreme obesity and additional hormonal disorders, e.g., central hypothyroidism and hypogonadotropic hypogonadism. Central hypothyroidism can be explained by the impairment of melanocortin signaling; they are necessary to activate cells that produce thyrotropin-releasing hormone, the hormone that releases thyroid-stimulating hormone. Hypogonadotropic hypogonadism can present as part of leptin receptor deficiency since leptin signaling is essential in the onset of activating the hypothalamic-pituitary-gonadal axis (Israel et al. 2012). It is still unknown why some patients have all these hormonal disturbances, while others only suffer from the early-onset obesity. Impaired T-cell immunity has been described in leptin-deficient patients. These children have more frequent and serious infections because of reduced amounts of T-cells or reduced functioning of T-cells. In 1998, the first patients with leptin receptor deficiency were identified. Parents of these patients were consanguineous. The phenotype is similar to leptin deficiency and growth hormone deficiency has been described. Moreover, some of the patients have reduced height as adults, probably because their pubertal growth spurt was absent.

19.4.2 MC4R Melanocortin 4 Receptor Mutations

MC4R mutations are the most common cause of non-syndromic genetic obesity disorders, with a prevalence of 2–5% in European obese populations (Hinney et al. 2013). The main feature of MC4R deficiency is hyperphagia, which leads to early-onset obesity. This phenotype is more severe in patients with homozygous or compound heterozygous *MC4R* mutations. People with a heterozygous mutation in *MC4R* will develop obesity later than individuals with homozygous or compound heterozygous mutations. Hyperphagia is the result of the defective MC4R. Normally agouti-related protein (AGRP) and α-melanocyte-stimulating hormone (α-MSH) compete to bind to the melanocortin 4 receptor. α-MSH activates the receptor, leading to a decrease in food intake. AGRP deactivates MC4R, leading to an increase in energy intake. When the MC4 receptor does not work, hyperphagic obesity occurs. Hyperinsulinemia and accelerated growth during childhood are described in these patients as well.

19.4.3 POMC (Proopiomelanocortin) Mutations

The first POMC-deficient patients have been described in 1998 (Krude et al. 1998). These children have adrenal insufficiency in early life due to ACTH deficiency. Biallelic *POMC* mutations further lead to early-onset severe obesity, red hair, and pale skin. Patients with homozygous or compound heterozygous mutations in *POMC* have a defect in the leptin-melanocortin pathway. In healthy individuals, when leptin binds to the proopiomelanocortin (POMC) neurons, they are stimulated to produce POMC. This precursor peptide is cleaved into different hormones, adrenocorticotropic hormone (ACTH) which stimulated the adrenal gland to the production of cortisol and the melanocyte-stimulating hormones (MSH). MSH stimulates the different melanocortin receptors including MC1R, MC2R, MC3R, and MC4R. MC1R is associated with pigmentation, explaining the pale skin and red hair in affected individuals. Low levels of ACTH lead to adrenal insufficiency in POMC patients, which can be lethal without early treatment. The hormones α- and β-MSH bind to the melanocortin 4 receptor (MC4R). MC4R activity results in anorexigenic signals. POMC deficiency therefore causes hyperphagic obesity, which is another main symptom of POMC deficiency. MC3R is likely to be involved in obesity as well. Notably, patients with a heterozygous mutation in *POMC* can have the hyperphagic obesity phenotype, without the other symptoms.

19.4.4 Other Leptin-Melanocortin Pathway Disorders

Table 19.1 shows the features and inheritance modes of non-syndromic genetic obesity disorders. Over the last decade, several other genetic obesity disorders caused by a defective leptin-melanocortin pathway have been identified. Proprotein convertase-1 deficiency is an autosomal recessive condition, caused by biallelic mutations in *PCSK1*. *PCSK1* is important for the cleavage of polypeptide POMC into the different peptide hormones. Moreover, *PCSK1* is involved in cleaving of other prohormones such as proinsulin or gut hormones leading to typical presentation of intractable diarrhea in the first year of life. The progressive severe obesity presents during early childhood. *PCSK1* heterozygosity appears to be a risk factor for obesity. Other genes involved in the leptin-melanocortin pathway of which defects lead to syndromic obesity (with intellectual disability or organ anomalies), such as *BDNF*, *CPE* and *TUB*, are mentioned in Table 19.2.

Table 19.1 Genetic obesity disorders (non-syndromic obesity disorders) without intellectual disability (ID), without developmental delay, without congenital anomalies, and/or without organ dysfunction

Name of the syndrome/ gene defect	Features	Inheritance	Chromosomal location	OMIM number
ADCY3	Severe early-onset obesity, hyperphagia, anosmia	AR	2	*600291
DYRK1B	Early-onset coronary artery disease, abdominal obesity, metabolic syndrome	AD	19	*604556
KSR2	Obesity, mild hyperphagia, and reduced metabolic rate	AD	12	*610737
LEP	Extreme early-onset severe obesity, hyperphagia, hyperinsulinemia, hypogonadotropic hypogonadism, central hypothyroidism, frequent infections	AR	7	*164160
LEPR	Extreme early-onset severe obesity, hyperphagia, hypogonadotropic hypogonadism, hypothyroidism, growth hormone deficiency, frequent infections	AR	1	*601007
MC4R	Recessive: extreme early-onset severe obesity, hyperphagia, hyperinsulinemia Dominant: early-onset obesity, less penetrant and later onset, hyperphagia, hyperinsulinemia Accelerated linear growth in childhood	AR/AD	18	*155541
PCSK1	Early-onset severe obesity, hyperphagia, central adrenal insufficiency, hypogonadotropic hypogonadism, neonatal malabsorptive diarrhea with failure to thrive, hyperproinsulinemia, abnormal glucose homeostasis, (partial) diabetes insipidus	AR AD risk factor for obesity	5	*162150
POMC	Extreme early-onset severe obesity, hyperphagia, red hair and fair skin in Caucasians, adrenal insufficiency	AR AD risk factor for obesity	2	*176830

OMIM number: * indicates a gene

19.5 Syndromic Genetic Obesity Disorders

Patients with syndromic obesity have, apart from obesity, intellectual disability (ID), developmental delay, congenital anomalies, and/or organ dysfunction. Their obesity often starts later in life than in patients with non-syndromic obesity. Table 19.2

Table 19.2 syndromic obesity disorders: genetic obesity disorders with intellectual disability (ID), developmental delay, congenital anomalies, and/or organ dysfunction

Name of the syndrome/gene	Features: childhood-onset severe obesity +	Inheritance	Chromosomal location	OMIM number
16p11.2 deletion (proximal and distal) *SH2B1*	Developmental delay (mostly speech), autism, macrocephaly, epilepsy	AD	16	#611913; #613444
Albright hereditary osteodystrophy/ pseudohypoparathyroidism type Ia (AHO/ PHP1a) *GNAS*	Mild ID, round facies, short stature, short fourth/fifth metacarpalia, PHP1a: multiple hormone resistance (TSH, PTH)	AD (imprinted)	20	#103580
Alström syndrome*ALMS1*	Cone-rod dystrophy/retinitis pigmentosa, progressive sensorineural hearing impairment, cardiomyopathy, childhood-onset type 2 diabetes, organ failure (liver, kidney, lung)	AR	2	*606844
Bardet-Biedl syndrome BBS genes (>20)	ID, retinal dystrophy, renal abnormalities, polydactyly, behavioral problems, hypogonadism	Typically AR, some cases of multiallelic inheritance	>20 genes on several chromosomes; majority *BBS1* 11, *BBS10* 12	*BBS1* *209901; *BBS10* *610148
BDNF	Memory and concentration problems, disturbed pain sensation, hyperphagia	AD	11	*113505
Börjeson-Forssman-Lehmann syndrome *PHF6*	ID, seizures, hypogonadism, and distinctive facial features	X-linked	X	*300414
Carpenter syndrome *RAB23* *MEGF8*	*RAB23:* acrocephaly, syndactyly, cardiac defects, short stature, genital abnormalities (most frequently	AR	*RAB23* 6*MEGF8* 19	*606144; *604267

(continued)

Table 19.2 (continued)

Name of the syndrome/gene	Features: childhood-onset severe obesity +	Inheritance	Chromosomal location	OMIM number
	cryptorchidism) *MEGF8:* cranio-synostosis, polysyndactyly			
CHOPS syndrome *AFF4*	ID, coarse facies, heart defects, pulmonary involvement, short stature, and skeletal dysplasia	AD	5	*604417
Cohen syndrome*VPS13B*	ID, failure to thrive in infancy and childhood, hypotonia and hyperextension of joints, microcephaly, progressive retinal dystrophy and high myopia at a young age, periodic neutropenia	AR	8	*607817
CPE	ID, hypogonadism (1 reported patient)	AR	4	*114855
CUL4B	Central obesity, delayed puberty, hypogonadism, relative macrocephaly, moderate short stature, unprovoked aggressive outbursts, fine intention tremor, and abnormalities of the toes	X-linked	X	*300304
IGSF1	Congenital central hypothyroidism and macroorchidism, variable prolactin deficiency, occasional growth hormone deficiency, delayed pubertal testosterone secretion	X-linked	X	*300137

(continued)

Table 19.2 (continued)

Name of the syndrome/gene	Features: childhood-onset severe obesity +	Inheritance	Chromosomal location	OMIM number
INPP5E	MORM (mental retardation, obesity, retinal dystrophy, and micropenis)	AR	9	*613037
KIDINS220	SINO syndrome (spastic paraplegia, intellectual disability, nystagmus, obesity)	AD	2	*615759
Kleefstra syndrome *EHMT1*	ID, seizures, hypotonia, brachycephaly, dysmorphic features	AD	9	*607001
MYT1L	ID, autism, speech delay, behavioral problems	AD	2	*613084
NTRK2	ID, hyperphagia	AD	9	*600456
PHIP	ID, overweight or obesity	AD	6	*612870
Prader-Willi syndrome	Neonatal hypotonia and feeding problems (often requiring tube feeding), followed by hyperphagia and obesity. ID, behavioral problems, short stature, hypothalamic hypogonadism	Methylation defect paternal 15q11.2, mostly sporadic	15	#176270
Schaaf-Yang syndrome *MAGEL2*	Intellectual disability, hypotonia, behavioral abnormalities, contractures/ arthrogryposis/fetal akinesia, sleep apnea	AD (imprinted, paternal allele)	15	*605283
SIM1	Autism, behavioral problems, hyperphagia	AD	6	*603128
Smith-Magenis syndrome 17p11.2 interstitial deletion or, less frequently, heterozygous mutations *RAI1*	Obesity phenotype most prominent in patients with *RAI1* mutationsID,	AD	17	#182290

(continued)

Table 19.2 (continued)

Name of the syndrome/gene	Features: childhood-onset severe obesity +	Inheritance	Chromosomal location	OMIM number
	behavioral problems (sleep disturbances, self-harm). Neonatal hypotonia and feeding problems. Square face, synophris, broad hands and feet			
Temple syndrome (mUPD14 or methylation abnormalities chromosome 14)	Neonatal hypotonia and feeding problems, followed by hyperphagia and obesity. Premature puberty, short stature, mild to no ID	Isolated cases, low recurrence risk (<1%)	14	#616222
TUB	Retinal dystrophy	AR	11	∗601197

OMIM number: ∗ indicates a gene; # indicates a syndrome or phenotype

shows the features and inheritance modes of syndromic genetic obesity disorders, of which several are discussed in more detail later in this paragraph.

19.5.1 Bardet-Biedl Syndrome

Bardet-Biedl syndrome is a ciliopathy, a disease of the cilia. Affected patients have, apart from the obesity, intellectual disability, visual problems, postaxial polydactyly, and renal problems. There are currently 22 genes associated with BBS, but the majority of patients have mutations in *BBS1* or *BBS10* (Geets et al. 2019). The obesity in Bardet-Biedl syndrome has multiple causes. The BBSome, the complex of several important BBS proteins, interacts with the leptin receptor and therefore probably plays a role in the leptin-melanocortin satiety system. Physical activity is often reduced in patients with BBS, possibly due to their visual problems and developmental delay. Energy expenditure is probably low in these patients. There are several other cilia disorders that include obesity such as Alström syndrome and Carpenter syndrome.

19.5.2 16p11.2 Deletion Syndrome

16p11.2 deletion syndrome is a common chromosomal microdeletion syndrome, which occurs in 3 per 10,000 individuals (Weiss et al. 2008). There is a broad variety of phenotypic features among 16p11.2 deletion patients. The majority has developmental delay (often more severe speech problems) and autism. Besides, there is an increased risk of developing overweight or obesity, macrocephaly, and epileptic seizures. Half of the 7-year-olds with a 16p11.2 deletion are obese (Maillard et al. 2016).

Overweight or obesity often starts between the ages of five and ten, remarkably later than in other genetic obesity disorders. The 16p11.2 deletion syndrome has a remarkable counterpart: 16p11.2 duplication syndrome. Individuals with a duplication are at risk of developing underweight and microcephaly, whereas individuals with a deletion are more often obese and macrocephalic. The SH2B1 gene is located in the distal 16p11.2 deletion and is most likely the cause of the obesity phenotype, because of its association with hypothalamic leptin sensitivity. SH2B1-deficient mice show a decreased leptin signaling and develop a hyperphagic obesity phenotype. For the more common proximal deletion, there is no candidate gene for the obesity within the deleted region, but genomic interaction between the 16p11.2 regions are suggested (Loviglio et al. 2017).

19.6 Genomic Imprinting Disorders Causing Obesity

Genomic imprinting causes genes to be expressed from only one allele instead of both. Maternally imprinted genes are turned off during the formation of the oocyte. Paternally imprinted genes are turned off during the spermatogenesis. Normally, a person inherits an inactive imprinted allele from one parent and an active non-imprinted allele from the other parent. In the case of a uniparental disomy, the fetus inherits two active regions or two inactive regions from one parent.

19.6.1 Prader-Willi Syndrome

Prader-Willi syndrome (PWS) is the best-known genetic obesity syndrome among many doctors. PWS has a prevalence of one in 10,000–30,000 people. Patients have, apart from their obesity, intellectual disability (average IQ 65), hypogonadism, and dysmorphic features (almond-shaped eyes, thin upper lip with downturned corners of the mouth). PWS is caused by a lack of paternal copies within the Prader-Willi region of chromosome 15. There are three mechanisms that can lead to this loss: a paternal deletion of the PWS region, maternal uniparental disomy of the region, and in rare cases imprinting defects of this region (Fig. 19.3). Nowadays, the diagnosis PWS is often established in the neonatal period, when the newborn shows severe feeding difficulties requiring nasal tube feeding and hypotonia. The turning point occurs around the age of 1 year, when children start to show an increasing appetite and consequently increasing weight. At the age of 8 years, almost all children with Prader-Willi syndrome are extremely hyperphagic and obese. The clinical phenotype

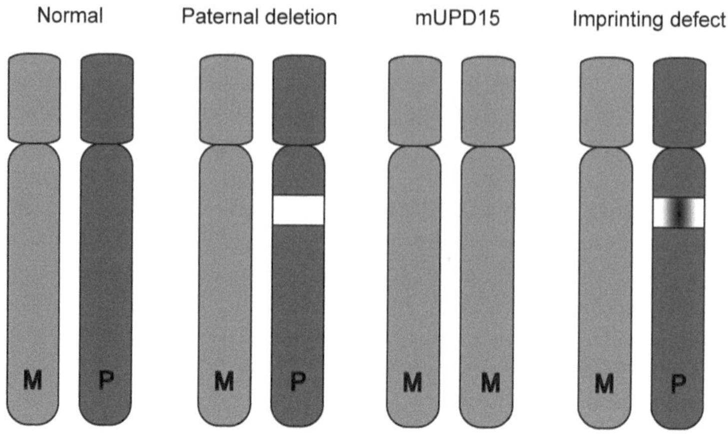

Fig. 19.3 Genetic mechanisms behind Prader-Willi syndrome. *M* maternal chromosome 15, *P* paternal chromosome 15, *mUPD15* maternal uniparental disomy of chromosome 15

of Prader-Willi syndrome is quite clear and the disease is studied extensively, but the exact mechanisms behind the hyperphagia and obesity remain obscure. One of the candidate genes in the PWS-critical region is *SNORD116*, which may be involved in prohormone processing. Many PWS patients also have a reduced energy expenditure, because of their physical disability and low amounts of muscle. Growth hormone therapy might help to improve this apart from the positive effect on the short stature. PWS is discussed in detail in Chap. 20.

19.6.2 Albright Hereditary Osteodystrophy

Just like Prader-Willi syndrome, Albright hereditary osteodystrophy (AHO) is a genetic imprinting disorder. It is caused by maternally inherited mutations in the *GNAS1* gene. GNAS1 produces many different transcripts, but an important one is Gs-α that encodes a specific part of G-proteins needed for signal transduction processes. *GNAS1* mutations are also involved in the pathogenesis of McCune-Albright's syndrome (MAS) discussed in Chap. 7. Whereas gain-of-function *GNAS1* mutations of postzygotic origin are involved in MAS, here, inactivating *GNAS1* mutations are pathogenic.

Patients with AHO often have a short stature, a round face, subcutaneous calcifications, and short fourth and/or fifth metacarpals. Mild intellectual deficiency can also be present. The AHO phenotype is typical for pseudohypoparathyroidism type 1a (PHP 1a), which refers to resistance to the parathyroid hormone. Patients with AHO have manifestations of hypoparathyroidism like hypocalcemia. The expression of *GNAS1* is tissue specific, with biallelic expression in some tissues and maternal expression only in others. The multi-hormone resistance can only occur when the Gs (alpha) mutations are maternally transmitted. Paternal transmission of the *GNAS1* mutation therefore only leads to pseudopseudohypoparathyroidism, without the classical phenotype of AHO (Weinstein et al. 2002).

The obesity in PHP1a most often starts in the first year of life. Several mechanisms for the development of obesity in AHO have been suggested. The reduced G-protein activity in AHO could lead to an underactive MC4 receptor, since the MC4 receptor is a G-protein-coupled receptor. Moreover, patients with PHP1a have remarkably low norepinephrine levels, suggesting that the central nervous system is a key factor in the energy metabolism of PHP1a patient as well (Carel et al. 1999).

19.6.3 Maternal Uniparental Disomy of Chromosome 14

Another genetic imprinting disorder causing obesity is maternal uniparental disomy of chromosome 14 (mUPD14). In uniparental disomy, the patient inherits two homologous chromosomes from one parent. This often occurs as "trisomic rescue": a situation where an initial trisomy is corrected by the elimination of the third chromosome (Fig. 19.4). The two remaining chromosomes can then derive from the same parent. This leads to problems if the uniparental disomy affects chromosomes that harbor imprinted regions. The clinical phenotype of a patient with mUPD14 includes, comparable to PWS, initially neonatal hypotonia and feeding difficulty later changing to hyperphagia, short stature, premature puberty, mild developmental delay, and truncal obesity. The cause of the obesity in mUPD14 patients might be the absence of paternally expressed DLK1, or preadipocyte factor 1. Lack of paternally inherited Pref-1/Dlk1 in knockout mice leads to obesity, growth retardation, and congenital anomalies like eyelid and skeletal abnormalities (Moon et al. 2002).

19.7 Common or Polygenic Obesity

Multifactorial obesity is caused by both genetic factors, hormonal and external factors. Two external players in obesity that are well known are diet and physical activity, but other environmental influences are important too. Stress, sleep disturbance, and chronic pain are all associated with obesity, possibly partly mediated by an increase in cortisol. Elevated cortisol levels can result in higher appetite and induce central adiposity (van Rossum 2017). Drugs like antidepressants, antipsychotics, and glucocorticoids are also known to be obesogenic. Sex differences are likely involved in the development of obesity as well, since females are at higher risk for obesity. This is probably due to both environmental and genetic differences between men and women. The genetic factors that play a role in multifactorial diseases or traits are small variations in genes. The effects of the obesogenic environment are probably enlarged by the genetic variants that make people more susceptible to develop obesity, also described as gene-environment interaction. The

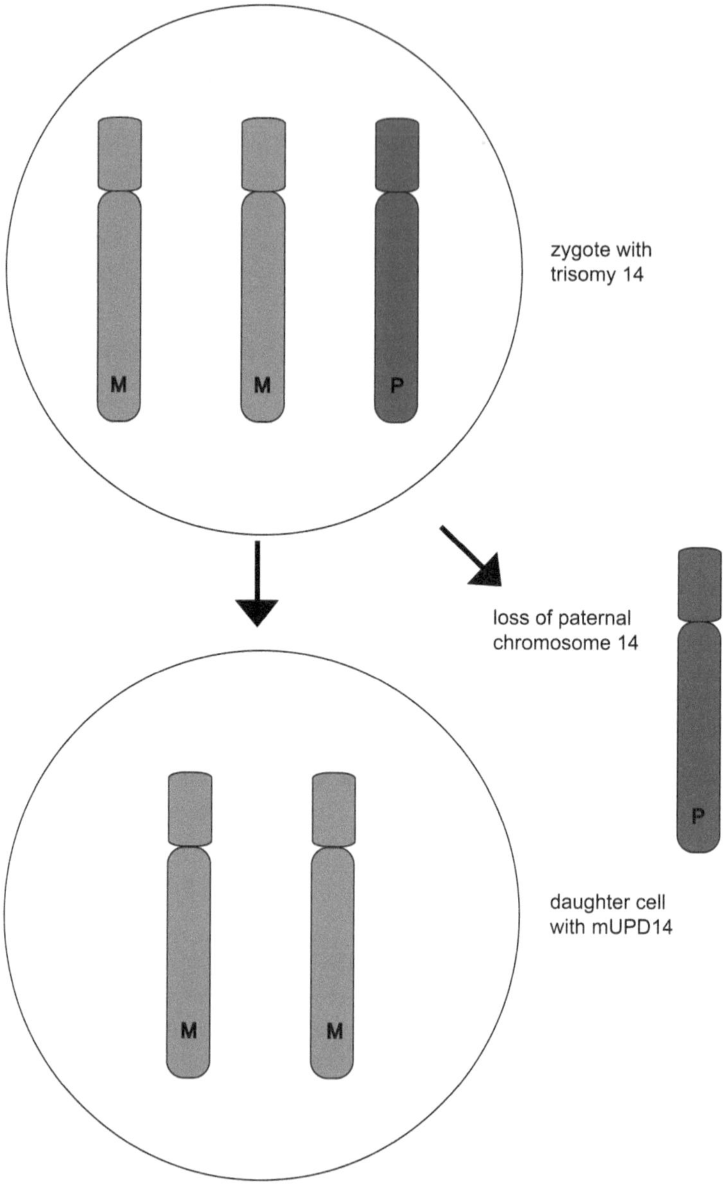

Fig. 19.4 Trisomy rescue resulting in maternal uniparental disomy of chromosome 14

first reported and most important contributor to polygenic obesity is the *FTO* gene. It is thought that variants in this gene influence the ability to feel hunger and satiety, but little is known about FTO's exact function. Common variants in *FTO* are responsible for around 0.35% of BMI variance in European Caucasians (Speliotes et al. 2010). People with heterozygous loss-of-function mutations, however, can be lean or obese. *FTO* is therefore not considered a monogenic obesity gene. Homozygous pathogenic *FTO* mutations however lead to an extremely severe, often lethal, malformation syndrome in humans.

Interestingly, known monogenic obesity genes such as *MC4R* are also playing a role in complex obesity. Small variations (a substitution of one base for another) in the *MC4R* gene can change one's obesity risk. These variations are called single-nucleotide polymorphisms (SNPs). Hundreds of SNPs in many different genes have been identified by genome-wide association studies performed in impressive numbers of individuals. All these SNPs together explain around 6% of the variance of BMI in Europeans (Yengo et al. 2018). Gene-gene interactions may also play a role in common obesity, but future studies are needed to further evaluate the exact mechanism. The way we look at polygenic/common obesity will probably further develop in the following years. Currently, several commercial companies offer direct to consumer genetic tests to gain insight in multiple lifestyle-related genetic factors. The reliability and usefulness of these test results are highly debatable. Moreover, it is still unclear whether knowledge of polygenic obesity risk is beneficial at the present moment. A recent study showed negative effects of counseling about reduced satiety and ability to exercise, independent of their actual genetic risks (Turnwald et al. 2019). But in the future, genetic risk estimation based on common variants might become useful in identifying individual response to specific treatment programs or surgical operations.

19.8 Genetic Counseling, Treatment, and Future Prospective

Genetic counseling is an essential part of care for patients with genetic obesity and their families. Often, patients have undertaken a long and burdening journey to reach an etiological diagnosis. Establishing a genetic diagnosis may end this period of uncertainty. Genetic counseling allows for early intervention in young children and supports patients and their social network in understanding the disease, which aids patients in coping with their lifelong weight problem. After the diagnosis is established, monitoring or screening for the other symptoms of the disorder is possible. Understanding the genetic cause of a rare obesity disorder can also be important for family members of the affected patient. The mode of inheritance and recurrence risk for specific family members of the proband are assessed after molecular confirmation of the clinical diagnosis. Family members can be offered genetic counseling, and, if they wish, they can undergo genetic testing. Depending on the molecular mechanism, prenatal testing and preimplantation genetic testing might be possible as well.

For all these reasons, genetic testing of patients with early-onset, hyperphagic, or syndromic obesity is of value. The current international guideline for obesity in children and adolescents of the Endocrine Society suggests genetic testing in children with extreme early-onset obesity before the age of 5 years (Styne et al. 2017).

Previously, genetic testing for specific obesity syndromes was only available as single-gene Sanger sequencing. Nowadays, with gene panel analysis or whole exome sequencing, multiple genes can be analyzed at the same time. But not all obesity syndromes can be identified using these techniques, for example, imprinting disorders like Prader-Willi syndrome or Temple syndrome request specific DNA methylation-specific testing. In patients with obesity and intellectual disability or developmental delay, microarray analysis is currently also recommended. A genetic diagnosis facilitates personalized medical treatment and expert healthcare. It can also support decision-making in bariatric surgery and lead to specific drug treatment. In general, it is difficult to achieve long-term weight loss. When people reduce their calorie intake, metabolism slows down and less calories are burnt. To lose more weight, a person has to decrease intake even more. Low-calorie diets also lead to changes in satiety hormones. One year after weight loss, the circulating levels of ghrelin are still higher than before weight loss and the levels of satiety hormones like leptin and PYY are lower, as if the body tries to regain its old weight (Sumithran et al. 2011). Patients with genetic obesity have to work even harder to achieve weight loss or weight stabilization. Since patients with monogenic obesity disorders are often hyperphagic, food access restriction seems the most promising prevention method or treatment strategy for them. Whether this is feasible depends on environmental circumstances as well. To date, there are no therapies to cure the primary causes of genetic obesity disorders. Leptin is a satiety hormone for which replacement therapy is available. Recombinant human leptin was first tested in a trial which included one patient, a 9-year-old girl with congenital leptin deficiency (Farooqi et al. 1999). The therapy is highly efficient in achieving weight loss (by reducing hyperphagia and increasing energy expenditure) and also in correcting the hormonal abnormalities in leptin-deficient patients. Leptin therapy is unfortunately not effective to treat other types of obesity, because most people with obesity are leptin resistant. New drugs are developed to treat common obesity or rare genetic obesity disorders, among which are melanocortin 4 receptor agonists. Since MC4R agonists replace MSH, they can be effective in several disorders with a defective leptin-melanocortin pathway. Clinical trials in *POMC* deficiency and *LEPR* deficiency have shown impressive reductions of hyperphagia and body weight (Clement et al. 2018; Kuhnen et al. 2016). A mechanistically interesting side effect is that the patients' skin and hair color become darker during treatment, which is likely caused by stimulation of MC1R. Several other new pharmacological agents might be useful in patients with genetic obesity as well, for example, analogs of GLP1, which decreases appetite (Bocarsly 2018). Many other clinical trials are focusing on Prader-Willi syndrome, since this is the most common syndromic obesity condition. Growth hormone therapy, initially prescribed for short stature, can be beneficial in patients with PWS for their body composition by increasing muscle mass and reducing fat mass. Multiple clinical trials are currently underway for new drugs in PWS patients, including intranasal oxytocin treatment and unacylated ghrelin analogs. The majority of studies with oxytocin treatment in PWS patients have not shown significant improvement in food-related behavior. Whether bariatric surgery is an appropriate treatment for PWS patients is highly debatable. PWS patients are at high risk for complications. Especially gastric rupture is a very dangerous complication. Gastric necrosis following an episode of binge-eating is a known cause of death in PWS. In the general population, bariatric surgery is the most effective obesity treatment option. Whether this is as effective for genetic obesity as well is unsure, especially because data on follow-up are lacking for most disorders. It is known that gastric bypass surgery leads to changes in gut hormones that influence satiety. Patients with heterozygous *MC4R* mutations who underwent a Roux-en-Y gastric bypass seem to have similar short-term follow-up results as patients without *MC4R* mutations (Valette et al. 2012). It is difficult to study this for other genetic obesity disorders because of their rarity, but future collaborative research might elucidate the effectiveness of different treatment options in rare genetic obesity disorders.

19.9 Genetic Obesity: Key Messages

- The body's energy balance is controlled by a complex system in the hypothalamus called the leptin-melanocortin pathway. It controls both energy intake (including hunger and satiety) and energy expenditure. Defects in genes regulating this pathway often lead to hyperphagic obesity.
- Most cases of obesity have a multifactorial cause; in a minority of patients, specific genetic aberrations can be identified that cause their severe obesity.
- Genetic obesity reflects a heterogeneous group of conditions. They are often divided into non-syndromic and syndromic obesity.
  The onset of obesity in syndromic obesity disorders often occurs later in childhood compared to early infancy in patients with genetic (non-syndromic) obesity disorders affecting the leptin-melanocortin pathway.
- Understanding rare genetic obesity disorders helps us in understanding common/polygenic obesity. Moreover, it helps us in finding novel targets for therapy. Current development in personalized medicine looks promising for patients with a disturbed leptin-melanocortin pathway.

References

Bocarsly ME (2018) Pharmacological interventions for obesity: current and future targets. Curr Addict Rep 5:202–211. https://doi.org/10.1007/s40429-018-0204-0

Carel JC, Le Stunff C, Condamine L et al (1999) Resistance to the lipolytic action of epinephrine: a new feature of protein Gs deficiency. J Clin Endocrinol Metab 84:4127–4131. https://doi.org/10.1210/jcem.84.11.6145

Clement K, Biebermann H, Farooqi IS et al (2018) MC4R agonism promotes durable weight loss in patients with leptin receptor deficiency. Nat Med 24:551–555. https://doi.org/10.1038/s41591-018-0015-9

Dykens EM, Maxwell MA, Pantino E, Kossler R, Roof E (2007) Assessment of hyperphagia in Prader-Willi syndrome. Obesity (Silver Spring) 15:1816–1826. https://doi.org/10.1038/oby.2007.216

Farooqi IS, Jebb SA, Langmack G et al (1999) Effects of recombinant leptin therapy in a child with congenital leptin deficiency. N Engl J Med 341:879–884. https://doi.org/10.1056/NEJM199909163411204

Geets E, Meuwissen MEC, Van Hul W (2019) Clinical, molecular genetics and therapeutic aspects of syndromic obesity. Clin Genet 95:23–40. https://doi.org/10.1111/cge.13367

Hall KD (2018) Did the food environment cause the obesity epidemic? Obesity (Silver Spring) 26:11–13. https://doi.org/10.1002/oby.22073

Hinney A, Volckmar AL, Knoll N (2013) Melanocortin-4 receptor in energy homeostasis and obesity pathogenesis. Prog Mol Biol Transl Sci 114:147–191. https://doi.org/10.1016/B978-0-12-386933-3.00005-4

Ignatieva EV, Afonnikov DA, Saik OV, Rogaev EI, Kolchanov NA (2016) A compendium of human genes regulating feeding behavior and body weight, its functional characterization and identification of GWAS genes involved in brain-specific PPI network. BMC Genet 17:158. https://doi.org/10.1186/s12863-016-0466-2

Israel DD, Sheffer-Babila S, de Luca C et al (2012) Effects of leptin and melanocortin signaling interactions on pubertal development and reproduction. Endocrinology 153:2408–2419. https://doi.org/10.1210/en.2011-1822

Kleinendorst L, Massink MPG, Cooiman MI et al (2018) Genetic obesity: next-generation sequencing results of 1230 patients with obesity. J Med Genet 55:578–586. https://doi.org/10.1136/jmedgenet-2018-105315

Krude H, Biebermann H, Luck W, Horn R, Brabant G, Gruters A (1998) Severe early-onset obesity, adrenal insufficiency and red hair pigmentation caused by POMC mutations in humans. Nat Genet 19:155–157. https://doi.org/10.1038/509

Kuhnen P, Clement K, Wiegand S et al (2016) Proopiomelanocortin deficiency treated with a melanocortin-4 receptor agonist. N Engl J Med 375:240–246. https://doi.org/10.1056/NEJMoa1512693

la Fleur SE, Serlie MJ (2014) The interaction between nutrition and the brain and its consequences for body weight gain and metabolism; studies in rodents and men. Best Pract Res Clin Endocrinol Metab 28:649–659. https://doi.org/10.1016/j.beem.2014.06.001

Loviglio MN, Leleu M, Männik K et al (2017) Chromosomal contacts connect loci associated with autism, BMI and head circumference phenotypes. Mol Psychiatry 22:836–849. https://doi.org/10.1038/mp.2016.84

Maillard AM, Hippolyte L, Rodriguez-Herreros B et al (2016) 16p11.2 Locus modulates response to satiety before the onset of obesity. Int J Obes 40:870–876. https://doi.org/10.1038/ijo.2015.247

Meguid MM, Fetissov SO, Varma M, Sato T, Zhang L, Laviano A, Rossi-Fanelli F (2000) Hypothalamic dopamine and serotonin in the regulation of food intake. Nutrition 16:843–857

Montague CT, Farooqi IS, Whitehead JP et al (1997) Congenital leptin deficiency is associated with severe early-onset obesity in humans. Nature 387:903–908. https://doi.org/10.1038/43185

Moon YS, Smas CM, Lee K, Villena JA, Kim KH, Yun EJ, Sul HS (2002) Mice lacking paternally expressed Pref-1/Dlk1 display growth retardation and accelerated adiposity. Mol Cell Biol 22:5585–5592

NCD Risk Factor Collaboration (2016) Trends in adult body-mass index in 200 countries from 1975 to 2014: a pooled analysis of 1698 population-based measurement studies with 19.2 million participants. Lancet 387:1377–1396. https://doi.org/10.1016/S0140-6736(16)30054-X

Polderman TJ, Benyamin B, de Leeuw CA, Sullivan PF, van Bochoven A, Visscher PM, Posthuma D (2015) Meta-analysis of the heritability of human traits based on fifty years of twin studies. Nat Genet 47:702–709. https://doi.org/10.1038/ng.3285

Speliotes EK, Willer CJ, Berndt SI et al (2010) Association analyses of 249,796 individuals reveal 18 new loci associated with body mass index. Nat Genet 42:937–948. https://doi.org/10.1038/ng.686

Styne DM, Arslanian SA, Connor EL, Farooqi IS, Murad MH, Silverstein JH, Yanovski JA (2017) Pediatric obesity-assessment, treatment, and prevention: an endocrine society clinical practice guideline. J Clin Endocrinol Metab 102:709–757. https://doi.org/10.1210/jc.2016-2573

Sumithran P, Prendergast LA, Delbridge E, Purcell K, Shulkes A, Kriketos A, Proietto J (2011) Long-term persistence of hormonal adaptations to weight loss. N Engl J Med 365:1597–1604. https://doi.org/10.1056/NEJMoa1105816

Turnwald BP, Goyer JP, Boles DZ, Silder A, Delp SL, Crum AJ (2019) Learning one's genetic risk changes physiology independent of actual genetic risk. Nat Hum Behav 3:48–56. https://doi.org/10.1038/s41562-018-0483-4

Valette M, Poitou C, Le Beyec J, Bouillot JL, Clement K, Czernichow S (2012) Melanocortin-4 receptor mutations and polymorphisms do not affect weight loss after bariatric surgery. PLoS One 7:e48221. https://doi.org/10.1371/journal.pone.0048221

van Galen KA, Ter Horst KW, Booij J, la Fleur SE, Serlie MJ (2018) The role of central dopamine and serotonin in human obesity: lessons learned from molecular neuroimaging studies. Metabolism 85:325–339. https://doi.org/10.1016/j.metabol.2017.09.007

van Rossum EF (2017) Obesity and cortisol: new perspectives on an old theme. Obesity (Silver Spring) 25:500–501. https://doi.org/10.1002/oby.21774

Wang GJ, Tomasi D, Convit A et al (2014) BMI modulates calorie-dependent dopamine changes in accumbens from glucose intake. PLoS One 9:e101585. https://doi.org/10.1371/journal.pone.0101585

Weinstein LS, Chen M, Liu J (2002) Gs(alpha) mutations and imprinting defects in human disease. Ann N Y Acad Sci 968:173–197

Weiss LA, Shen Y, Korn JM et al (2008) Association between microdeletion and microduplication at 16p11.2 and autism. N Engl J Med 358:667–675. https://doi.org/10.1056/NEJMoa075974

Williams EP, Mesidor M, Winters K, Dubbert PM, Wyatt SB (2015) Overweight and obesity: prevalence, consequences, and causes of a growing public health problem. Curr Obes Rep 4:363–370. https://doi.org/10.1007/s13679-015-0169-4

World Health Organization (2018) Obesity and overweight. https://www.who.int/news-room/fact-sheets/detail/obesity-and-overweight. Accessed 12 Feb 2019

Yengo L, Sidorenko J, Kemper KE et al (2018) Meta-analysis of genome-wide association studies for height and body mass index in approximately 700000 individuals of European ancestry. Hum Mol Genet 27:3641–3649. https://doi.org/10.1093/hmg/ddy271

Chapter 20
Chromosomal Aberrations with Endocrine Relevance (Turner Syndrome, Klinefelter Syndrome, Prader-Willi Syndrome)

Irén Haltrich

Abstract Turner and Klinefelter syndromes are the most common chromosome abnormalities compatible with life. Prader-Willi syndrome is a complex multisystem imprinting disorder characterized by hypothalamic dysfunction, neurological implications, and psychiatric disturbances. All three conditions are associated with progressively increasing risk for metabolic and autoimmune morbidity and mortality. This chapter focuses on the endocrine aspects of these syndromes and recent discoveries based on epigenetics and gene expression studies that have broadened our understanding of their extensive phenotypic variability and heterogeneous comorbidities.

Keywords Turner syndrome · Klinefelter syndrome · Prader-Willi syndrome · Autoimmune disease · Hypothyroidism · Infertility · Chromosomal aberration · Imprinting disorder · Gene expression · Methylation

List of Abbreviations

AKAP17A	A-kinase anchoring protein 17A
AMOT	*Angiomotin*
AS	Angelman syndrome
ASD	Autism spectrum disorder
ATP10C	ATPase phospholipid transporting 10A
BMD	Bone mineral density
BP1, BP2, BP3	Breakpoint 1, 2, 3
CAI	Central adrenal insufficiency
CD99	T-cell adhesion molecule
CNR1	Cannabinoid receptor 1
CSF2RA	Colony-stimulating factor 2 receptor

I. Haltrich (✉)
Faculty of Medicine, 2nd Department of Pediatrics, Semmelweis University, Budapest, Hungary
e-mail: haltrich.iren@med.semmelweis-univ.hu

P. Igaz, A. Patócs (eds.), *Genetics of Endocrine Diseases and Syndromes*, Experientia Supplementum 111, https://doi.org/10.1007/978-3-030-25905-1_20

CYFIP1	Cytoplasmic FMR1 interacting protein 1
DACT1	Dishevelled binding antagonist of beta catenin 1
DM	Diabetes mellitus
DOCK1, 7	Dedicator of cytokinesis 1, 7
DVT	Deep vein thrombosis
EIF2S3	Eukaryotic translation initiation factor 2 subunit gamma
FIGNL1	Fidgetin-like 1
FISH	Fluorescence in situ hybridization
FSH	Follicle-stimulating hormone
G3BP1	Stress granule assembly factor 1
GHD	Growth hormone deficiency
GH	Growth hormone
HERC2	HECT and RLD domain containing E3 ubiquitin protein ligase 2
i(X)	isoXq chromosome
IC	Imprinting center
ID	Imprinting defects
IL3RA	Receptor for interleukin-3
IVF-ET	In vitro fertilization-embryo transfer
JPX-JPX	Transcript, XIST activator
KANK1	KN motif and ankyrin repeat domains 1
KDM6A	Lysine demethylase 6A
KS	Klinefelter syndrome
LGALS1	Lectin galactoside-binding soluble 1
LH	Luteinizing hormone
M-GCTs	Mediastinal germ cell tumors
MAGEL2	MAGE family member L2
matUPD	Maternal uniparental disomy
MKRN3	Makorin ring finger protein 3
MS-MLPA	Methylation-specific multiplex-ligation probe amplification
NDN	Necdin, MAGE family member
NIPA1, 2	NIPA magnesium transporter 1, 2
NPAP1	Nuclear pore-associated protein 1
NSD1	Nuclear receptor-binding SET domain protein 1
PEX 10	Peroxisomal biogenesis factor 10
PIN4	Peptidylprolyl cis/trans isomerase, NIMA-interacting 4
POF	Premature ovarian failure
PRKX	Protein kinase X-linked
PWS	Prader-Willi syndrome
R1FM	Fragile X mental retardation 1
RPS4X	Ribosomal protein S4 X-linked
RSPO1	R-Spondin 1
SCA	Sex chromosomal aneuploidy
SHOX	Short stature homeobox
SHROOM2	Shroom family member 2

SLC25A6	Solute carrier family 25 member 6
SMARCA1	SWI/SNF related, matrix associated, actin dependent regulator of chromatin, subfamily A, member 1
snoRNAs	Small nucleolar RNAs
SNRPN	Small nuclear ribonucleoprotein polypeptide N
SNURF	SNRPN upstream reading frame
SOX3, 9	SRY-box 3, 9
TRT	Testosterone replacement therapy
TSC22D3	TSC22 Domain family member 3
TS	Turner syndrome
TUBGCP5	Tubulin gamma complex associated protein 5
TXLNG	Taxilin gamma
UBE3A	Ubiquitin protein ligase E3A
USP9X	Ubiquitin-specific peptidase 9 X-linked
VGLL1	Vestigial-like family member 1
WNT4	Wnt family member 4
XIAP-X	Linked inhibitor of apoptosis
XIST-X	Inactive specific transcript
ZFYVE9	Zinc finger FYVE-type containing

20.1 Turner Syndrome

Turner syndrome (TS) is a chromosomal disorder that affects phenotypic females who have one intact X chromosome and complete or partial absence of the second sex chromosome. TS affects 25–50 per 100,000 females. In contrast to other numerical chromosomal anomalies, the incidence of TS does not increase with maternal age. Clinical manifestations of TS include linear growth failure, ovarian insufficiency, early sensorineural hearing loss, a specific neurodevelopmental profile, and distinctive congenital cardiovascular, skeletal, digital, and renal anomalies. In addition, the condition is often associated with neuropsychiatric, metabolic, endocrine, and immune-related diseases. Patients usually have normal intelligence but may have problems with nonverbal, social, and psychomotor skills.

20.1.1 Diagnosis and Clinical Manifestation

The comprehensive clinical spectrum of TS ranges from a typical appearance with common findings such as short stature, webbed neck, broad chest with widely spaced nipples, pubertal delay, and cardiac anomalies to individuals who have minimal observable features. Because of these TS is diagnosed in females of all ages with peaks during fetal life, infancy, adolescence, and early adulthood (Lee and Conway 2014).

The current clinical practice guideline (Gravholt et al. 2017) suggests a new indication approach for the diagnosis of TS. Chromosomal analysis is recommended if at least one of the following clinical features is present: fetal cystic hygroma or hydrops, idiopathic short stature, obstructive left-sided congenital heart defect (typically bicuspid aortic valve, coarctation, aortic stenosis, mitral valve anomalies, and hypoplastic left heart syndrome), unexplained delayed puberty/menarche, infertility, and characteristic facial features (down-slanted palpebral fissures, epicanthal folds, low-set anomalous pinnae, micrognathia, narrow palate, short, broad neck, and webbing). Karyotype analysis would also be recommended in the presence of at least two of the following clinical criteria: renal anomaly (horseshoe, absence, or hypoplasia), Madelung deformity, neuropsychologic problems and/or psychiatric issues, multiple typical or melanocytic naevi, dysplastic or hyperconvex nails, hearing impairment in women less than 40 years of age together with short stature, and congenital heart defects (partial anomalous pulmonary venous return, secundum-type atrial septal defect, muscular or membranous ventricular septal defects).

The diagnosis of TS is usually carried out by standard karyotyping based on chromosomal analysis of 20–30 peripheral lymphocyte metaphases. This technique identifies mosaicism of at least 10% with 95% confidence. If mosaicism is strongly suspected, interphase fluorescence in situ hybridization (FISH) studies and/or genotyping of additional tissues (buccal swabs, fibroblast) may be performed. Fluorescence in situ hybridization (FISH) of buccal cells may detect X or Y chromosome mosaicisms that are not present in peripheral blood.

Approximately 5–10% of patients may have an abnormal Y chromosome or mosaicism characterized by the coexistence of a 45,X cell line with another cell line in which all or part of chromosome Y is present. The presence of Y chromosome material is suggested to be a risk factor for gonadoblastoma in patients with Turner syndrome. The risk of gonadoblastoma in patients with Y chromosome sequences is approximately 10% (Gravholt et al. 2017; Sallai et al. 2010; Changchien et al. 2012). However, the rate of gonadoblastoma among all TS patients is low (1%). Current guidelines recommend gonadectomy in all female individuals with Y chromosome material identified on standard karyotyping. Molecular screening to detect Y chromosomal sequences is recommended only in TS cases exhibiting virilization (Gravholt et al. 2017). Real-time polymerase chain reaction (PCR) with multiple Y-specific probes has good sensitivity for the detection of cryptic Y chromosome material in various tissues. Microarray-based analysis might be a useful complementary test to reveal submicroscopic copy number variations or complex rearrangements of X or Y chromosomes (Haltrich et al. 2015).

Retrospective analyses have shown that there is often a delay in the diagnosis of TS. Lymphedema and webbed neck are the most common reasons to screen for TS during infancy. In the absence of these symptoms, the diagnosis is made at the average of 5 years of age once growth failure has become apparent (below the fifth percentile). Early diagnosis could facilitate treatment of growth failure and allows for the optimal management of renal and cardiac abnormalities, hearing loss, and other associated conditions.

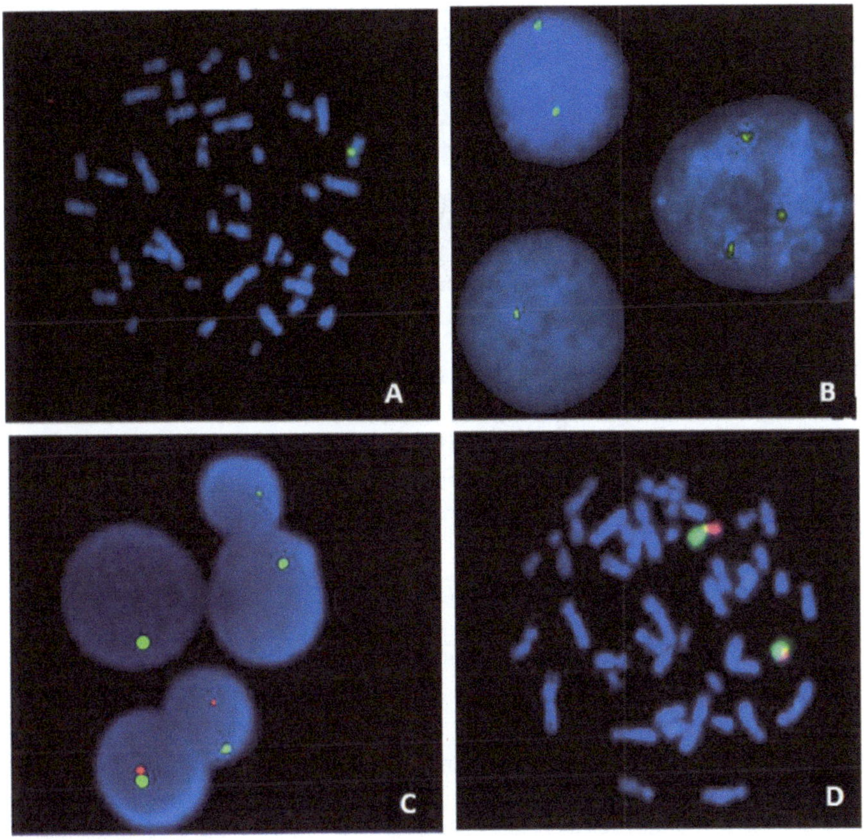

Fig. 20.1 Genetic subtypes of Turner syndrome. X centromere (green) and Y centromere (red) FISH probes identified X chromosome monosomy (**a**), 45,X/46XX/47,XXX mosaic karyotype (**b**), and 45,X/46,XY mosaicism (**c**); Xq-arm (green) and Xp-arm (red) probes identified one normal and one ring X chromosome (**d**)

20.1.2 Cytogenetic and Molecular Basis of TS Phenotype

Approximately one-half of TS patients have X monosomy (45,X) in all studied cells, a group of patients have mosaic karyotypes, and another group has different sex chromosome structural anomalies such as isochromosome Xq, partial deletion/duplication of the second X, ring X, or an abnormal Y chromosome. The most common form of mosaicism is 45,X/46,XX, while the rest of the mosaic TS karyotypes shows different combinations of X monosomy, normal 46,XX cells, and trisomy X (Figs. 20.1 and 20.2). Smaller X chromosome deletions cause distinct phenotypes and are classified into other disease groups, such as **SHOX-related short stature** in the case of Xp22.3 microdeletion or **premature ovarian failure**

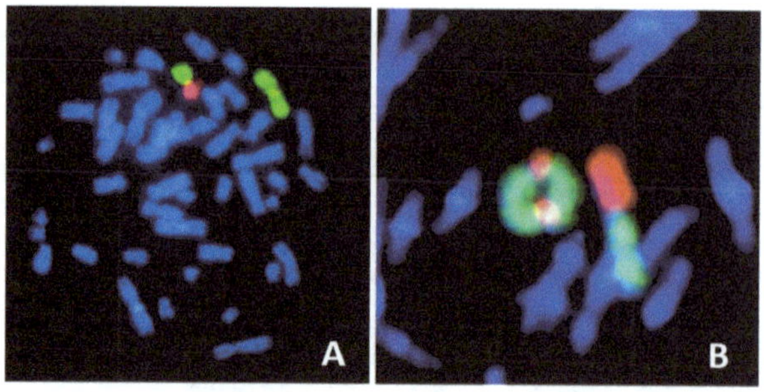

Fig. 20.2 Turner syndrome with iso(Xq) chromosome. The Xq arm (green) and Xp arm (red) FISH probes identified one normal X chromosome and another X formed only from two Xq arms (**a**) as well as one normal X and one ring iso (Xq) chromosome (**b**)

Table 20.1 Types and frequencies of chromosome abnormalities in TS (based on Gravholt et al. 2017)

Description	Karyotype	(%)
Monosomy X	45,X	40–50
Mosaicism	45,X/46,XX	15–25
Mosaicism with triple X	45,X/47,XXX; 45,X/46,XX/47,XXX	3
Mixed gonadal dysgenesis	45,X/46,XY	10–12
Deletion Xp22.3	46,XX,del(22p23)	
Ring X chromosome	46,X,r(X)/46,XX	
Isochromosome Xq; isodicentric Xp	46,X,i(Xq); 46,X,idic(Xp)	10

(POF) in the case of Xq24 distal deletion. Women over the age of 50 years with less than 5% X mosaicism should not be considered to have TS (Gravholt et al. 2017).

The types and frequencies of chromosome abnormalities in TS are summarized in Table 20.1.

Comparative analysis of the karyotype and phenotype is difficult because: (1) mosaicism varies with tissue type and (2) karyotyping only investigates lymphocytes and will not provide information regarding the level of mosaicism in other, more relevant tissues (brain, ovaries). Thus, a mosaic result does not necessarily predict severity. However, 45,X/46,XX and 45,X/47,XXX lymphocyte mosaicisms could be associated with milder phenotypes, spontaneous pregnancy, and less severe congenital heart disease. Ring X chromosome is sometimes associated with variable intellectual disability.

Although it has been known for the past 60 years that TS is caused by the deletion of the second sex chromosome, the mechanism by which X chromosome monosomy disrupts development is still not well understood. Researchers have attempted to explain the clinical findings in TS based on cytogenetic and gene dosage changes. This hypothesis, known as "Gene Dosage Effect," explains the clinical and metabolic features of TS based on the absence of a limited number of dosage-sensitive genes mapped to specific regions of sex chromosomes (Zinn and Ross 1998). The well-known dosage-sensitive gene that have been proven to be associated with skeletal anomalies and the short stature phenotype of TS patients is the highly conserved *SHOX* (Rappold et al. 2007).

By analyzing 224 TS women, Bakalov et al. found that haploinsufficiency of Xp genes increases, and excess dosage of Xq genes compounds the risk of type 2 DM, which has significantly a higher prevalence (43%) in the case of i(Xq) vs. X monosomy (24%). By comparing the gene expression profiles of X chromosomes in these two groups, they identified several overexpressed Xq genes involved in gene expression regulation (*XIST, RPS4X, PIN4, VGLL1, SMARCA1*) in i(Xq) patients and a few downregulated Xq genes with roles in immune system functions (anti-inflammatory transcription factor gene *TSC22D3* and *XIAP* which encodes the X-linked inhibitor of apoptosis that protects β-cells from cytokine- and ER stress-induced programmed cell death) (Bakalov et al. 2009). There have been several reports on the role of X chromosome gene dosage through inactivation or duplication in women with autoimmune diseases (Jørgensen et al. 2010; Bianchi et al. 2012; Bakalov et al. 2012; Grossi et al. 2013). However, the gene dosage theory could not elucidate the mechanisms underlying the increased frequency and striking diversity (with some individuals left untouched, while others suffer from severe cardiovascular, renal, and autoimmune disease) of morbidity and mortality seen in TS.

Current studies suggest that TS features could be caused by the altered regulation and complex interrelations of many genes both on and outside the sex chromosomes and that the epigenetic machinery has regulatory impact on gene transcription. Trolle et al. recently investigated leukocyte DNA methylation- and RNA-expression profiles in a cohort of individuals with 45,X monosomy and compared them to age-matched karyotypically normal female and male controls. They found that Turner syndrome patients are clearly distinguishable from controls based on genome-wide X chromosome RNA-expression profiles, autosomal DNA methylation profiles, and X chromosome methylation profiles. They identified candidate genes possibly involved in TS comorbidity both on the X chromosomes (escape genes, pseudoautosomal regions genes, as well as X–Y gene pairs) and on the autosomes (Trolle et al. 2016).

One such candidate gene is RPS4X, mapping to the long arm of the X chromosome, where no other genes are known to escape X inactivation, near the site from which the X-inactivating signal is thought to emanate. Ribosomal protein S4 is the only ribosomal protein known to be encoded by more than one gene. As is typical for genes encoding ribosomal proteins, there are multiple processed pseudogenes of this gene dispersed through the genome. Its related pathways are potentially associated with the pathophysiology of Turner syndrome (Fisher et al. 1990).

The other X inactivation escape gene *JPX,* affiliated with the noncoding RNA class, is a molecular switch for X chromosome inactivation. In TS, *JPX* and likewise *XIST* are downregulated, mirroring the similarities in the two genes' biological functions (Tian et al. 2010).

Three of the differentially expressed genes of the pseudoautosomal region code for proteins involved in immune responses (*CD99*, *IL3RA*, *CSF2RA*) and thus may play a role in the predisposition to autoimmune disease observed in TS. *CSF2RA* was suggested as a candidate gene explaining the early lethality of TS embryos (Urbach and Benvenisty 2009).

Several differentially expressed autosomal genes that could be involved in comorbidity have also been identified in TS: *ZFYVE9* (aortic aneurysm), *CNR1* (obesity), *PRKX* (congenital urinary malformations), *KDM6A* (premature ovarian failure), and *DOCK1* (melanocytic naevi).

The chromosome X of TS has a distinct methylation profile when compared to the chromosome X of 46,XY males and XX females; the most pronounced differences were seen in the TS vs. 46,XX comparison. 45,X monosomy is associated with global hypomethylation of the genome with predominantly proximal promoter hypomethylation and, to a lesser extent, areas of hypermethylation (Trolle et al. 2016; Sharma et al. 2015). Such a hypomethylated gene, the *USP9X* is a member of the peptidase C19 family with a role in chromosome alignment and segregation in mitosis, neuronal migration, and axonal growth; its loss of function germline mutations cause X-linked female-restricted facial dysmorphism, short stature, choanal atresia, and non-syndromic intellectual disability.

Another example, the Y homolog *KDM6A* gene belongs to the homeobox gene family and its protein catalyzes the demethylation of the tri-/dimethylated histone H3. *KDM6A* helps direct tissue differentiation in cardiac cells as well as myogenesis and is potentially involved in the abnormal cardiovascular development in TS. Interestingly, *KDM6A* and overlapping congenital cardiovascular abnormalities are a common denominator in TS and Kabuki syndrome 2, where this gene is mutated. *KDM6A* is also important for the reestablishment of pluripotency and germ cell development, making it a potential candidate gene in the ovarian failure in TS (Adam et al. 2018).

20.1.3 Genetic Counseling and Management of TS

Given the complexity and multisystem nature of TS, pediatricians, endocrinologists, and family physicians play an important role in coordinating multidisciplinary management and health surveillance for comorbidities throughout the lifespan of TS patients.

Prenatal counseling is important because the rate of spontaneous fetal loss for 45, X fetuses with an ultrasound finding is high. TS may cause up to 10% of all miscarriages, with 99% of conceptuses terminating spontaneously during the first and second trimesters. Abnormal maternal serum markers and ultrasound findings such as coarctation of the aorta, left-sided cardiac defects, brachycephaly, renal anomalies, polyhydramnios, and oligohydramnios (Bronshtein et al. 2003) suggest an increased likelihood of TS, but these tests are not diagnostic, and karyotype confirmation of TS by chorionic villous sampling or amniocentesis is obligatory. The current TS clinical practice guideline (Gravholt et al. 2017) does not recommend the recently developed noninvasive prenatal testing (NIPT) (sequencing and single-nucleotide polymorphism array analysis of cell-free fetal DNA [cfDNA]) in maternal blood for fetal karyotype assessment because detection rates and positive predictive values of these investigations are relatively low.

Regardless of specific results, genetic counseling should be provided before and after any prenatal diagnostic procedure. Pre- and postnatal genetic counselors should be fully informed about the pathogenesis, phenotypic variability, and comorbidities of TS in order to inform parents according to the highest scientific standards. A straightforward conversation with the family about all possible medical and psychological aspects of TS is usually very helpful for the parents to make an informed decision.

The prenatal TS karyotype could be based on fibroblast analysis; therefore constitutional karyotypes should be determined postnatally in all patients. In childhood, the key aspects of TS management are cardiovascular monitoring and treatment of congenital heart disease, growth hormone therapy, supplemental estrogen therapy for sexual development, and preservation of bone mineral density. The mean adult height in patients who have received growth hormone (GH) and estrogen therapy is 150 cm, and about 1 cm height gain per year is a reasonable expectation of GH therapy. GH treatment should be initiated early (around 4–6 years of age and preferably before 12–13 years) and discontinued after the patient reaches a bone age of 14 years; sex hormone therapy is generally continued throughout life (Gravholt et al. 2017).

Patients with TS require audiometry at diagnosis and periodically thereafter to differentiate between sensorineural or conductive hearing loss and recurrent otitis media. Early recognition and appropriate management of hearing impairment are crucial to avoid hearing-related speech pathology and the risk of social isolation (Kubba et al. 2017). Renal ultrasound should also be performed at the time of diagnosis to assess for congenital renal malformations. A comprehensive ophthalmological examination between 12 and 18 months and dental-orthodontic as well as orthopedic (congenital hip dislocation, kyphosis, scoliosis, osteoporosis) evaluations are also important aspects of therapy. Keeping in mind the increased risk of atherosclerosis and cardiovascular disease across the patient's lifespan, a wide spectrum of cardiometabolic risk factors (overweight, hypertension, impaired glucose metabolism, hypercholesterolemia, and dyslipidemia) should also be monitored in childhood (Lebenthal et al. 2018). Early assays of autoantibodies and immunoglobulins and monitoring of thyroid hormones and liver function are fundamental for anticipatory detection of autoimmune diseases and implementation of adequate treatment.

Fertility and sexual development issues often create major anxiety for adult TS patients. Advances in reproductive medicine involving in vitro fertilization-embryo transfer (IVF-ET) have increased the possibility of childbearing in TS women, but pregnancy remains particularly challenging due to the high prevalence of cardiovascular complications such as aortic dissection or aortic valve stenosis (Lucaccioni et al. 2015). An age-appropriate counseling about infertility treatments can markedly mitigate the adverse psychological impact of the diagnosis. The likelihood of spontaneous conception decreases with age, and oocyte cryopreservation should accordingly be counselled only in the cases of young mosaic TS women with persistent ovarian function. The psychosocial burden of TS (infertility, short stature, lack of libido) may be substantial; therefore, neuropsychologic and behavioral health services should be integrated into the care for girls and women with TS. The counselor should consider advising TS individuals to join patient organizations because belonging to a peer support group generally improves the quality of life and diminishes the risk of isolation (Sylvén et al. 1993).

Recently published comprehensive management guidelines of the International Turner Syndrome Consensus Group (Gravholt et al. 2017), based on collective expert opinion and a review of existing literature, contain recommendations regarding the most optimal treatment options of short stature, infertility, hypertension, and hormonal replacement therapy and provide a practical clinical guideline focusing on operational recommendations for daily management.

20.2 Klinefelter Syndrome

Klinefelter syndrome (KS) is a condition in which a male patient has one Y chromosome and one or more extra X chromosomes (Fig. 20.3). Typical characteristics of KS include hypergonadotropic hypogonadism, small testes, infertility, and cognitive impairment.

KS was first described by H. F. Klinefelter, E. C. Reifenstein, and F. Albright in Boston in 1942 (Klinefelter et al. 1942). They reported nine men with bilateral gynecomastia, absence of spermatogenesis, normal to moderately reduced function of the Leydig cells, and high follicle-stimulating hormone (FSH) levels. In 1959, two Scottish researchers, P. A. Jacobs and J A. Strong, described the chromosomal abnormality responsible for KS: 47,XXY karyotype. Standard karyotyping remains the most common diagnostic method for KS to this day.

Due to the great age-dependent phenotypic variability and the high rate of associated morbidity, KS continues to impose significant diagnostic challenges for clinicians. The prepubertal phenotype is usually atypical and often unremarkable. Infant boys with KS may have decreased muscle tone, cryptorchidism, and smaller testicular and penile size (Davis et al. 2016), and head circumference beginning at the age of 4 years tends to be below the mean for age. During childhood, delayed speech and language skills and learning difficulties may be present. Children can develop attention deficit disorders, and development of social skills is problematic. Hypergonadotropic hypogonadism becomes clinically evident in KS at the onset of puberty, which occurs at the same time as in normal young men, but with some enlargement of the testes. Starting in midpuberty the testes shrink again and the androgen levels remain low despite of FSH and luteinizing hormone (LH) levels increasing to reach the hypergonadotropic levels seen in adult KS. Symptoms developed in adult KS are indicative of testosterone deficiency: firm, very small testes with an average size of 2 to 4 ml (normal range: 15–30 ml) and infertility. The severity of hypogonadism depends somewhat on testosterone levels, which typically vary in the subnormal to low normal range (Gravholt et al. 2018). Estrogen levels are elevated in early puberty and remain slightly increased in comparison with controls but can also be normal. However, the clinical symptoms often remain subtle and resembles that of normal 46,XY males.

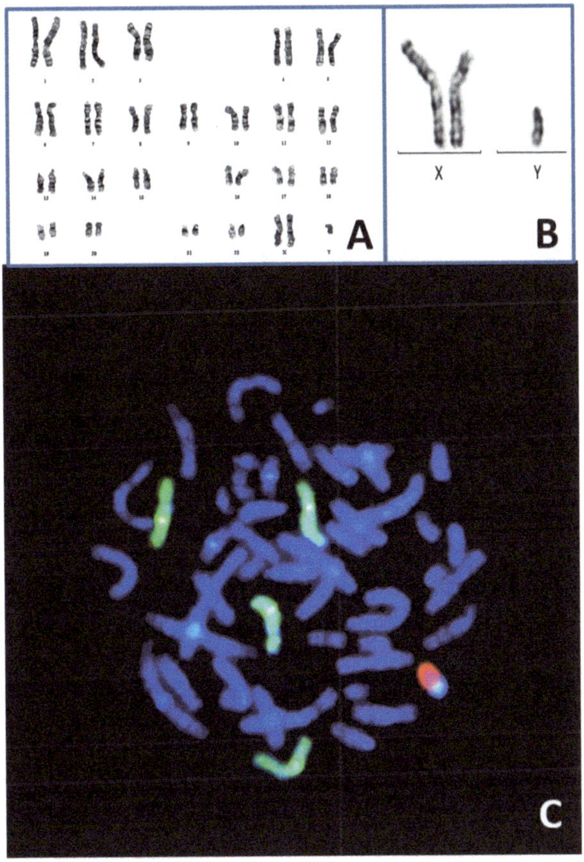

Fig. 20.3 Genetic forms of Klinefelter syndrome. Karyotype of the common form (**a**), partial karyotype with iso(Xq) chromosome (**b**), and rare variant Klinefelter syndrome with 48,XXXXY karyotype (the four X chromosomes are shown in green and the Y in red) (**c**)

20.2.1 Prevalence and Diagnosis

KS is the most common male sex chromosomal aneuploidy (SCA) with an incidence of 0.1% to 0.2% of male neonates corresponding to approximately one in every 600 males being affected.

Epidemiological studies show that only 10% of patients are identified during childhood, and the majority are diagnosed in adulthood typically in the course of infertility investigations. A minority are diagnosed after the age of 50 years and the bulk of patients (60–75%) might never be diagnosed (Samplaski et al. 2014).

Based on a number of large cytogenetic chromosome analyses in various countries around the world, there is a significant incidence divergence depending on the time of diagnosis. Updated data have revealed that prenatal prevalence is generally higher than postnatal and a higher prevalence among Asians has been described, suggesting that ethnicity might have an influence on the prevalence of KS.

The genetic diagnosis of KS is based on karyotype determination. About 80% of KS patients show a 47,XXY karyotype; the remaining 20% have either mosaic karyotypes, numeric, or structural sex chromosome abnormalities.

20.2.2 *Mosaic KS Form*

Mosaicism arises from postfertilization nondisjunction of paired X chromosomes. 46,XY/47,XXY mosaicism has been described in 6% to 7% of KS patients, but the true prevalence of mosaic forms may be greatly underestimated, even compared to the non-mosaic form. In principle, mosaic KS patients are reported to be less affected than non-mosaic KS patients, but the severity of the phenotype depends on the degree of mosaicism (Samplaski et al. 2014). Men with mosaic KS appear to be more androgenized; they have larger testicular volumes, lower levels of LH, higher mean total sperm counts, and higher proportions of sperm in the ejaculate than their non-mosaic counterparts. Mosaicism can be present in the testes only, while the karyotype of peripheral leukocytes remains normal.

47,XXY/46,XX mosaicism with characteristics suggesting KS is very rare: at present, only eight cases have been reported in the literature (Gravholt et al. 2018).

20.2.3 *Numerical X Chromosome Variants of Klinefelter Syndrome*

The presence of additional X chromosomes in males leads to the same longitudinal hormonal pattern changes, testicular fibrosis with subsequent testosterone deficiency, infertility, and hypergonadotropic hypogonadism as in 47,XXY. Because of these shared features 48,XXYY, 48,XXXY, and 49,XXXXY syndromes are considered "variants" of KS. In rarer KS variants patients display structurally abnormal X or Y chromosomes.

Besides hypergonadotropic hypogonadism, common medical problems associated with XXYY, XXXY, and XXXXY are intention and postural tremor, asthma/reactive airway disease, seizure disorder, food/environmental allergies, congenital heart defects, type 2 DM, radioulnar synostosis, congenital elbow dislocation, congenital hip dislocation, pes planus, clubfoot, scoliosis, osteoporosis, peripheral vascular disease, deep vein thrombosis (DVT), pulmonary embolism, strabismus, recurrent otitis, gastroesophageal reflux, obstructive sleep apnea, constipation, dental problems, and inguinal hernia/undescended testicles (Visootsak et al. 2007; Tartaglia et al. 2011). Some medical features can be present from birth, others emerge and increase in adolescence and/or in young adulthood, but not all patients have all of the findings listed above.

20.2.3.1 48,XXYY

The estimated incidence of 48,XXYY karyotype is 1:17,000–1:40,000 males and represents approximately 2.3% of KS individuals (Borja-Santos et al. 2010).

Although the phenotypic features are similar to 47,XXY (tall stature, hypergonadotropic hypogonadism, and infertility), XXYY is associated with additional medical problems and more significant neurodevelopmental and psychological characteristics. These are mild craniofacial dysmorphism, skeletal abnormalities such as radioulnar synostosis, clinodactyly, poor dentition, pes planus, and lower IQ (typically between 70 and 80) with profiles showing significantly lower verbal IQ than performance IQ. In infants, early feeding problems (weak suck, slow feeding) were noted. The common facial features in childhood are mild hypertelorism, narrow and upslanting palpebral fissures, and full lips. In adulthood a long face, prominent brows and bitemporal narrowing are common. Tall stature is a characteristic feature, the mean final adult height (192.4 cm) falling almost two-thirds above the 90th centile (Tartaglia et al. 2008). Affected males seem to perform better at tasks focused on math, visual-spatial skills such as puzzles, and memorization of locations or directions.

20.2.3.2 48,XXXY

This sex chromosome aneuploidy is characterized by the presence of two extra X chromosomes in males, and the incidence is 1:17,000 to 1:50,000 in male births (Frühmesser and Kotzot 2011).

However, the 48,XXXY syndrome differs from KS by the presence of mild intellectual disability (Visootsak et al. 2007), more marked genital hypoplasia (microorchidism, micropenis, hypoplasia of the scrotum) and by more frequently observed facial dysmorphisms (hypertelorism, epicanthal folds, upslanting palpebral fissures, flat nose, simplified ears, mild prognathism, facial asymmetry, short neck). Congenital skeletal malformations and other dysmorphic characteristics such as fifth-digit clinodactyly, short nail beds, and prominent elbows with hyperextensibility are often associated with this syndrome. Behavioral problems (hyperactivity, irritability, anxiety, immaturity, passivity, anger, communication and socialization problems) and language retardation may become more pronounced with age.

20.2.3.3 49,XXXXY

The 49, XXXXY syndrome (Fig. 20.3c) with an incidence of 1:85,000 to 1:1,00,000 in male births has become known as a severe variant of KS due to its characteristic features including central nervous system dysfunction, congenital anomalies, and global developmental delays (Gropman et al. 2010). Compared with 48,XXYY and 48,XXXY, the degree of facial dysmorphism is more pronounced, and congenital anomalies (persistent ductus arteriosus, atrial septal defect, tetralogy of Fallot, bifid uvula, cleft palate and skeletal abnormalities) are more common (50–100%). Furthermore, intellectual and learning disabilities as well as speech and motor delays affect 95–100% of XXXXY patients. Common features include low birth weight, hypotonia, short stature, round face in infancy, coarsening of features in older age, prognathism, microcephaly, short, broad neck, hyperextensible joints, and hypoplastic genitalia. Behavior has been described as timid and shy to friendly; however, anxiety, irritability, and bouts of temper can also occur.

20.2.4 Structural Variants of Klinefelter Syndrome

In this class, patients display structurally abnormal X or Y chromosomes; these forms are even less frequent than numerical variants.

The 47,X,i(X)(q10),Y variant of KS (only 25 reported cases in the literature) is characterized by an additional isochromosome made of the long arm of the X chromosome (Fig. 20.3b). Its prevalence is calculated to be between 0.3 and 0.9% in males with KS phenotype. It has been suggested that the cause of the formation of Xq isochromosome is a misdivision of the centromere or sister chromatids during meiotic division. The patients share many aspects with classical KS (infertility, increased plasma LH and FSH levels, and in most cases azoospermia), but the typical tall stature seen in KS is absent; in fact the patients are usually shorter than average height. 47,X,i(Xq),Y patients have normal intelligence; the intellectual disability seen in other KS variants has not been described in the reported cases (Frühmesser and Kotzot 2011; Kondo et al. 2018).

Additional aberrations on the X or on the Y chromosome might also be associated with the phenotype of KS. Regarding the structural rearrangements of the Y microdeletions, ring Y and dicentric Y chromosome have been described in some patients showing signs of KS. The new consensus statement of disorders of sex development (DSD) defined individuals with 46,XX maleness as 46,XX DSD (Houk et al. 2006). The common cause of 46,XX DSD is the translocation of a normal SRY gene from the Y chromosome onto an X chromosome.

These SRY-positive XX patients present with gynecomastia, small testes, and azoospermia-related sterility, but are otherwise normal men with regular pubic hair and penile size. Contrary to KS, they are usually short which often causes difficulties in differential diagnosis.

Long-term complications of male hypogonadism include low libido, erectile dysfunction, decreased secondary sexual characteristics, osteopenia, and depression. Usually the phenotype of SRY-negative individuals is more severe and less remindful of KS, and it is influenced more by the implicated genes (SOX9, SOX3, RSPO1, and WNT4).

Based on literature data, KS with X chromosome structural aberrations is very rare, the phenotype is usually nearly identical to typical KS, and body height is variable depending on the number of SHOX gene copies present on the X chromosomes (Frühmesser and Kotzot 2011).

20.2.5 Morbidity and Mortality

KS is associated with a significantly elevated risk of morbidity and mortality affecting almost all organ systems and leading to a life expectancy 11.5 years below that of the male population as a whole (Nieschlag 2013).

KS is often accompanied by circulatory diseases (ischemic heart disease, DVT, pulmonary embolism, heart malformations), pulmonary diseases (pneumonia, chronic obstructive pulmonary disease, asthma), gastrointestinal diseases (ulcus, cirrhosis of liver), urogenital system diseases (infections, retention of testes), musculoskeletal system diseases (osteoarthritis, osteopenia, osteoporosis, hip fracture), and neurologic and psychiatric diseases (epilepsy, autism spectrum disorder, attention deficit hyperactivity disorder, psychoses, neuroses, learning difficulties, neurocognitive deficits, depression, anxiety, personality and language disorders) (Green et al. 2019). People with KS have increased risk for a number of autoimmune diseases, particularly those that are female-predominant (Sjogren's syndrome, systemic lupus erythematosus, Addison's disease, multiple sclerosis, rheumatoid arthritis, celiac disease, autoimmune hypothyroidism, psoriasis, ulcerative colitis, diabetes mellitus type I) (Seminog et al. 2015).

Breast cancer, mediastinal nonseminomatous germ cell tumors, non-Hodgkin lymphoma, and hematological cancers occur with a higher incidence than in men with normal karyotypes, whereas the risk of prostate cancer is lower. Endocrine diseases (hypogonadism, hypothyroidism) are seen more frequently as well. The often observed central obesity with reduced glucose tolerance usually leads to metabolic syndrome and type 2 DM.

20.2.6 Molecular Basis of KS

Although the genetic background of KS was identified over 70 years ago, the molecular basis for the phenotypic traits and morbidity are not well understood. Thus far, only CAG repeat length and SHOX gene copy number have been convincingly connected to the phenotype in KS. The existing literature demonstrates that CAG repeat length in exon 1 of the androgen receptor gene is related to different anthropometric measurements showing a positive correlation with height, arm span, and arm and leg length (Bojesen et al. 2011; Chang et al. 2015). The SHOX gene is localized in the pseudoautosomal region of the sex chromosome and thus escapes X-linked inactivation, which explains the excess height seen in KS.

Recent studies based on genome-wide RNA sequencing and DNA methylation profile analysis enhance the understanding of molecular mechanisms and pathophysiology underlying the KS phenotype and the increased risk of comorbidities. A recent study carried out the comprehensive characterization of the methylome and the transcriptome of both coding and noncoding genes in KS as well as 46,XY and 46,XX controls. It was demonstrated that the methylome and the transcriptome of both the autosomes and the X chromosome are altered in leukocytes from KS subjects, which therefore exhibit a unique epigenetic and genetic landscape compared to both male and female normal karyotypes. The KS methylation signature is predominantly characterized by hypermethylation (Skakkebak et al. 2018), exactly the opposite of the hypomethylation seen in Turner syndrome, which demonstrates that epigenetic alteration may be implicated in the phenotypes seen in SCA.

Although the X chromosome inactivation process in KS is comparable to that seen in women, the X chromosomal gene expression profile is more reminiscent of 46,XY males. Differentially expressed gene set analyses revealed enrichment for genes involved in the immune system, neuron development, and the Wnt signaling pathway. Deregulated Wnt signaling may be involved in cognitive deficit, vascular comorbidities, higher cancer risk, and embryonal development and congenital malformations (Skakkebak et al. 2018; Belling et al. 2017). Aberrant expression of escape genes and/or differentially methylated genes has been suggested to be responsible for some phenotypic and comorbidity traits of KS such as cognitive dysfunction (*EIF2S3*, *G3BP1*, *NSD1*, *PEX 10*, *DACT1*, *KANK1*, *LGALS1*), decreased bone density and osteoporosis (*FIGNL1*, *TXLNG*), dyslipidemia and obesity (*DOCK7*, *EIF2S3*), tic disorders (*AKAP17A*), and endothelial cell dysfunction (*SHROOM2*, *AMOT*). Upregulated pseudoautosomal genes such as *SLC25A6*, playing a fundamental role in cellular energy metabolism, may also be implicated in KS phenotype.

Data from a large cohort of individuals with SCA syndromes provided evidence that sex chromosome dosage could have a complex regulatory effect on large autosomal gene networks with key roles in cellular functioning. Downregulation of protein trafficking genes, upregulation of cell cycle progression, and a significant upregulation of immune system genes were seen in KS patients, which is congruent with their 18-fold elevated risk for autoimmune disease (Raznahan et al. 2018).The phenotypic consequence of X-supernumerary chromosome(s) is more severe in males than in females: the increasing X chromosome count decreases expression of X-linked genes that undergo X chromosome inactivation. Sex chromosome dosage regulates large-scale gene expression networks and broadly influences differences in phenotypic severity.

20.2.7 Treatment, Management, and Genetic Counseling

KS is a chromosomal disorder with a large spectrum of clinical manifestations, with "no standardized set of guidelines for appropriate management"; each patient should be treated in an individualized manner depending on the degree of presented symptoms (Bearelly and Oates 2019). However, KS usually requires complex treatment and management conducted by a health care team including endocrinologist, genetic counsellor, speech therapist, pediatrician, physical therapist, reproductive medicine specialist, and psychologist.

Several studies demonstrated that KS is the second most frequent chromosome abnormalities associated with terminating pregnancy, yielding an average termination rate of 61% (Jeon et al. 2012). The parents' main concerns about the children's future are the potential infertility and cognitive impairments. Generally nondirective counseling leads to better-informed decision making and genetic counselors updated with all aspects of KS could provide the most appropriate quality information. A proper education about the sex chromosome, a discussion about the possible abnormalities and treatment options, and connection to support groups of families with KS affected children could diminish the parents' anxieties and might prove useful for dealing with uncertainty. The genetic counselor should provide a culturally sensitive counseling for marital status; ethnicity and religion could also play a role in decisions around pregnancy.

In childhood there are no distinct phenotype feature; the children usually are diagnosed on the bases of prenatal XXY karyotype, which should be confirmed postnatally.

In adolescents, early recognition and anticipatory guidance are extremely helpful in the management of KS patients. The treatment should focus on the three major traits of the syndrome: hypogonadism, gynecomastia, and psychosocial problems. Lifelong replacement therapy with testosterone should commence at puberty for proper masculine development of sexual characteristics, muscle bulk, and bone structure and to avoid the long-term deleterious consequences of hypogonadism (Seminog et al. 2015). Testosterone therapy will not have any positive effect on spermatogenesis and infertility. Aromatase inhibitor therapy may be useful in males with gynecomastia. If gynecomastia is cosmetically problematic, mastectomy should be performed by surgeons with experience in this area as this can be a challenge for the patients especially during puberty and young adulthood. Erectile function is not commonly impacted, but infertility is close to 100% in non-mosaic KS patients. Educational and psychological support should be given to prevent difficulties and improve life quality. Although spontaneous pregnancy in partners of KS patients remains extremely rare, treatment for infertility has changed drastically in the last 20 years (Gravholt et al. 2018). Using the latest fertilization techniques such as microTESE (testicular sperm extraction) followed by intracytoplasmic sperm injection (ISCI), pregnancy and live birth were achieved in approximately half of the published cases.

In KS patients, there is an increase incidence in extragonadal—almost exclusively mediastinal—germ cell tumors (M-GCTs) that present at young age as precocious puberty, whereas the older ones show thorax-associated symptoms. Therefore, a karyotype analysis should be included in the clinical workup of boys with M-GCTs (Williams et al. 2018).

In adulthood, the higher-risk comorbidities such as cardiovascular, cerebrovascular, and metabolic syndrome require closer medical control. It is reasonable for practitioners to consider a diagnostic echocardiogram and glucose tolerance monitoring. In a recent study, Glueck et al. suggested that long-term testosterone replacement therapy (TRT) with previously undiagnosed familial thrombophilia may be an interaction that results in higher prevalence of thromboembolism in KS patients.

They recommend thrombophilia screening before starting TRT to delineate the KS individuals at increased risk for DVT (Glueck et al. 2017).

Recently and future research will likely help to understand the phenotypic diversity of KS, to better delineate the associated mortality and morbidity, and also to devise more efficient and effective treatment strategies.

20.3 Prader-Willi Syndrome

Prader-Willi syndrome (PWS, OMIM 176270) is a complex multisystem genetic disorder caused by the absent expression of paternally active genes on chromosome 15q11.2–q13, the PWS critical region. PWS was the first recognized genomic imprinting disorder in humans and is characterized by hypothalamic and severe metabolic dysfunction, neurological implications, and psychiatric disturbances. PWS affects an estimated 1 in 10,000 to 30,000 people worldwide.

20.3.1 Clinical Manifestations of PWS

Clinical diagnosis remains a challenge for most practitioners because the majority of clinical manifestations of PWS change with age, others evolve over time, and many features are nonspecific or subtle. During the neonatal period, PWS is characterized by unexplained muscle hypotonia and failure to thrive. Other features noted include feeding difficulties, lethargy, thick saliva, small genitalia in both males and females, and cryptorchidism in males. In later infancy or early childhood, the symptoms change dramatically: excessive appetite and gradual development of central obesity become the predominant clinical problem. As the PWS individual ages, developmental delay, intellectual disabilities, typical behavior problems (temper tantrums, obsessive-compulsive features such as food seeking, outbursts, skin picking) become more and more prominent. Sleep abnormalities and scoliosis are common; GH deficiency is frequent. The phenotype of adult PWS is mostly determined by hypothalamic dysfunction which may lead to several endocrinopathies, including growth hormone deficiency, hypogonadism, hypothyroidism, central adrenal insufficiency (CAI), and poor bone mineral density (BMD). The endocrine dysfunction is usually complicated by metabolic syndrome and type 2 DM (Heksch et al. 2017).

The major and minor clinical diagnostic criteria were established by a consensus in 1993 (Holm et al. 1993). Subsequently, decisive molecular genetic testing became available for laboratory diagnosis of PWS. Accordingly, an age-related, less strict clinical scoring system was accepted to help define appropriate patients for PWS diagnostic testing (Table 20.2) (Gunay-Aygun et al. 2001).

Table 20.2 New criteria to prompt genetic testing for PWS (adapted from Gunay-Aygun et al. 2001)

Age at assessment	Features to prompt DNA testing for PWS
Birth to 2 years	1. Severe hypotonia, weak suck
2–6 years	1. Hypotonia with history of weak suck 2. Global developmental delay 3. Short stature and/or decreased growth 4. Hypogenitalism/hypogonadism
6–12 years	1. History of hypotonia with weak suck 2. Global developmental delay 3. Excessive eating with central obesity, if uncontrolled 4. Hypogenitalism/hypogonadism
13 years–adulthood	1. Cognitive impairment; usually mild intellectual disability 2. Excessive eating (hyperphagia; obsession with food) with central obesity, if uncontrolled 3. Hypogonadism and/or typical behavior problems (temper tantrums, obsessive-compulsive features) 4. Short stature; small hands and feet

20.3.2 Genetics of PWS

The human chromosome 15q11–q13 region contains four distinct gene areas: (1) a proximal region with non-imprinted genes expressed biallelically, (2) a PWS region with paternally expressed imprinted genes, (3) an Angelman syndrome (AS) region with maternally expressed imprinted genes, and (4) a distal region with non-imprinted genes expressed with paternal bias. These gene areas are delineated by three common breakpoint cluster regions (BP1, BP2, BP3) (Fig. 20.4) lying within segmental duplications.

The proximal non-imprinted region located between breakpoints BP1 and BP2 contains four biparentally expressed genes: two genes (*NIPA1* and *NIPA2*) with magnesium ion transmembrane transporter activity, the cytoplasmic FMR1 interacting protein 1 (*CYFIP1*), and the microtubule-binding *TUBGCP5* gene. Individuals with a microdeletion/microduplication of this proximal region are reported with neurological dysfunction and autistic features (Chai et al. 2003).

The PWS region has only paternally expressed genes: five protein coding genes (*MKRN3*, *MAGEL2*, *NDN*, and the bicistronic *SNURF-SNRPN*), a cluster of snoRNAs (C/D box small nucleolar RNAs), and a long noncoding RNA. The protein coding genes of the PWS critical region are located proximally to the imprinting center (IC) and are involved in neural development and brain function. *MKRN3* encodes a zinc finger protein involved in hormone regulation and precocious puberty [OMIM 603856] (Abreu et al. 2015; Macedo et al. 2014).

MAGEL2 (OMIM * 605283), an intronless gene with protein expression mainly in the hypothalamus, has been reported to have functions in circadian rhythm, leptin sensitivity, and human reproduction and fertility (Fountain and Schaaf 2015; Pravdivyi et al. 2015). Recently, subjects with truncating mutations on the paternal

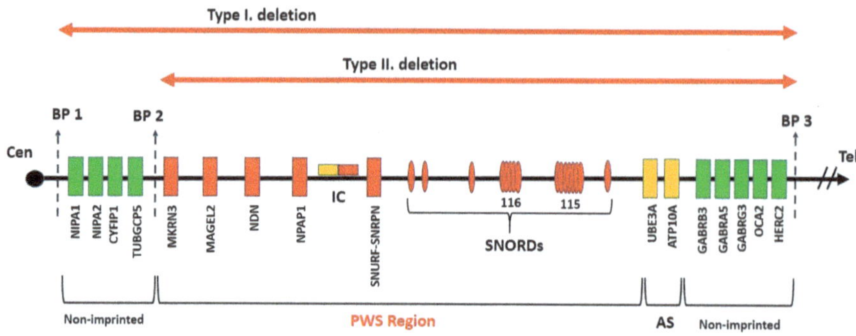

Fig. 20.4 Schematic presentation of the chromosome region 15q11.2–q13. The Prader-Willi syndrome (PWS) critical region (shown in red) contains four paternally-only expressed protein-coding genes (*MKRN3, MAGEL2, NDN,* and *SNURF-SNPRN*) and a family of paternally-only expressed small nuclear RNA species (SNORDs). The protein coding *NPAP1* (nuclear pore-associated protein 1) gene is biallelically expressed in adult testis and brain but is paternally imprinted in fetal brain. The imprinting center (IC) has a bipartite structure with a maternal component implicated in Angelman syndrome (AS, shown in orange) and a paternal component implicated in PWS (shown in red). The biparentally expressed, not imprinted genes are displayed in green color. The dashed vertical lines denote the three common PWS-AS deletion breakpoints (BP1, BP2, BP3) delineating Type I and Type II deletions (shown in red horizontal lines)

allele of MAGEL2 have been reported to have autism spectrum disorder (ASD) and, to a variable extent, aspects of the PWS phenotype (Schaaf et al. 2013). This phenotypically distinct form of PWS was named Schaaf-Yang syndrome.

The intronless gene product, functionally similar to the retinoblastoma protein, is a growth suppressor that facilitates the entry of the cell into cell cycle arrest and may suppress growth in postmitotic neurons. Necdin is highly expressed in mature hypothalamic neurons; lack of necdin during development may contribute to hypogonadotropic hypogonadism in individuals with PWS (Miller et al. 2009). The intronless *NPAP1* gene is biallelically expressed in the adult testis and brain but is paternally imprinted in the fetal brain. Defects in this gene may also be associated with PWS phenotype.

In the center of the PWS region, the extremely complex bicistronic SNURF-SNRPN gene encodes two different proteins: one involved in the genomic imprinting process (encoded by exons 1 through 3) and another involved in RNA processing (exons 4 to 10). The promoter region and exon 1 at the 5′ end of the *SNURF-SNRPN* locus overlap with the paternal PWS imprinting center (IC) and play a critical role in the initiation of imprint switching during spermatogenesis. The IC has a bipartite structure displaying a maternal component implicated in AS alongside the paternal component implicated in PWS. PWS IC mutations block the normal maternal-to-paternal imprint switch in the male germ line, and AS IC mutations block the paternal-to-maternal imprint switch in the female germ line (Ohta et al. 1999; Buiting 2010).

The IC-*SNURF-SNRPN* transcript serves as a host for multiple small nuclear RNA species. These RNA genes named SNORDs, present in a single copy (*SNORD*

64, *SNORD 107*, *SNORD 108*, *SNORD 109A*, *SNORD 109B*) or in gene clusters (*SNORD 115* and *SNORD 116*), are encoded by a large transcript from the complex SNURF-SNRPN and are not translated into protein. The SNORDs function in pre-mRNA processing and may contribute to tissue-specific alternative splicing. Several case studies have revealed that microdeletion of SNORDs may be responsible for several features of PWS and that lack of the paternal SNORD116 gene cluster has a determinant role in the pathogenesis of PWS (Bieth et al. 2015).

The intronless *NPAP1* gene is biallelically expressed in the adult testis and brain but is paternally imprinted in the fetal brain. Defects in this gene may also be associated with PWS phenotype.

The vicinity of the PWS region contains several antisense transcripts complementary to DNA sequences of other genes in a reverse direction, including the antisense transcript to *UBE3A* (ubiquitin protein ligase E3A). The maternally expressed imprinted UBE3A and *ATP10C* (ATPase phospholipid transporting 10A) genes are located in the AS region. UBE3A encodes a ubiquitin ligase required for long-term synaptic potentiation and is maternally expressed in the brain but biallelically expressed in other tissues. Maternally inherited deletion/mutation of this gene causes AS (OMIM 105830), characterized by severe motor and intellectual retardation, ataxia, hypotonia, epilepsy, absence of speech, and characteristic facies (Buiting 2010).

The cluster of *GABA* receptor genes (*GABRB3*, *GABRA5*, and *GABRG3*), the *P locus* for oculocutaneous albinism type 2 (*OCA2*) and *HERC2* genes are found in the distal non-imprinted 15q11–q13 area delineated by the BP3 common distal breakpoint. The GABA receptor subunit genes are expressed unequally, with more expression from the paternal allele than the maternal one. GABA is a major inhibitory neurotransmitter in the brain; alteration in its expression may be associated with appetite and memory changes and visual perception disturbances (Cassidy et al. 2012).

20.3.3 Genetic Subtypes of PWS

There are three main classes of chromosomal abnormalities that lead to PWS: paternal 15q11–q13 deletion (65–75%), maternal uniparental disomy (matUPD) of chromosome 15 (20–30%), and imprinting defects (ID) (5%). Rarely (0.1%) gene mutations or balanced translocations are accountable (Angulo et al. 2015).

20.3.3.1 Paternal Deletion

Paternal deletions are subdivided into three subtypes: the larger Type I, the smaller Type II, and atypical deletion. The typical deletions are almost always de novo events, involving three BPs flanked by low copy repeats (LCRs) which can cause nonhomologous pairing during meiosis. Type I deletion (40%), approximately 6 Mb

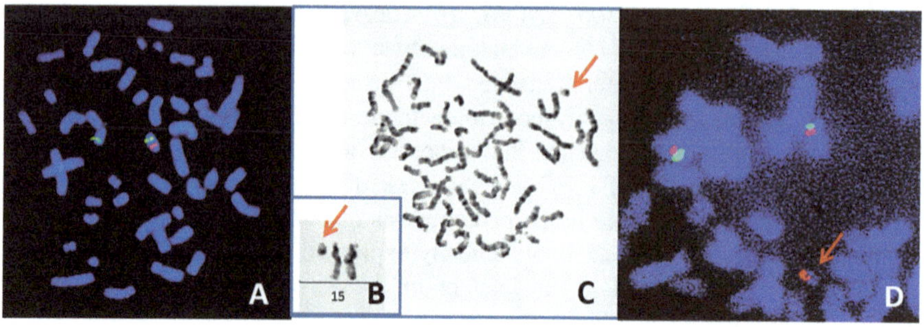

Fig. 20.5 Cytogenetic and FISH pattern of Prader-Willi syndrome. (**a**) Paternal deletion form of Prader-Willi syndrome; chromosomes 15 are identified by the control region (PML—green). The white arrow shows the absence of the SNRPN critical region (red) from one of the chromosomes 15. (**b**, **c**) The red arrows mark a small supernumerary chromosome 15 marker (sSMC15) in a partial karyotype (**b**) and a metaphase cell (**c**). (**d**) The white arrow points to the SNRPN critical region (red) identified by FISH on sSMC 15. The presence of sSMC15 is usually associated with the matUPD form of PWS

in size, extends from proximal BP1 to distal BP3, and the most common Type II deletion (60%) spans 5.3 Mb between BP2 and BP3 (Fig. 20.5) (Manzardo et al. 2018). Atypical deletions that vary in size and breakpoints are reported in about 5% of PWS individuals (Kim et al. 2012). The shortest microdeletions implicated in PWS include the paternally expressed noncoding snoRNAs (Bieth et al. 2015).

The Type I larger deletion affects the non-imprinted ASD prone genes as well. PWS individuals with Type 1 deletions have been reported to have more compulsions, poorer adaptive behavior, and impairment of visual perception more frequently. Patients with the smaller Type II deletion show higher academic achievement scores than Type I PWS patients which may reflect a difference in intellectual functioning as well as differences in visual perception potentially affecting reading ability (Butler et al. 2019).

20.3.3.2 Maternal Uniparental Disomy

The second most common genetic abnormality—accounting for 20–30% of individuals with PWS—is matUPD, the situation in which both chromosomes 15 have been inherited from the mother and none from the father. MatUPD has three different subclasses: heterodisomy, total isodisomy, and segmented isodisomy. Heterodisomy is generated by the non-disjunction of maternal chromosome 15 homologues in meiosis I followed by the loss of the paternal chromosome 15 in the fertilized egg, a mechanism referred to as a trisomy 15 rescue event. Robertsonian translocation of chromosome 15 would also lead to heterodisomy in 50% of cases (Cassidy et al. 2012). In the case of isodisomy, the two completely identical maternal chromosomes 15 are originated from non-disjunction in meiosis II. Segmental isodisomies occur as a result of crossing-over errors in maternal meiosis I or somatic chromosome recombination in early pregnancy (Manzardo et al. 2018). UPD can also be associated with small supernumerary chromosome 15 markers (sSMC) (Fig. 20.5b, c, d) (Liehr et al. 2005). Maternal UPD has been shown to be associated with advanced maternal age. PWS individuals with matUPD 15 often have a milder phenotype, higher verbal IQ scores, milder behavior problems, and better social reasoning skills than those with Type I and Type II deletions but are more prone to increased episodes of psychosis and autistic spectrum disorders (Gold et al. 2018).

20.3.3.3 Imprinting Defect

ID affects the imprinting process on the paternally inherited chromosome 15 and only accounts for approximately 1–3% of PWS cases. The majority of IDs are produced by random imprinting errors on chromosome 15 during paternal spermatogenesis or in the cases of somatic mosaicism during early embryogenesis (Ohta et al. 1999). In these cases, both parental alleles are present, DNA sequence changes are not found, the ID is caused by an epigenetic failure (epimutation), and both paternal and maternal chromosomes 15 exhibit a maternal-only DNA methylation pattern. About 15% of individuals with ID are found to have very small deletions (7.5–100 Kb) in the PWS IC region located at the 5′ end of the SNRPN gene and promoter. In most cases, IC deletions are familial mutations transmitted from the paternal grandmother to the father and are associated with a 50% recurrence risk. However, in some cases the IC deletion is de novo or the consequence of parental germ line mosaicism in the parents (Cassidy et al. 2012; Angulo et al. 2015).

20.3.4 Diagnostic Strategies of PWS

The type and accuracy of genetic testing for PWS has progressed substantially over the last ten years. The deletion form of PWS has traditionally been diagnosed with FISH with SNRPN-specific probes (Fig. 20.5a). Currently DNA methylation analysis (Fig. 20.6) targeting the 5′ CpG island of the SNURF-SNRPN locus is the gold standard technique for detecting PWS (Ács et al. 2018). Although this method correctly diagnoses PWS in more than 99% of cases, it cannot distinguish between a deletion, matUPD, or ID. The newly developed, methylation-specific multiplex-ligation probe amplification (MS-MLPA) kits have particularly dense probe coverage for dosage and methylation analysis of the PWS critical region. Therefore, MS-MLPA analysis might be considered as the first-tier test for screening patients with suspected PWS. The advantage of high-resolution chromosomal microarray compared to FISH is that it will detect not only the precise PWS deletion size, but also additional chromosomal copy number alterations elsewhere in the genome. For genetic counseling purposes, a classical karyotype analysis is also recommended in the proband to discern rare familial balanced chromosomal rearrangements

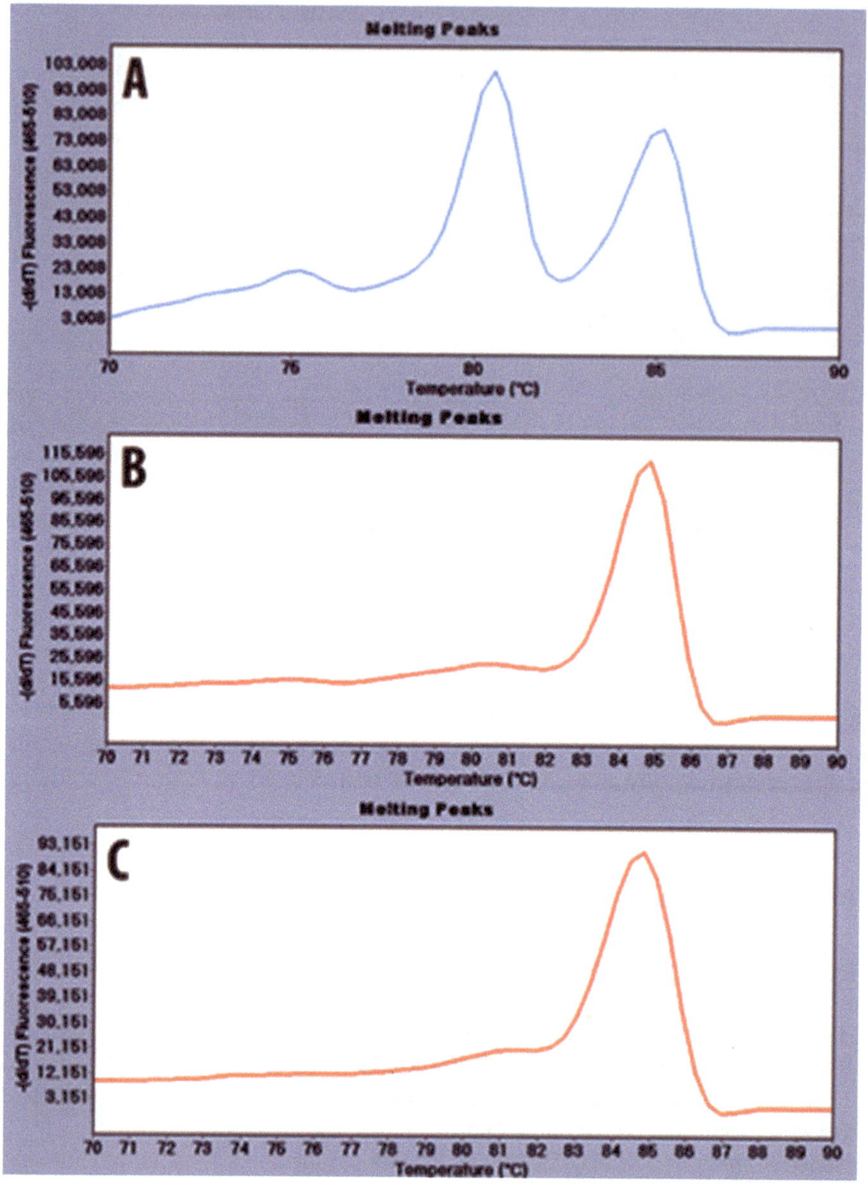

Fig. 20.6 DNA methylation analysis of the promoter region of locus SNRPN (originally published as Open Access in Orv Hetil (2018) 159:64–69). (**a**) Two amplicon melting peaks detected in normal sample (paternal non-methylated T_m 80.63 ± 0.24 °C; maternal methylated T_m 84.97 ± 0.35 °C); (**b**) PWS with paternal deletion (T_m 84.48 ± 0.99 °C); (**c**) PWS with matUPD or ID (T_m 84.5 ± 0.6 °C). T_m melting temperature, *matUPD* maternal uniparental disomy, *ID* imprinting defect

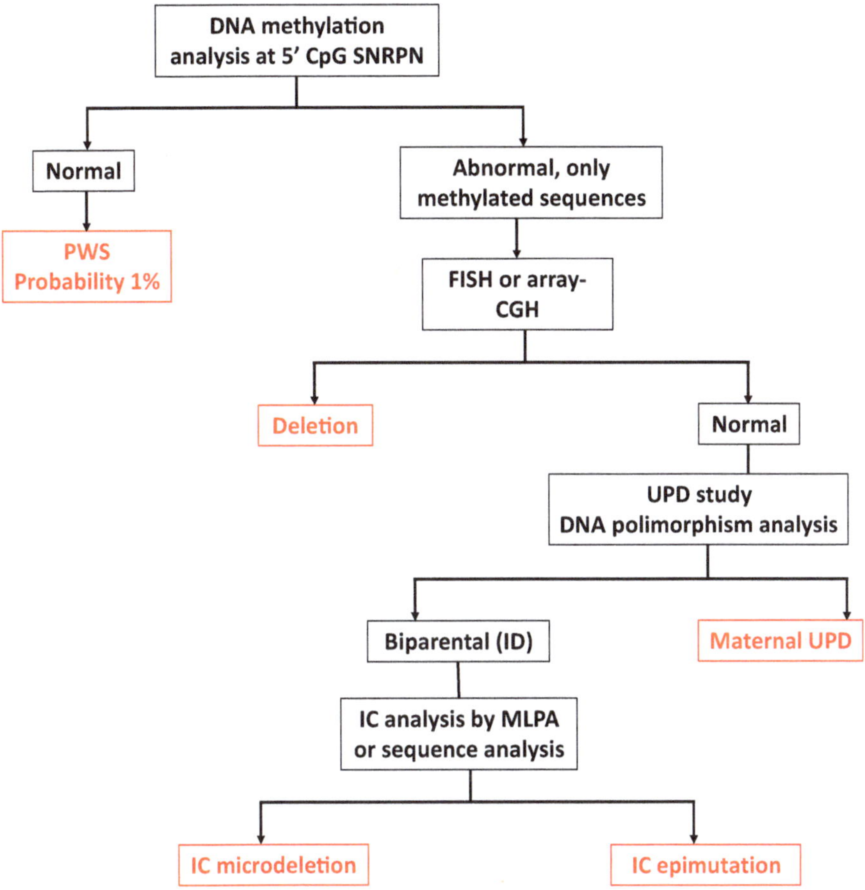

Fig. 20.7 Recommended genetic testing algorithm for Prader-Willi syndrome (PWS). *FISH* fluorescence in situ hybridization, *array-CGH* array comparative genomic hybridization, *UPD* uniparental disomy, *ID* imprinting defect, *IC* imprinting center, *MLPA* multiplex ligation probe amplification

(translocations, inversions) from an interstitial de novo deletion. For the accurate diagnosis of PWS, further testing will be necessary in about 30% of patients (Ramsden et al. 2010). The possible testing strategies for rapid and correct PWS diagnosis are summarized in Fig. 20.7.

Table 20.3 Frequency and recurrence risk of PWS depending on the genetic etiology

Genetic subtypes		Frequency	Recurrence risk
Paternal deletion		70%	<1%
matUPD	de novo	25%	<1%
	rob(15;15)	Extremely rare	50–100%
	sSMC(15)	<1%	50%
ID	epimutation	2%	<1%
	IC deletion	<0,5%	50% if familial
Paternal 15q11 rearrangements		Extremely rare	50%

matUPD maternal uniparental disomy, *ID* imprinting defect, *IC* imprinting deletion, *sSMC15* small supernumerary marker chromosome 15

20.3.5 Management and Genetic Counseling

Management of PWS patients is age dependent and should include addressing the consequences of the syndrome along with anticipatory guidance. Patient monitoring is best navigated by endocrinologists experienced in this complex disorder, but only a multidisciplinary team approach (clinical geneticist, psychiatrist, neurologist, dietician, dentist, orthopedist) can provide the optimal care for the affected population. Growth hormone replacement therapy provides improvement in growth, body composition, and physical attributes (Grugni et al. 2016). Dietary restriction, physical activity, and behavior management are fundamental in the prevention and management of obesity. In spite of all available therapeutic tools, however, successful weight loss and maintenance are hardly ever accomplished (Crinò et al. 2018). Clinical trials with novel drugs have been initiated in order to find new therapeutic possibilities for obesity in PWS patients and preliminary results seem to be encouraging. On the other hand, until well-proven medical treatments are available, bariatric surgery can be taken into consideration, especially in PWS patients with life-threatening comorbidities.

Genetic counseling for parents of an affected child should be provided by an expert diagnostician geneticist who is well-informed about the genetic background of PWS and in the latest advancements in testing. Knowledge of the genetic etiology is essential for appropriate counseling because the recurrence risk depends on the underlying genetic defect (Ramsden et al. 2010) (Table 20.3).

The most common form of PWS is usually sporadic and is caused by a microdeletion of paternal origin of the 15q11.2–q13 region; the chance of recurrence of these interstitial deletions is less than 1%. Occasionally, paternal atypical microdeletions or chromosomal rearrangements (inversion, cryptic translocation) with breakpoints within the PWS critical region could also cause PWS in the offspring (Flori et al. 2004). In these rare familial cases the risk of having another affected child is much higher (50%); therefore, fathers of children with deletions should be offered karyotype and FISH analysis with multiple adequate probes to detect possible cryptic chromosomal rearrangements (Cassidy et al. 2012).

MatUPD15 is typically de novo with a recurrence risk less than 1%. In rare cases matUPD15 is originated from a parental Robertsonian translocation or sSMC15 and thus the theoretical recurrence risk of these genetic subtypes is as high as 50%–100%. Karyotype analysis of the proband and their parents is indicated in all matUPD cases. Older maternal age may increase the risk of nondisjunction events and therefore matUPD occurs more often in older mothers' babies, accompanied by a higher risk of having additional genetic defects. These co-occurring genetic conditions are especially likely in the case of chromosome 15 isodisomy.

ID represents only a small subgroup of PWS and in the majority of cases (85%) arises from epimutations (errors in methylation-based imprinting processing), which have a recurrence risk of <1%. Approximately 15% of those with an ID have a microdeletion in the IC, which can appear de novo or could be familial; in this latter situation IC deletion carries a potential 50% recurrence risk. The IC microdeletion can be contributed by the paternal grandmother to the father. The father with the IC deletion on his maternal chromosome 15 would not have PWS himself but could pass on the mutation to his children. This applies to the father's siblings as well. Therefore, if an IC deletion is found in a proband, then the father and his siblings (in proved familial IC deletion) should have MS-MLPA analysis, which can pick up all cases of PWS-IC deletions.

When the molecular cause of PWS has been established, prenatal diagnosis can be performed.

In familial cases prenatal testing should always be offered, as the recurrence risk is high. The risk of having a second child with PWS is very low in de novo deletions and matUPD cases; prenatal testing can nonetheless provide reassurance to the family that their next child is not affected. Prenatal testing might also be done in cases where a genetic study of the fetus shows abnormalities that raise suspicion of PWS. Laboratories typically prefer to use amniocytes for analysis because tissue derived from the chorionic villi is known to be hypomethylated.

Fertility in PWS individuals is very rare; only a few female cases have been reported in the literature. The risk to the child of an affected individual depends on the sex of the affected parent and their genetic cause of PWS. If the proband is female and has the deletion form of PWS, the offspring have a 50% risk of having AS (Ostergaard 2015).

References

Abreu AP, Macedo DB, Brito VN et al (2015) A new pathway in the control of the initiation of puberty: the MKRN3 gene. J Mol Endocrinol 54:R131–R139. https://doi.org/10.1530/JME-14-0315

Ács OD, Péterfia B, Hollósi P et al (2018) Rapid first-tier genetic diagnosis in patients with Prader-Willi syndrome. Orv Hetil 159:64–69. https://doi.org/10.1556/650.2018.30918

Adam MP, Banka S, al BHT (2018) Kabuki Syndrome Medical Advisory Board Kabuki syndrome: international consensus diagnostic criteria. J Med Genet 56:89–95. https://doi.org/10.1136/jmedgenet-2018-105625

Angulo MA, Butler MG, Cataletto ME (2015) Prader-Willi syndrome: a review of clinical, genetic, and endocrine findings. J Endocrinol Investig 38:1249–1263. https://doi.org/10.1007/s40618-015-0312-9
Bakalov VK, Cheng C, Zhou J et al (2009) X-chromosome gene dosage and the risk of diabetes in Turner syndrome. J Clin Endocrinol Metab 94:3289–3296. https://doi.org/10.1210/jc.2009-0384
Bakalov VK, Gutin L, Cheng CM et al (2012) Autoimmune disorders in women with Turner syndrome and women with karyotypically normal primary ovarian insufficiency. J Autoimmun 38:315–321. https://doi.org/10.1016/j.jaut.2012.01.015
Bearelly P, Oates R. (2019) Recent advances in managing and understanding Klinefelter syndrome. F1000Res 8. pii: F1000 Faculty Rev-112. doi:https://doi.org/10.12688/f1000research.16747.1
Belling K, Russo F, Jensen AB et al (2017) Klinefelter syndrome comorbidities linked to increased X chromosome gene dosage and altered protein interactome activity. Hum Mol Genet 26:1219–1229. https://doi.org/10.1093/hmg/ddx014
Bianchi I, Lleo A, Gershwin ME et al (2012) The X chromosome and immune associated genes. J Autoimmun 38:J187–J192. https://doi.org/10.1016/j.jaut.2011.11.012
Bieth E, Eddiry S, Gaston V et al (2015) Highly restricted deletion of the SNORD116 region is implicated in Prader-Willi syndrome. Eur J Hum Genet 23:252–255. https://doi.org/10.1038/ejhg.2014.103
Bojesen A, Hertz JM, Gravholt CH (2011) Genotype and phenotype in Klinefelter syndrome - impact of androgen receptor polymorphism and skewed X inactivation. Int J Androl 34:e642–e648. https://doi.org/10.1111/j.1365-2605.2011.01223.x
Borja-Santos N, Trancas B, Santos Pinto P et al (2010) 48,XXYY in a General Adult Psychiatry Department. Psychiatry (Edgmont) 7:32–36
Bronshtein M, Zimmer EZ, Blazer S (2003) A characteristic cluster of fetal sonographic markers that are predictive of fetal Turner syndrome in early pregnancy. Am J Obstet Gynecol 188:1016–1020
Buiting K (2010) Prader-Willi syndrome and Angelman syndrome. Am J Med Genet C Semin Med Genet 154C:365–376. https://doi.org/10.1002/ajmg.c.30273
Butler MG, Hartin SN, Hossain WA et al (2019) Molecular genetic classification in Prader-Willi syndrome: a multisite cohort study. J Med Genet 56(3):149–153. https://doi.org/10.1136/jmedgenet-2018-105301
Cassidy SB, Schwartz S, Miller JL et al (2012) Prader-Willi syndrome. Genet Med 14:10–26. https://doi.org/10.1038/gim.0b013e31822bead0
Chai JH, Locke DP, Greally JM et al (2003) Identification of four highly conserved genes between breakpoint hotspots BP1 and BP2 of the Prader-Willi/Angelman syndromes deletion region that have undergone evolutionary transposition mediated by flanking duplicons. Am J Hum Genet 73:898–925
Chang S, Skakkebak A, Gravholt CH (2015) Klinefelter syndrome and medical treatment: hypogonadism and beyond. Hormones 14:531–548. https://doi.org/10.14310/horm.2002.1622
Changchien YC, Haltrich I, Micsik T et al (2012) Gonadoblastoma: case report of two young patients with isochromosome 12p found in the dysgerminoma overgrowth component in one case. Pathol Res Pract 208:628–632. https://doi.org/10.1016/j.prp.2012.07.006
Crinò A, Fintini D, Bocchini S et al (2018) Obesity management in Prader-Willi syndrome: current perspectives. Diabetes Metab Syndr Obes 11:579–593. https://doi.org/10.2147/DMSO.S141352
Davis S, Lahlou N, Bardsley M et al (2016) Gonadal function is associated with cardiometabolic health in pre-pubertal boys with Klinefelter syndrome. Andrology 4:1169–1177. https://doi.org/10.1111/andr.12275
Fisher EMC, Beer-Romero P, Brown LG, Ridley A, McNeil JA, Lawrence JB, Willard HF, Bieber FR, Page DC (1990) Homologous ribosomal protein genes on the human X and Y chromosomes: escape from X inactivation and possible implications for turner syndrome. Cell 63 (6):1205–1218

Flori E, Biancalana V, Girard-Lemaire F, Favre R, Flori J, Doray B, Louis Mandel J (2004) Difficulties of genetic counseling and prenatal diagnosis in a consanguineous couple segregating for the same translocation (14,15) (q11;q13) and at risk for Prader–Willi and Angelman syndromes. Eur J Hum Genet 12(3):181–186

Fountain MD Jr, Schaaf CP (2015) MAGEL2 and oxytocin-implications in Prader-Willi syndrome and beyond. Biol Psychiatry 78:78–80. https://doi.org/10.1016/j.biopsych.2015.05.006

Frühmesser A, Kotzot D (2011) Chromosomal variants in Klinefelter syndrome. Sex Dev 5:109–123. https://doi.org/10.1159/000327324

Glueck CJ, Jetty V, Goldenberg N et al (2017) Thrombophilia in Klinefelter syndrome with deep venous thrombosis, pulmonary embolism, and mesenteric artery thrombosis on testosterone therapy: a pilot study. Clin Appl Thromb Hemost 23:973–979. https://doi.org/10.1177/1076029616665923

Gold JA, Mahmoud R, Cassidy SB et al (2018) Comparison of perinatal factors in deletion versus uniparental disomy in Prader-Willi syndrome. Am J Med Genet A 176:1161–1165. https://doi.org/10.1002/ajmg.a.38679

Gravholt CH, Andersen NH, Conway GS et al (2017) Clinical practice guidelines for the care of girls and women with Turner syndrome: proceedings from the 2016 Cincinnati international Turner syndrome meeting. Eur J Endocrinol 177(3):G1–G70. https://doi.org/10.1530/EJE-17-0430

Gravholt CH, Chang S, Wallentin M et al (2018) Klinefelter syndrome: integrating genetics, neuropsychology, and endocrinology. Endocr Rev 39:389–423. https://doi.org/10.1210/er.2017-00212

Green T, Flash S, Reiss AL (2019) Sex differences in psychiatric disorders: what we can learn from sex chromosome aneuploidies. Neuropsychopharmacology 44:9–21. https://doi.org/10.1038/s41386-018-0153-2

Gropman AL, Rogol A, Fennoy I et al (2010) Clinical variability and novel neurodevelopmental findings in 49,XXXXY syndrome. Am J Med Genet A 152A:1523–1530. https://doi.org/10.1002/ajmg.a.33307

Grossi A, Crinò A, Luciano R et al (2013) A. Endocrine autoimmunity in Turner syndrome. Ital J Pediatr 39:79. https://doi.org/10.1186/1824-7288-39-79

Grugni G, Sartorio A, Crinò A (2016) Growth hormone therapy for Prader-willi syndrome: challenges and solutions. Ther Clin Risk Manag 12:873–381. https://doi.org/10.2147/TCRM.S70068

Gunay-Aygun M, Schwartz S, Heeger S et al (2001) The changing purpose of Prader-Willi syndrome clinical diagnostic criteria and proposed revised criteria. Pediatrics 108:E92

Haltrich I, Pikó H, Pamjav H et al (2015) Complex X chromosome rearrangement associated with multiorgan autoimmunity. Mol Cytogenet 8:51. https://doi.org/10.1186/s13039-015-0152-5

Heksch R, Kamboj M, Anglin K et al (2017) Review of Prader-Willi syndrome: the endocrine approach. Transl Pediatr 6:274–285. https://doi.org/10.21037/tp.2017.09.04

Holm VA, Cassidy SB, Butler MG et al (1993) Prader-Willi syndrome: consensus diagnostic criteria. Pediatrics 91:398–402

Houk CP, Hughes IA, Ahmed SF et al (2006) Writing Committee for the International Intersex Consensus Conference Participants. Summary of consensus statement on intersex disorders and their management. International Intersex Consensus Conference. Pediatrics 118:753–757

Jeon KC, Chen LS, Goodson P (2012) Decision to abort after a prenatal diagnosis of sex chromosome abnormality: a systematic review of the literature. Genet Med 14:27–38. https://doi.org/10.1038/gim.0b013e31822e57a7

Jørgensen KT, Rostgaard K, Bache I et al (2010) Autoimmune diseases in women with Turner's syndrome. Arthritis Rheum 62:658–666. https://doi.org/10.1002/art.27270

Kim SJ, Miller JL, Kuipers PJ et al (2012) Unique and atypical deletions in Prader-Willi syndrome reveal distinct phenotypes. Eur J Hum Genet 20:283–290. https://doi.org/10.1038/ejhg.2011.187

Klinefelter HF, Reifenstein EC, Albright F (1942) Syndrome characterized by gynecomastia, spermatogenesis without A-Leydigism, and increased excretion of follicle-stimulating hormone. J Clin Endocrinol 11:615–627

Kondo T, Kuroda S, Usui K et al (2018) A case of a rare variant of Klinefelter syndrome, 47,XY,i (X)(q10). Andrologia 50:e13024. https://doi.org/10.1111/and.13024

Kubba H, Smyth A, Wong SC et al (2017) Ear health and hearing surveillance in girls and women with Turner's syndrome: recommendations from the Turner's Syndrome Support Society. Clin Otolaryngol 42:503–507. https://doi.org/10.1111/coa.12750

Lebenthal Y, Levy S, Sofrin-Drucker E et al (2018) The natural history of metabolic comorbidities in turner syndrome from childhood to early adulthood: comparison between 45,x monosomy and other karyotypes. Front Endocrinol 9:27. https://doi.org/10.3389/fendo.2018.00027

Lee MC, Conway GS (2014) Turner's syndrome: challenges of late diagnosis. Lancet Diabetes Endocrinol 2:333–338. https://doi.org/10.1016/S2213-8587(13)70153-0

Liehr T, Brude E, Gillessen-Kaesbach G et al (2005) Prader-Willi syndrome with a karyotype 47, XY,+min(15)(pter->q11.1:) and maternal UPD 15-case report plus review of similar cases. Eur J Med Genet 48:175–181

Lucaccioni L, Wong SC, al SA (2015) Turner syndrome – issues to consider for transition to adulthood. Br Med Bull 113:45–58. https://doi.org/10.1093/bmb/ldu038

Macedo DB, Abreu AP, Reis AC (2014) Central precocious puberty that appears to be sporadic caused by paternally inherited mutations in the imprinted gene makorin ring finger 3. J Clin Endocrinol Metab 99:E1097–E1103. https://doi.org/10.1210/jc.2013-3126

Manzardo AM, Weisensel N, Ayala S et al (2018) Prader-Willi syndrome genetic subtypes and clinical neuropsychiatric diagnoses in residential care adults. Clin Genet 93:622–631. https://doi.org/10.1111/cge.13142

Miller NL, Wevrick R, Mellon PL (2009) Necdin, a Prader-Willi syndrome candidate gene, regulates gonadotropin-releasing hormone neurons during development. Hum Mol Genet 18:248–260. https://doi.org/10.1093/hmg/ddn344

Nieschlag E (2013) Klinefelter syndrome: the commonest form of hypogonadism, but often overlooked or untreated. Dtsch Arztebl Int 110:347–353. https://doi.org/10.3238/arztebl.2013.0347

Ohta T, Gray TA, Rogan PK et al (1999) Imprinting mutation mechanisms in Prader-Willi syndrome. Am J Hum Genet 64:397–413

Ostergaard JR (2015) Phenotype of a child with Angelman syndrome born to a woman with Prader–Willi syndrome. Am J Med Genet Part A 167A:2138–2144. https://doi.org/10.1002/ajmg.a.37080

Pravdivyi I, Ballanyi K, Colmers WF et al (2015) Progressive postnatal decline in leptin sensitivity of arcuate hypothalamic neurons in the Magel2-null mouse model of Prader-Willi syndrome. Hum Mol Genet 24:4276–4278. https://doi.org/10.1093/hmg/ddv159

Ramsden SC, Clayton-Smith J et al (2010) Practice guidelines for the molecular analysis of Prader-Willi and Angelman syndromes. BMC Med Genet 11:70. https://doi.org/10.1186/1471-2350-11-70

Rappold G, Blum WF, Shavrikova EP et al (2007) Genotypes and phenotypes in children with short stature: clinical indicators of SHOX haploinsufficiency. J Med Genet 44:306–313

Raznahan A, Parikshak NN, Chandran V et al (2018) Sex-chromosome dosage effects on gene expression in humans. Proc Natl Acad Sci U S A 115:7398–7403. https://doi.org/10.1073/pnas.1802889115

Sallai A, Sólyom J, Dobos M et al (2010) Y-chromosome markers in Turner syndrome: screening of 130 patients. J Endocrinol Investig 33:222–227. https://doi.org/10.3275/6442

Samplaski MK, Lo KC, Grober ED et al (2014) Phenotypic differences in mosaic Klinefelter patients as compared with non-mosaic Klinefelter patients. Fertil Steril 101:950–955. https://doi.org/10.1016/j.fertnstert.2013.12.051

Schaaf CP, Gonzalez-Garay ML, al XF (2013) Truncating mutations of MAGEL2 cause Prader-Willi phenotypes and autism. Nat Genet 45:1405–1408. https://doi.org/10.1038/ng.2776

Seminog OO, Seminog AB, Yeates D et al (2015) Associations between Klinefelter's syndrome and autoimmune diseases: English national record linkage studies. Autoimmunity 48:125–128. https://doi.org/10.3109/08916934.2014.968918

Sharma A, Jamil MA, Nuesgen N et al (2015) DNA methylation signature in peripheral blood reveals distinct characteristics of human X chromosome numerical aberrations. Clin Epigenetics 7:76. https://doi.org/10.1186/s13148-015-0112-2

Skakkebak A, Nielsen MM, Trolle C et al (2018) DNA hypermethylation and differential gene expression associated with Klinefelter syndrome. Sci Rep 8:13740. https://doi.org/10.1038/s41598-018-31780-0

Sylvén L, Magnusson C, Hagenfeldt K et al (1993) Life with Turner's syndrome-a psychosocial report from 22 middle-aged women. Acta Endocrinol 129:188–194

Tartaglia N, Davis S, Hench A et al (2008) A new look at XXYY syndrome: medical and psychological features. Am J Med Genet A 146A:1509–1522. https://doi.org/10.1002/ajmg.a.32366

Tartaglia N, Ayari N, Howell S et al (2011) 48,XXYY, 48,XXXY and 49,XXXXY syndromes: not just variants of Klinefelter syndrome. Acta Paediatr 100:851–860. https://doi.org/10.1111/j.1651-2227.2011.02235.x

Tian D, Sun S, Lee JT (2010) The long noncoding RNA, Jpx, is a molecular switch for X chromosome inactivation. Cell 143:390–403. https://doi.org/10.1016/j.cell.2010.09.049

Trolle C, Nielsen MM, Skakkebæk A et al (2016) Widespread DNA hypomethylation and differential gene expression in Turner syndrome. Sci Rep 30(6):34220. https://doi.org/10.1038/srep34220

Urbach A, Benvenisty N (2009) Studying early lethality of 45,XO (Turner's syndrome) embryos using human embryonic stem cells. PLoS One 4:e4175. https://doi.org/10.1371/journal.pone.0004175

Visootsak J, Rosner B, Dykens E et al (2007) Behavioral phenotype of sex chromosome aneuploidies: 48,XXYY, 48,XXXY, and 49,XXXXY. Am J Med Genet A 143A:1198–1203

Williams LA, Pankratz N, Lane J et al (2018) Klinefelter syndrome in males with germ cell tumors: a report from the Children's Oncology Group. Cancer 124:3900–3908. https://doi.org/10.1002/cncr.31667

Zinn AR, Ross JL (1998) Turner syndrome and haploinsufficiency. Curr Opin Genet Dev 8:322–327

FSC
www.fsc.org
MIX
Papier | Fördert
gute Waldnutzung
FSC® C083411

Kolibri 360 GmbH
Ferdinand-Jühlke-Straße 7
99095 Erfurt, Deutschland
produktsicherheit@kolibri360.de